Emergency EC

Case-Based Review and Interpretations

Editors-in-Chief

Jeremy Berberian, MD | ChristianaCare

William J. Brady, MD | University of Virginia

Amal Mattu, MD | University of Maryland

ISBN 978-1-929854-64-6 (Kindle)
ISBN 978-1-929854-66-0 (Print)
4950 W. Royal Lane | Irving, TX 75063
972.550.0920 | www.emra.org

Disclaimer

This handbook is intended only as a general guide. While the editors have taken reasonable measures to ensure the accuracy of the information presented herein, the user is encouraged to consult other resources when necessary to confirm appropriate treatment, side effects, interactions, and contraindications. The publisher, authors, editors, and sponsoring organizations specifically disclaim any liability for omissions or errors found in this handbook, for appropriate use, or for treatment errors. Further, although this handbook is as comprehensive as possible, the vast differences in emergency practice settings may necessitate treatment approaches other than those presented here. Refer to your institution's protocols.

Resident Reviewers

Salman Aziz, MD
Matt Baltz, MD

Lauren Briskie, MD
Alicia "Piper Lou" Cox, DO

Parth Gandhi, DO
Emily Luvison, MD

Matt Rizzotti, DO
W. Brandon White, DO

Kindle Design/Development

Jurie Pieterse, Pebbles Marketing

EMRA Staff Contributor

Managing Editor Valerie Hunt

TABLE OF CONTENTS

CASES BY TOPIC

FOREWORD

JUDITH TINTINALLI, MD, MS

Professor and Chair Emeritus
University of North Carolina
Chapel Hill, North Carolina

Three of our emergency medicine master educators - **Amal Mattu, William Brady, and Jeremy Berberian** - have assembled this brand-new ECG series. The collection includes 102 high-yield case descriptions and an analytic description of each ECG itself. Cases are followed by a detailed differential diagnosis, concise learning points, and key references sprinkled throughout. These are so many good aspects for expanding your knowledge base.

For students and residents who want to move up to the top in ECG interpretation, this collection will knock your socks off. Clinicians who want to stay sharp (at least as sharp as their residents) will the collection interesting and challenging! It's just never too often to test your ECG wits.

I'd encourage paramedics, EMTs, nurse practitioners, and physician assistants to check this collection out. The increasing expectations and scope of care of all those who practice in an emergency department or urgent care setting make ECG expertise an essential skill for everyone.

This resource can be used for self-study, for teaching and learning during slow shifts, and even for the "heart-stopper" case that unexpectedly presents itself in the ED. Pack it up in your doctor bag for work, along with your other tools! Or, get the interactive Kindle version to give you a more complete experience.

For students and residents who want to move up to the top in ECG interpretation, this collection will knock your socks off. Clinicians who want to stay sharp (at least as sharp as their residents) will the collection interesting and challenging!

It's just never too often to test your ECG wits.

PREFACE

JEREMY BERBERIAN, MD
WILLIAM J. BRADY, MD
AMAL MATTU, MD

"Cogito, ergo sum"

The term electrocardiogram was first used by Willem Einthoven in 1893. Using a refined capillary electrometer, he recorded a tracing with four deflections, which he labeled ABCD. In 1895, he published a corrected tracing with five deflections that accounted for the inertia and friction of the mercury in the capillary electrode.1 Einthoven superimposed the two tracings to illustrate the differences ***(see Figure 1),*** so he needed to label the deflections in the corrected tracing with different letters. He chose PQRST, which is the labeling system still used today. There are many theories on why Einthoven chose PRQST (as opposed to QRSTU or HIJKL), the most popular being that he was influenced by the work of Rene Descartes. Two famous instances of Descartes' use of the PQRST labeling system include his diagram of light refraction in his 1637 publication La Dioptrique and his diagram of nerve function in his 1662 publication *De Homine*[2] and 1692 publication *Opera Philosophica. [Editor's note: While this makes for a good story, there is no mathematical convention that dictates the use of PQRST exclusive of other letters.]*

Rene Descartes was a 17th century French mathematician and philosopher. He is credited with inventing analytic geometry, including what we now call Cartesian coordinates, as well as being the father of modern/western philosophy. Descartes developed what is now called Cartesian doubt, which is a way of searching for what is true by systematically doubting everything [Editor's note: This is a gross oversimplification]. He believed that if the foundations of knowledge were not completely solid, anything built upon them would inevitably collapse. It was with this in mind that he famously wrote, "I think, therefore I am," which he described as a truth that is certain and irrefutable. *[Editor's note: Descartes was French, so he actually wrote "je pense, donc je suis." In a subsequent publication in Latin he wrote, "***cogito, ergo sum***." These phrases can be translated to "I think, therefore I am" or "I am thinking, therefore I exist."]*

Figure 1. Einthoven's corrected ECG tracing PQRST superimposed over the uncorrected ECG tracing ABCD

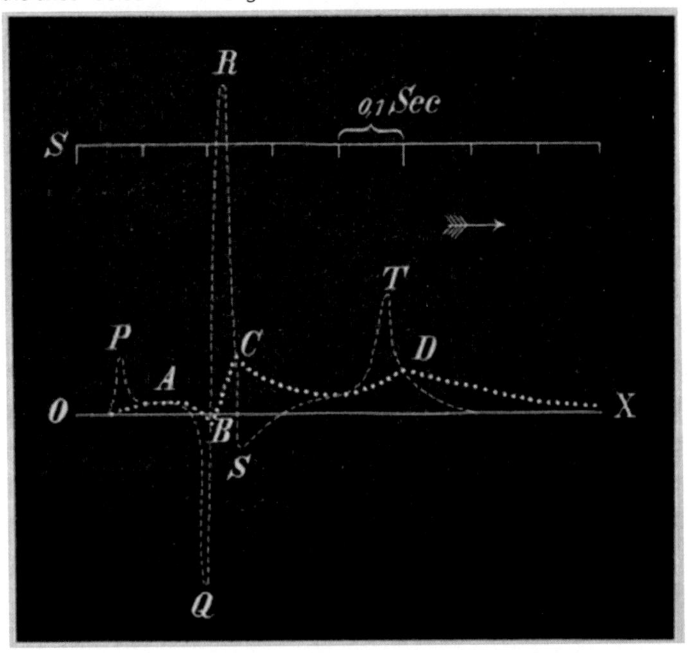

While it may sound a little pretentious, this book was written in the spirit of Cartesian doubt [*Editor's note: this definitely sounds pretentious*] with the goal of providing a "certain and irrefutable" foundation of ECG knowledge [*Editor's note: this sounds even more pretentious*]. The cases have detailed explanations based on the most recent AHA Guidelines, landmark publications on ECGs, and Chou's Electrocardiography in Clinical Practice. Whenever possible, ECG dogmata is discussed and refuted. And as with any good picture book, each image is designed to be worth 1000 words. We hope you enjoy this book.

- Jeremy Berberian, William Brady, and Amal Mattu

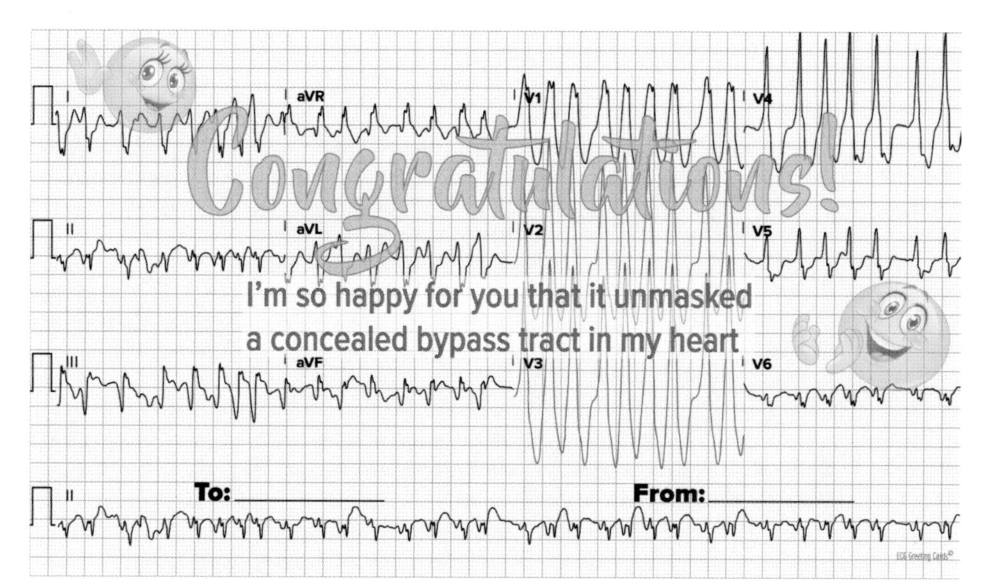

Congratulations!
I'm so happy for you that it unmasked
a concealed bypass tract in my heart
To:
From:
I aVR V1 V4
II aVL V2 V5
III aVF V3 V6
II
ECG Greeting Cards©

When times get *TOUGH*

I aVR V1 V4
II aVL V2 V5

Don't forget that mostly dead . . .

III aVF V3 V6

. . . is still slightly alive

II

To:

From:

ECG Greeting Cards©

DEDICATIONS

I would like to thank my wife Sejal and my children Nikhil, Eleena, and Kamran for always reminding me of my proper priorities in life; I thank my colleagues, the residents, and students at the University of Maryland School of Medicine for providing me the inspiration for the work I do every day; and my thanks to Dr. Berberian, Dr. Brady, and Valerie Hunt for their tireless work and commitment to this project.

- Amal Mattu, MD, FACEP

I would like to thank my wife, King, and children, Lauren, Anne, Chip, and Katherine, for being awesome; EM residents, for your interest, enthusiasm, and dedication to emergency medicine and our patients...thanks for being there every day; my co-editors, Drs. Berberian and Mattu, for their dedication to emergency medicine and partnership in furthering our specialty; and lastly, our production editor, Ms Valerie Hunt, for doing the heavy lifting on this, and so many other, projects.

- William Brady, MD, FACEP, FAAEM

I would like to thank my residents and colleagues for always sharing their interesting EKGs with me and making me a better clinician and educator; everyone at MPP for reminding me that play is essential to the pursuit of purrfection; Drs. Mattu and Brady for being the Miles and Coltrane of EM ECG interpretation; and EMRA for supporting this project, and Valerie Hunt for her attention to detail and dedication to making sure every P-wave looks perfect at 17,000% magnification. There are some people for whom no amount of thanks seems sufficient, so I would like to dedicate this book to Bob Gullotti, Len Samuels, Thelonious Monk Jr., and my pop for sharing their love of learning and teaching with me.

- Jeremy Berberian, MD

Thank you for reading

Emergency ECGs
Case-Based Review and Interpretations

You can shop for other EMRA publications:
https://www.amazon.com/emra

Jeremy Berberian, MD | ChristianaCare

William J. Brady, MD | University of Virginia

Amal Mattu, MD | University of Maryland

Print edition: v1.03

DISCLAIMERS

1. Every ECG was hand-traced from the original, so there may be natural variations between the lead II and lead II rhythm strip tracings.
2. The ECG grid was created by hand to allow for super high-resolution images. In full disclosure, the small boxes are not exactly square, as the height is approximately 12 microns more than the width. Further accuracy was limited by the width of the lines need to measure the boxes at 17,000% magnification.
3. When brackets are used, measurements are made from the middle of each leg as show in the image below.

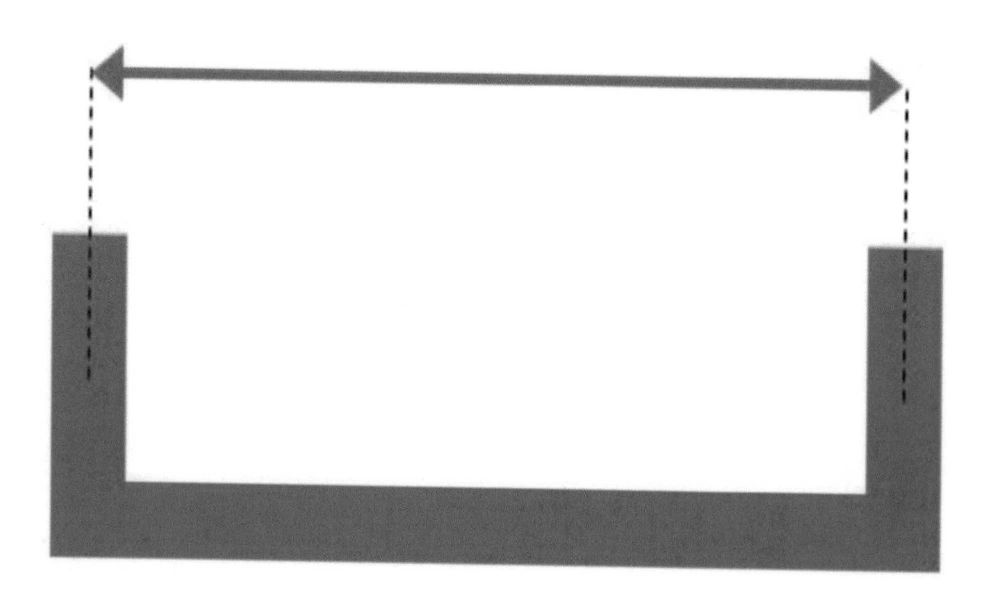

4. All measurements were made on the original ECGs then transferred to the redrawn images in order to respect the limitations of measuring ECGs in real life.
5. Even though proper grammar dictates that a hyphen should only be placed after a single letter when the term is used as an adjective (ie, "T-wave inversions" is hyphenated, but "inverted T waves" is not), we hyphenated all waves for the sake of simplicity. We beg forgiveness from the grammar gods.
6. A hidden P-wave is not visible while a buried P-wave is partially visible.
7. There are a handful of Easter Eggs, two of which involve images.
8. There is a bonus section of ECG greeting cards for you to use. Nothing says "heartwarming" like a hand-signed card that has a picture of fever-induced Brugada. Hallmark will be kicking themselves for not thinking of this first *[Editor's note: This is highly unlikely given Hallmark's ~$3.5 billion annual revenue.]*

References

1. Hurst JW. Naming of the Waves in the ECG, With a Brief Account of Their Genesis. *Circulation.* 1998;98:1937-1942.
2. Henson JR. Descartes and the ECG lettering series. *J Hist Med Allied Sci.* 1971;26(2):181–186.

NOTES:

Case 1: Presentation

A 39-year-old male with no past medical history presents with 3 days of palpitations and 2 episodes of syncope in the past 8 hours. What is your interpretation of his ECG?

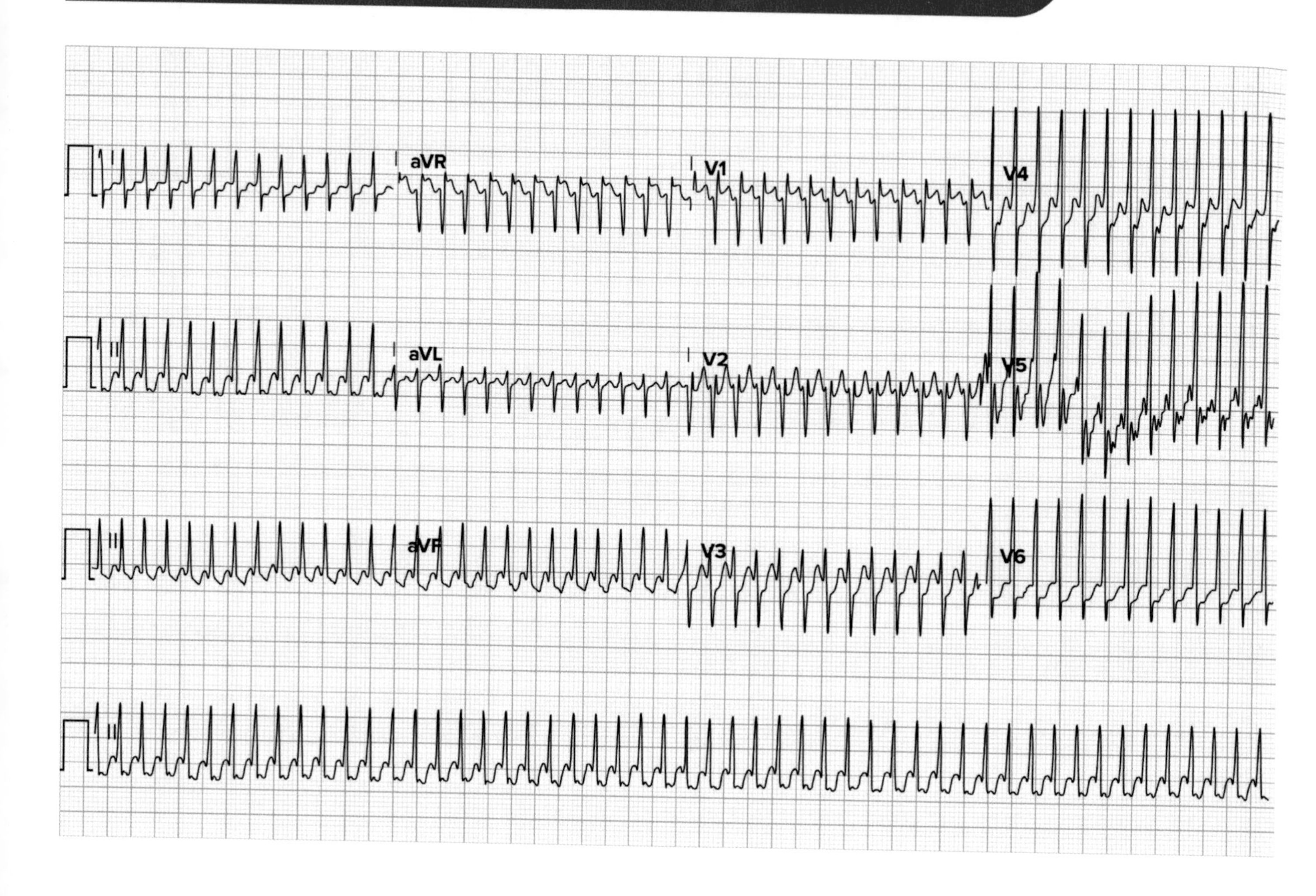

Case 1: Answer

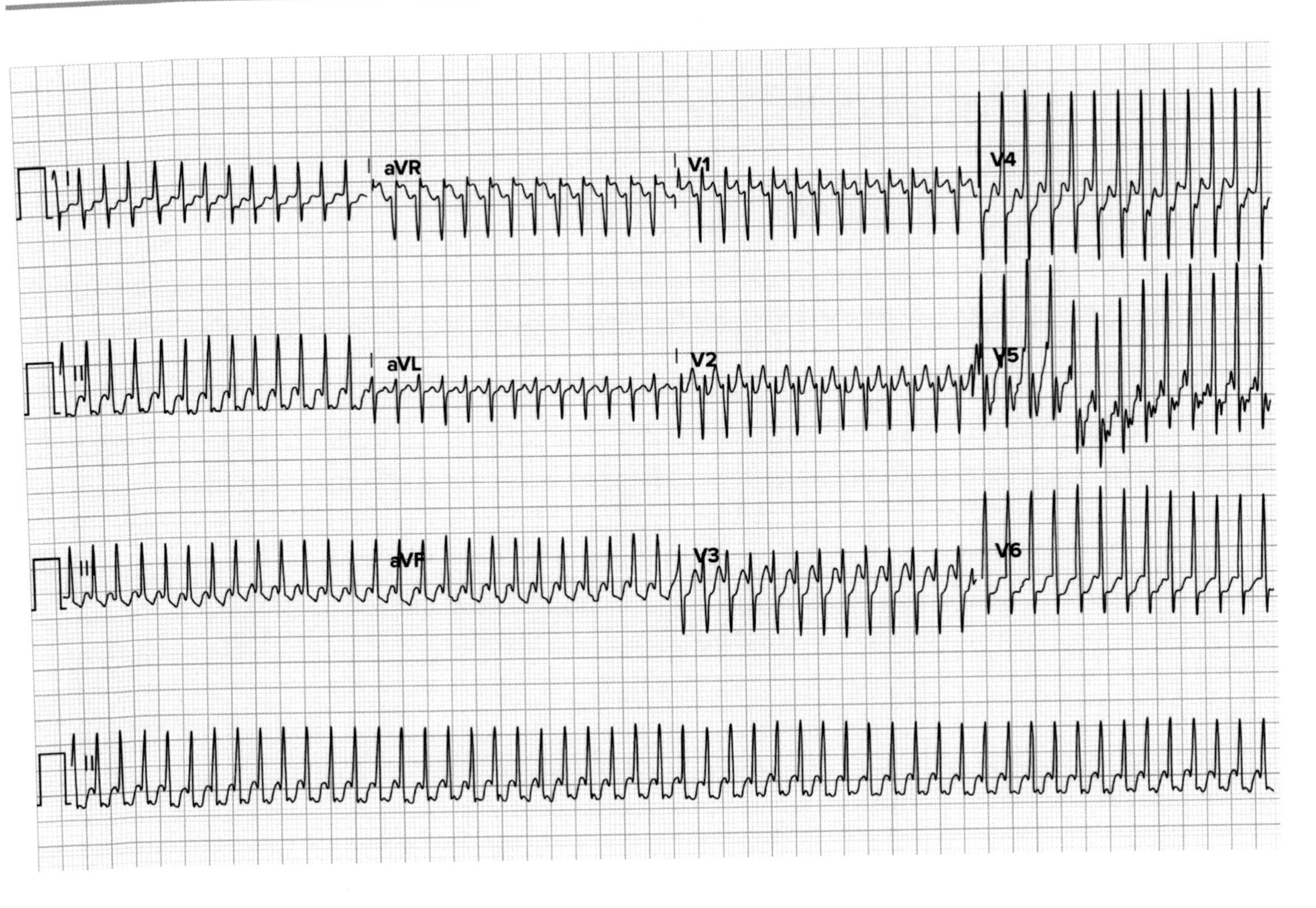

This ECG shows a regular narrow-complex tachycardia with a ventricular rate of 309 bpm, normal axis, STE in leads aVR and V1, and STD in leads I, II, III, aVF, and V2-V6.

The differential diagnosis for a regular narrow-complex tachycardia includes:

- Atrial flutter
- Atrial tachycardia
- AV nodal reentrant tachycardia
- AVRT (ie, WPW) with orthodromic conduction
- Junctional tachycardia
- Narrow complex VT
- Sinus tachycardia

The absence of P-waves rules out atrial tachycardia and sinus tachycardia. The rate is too fast for junctional tachycardia. The QRS complex duration is ~80 msec, so narrow complex VT is unlikely. Without more history, it is impossible to tell whether this AVNRT, orthodromic AVRT (ie, retrograde conduction via the AP), or atrial flutter with 1:1 conduction.

The most impressive finding in this ECG is the ventricular rate of 309 bpm. NCT with ventricular rates this high are rarely seen in the adult population, let alone in one that is walking and talking as this patient was. The AV node's intrinsic refractory period prevents ventricular rates from exceeding 220-240 bpm in the absence of any extrinsic factors that increase conduction velocity (see differential diagnosis below). In such cases, successful termination of the tachydysrhythmia will often be temporary at best until the underlying cause is identified and treated.

The differential diagnosis for causes of supraventricular tachycardias with rates > 220-240 bpm includes:

- Catecholamine surge
- Sympathomimetic toxicity
- Hyperthyroidism/thyroid storm

The differential diagnosis for the pattern of STE in lead aVR +/- lead V1 with diffuse STD includes both ACS and non-ACS etiologies:

ACS causes[1]	Non-ACS causes[2]
• LMCA insufficiency (can see STE aVR > V1) • Prox LAD insufficiency (can see STE V1 > aVR) • Triple vessel disease • Global cardiac ischemia • Prinzmetal angina	• Acute and/or severe anemia • Aortic dissection • LBBB and ventricular-paced rhythms • LVH with strain pattern • Pulmonary embolism • ROSC s/p epinephrine or defibrillation • Severe hypokalemia or hyperkalemia • Sodium channel blockade • Supraventricular tachycardia (especially with rapid rates)

Although the pattern of STE in lead aVR +/- lead V1 with diffuse STD is discussed in the cardiology literature, its clinical significance is not without some controversy. This is likely due to the broad differential diagnosis associated with this pattern that includes both ACS and non-ACS causes. The 2018 Fourth Universal Definition of MI states "ST-segment depression ≥ 1 mm in 6 or more leads, which may be associated with ST segment elevation in leads aVR and/or V1 and hemodynamic compromise, is suggestive of multivessel disease or left main disease" but does not provide specific management recommendations.

Treatment should be guided by the underlying etiology, and it is imperative to consider both ACS and non-ACS causes. For patients suspected of having an ACS cause, this ECG pattern is highly suggestive of LMCA insufficiency, proximal LAD insufficiency, or triple vessel disease. So, while this pattern does not meet "traditional" STEMI criteria, it can represent high-risk ACS, including possible acute coronary occlusion, in the correct clinical context, and immediate angiography should be considered. Whether this is done by emergent cardiology consultation or activation of the cardiac catheterization lab depends on local practice preferences.

The pattern of STE in leads aVR and V1 with diffuse STD seen in this ECG is likely due to the abnormal conduction associated with the supraventricular tachycardia. The ECG changes alone do not constitute a "failed stress test" and the decision to evaluate for ischemia that caused, or was caused by, the tachydysrhythmia should be a clinical one.

This patient's ED workup was consistent with thyroid storm. He was chemically cardioverted with adenosine after which he briefly went into sinus tachycardia before going into atrial fibrillation with RVR at ~140 bpm. Atrial fibrillation is commonly seen with thyroid storm and will often be refractory to rate control or cardioversion until the elevated thyroid hormones are treated.

This patient was treated with methimazole (propylthiouracil carries an FDA black box warning due to risk of acute liver failure and should be reserved for 1st trimester of pregnancy or patients unable to tolerate any other treatment), potassium iodide, and steroids, and admitted to the ICU.

Treatment with a beta-blocker, typically propranolol, was avoided due to concern for tachycardia-induced cardiomyopathy (TIC). The patient had been having palpitations for 3 days and TIC is one of the severe complications of any untreated tachydysrhythmia. TIC is a dilated cardiomyopathy induced by a persistent tachydysrhythmia. It is often reversible, and after cessation of the tachydysrhythmia, ventricular function typically returns to normal. In this case, the patient's EF was severely reduced on bedside echo so the tachycardic ventricular rates associated with the atrial fibrillation were likely necessary to maintain adequate cardiac output (note CO = HR x SV).

AV Nodal Reentrant Tachycardia (AVNRT) Learning Points

- Also called paroxysmal supraventricular tachycardia or SVT
- Caused by re-entrant circuit within or around the AV Node and typically triggered by a PAC
- ECG shows a regular narrow-complex tachycardia in the absence of concurrent conduction abnormalities (eg, bundle branch block)
- Ventricular rate typically 140-280 bpm
- Retrograde P-waves can appear before, after, or superimposed on the QRS complexes
- The fastest animals include black marlin (ocean), cheetah (4 legs on land), ostrich (2 legs on land), and peregrine falcon (air)

Atrioventricular Re-entry Tachycardia (AVRT) Learning Points

- Caused by re-entrant circuit involving AV node and an accessory pathway
  - Most common dysrhythmia seen in patients with pre-excitation syndrome (eg, WPW)
- Rate tends to be faster than AVNRT
- Orthodromic AVRT
  - Antegrade conduction through the AV node and retrograde conduction via the accessory pathway
  - ECG shows a regular narrow-complex tachycardia in the absence of concurrent conduction abnormalities (eg, bundle branch block)
- Antidromic AVRT
  - Antegrade conduction through the accessory pathway and retrograde conduction via the AV node
  - ECG shows a regular wide-complex tachycardia generally indistinguishable from VT

Lead aVR Learning Points

- Lead aVR views the right upper portion of the heart including the basal part of the septum
- STE in lead aVR +/- V1 with diffuse STD ≥ 1 mm in ≥ 6 leads can be due to ACS or non-ACS etiologies; therefore, always consider the clinical context when considering the differential diagnosis
- In ACS presentations, this pattern is highly suggestive of LMCA obstruction, proximal LAD obstruction, and triple vessel disease, and immediate angiography should be considered[3]
- In non-ACS causes, the ECG changes should resolve with treatment of non-ACS cause
- Anterior or inferior MI with STE > 1 mm in lead aVR are associated with an increased 30-day mortality[4]

Tachycardia-induced cardiomyopathy (TIC) Learning Points

- Dilated cardiomyopathy induced by a persistent tachydysrhythmia
- Severe (can lead to cardiogenic shock), but reversible, complication of any untreated tachydysrhythmia
- Treatment is cessation of the tachydysrhythmia which typically results in clinical improvement and recovery of ventricular function

References

1. Thygesen K, Alpert JS, Jaffe AS, et al. 2018 ESC/ACC/AHA/WHF Expert Consensus Document: Fourth Universal Definition of Myocardial Infarction (2018). Circulation. 2018;138:e618-e651.
2. Mattu A. ECG Weekly.
3. Writing Committee, et al. 2013 ACCF/AHA Guideline for the Management of ST-Elevation Myocardial Infarction: A Report of the American College of Cardiology Foundation/American Heart Association Task Force on Practice Guidelines. Circulation. 2013;127:e362-e425.
4. Wong CK, Gao W, Stewart RA, Benatar J, French JK, Aylward PE, White HD; HERO-2 Investigators. aVR ST elevation: an important but neglected sign in ST elevation acute myocardial infarction. Eur Heart J. 2010;31:1845–1853.

Case 2: Presentation

An 87-year-old female with history of chronic atrial fibrillation s/p AV node ablation and permanent implanted pacemaker presents with chest pain. What is your interpretation of her ECG?

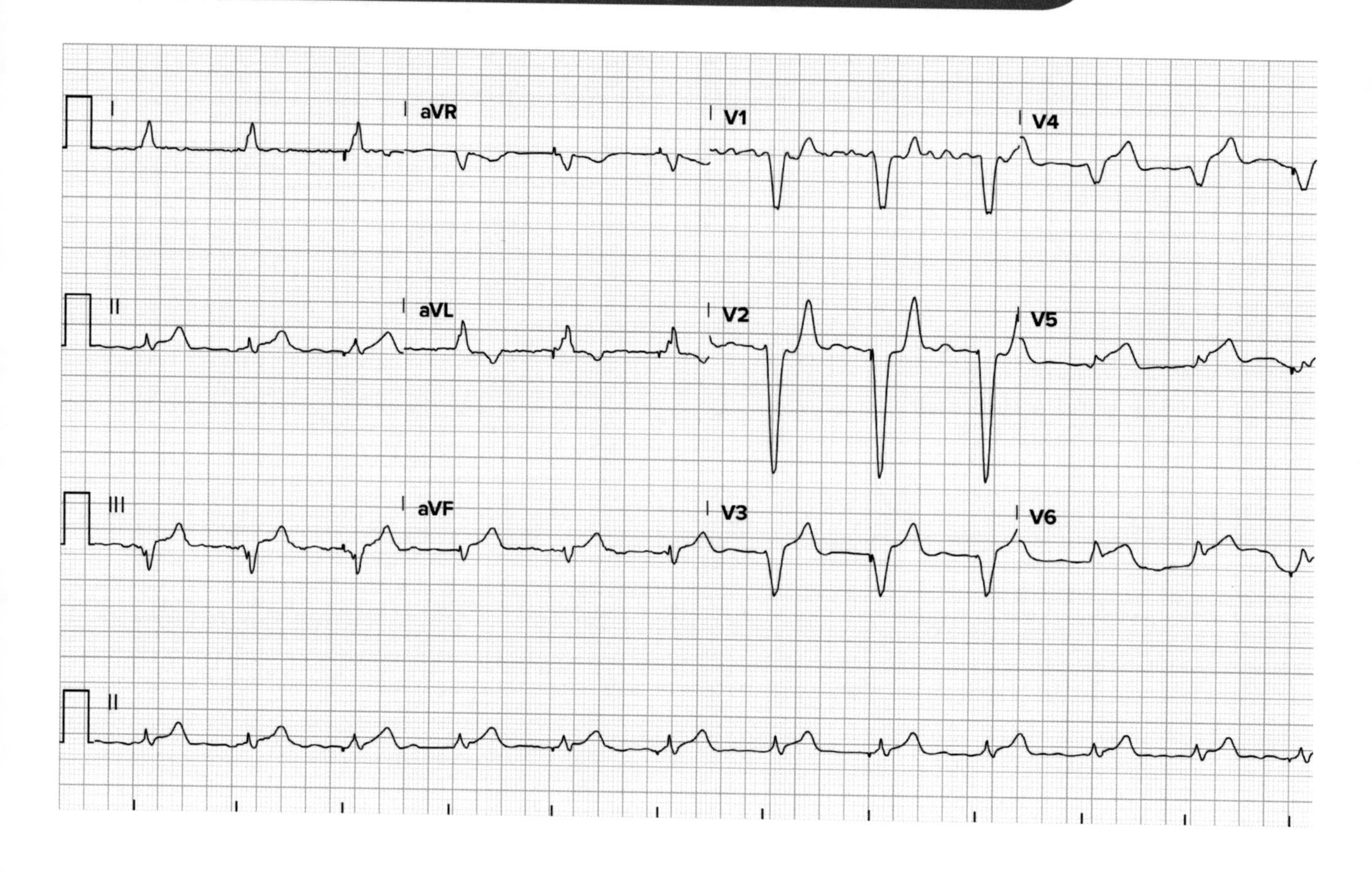

Case 2: Answer

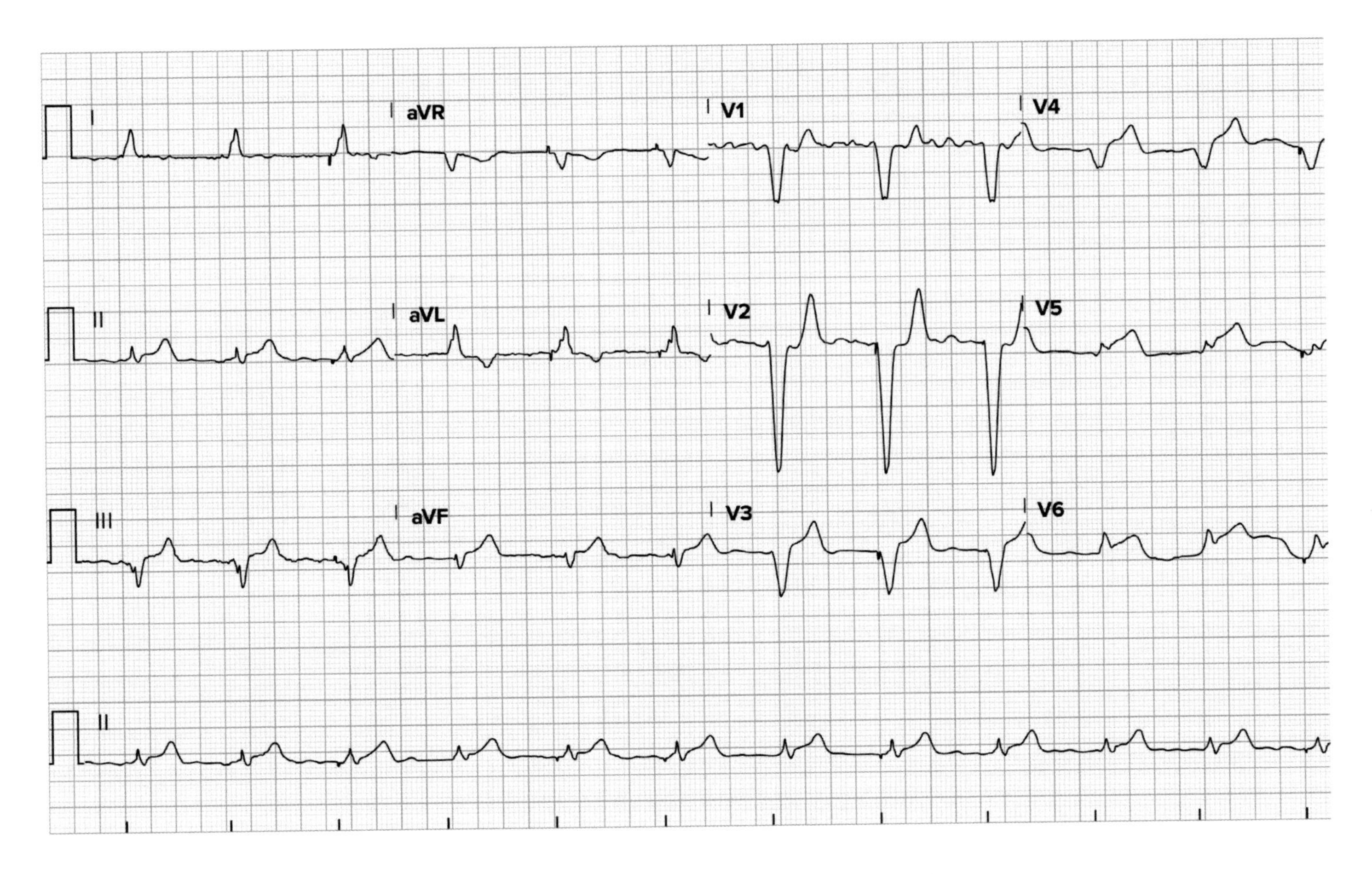

This ECG shows a ventricular-paced rhythm at 70 bpm, normal axis, prolonged QRS complex duration with a LBBB-like morphology, and concordant STE in leads II, V5, and V6 suggesting AMI. The STE in either lead II, V5, or V6 meets Sgarbossa criteria and the STE in leads V5-V6 meets traditional STEMI criteria.

The fundamentals of right ventricular pacing include:

- Depolarization is initiated in the apex of the right ventricle
- Produces an abnormal but predictable pattern that mimics an intrinsic LBBB except for leads V-V6, which will almost always have negatively oriented QRS complexes with a ventricular-paced rhythm
  - These repolarization abnormalities confound the ECG's ability to detect an AMI and/or other findings suggestive of ACS

As with an intrinsic LBBB, the expected repolarization abnormalities in a paced rhythm follow the "rule of appropriate discordance" which describes the relationship between the direction of the QRS complex and its ST-segment (and usually T-wave). In other words, if the main vector of the QRS complex points up, there will be STD (and often TWI), and if the QRS complex points down, there will STE (and often upright T-waves). These repolarization abnormalities confound the ECG's ability to detect an AMI and other ACS findings, so interpretation of the ECG in a presentation suggestive of ACS requires using the Sgarbossa criteria to diagnose an AMI. It is important to note that a significant number of patients with an AMI and a ventricular-paced rhythm will not have any abnormalities, Sgarbossa or otherwise, on their ECG.

The Sgarbossa criteria are based on the underlying principle that concordance and excessive discordance in a LBBB are abnormal. The criteria assign a point value for any concordant STE ***(see Figures 1a and 1b)*** or excessively discordant STE *(see Figure 1C)*. A score ≥ 3 is 98% specific for AMI, so the presence of criteria A or B are considered diagnostic of an AMI. Criterion C is only assigned 2 points, so the presence of just criterion C is not diagnostic of an AMI. However, in the setting of a right ventricular-paced rhythm, Sgarbossa criterion C was found to have 99% specificity for AMI.[1]

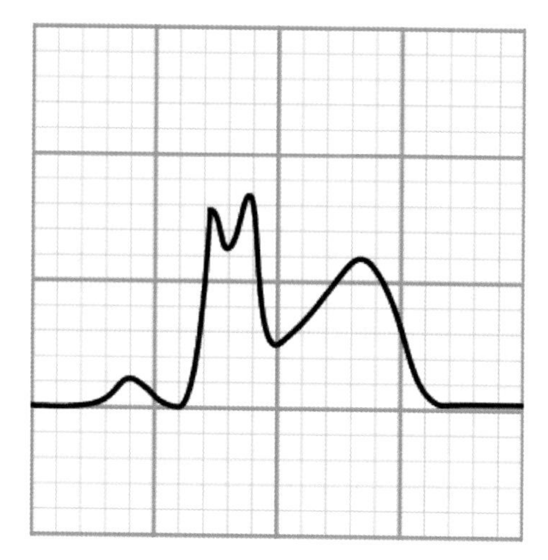

Figure 1a. Sgarbossa criterion A
Concordant STE ≥ 1 mm in ≥ 1 lead
(5 points = diagnostic of AMI)

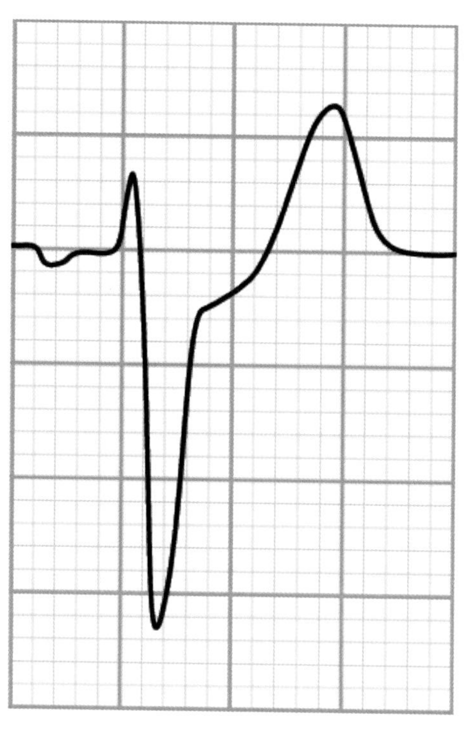

Figure 1b. Sgarbossa criterion B
STD ≥ 1 mm in V1, V2, or V3
(3 points = diagnostic of AMI)

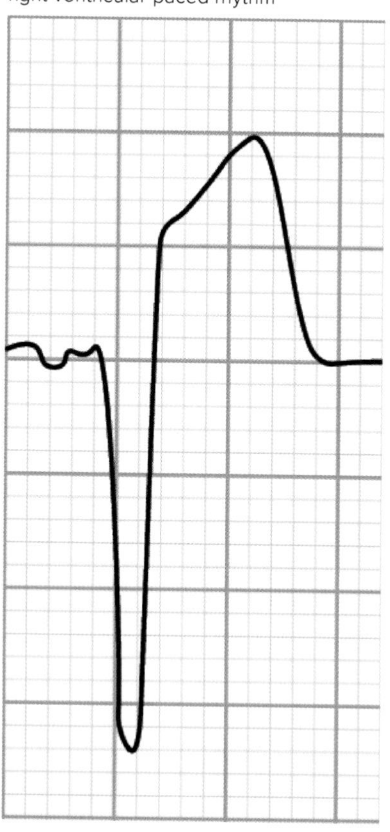

Figure 1c. Sgarbossa criterion C
Discordant STE ≥ 5 mm in ≥ 1 lead
(99% specific for AMI in the setting of a right ventricular-paced rhythm

The Modified Sgarbossa criteria includes Sgarbossa criteria A and B with a variation of criterion C. Instead of using a fixed cutoff of 5 mm for discordant STE, it uses a ratio of the STE height to the S-wave depth (***see Figure 2***). A STE/S ratio ≥ 0.25 in ≥ 1 lead is considered diagnostic of an AMI. This means that more than 5 mm of STE is permissible if there is a large S-wave, and less than 5 mm of STE may be diagnostic if the accompanying S-wave is small. The Modified Sgarbossa criteria are not mandated in the current AHA/ACC STEMI guidelines, and at the time of publication, there are no published studies on the use of the Modified Sgarbossa criteria in ventricular-paced rhythms.

Figure 2. Modified Sgarbossa criterion C
STE/S ratio ≥ 0.25 in ≥ 1 lead
(diagnostic of AMI but not mandated in current AHA/ACC STEMI guidelines)

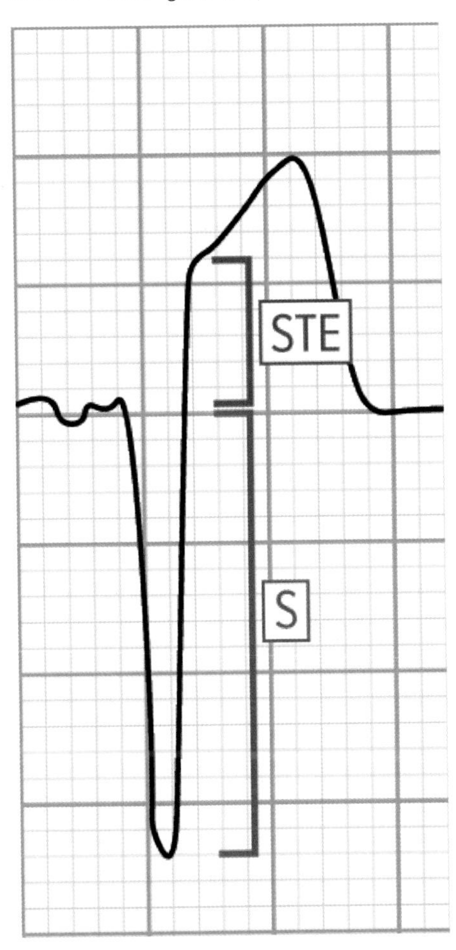

This patient was taken to the catherization laboratory, where a 100% occlusion of the 2nd obtuse marginal artery was successfully treated with a stent.

AMI in Right Ventricular-Paced Rhythms Learning Points

- In general, evaluate a paced ECG for ischemia as you would a LBBB, using Sgarbossa criteria
- Discordant STE ≥ 5 mm: 99% specificity[1] (note that this study had no cases with STE > 1 mm)
- Concordant STE ≥ 1 mm: 94% specificity[2]
- At the time of publication, there are no published studies on the use of the Modified Sgarbossa criteria in ventricular-paced rhythms

References

1. Maloy KR, Bhat R, Davis J, Reed K, Morrissey R. Sgarbossa Criteria Are Highly Specific for Acute Myocardial Infarction with Pacemakers. *West J Emerg Med.* 2010;11(4):354-357.
2. Sgarbossa EB, Pinski SL, Gates KB, Wagner GS, The GUSTO-1 Investigators. Early electrocardiographic diagnosis of acute myocardial infarction in the presence of ventricular-paced rhythm. *J Am Coll Cardiol.* 1996;77(5):423-424.

Case 3: Presentation

A 76-year-old male presents due to exertional chest pain that resolved immediately prior to arrival. What is your interpretation of his ECG?

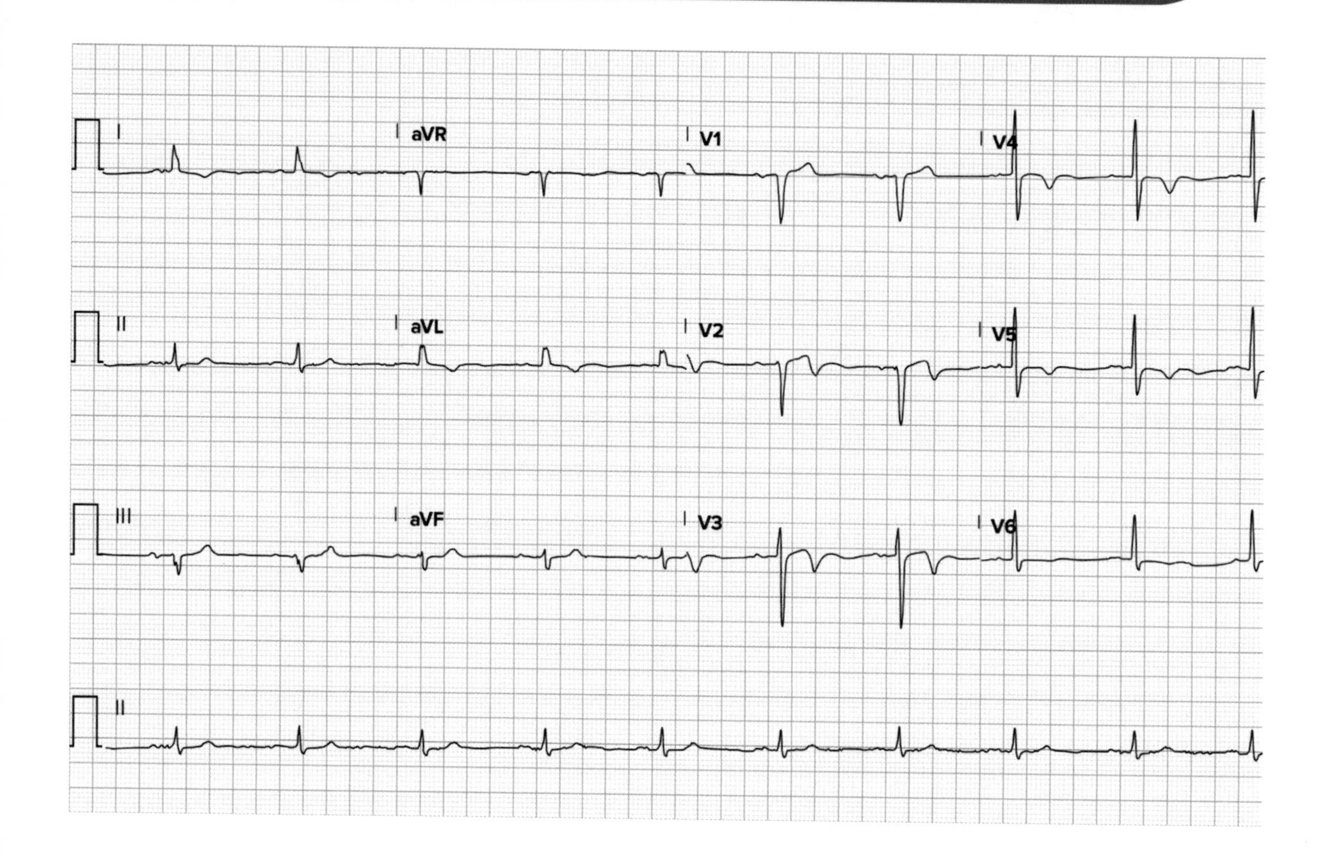

Prior ECG from 6 months ago

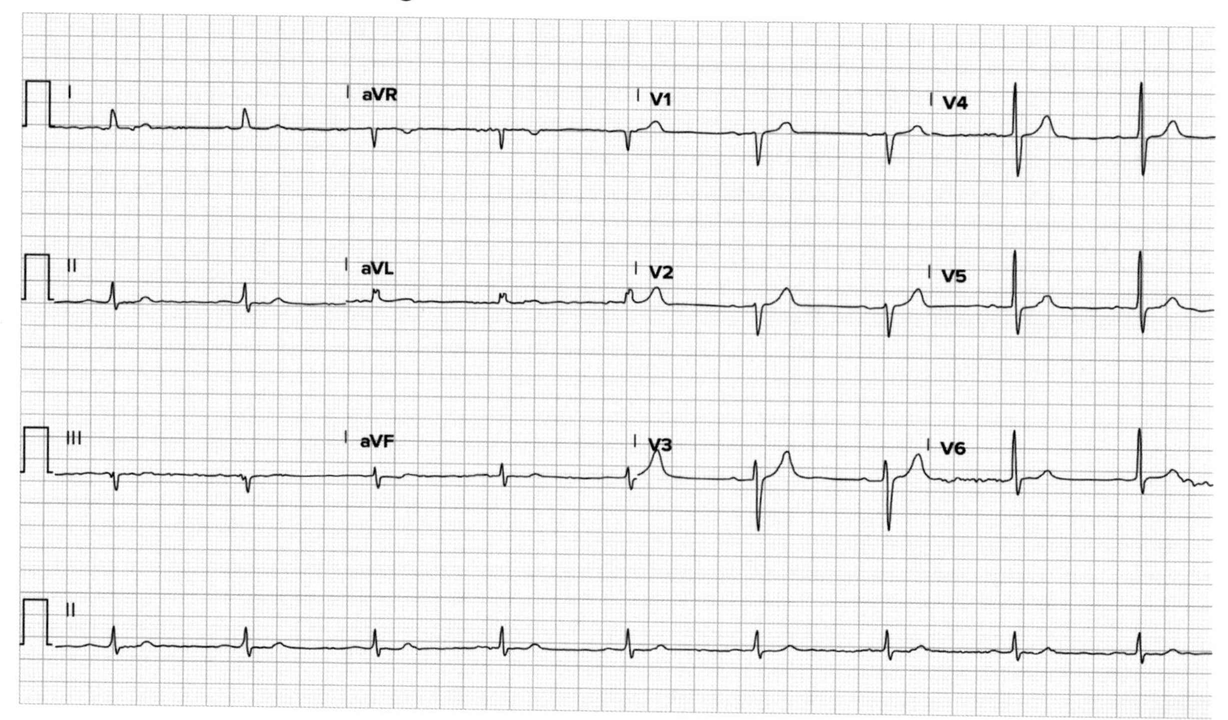

Case 3: Answer

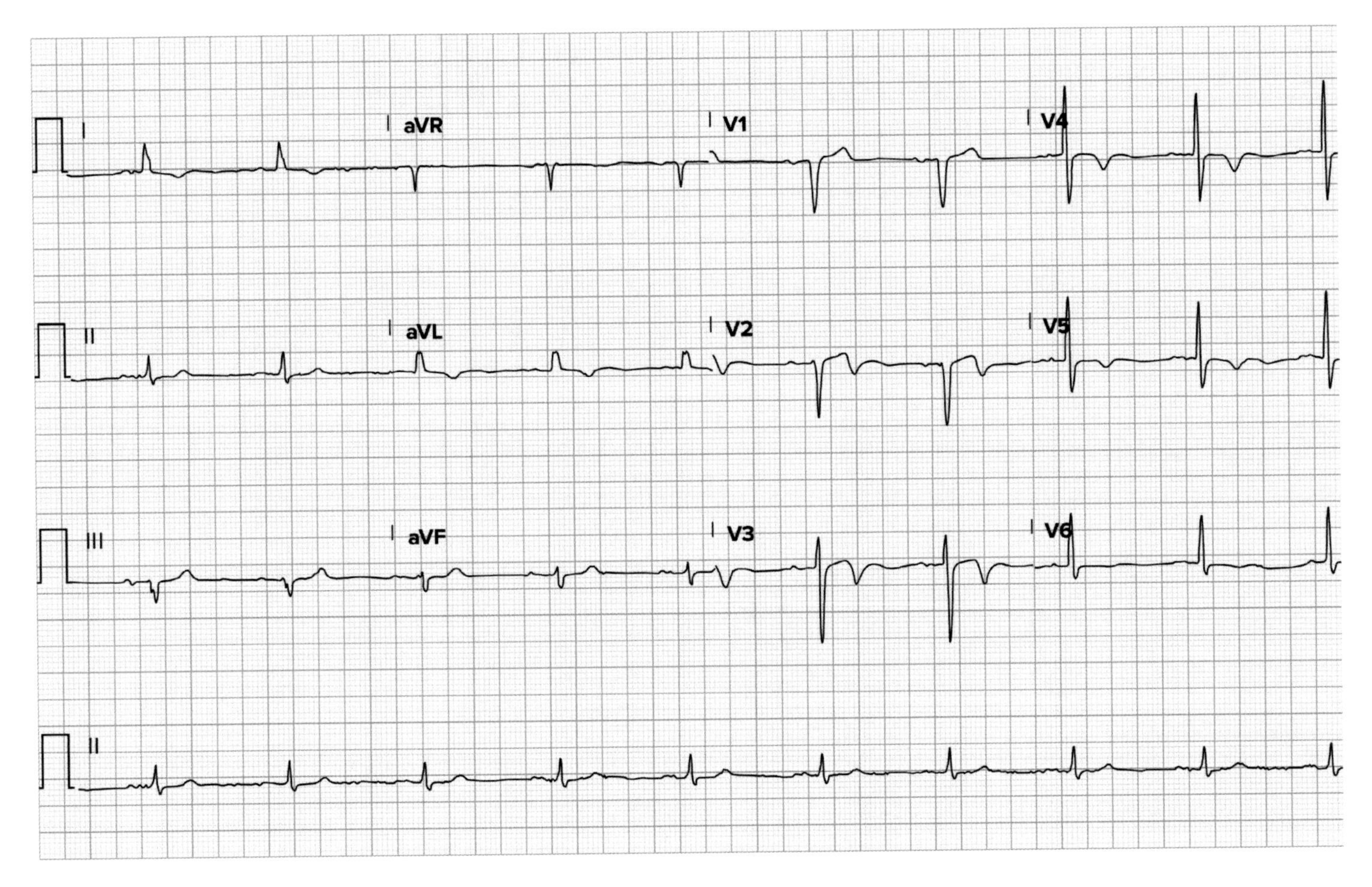

This ECG shows sinus bradycardia at 58 bpm, normal axis, normal QRS complex duration, TWI in leads I, aVL, V4-V5, and biphasic T-waves in V2-V3. The TWI and biphasic T-waves are new from the prior ECG six months ago ***(see figure on next page)***.

The morphology of the precordial TWI is typically seen in Wellens syndrome, also called "LAD coronary T-wave syndrome," which describes an abnormal T-wave pattern seen in a pain-free state with recent history of anginal symptoms. These characteristic ECG findings were first described in 1982 by Dr. Hein J.J. Wellens, a Dutch cardiologist, who found that 75% of patients with this syndrome developed an anterior MI within a few weeks of hospital admission if no intervention was performed.[1] The diagnostic criteria include:

- Biphasic (type A, as seen in this example) or deeply inverted (type B) T-waves in the mid-precordial leads, typically V2-V3 ***(see Figures 1a and 1b)***
- Isoelectric or minimally elevated ST-segment (< 1 mm)
- No precordial Q-waves
- Preserved precordial R-wave progression
- Normal or minimally elevated troponins

Prior ECG from 6 months ago

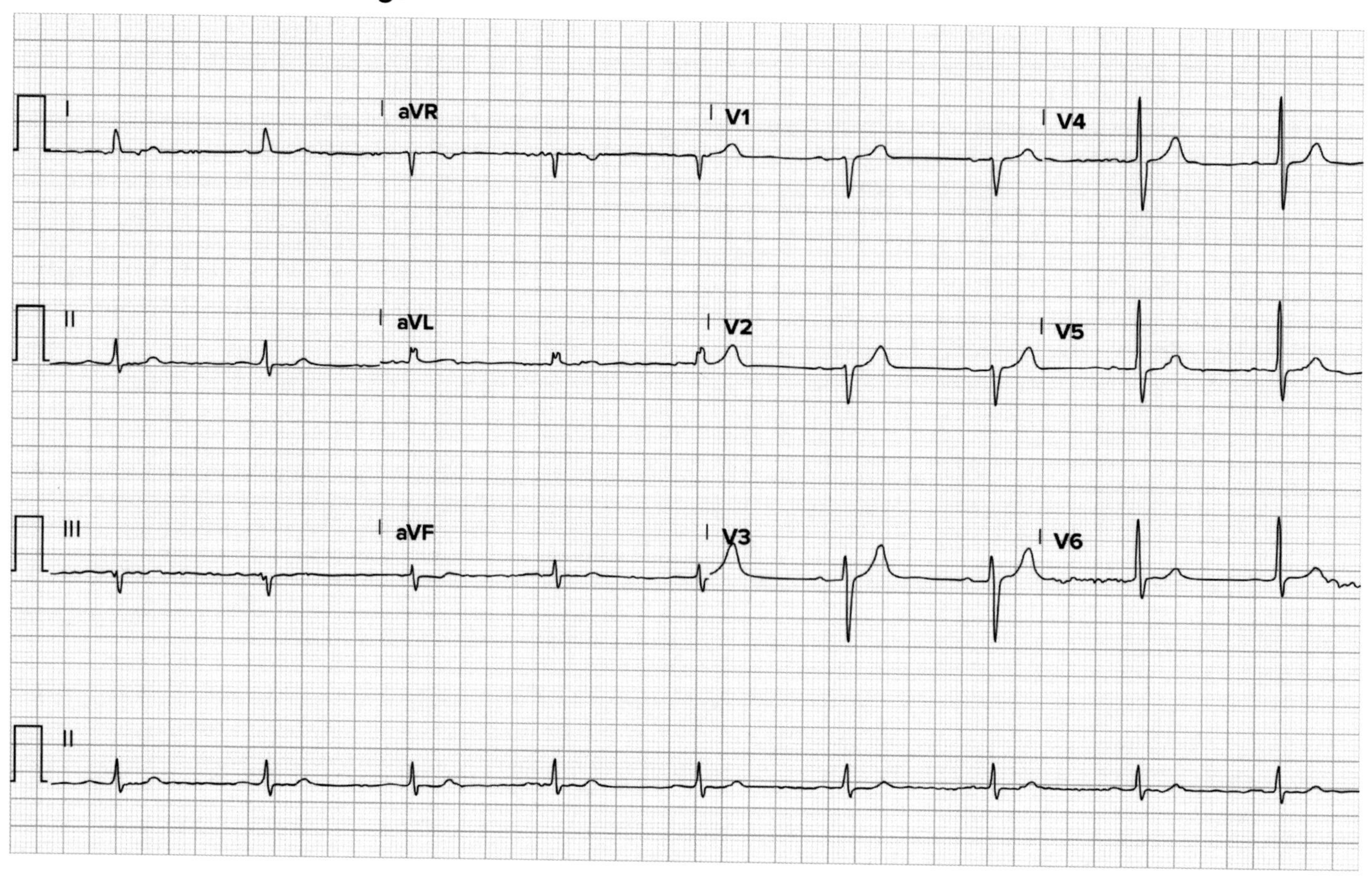

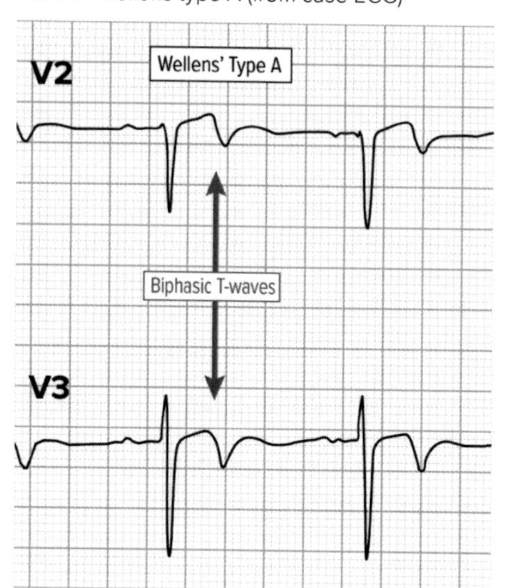

Figure 1a. Biphasic T-waves
Seen in Wellens type A (from case ECG)

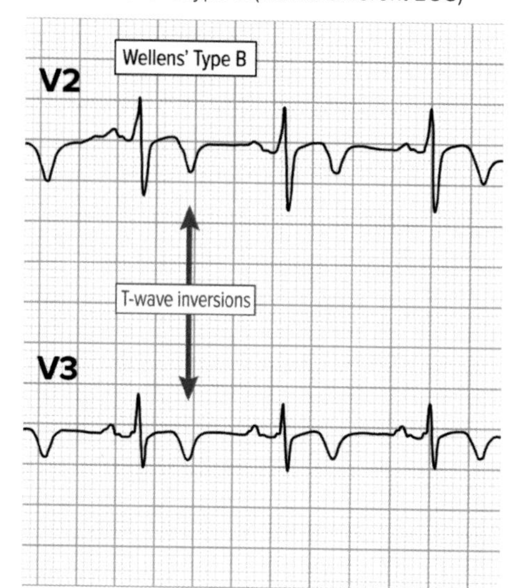

Figure 1b. TWI
Seen in Wellens type B (from a different ECG)

There is no universal definition for a preserved precordial R-wave progression, but common criteria include:

- R-wave > 2-4 mm in lead V3 or V4
- R-wave in lead V4 > lead V3 or lead V3 > lead V2
- R-wave in lead V3 ≥ 3 mm

This ECG pattern is concerning for a critical stenosis/lesion of the proximal LAD, and the T-wave abnormalities are thought to represent reperfusion after an ischemic event. Biphasic T-waves, also called Wellens type A, are an early finding, while deeply inverted T-waves, also called Wellens type B, are a later finding and more common (up to 75% of cases). Patients with these ECG findings in the appropriate clinical context have a high likelihood of developing an anterior MI within a short period of time1 and warrant admission for cardiac catheterization. Coronary angiography is required to evaluate the need for early angioplasty or coronary bypass surgery, and provocative testing, especially exercise stress testing, should be avoided as it could precipitate an AMI or cardiac arrest.[2,3,4]

It is important to recognize that these ECG findings were originally described in patients in a pain-free state. In fact, it is not unusual to see these ECG changes persist from the painful presentation into the pain-free state as the ECG changes do not resolve until the LAD lesion is successfully managed with either PCI or CABG.

The term "Wellens waves" is sometimes used to describe these ECG findings in symptomatic patients. In these cases, the ECG changes are due to active ischemia. The term "pseudo-Wellens" is commonly used to describe these ECG findings when associated with causes other than LAD stenosis such as LVH, PE, hypertrophic cardiomyopathy, intracranial hemorrhage, and RBBB. In these cases, the ECG changes are due to repolarization abnormalities.

This patient presented in the middle of the night and was ultimately admitted for an urgent, but not emergent, cardiac catheterization later that morning. He was found to have a 95% occlusion of the proximal LAD, which was successfully treated with a stent.

Wellens Syndrome Learning Points

- Wellens syndrome describes an abnormal T-wave pattern seen in the mid-precordial leads, typically V2-V3, in a pain-free state with recent history of anginal symptoms
  - Type A: biphasic T-waves seen immediately upon reperfusion
  - Type B: deeply inverted T-waves, later finding
- These findings represent critical stenosis of the proximal LAD and warrants admission for cardiac catheterization
  - Provocative testing should be avoided as it could precipitate an MI
- Associated with a high risk of an anterior MI if left untreated

References

1. de Zwaan C, Bär FW, Wellens HJ. Characteristic electrocardiographic pattern indicating a critical stenosis high in left anterior descending coronary artery in patients admitted because of impending myocardial infarction. *Am Heart J.* 1982;103(4 Pt 2):730-736.
2. de Zwann C, FW Bar, JH Janssen, et al. Angiographic and clinical characteristics of patients with unstable angina showing an ECG pattern indicating critical narrowing of the proximal LAD coronary artery. *Am Heart J.* 1989;117(3):657-665.
3. Rhinehardt J, Brady WJ, Perron AD, Mattu A. Electrocardiographic manifestations of Wellens syndrome. *Am J Emerg Med.* 2002;20(7):638-643.
4. Patel K, Alattar F, Koneru J, Shamoon F. ST-Elevation Myocardial Infarction after Pharmacologic Persantine Stress Test in a Patient with Wellens Syndrome. Case Rep Emerg Med. v2014; 2014:PMC4006572.

Case 4: Presentation

A 66-year-old male with history of only hypertension presents with exertional near syncope. What is your interpretation of his ECG?

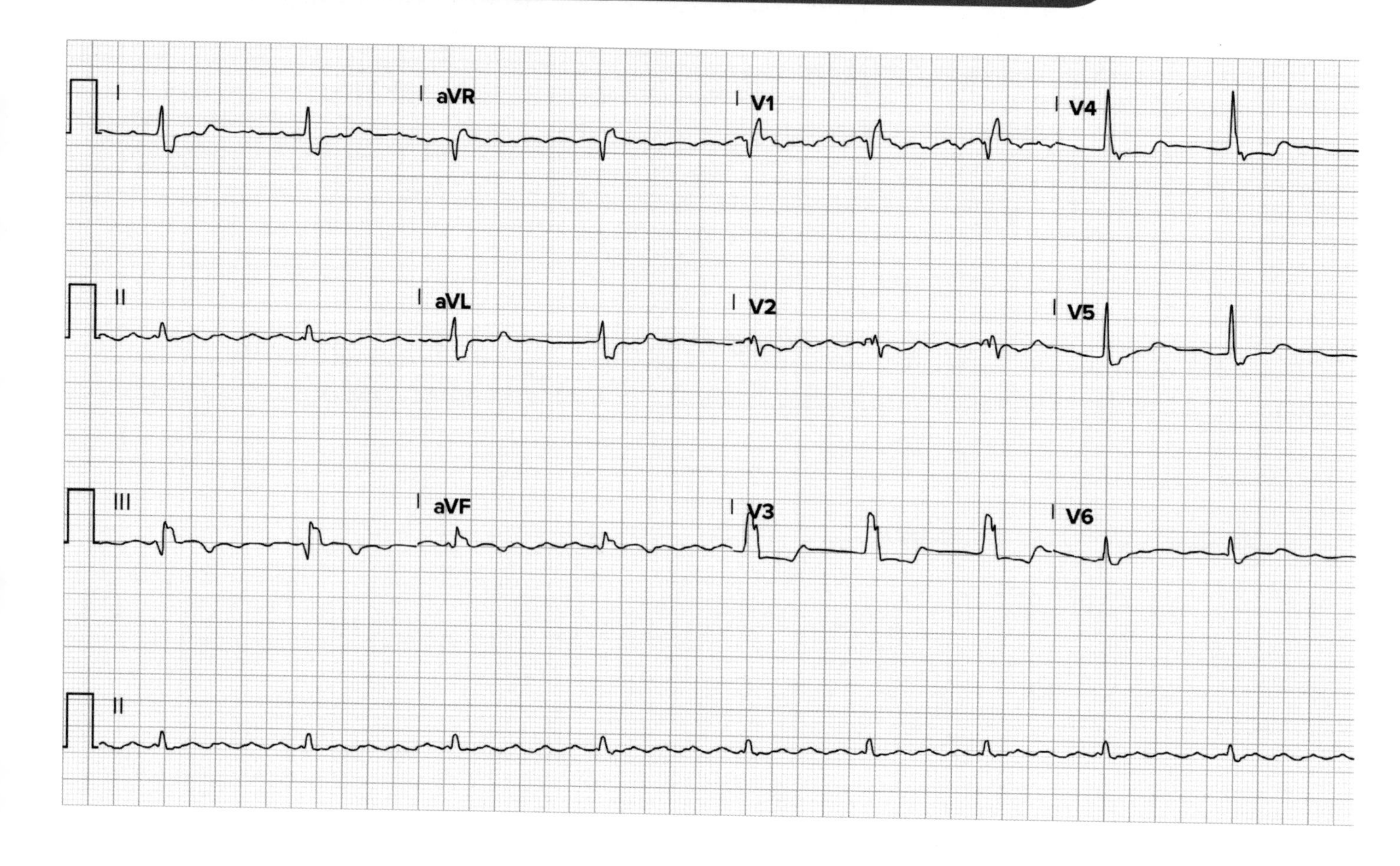

Case 4: Answer

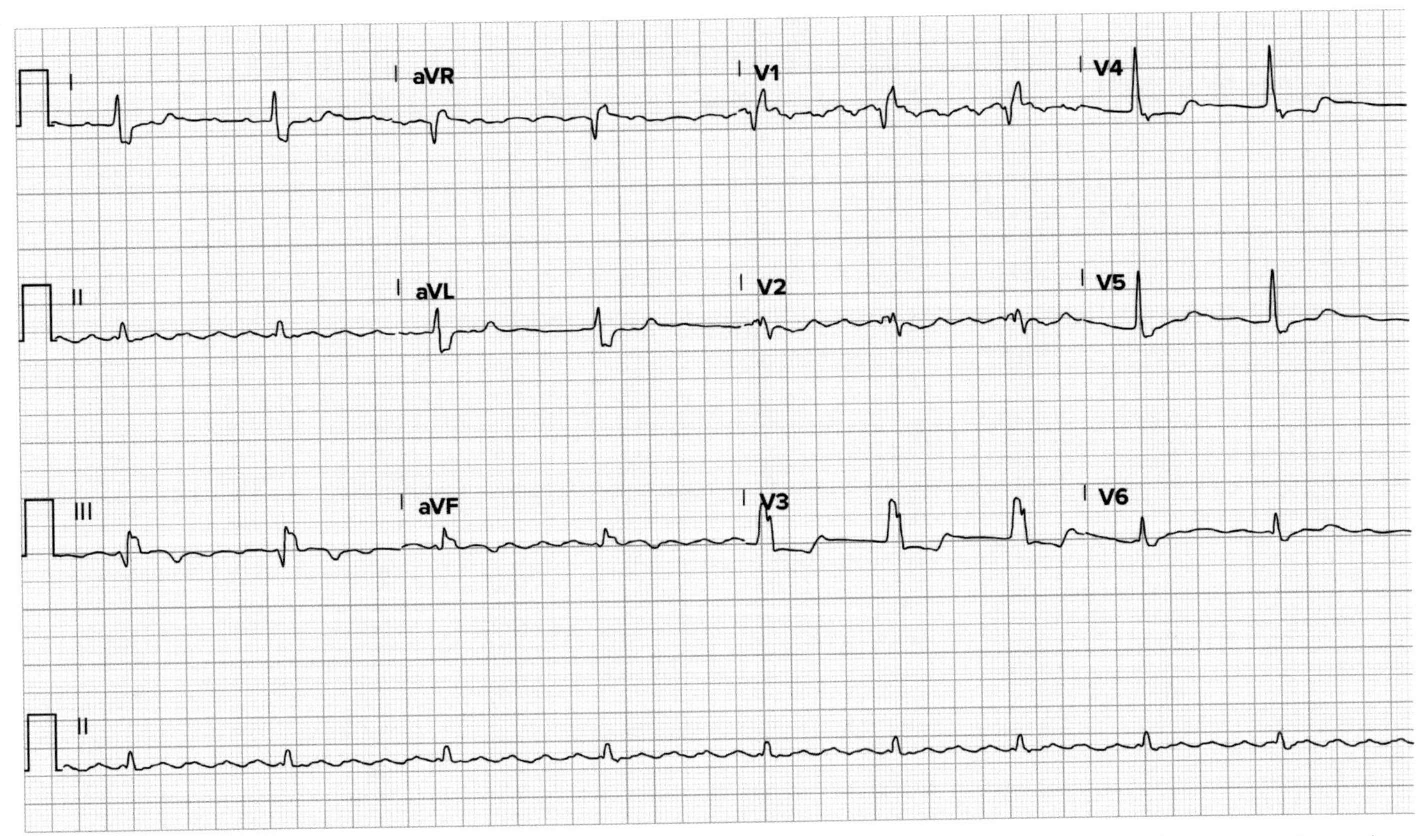

This ECG shows atrial flutter with variable block and an average ventricular rate of 57 bpm, normal axis, and a prolonged QRS complex duration with a RBBB.

This ECG shows flutter waves, also called F-waves, best seen in the inferior leads, that are diagnostic of atrial flutter. Atrial flutter is typically due to a right atrial re-entry circuit around the tricuspid ring. It is classified as a macro-reentry tachycardia because it revolves around a large obstacle, the right atrium, as opposed to a small obstacle like the AV node. This ECG shows atrial flutter with both 5:1 and 4:1 conduction ***(see Figure 1)***.

Figure 1. Atrial flutter

The lead II rhythm strip shows atrial flutter with both 5:1 and 4:1 conduction

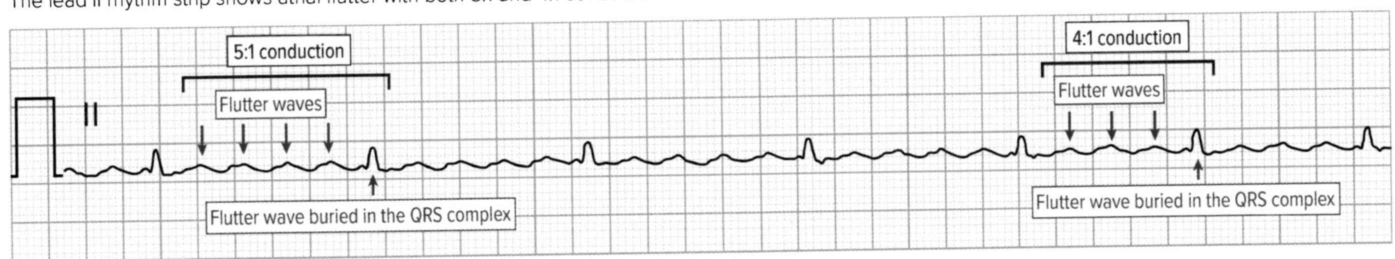

The flutter waves have a consistent FF interval of 230 msec which equates to ~260 bpm. Beats 1-4 and 9 show 5:1 flutter. Using beats 1 and 2 as an example ***(see Figure 2)***, the RR interval is 1150 msec which is exactly 5 times the FF interval of 230 msec. This is consistent with 5:1 flutter (ie, 5 flutter waves for every 1 QRS complex). Beats 5-8 ***(see Figure 3)*** show an RR interval of 920 msec which is exactly 4 times the FF interval and consistent with 4:1 flutter.

Figure 2.
The atrial rate is exactly five times the ventricular rate (seen here in the initial portion of the lead II rhythm strip), consistent with atrial flutter with 5:1 conduction

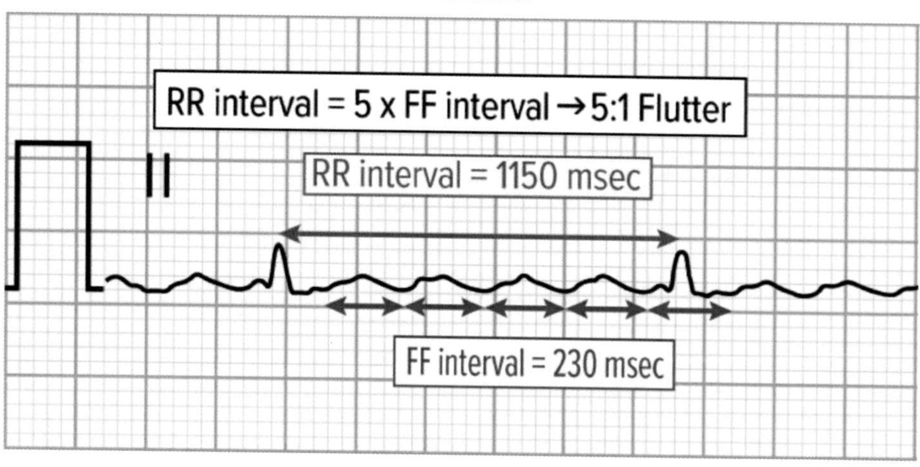

Figure 3.
The atrial rate is exactly four times the ventricular rate between the 5th and 7th QRS complexes (the 5th and 6th QRS complexes from the lead II rhythm strip are shown here), consistent with atrial flutter with 4:1 conduction

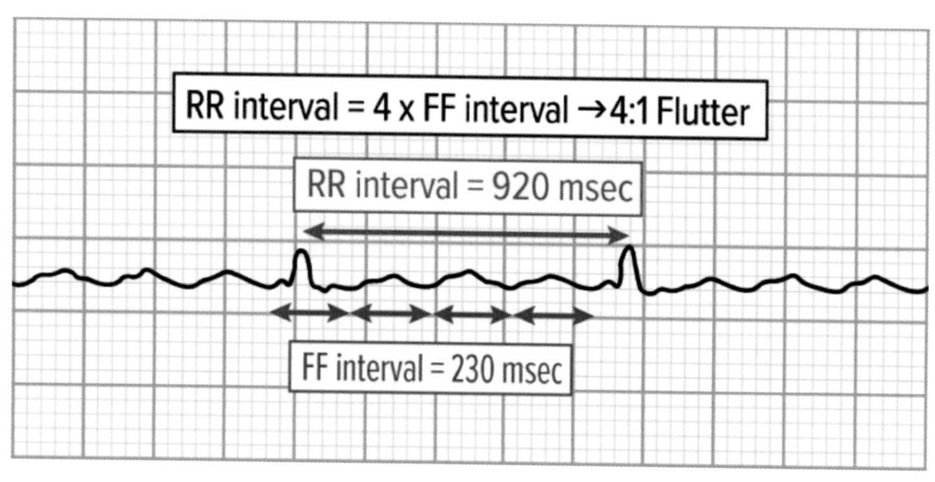

This ECG also shows a RBBB. The characteristic findings in a RBBB include:

- QRS complex duration ≥ 120 msec
- rsr', rsR', or rSR' pattern in lead V1 +/- V2 ***(see Figure 4)***
  - Variations in lead V1 include qR pattern or broad R-wave that is often notched
  - In lead V1, the initial upward deflection should always be smaller than the 2nd upward deflection ***(see Figure 4)***
- S-wave duration > R-wave or > 40 msec in leads I and V6 ***(see Figures 5 and 6)***
- Normal R-wave peak time in leads V5 and V6 but > 50 msec in lead V1 (only required if broad R-wave +/- notch is present in lead V1)
- Repolarization abnormalities include STD and TWI in lead V1 +/- lead(s) V2-V3 if they have an rsR' pattern, so STE and/or upright T-waves in those leads are concerning for ischemia

A RBBB will typically have STD and TWI in lead V1, and if leads V2-V3 have an rsR' pattern present, they will also typically have STD and TWI. Consequently, upright T-waves or STE in those leads with an rsR' pattern is concerning for ischemia, and even isoelectric or minimally elevated ST-segments can be a subtle indicator of early AMI. Otherwise, the presence of a RBBB does not confound the ECG evaluation of ACS as does a LBBB. This ECG also shows STD in lead V4, but this is unlikely to be clinically significant in this case.

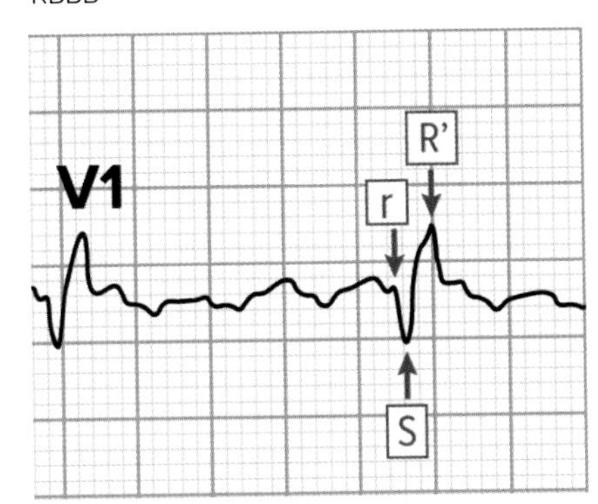

Figure 4.
rSR' pattern in lead V1, consistent with a RBBB

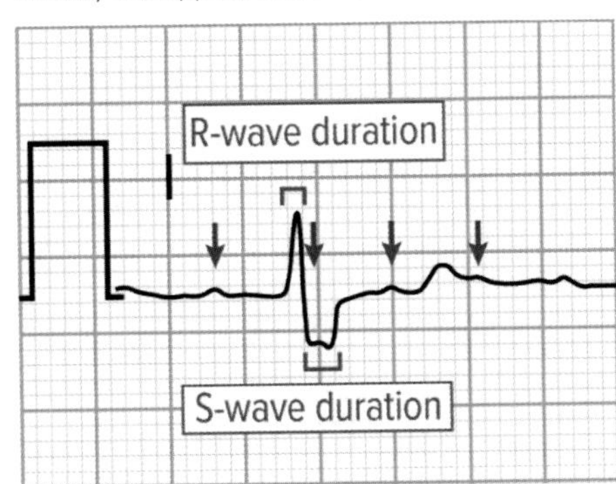

Figure 5.
S-wave duration > R-wave duration in lead I, consistent with a RBBB, and flutter waves (purple arrows) that appear similar to P-waves

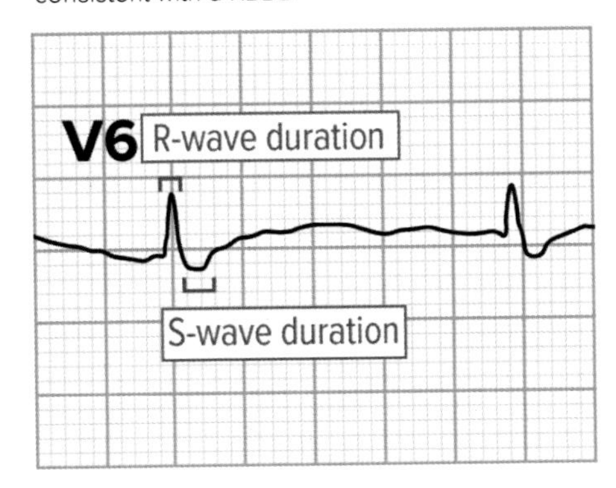

Figure 6.
S-wave duration > R-wave duration in lead V6, consistent with a RBBB

This patient had new onset atrial flutter that was likely rate-controlled by his use of metoprolol for hypertension. The time of onset was unclear and the patient remained hemodynamically stable, so there was no indication for immediate cardioversion. The patient was admitted to the cardiology service and spontaneously converted to sinus rhythm.

Atrial Flutter Learning Points

- Due to a re-entrant circuit in the right atrium
- Stereotypical 'sawtooth pattern' of P-waves seen best in the inferior leads
  - Absence of isoelectric baseline (eg, TP segment) in lead II
- Atrial rate is 250-350 bpm and typically fixed over time
  - Ventricular rate is a fraction of atrial rate (ie, for an atrial rate of 300 bpm, 2:1 conduction produces a ventricular rate of 150 bpm, 3:1 conduction produces a ventricular rate of 100 bmp, 4:1 conduction produces a ventricular rate of 75 bpm, etc.)
- Consider atrial flutter when ventricular rate is consistently around 150 bpm
- Vagal maneuvers or adenosine will slow ventricular rate but have no effect on flutter waves

RBBB Learning Points

- Delayed conduction through right ventricle with normal left ventricular conduction
- In lead V1, the initial upward deflection should always be smaller than the 2nd upward deflection
- Repolarization abnormalities include STD and TWI in lead V1 +/- lead(s) V2-V3 if they have an rsR' pattern, so STE and/or upright T-waves in those leads are concerning for ischemia
  - Otherwise, the presence of a RBBB does not confound the ECG evaluation of ACS as does a LBBB
- RBBB with axis deviation should prompt evaluation for a concurrent LAFB or LPFB

Case 5: Presentation

An 84-year-old male is sent to the emergency department due to an abnormal pre-op ECG. He has no complaints. What is your interpretation of his ECG?

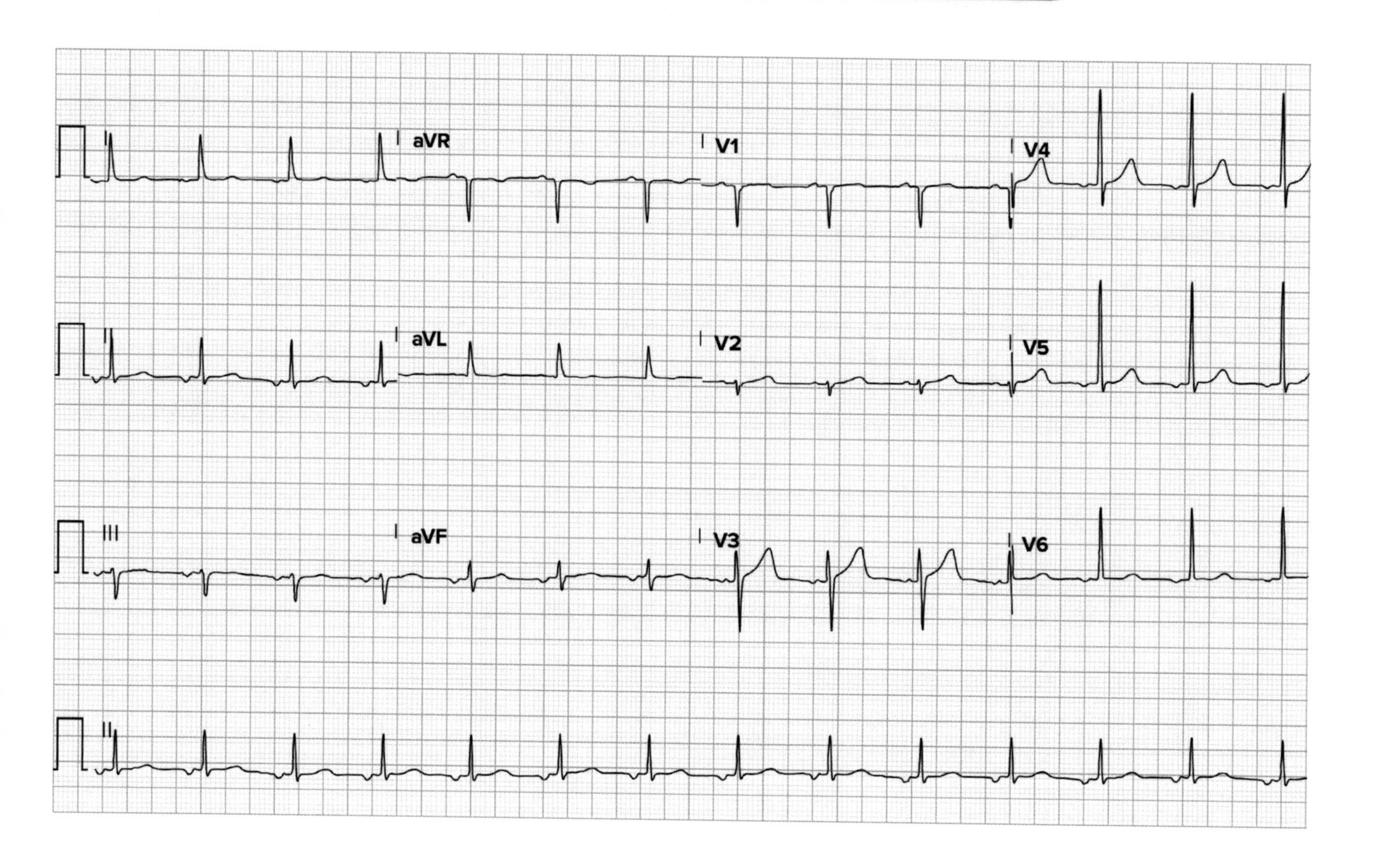

Case 5: Answer

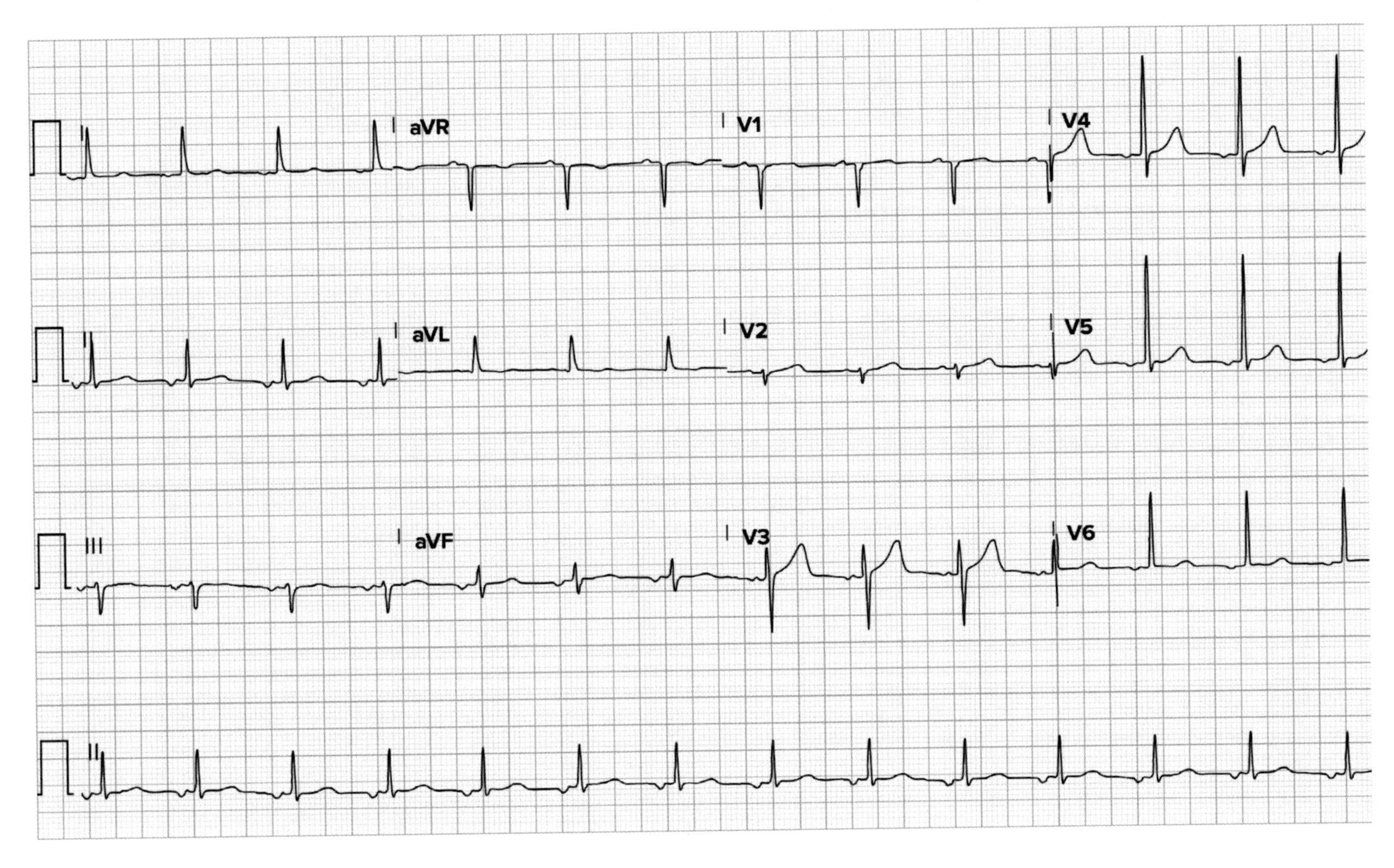

This ECG shows an ectopic atrial rhythm with a ventricular rate of 82 bpm, normal axis, normal intervals, negative P-waves in leads I, II, III, aVF, and V4-V6, and positive P-waves in lead aVR.

The key to interpreting this ECG is identifying the abnormal P-waves, in particular the negative P-wave in lead II which is never present in a normal sinus rhythm ***(see Figure 1)***. The characteristics of normal P-waves includes:

- Leads I and II: always upright and monophasic
- Lead III: upright, inverted, or biphasic (positive-negative)
- Lead aVR: always inverted and monophasic
- Lead aVL: upright, inverted, or biphasic (negative-positive)
- Lead aVF: usually upright but can be flat or biphasic
- Lead V1: usually biphasic (positive-negative) but can be entirely upright or inverted
- Lead V2: usually biphasic (positive-negative) but can be entirely upright (entirely inverted is rare)
- Leads V3-V6: always upright and monophasic
- The PR interval, which includes the time for atrial depolarization and conduction through the AV node, is 120-200 msec for adults and 70-180 msec for pediatric patients

Figure 1.
The P-wave in lead II should be upright in sinus rhythm

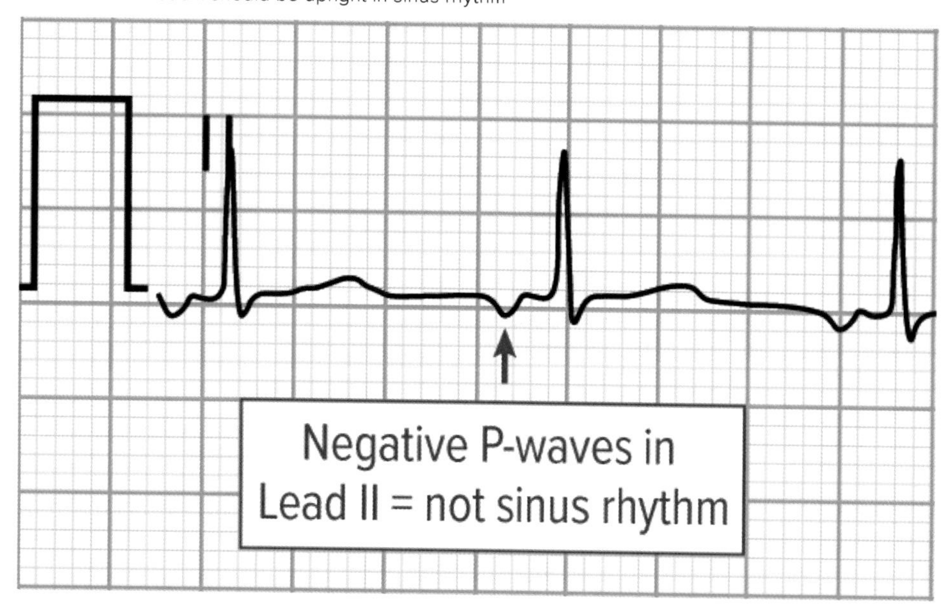

The differential diagnosis for inverted P-waves in a regular narrow complex rhythm with normal ventricular rates includes:

- Ectopic atrial rhythm
- Junctional rhythm with retrograde P-waves that precede the QRS complex

An ectopic atrial rhythm originates from a site in the atria other than the SA node with a rate of 60-100 bpm. Ectopic P-waves will differ from sinus P-wave in their morphology (ie, shape), axis (ie, positive or negative), or both. The PR interval is typically 120-200 msec but can be < 120 msec when the ectopic atrial focus is located near the AV node.

A junctional rhythm originates from the AV node or proximal Purkinje system with a rate of 40-60 bpm. It is called an accelerated junctional rhythm when the rate is 61-100 bpm. In junctional rhythms, the depolarization of the cardiac conduction system starts in the middle so there is anterograde conduction to the ventricles and retrograde conduction back to the atria. This retrograde conduction creates P-waves that are typically inverted when compared to the sinus P-waves. If the junctional focus initiates conduction in the AV node, the retrograde P-waves can appear before the QRS complex with a short PR interval. If the junctional focus is farther down the conduction system, the retrograde P-waves can appear after the QRS complex, be buried in the QRS complex, or be hidden in the QRS complex and not appear at all.

Ectopic atrial rhythms occur when the ectopic atrial rate exceeds the SA node rate or the SA node rate slows to below the ectopic atrial rate. In this patient's ECG, the normal PR interval suggests that the rhythm is an ectopic atrial rhythm. This patient had an unremarkable workup in the ED and was discharged.

Normal P-wave and T-wave Learning Points

- Normal P-wave and T-wave morphologies[1,2] in adults in normal sinus rhythm in the absence of conduction abnormalities, ischemia, structural abnormalities, etc. include:

I	aVR	V1	V4
P: always upright T: always upright	P: always inverted T: always inverted	P: usually biphasic (+/-) but can be entirely upright or inverted T: upright or inverted	P: upright T: almost always upright
II P: always upright T: always upright	**aVL** P: upright, inverted, or biphasic (-/+) T: upright or inverted	**V2** P: usually biphasic (+/-) but can be entirely upright (entirely inverted is rare) T: usually upright	**V5** P: upright T: always upright
III P: upright, inverted, or biphasic (+/-) T: upright or inverted	**aVF** P: usually upright but can be flat or biphasic T: usually upright	**V3** P: upright T: usually upright	**V6** P: upright T: always upright

- Inverted, flat, or positive-negative biphasic T-waves in lead V1 (less so in leads V2-V3) can be normal
- Positive-negative biphasic T-waves in leads V1-V3 can be abnormal or a normal variant
- T-wave amplitude is typically < 6 mm in limb leads and < 10 mm in precordial leads

Ectopic Atrial Rhythm Learning Points

- Ectopic focus from the atria other than the SA node
- ECG shows ventricular rate 60-100 bpm with normal QRS complex duration unless concurrent conduction abnormality (eg, bundle branch block)
- P-waves with have different morphology/axis than sinus P-waves
- PR interval typically normal at 120-200 msec but can be < 120 msec if the focus is near the AV node

Junctional Rhythm Learning Points

- Ectopic focus from AV node or proximal Purkinje system
  - Also called AV junctional rhythm, nodal rhythm, nodal escape rhythm, junctional escape rhythm, AV nodal rhythm
- ECG shows ventricular rate of 40-60 bpm with normal QRS complex duration unless concurrent conduction abnormality (eg, bundle branch block)
- May have retrograde P-waves that precede (with PR interval < 120 msec) or follow QRS complex, typically best seen in the inferior leads
- Variations include:
  - Junctional Bradycardia: ventricular rate < 40 bpm
  - Accelerated Junctional Rhythm: ventricular rate 61–100 bpm
  - Junctional Tachycardia: ventricular rate > 100 bpm
  - Normal variant, especially in young athletes

References

1. Knilans T, Surawicz B. Chou's Electrocardiography in Clinical Practice. Philadelphia, PA: Elsevier. 2020.
2. Berberian, JG. Normal P-waves and T-waves. In: Berberian JG, Brady WJ, Mattu A. EMRA EKG Guide, 2nd ed. Emergency Medicine Residents' Association. Dallas, TX:2022:1.

Case 6: Presentation

This is the preop ECG of a 74-year-old male being admitted for a hip fracture. What is your interpretation of his ECG?

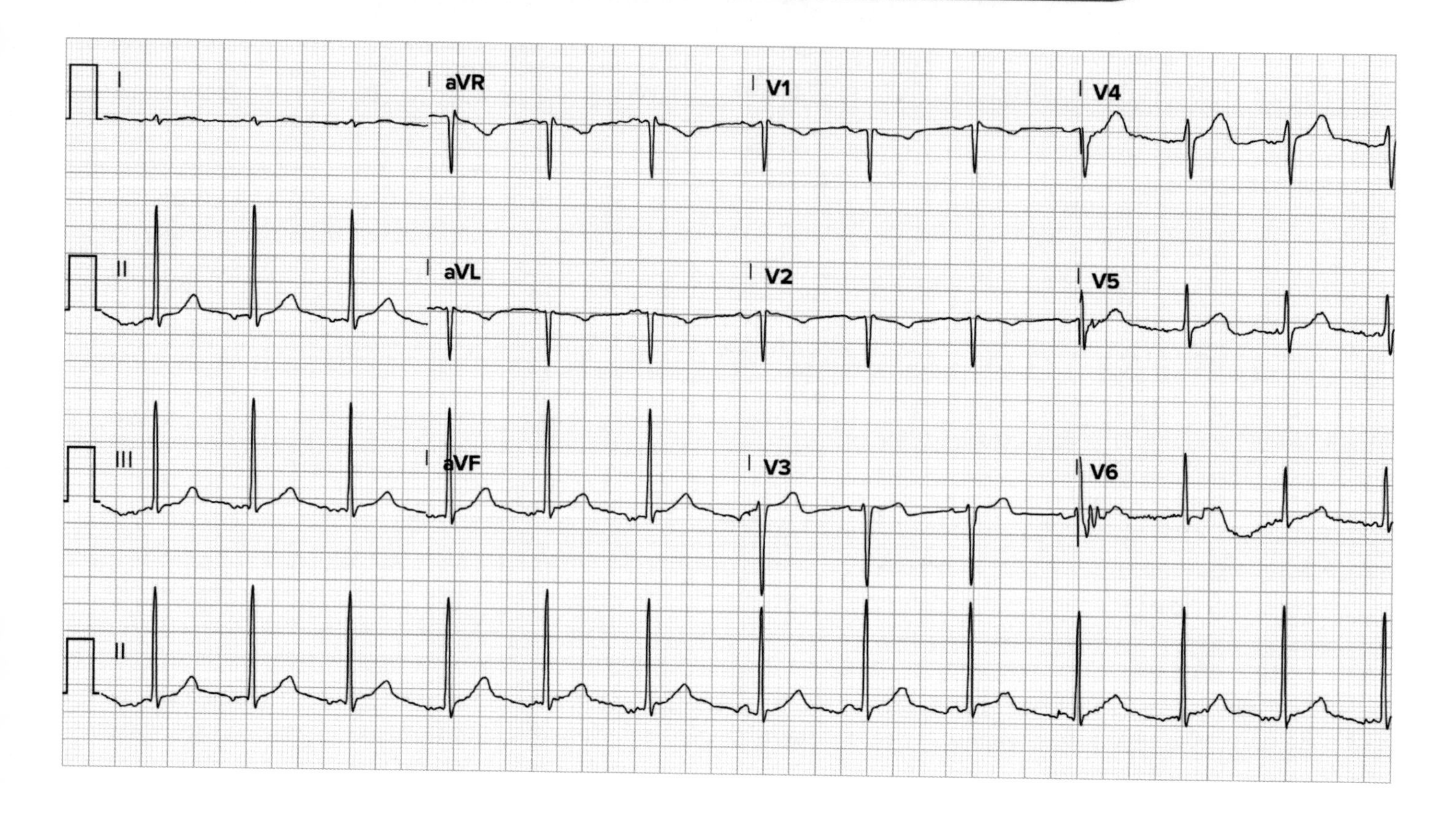

Case 6: Answer

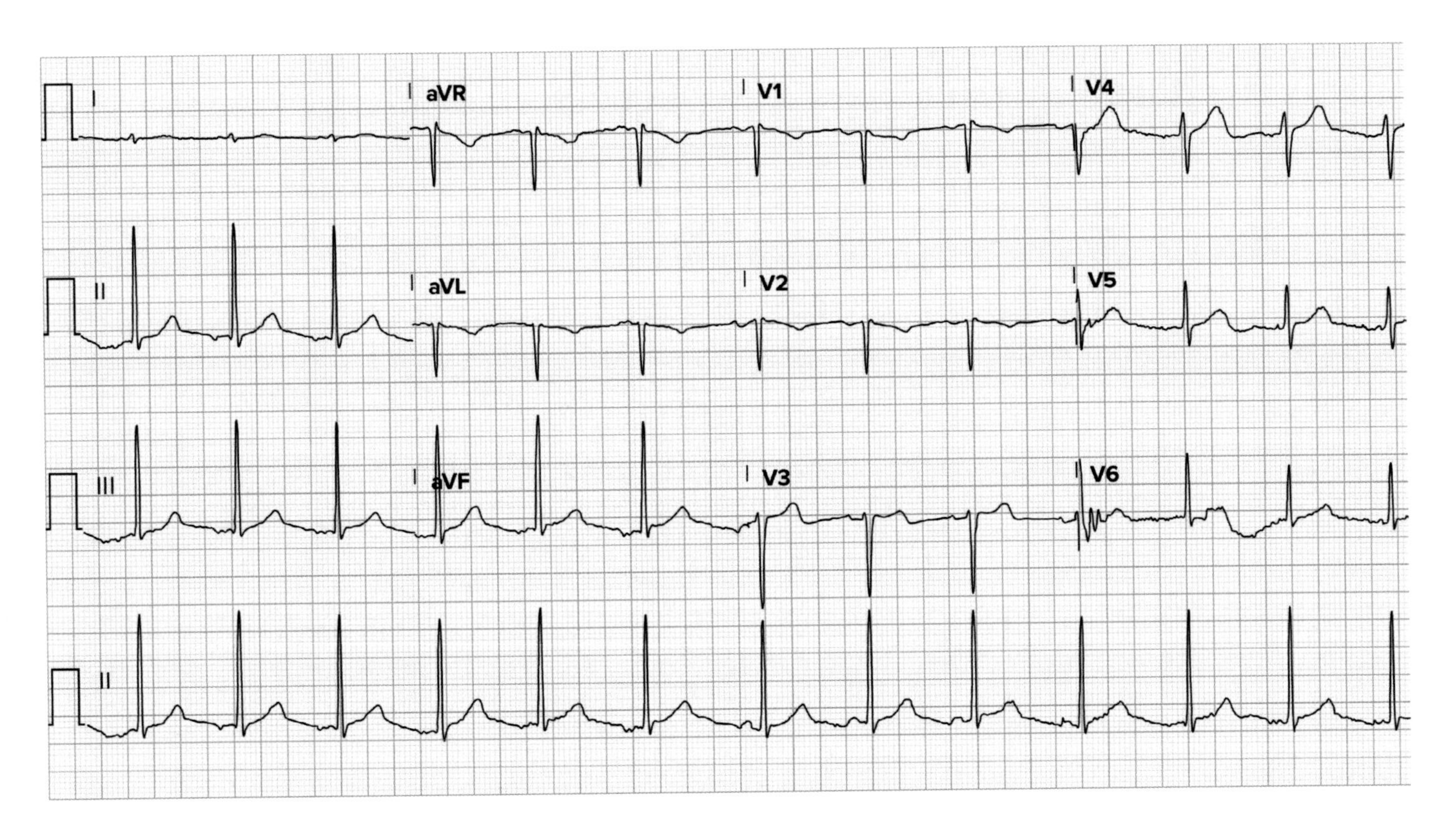

This ECG shows left arm-left leg (LA-LL) and right arm-right leg (RA-RL) lead reversal. The most easily recognizable abnormality in this ECG that should prompt concern for lead reversal is that lead I is almost "flatline" with barely discernible P-QRS-T complexes, often referred to as "pseudo-asystole."

ECG findings seen with LA-LL and RA-RL lead reversal include ***(see Figure 1)***:

- Lead I is almost a straight line with barely discernible P-QRS-T complexes
- Leads aVR and aVL are identical
- Lead III is inverted, meaning that the P-QRS-T complexes are all oriented in the opposite direction from the normal P-QRS-T complexes (ie, normal sinus rhythm with normal lead placement)
- Leads II, III, and aVF are identical

Figure 1.
Findings in LA-LL + RA-RL lead reversal

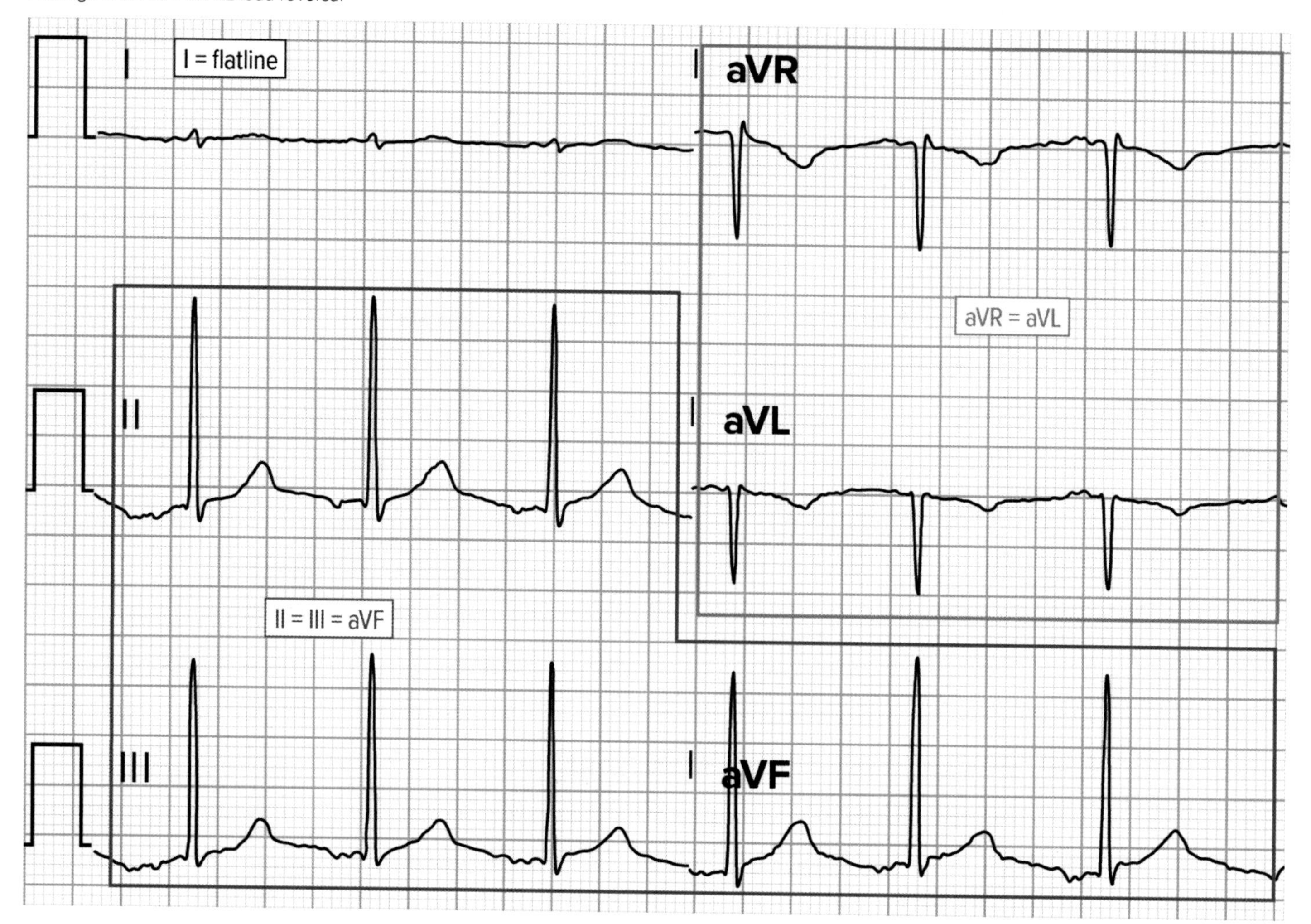

Lead Reversal Summary							
	I	II	III	aVR	aVL	aVF	V1-V6
LA-RA	Inverted	Switches with III	Switches with II	Switches with aVL	Switches with aVR	No change	No change
LA-LL	Switches with II	Switches with I	Inverted	No change	Switches with aVF	Switches with aVL	No change
LA-RL	Looks like II	Unchanged	Flatline	Looks like inverted II	Looks identical to aVF	Looks identical to aVL	No change
RA-LL	Switches with inverted III	Inverted	Switches with inverted I	Switches with aVF	No change	Switches with aVR	No change
RA-RL	Looks like inverted III	Flatline	Unchanged	Looks identical to aVF	Looks like inverted III	Looks identical to aVR	No change
LA-LL + RA-RL	Flatline	Looks like inverted III	Inverted	Looks identical to aVL	Looks identical to aVR	Looks like inverted III	No change
Dextrocardia	Inverted	Switches with III	Switches with II	Switches with aVL	Switches with aVR	No change	Dominant S-wave and poor R-wave progression

NOTE: *RL is a ground lead, so RL-LL reversal does not result in any significant changes*

Case 7: Presentation

A 76-year-old male presents with intermittent palpitations.
What is your interpretation of his ECG?

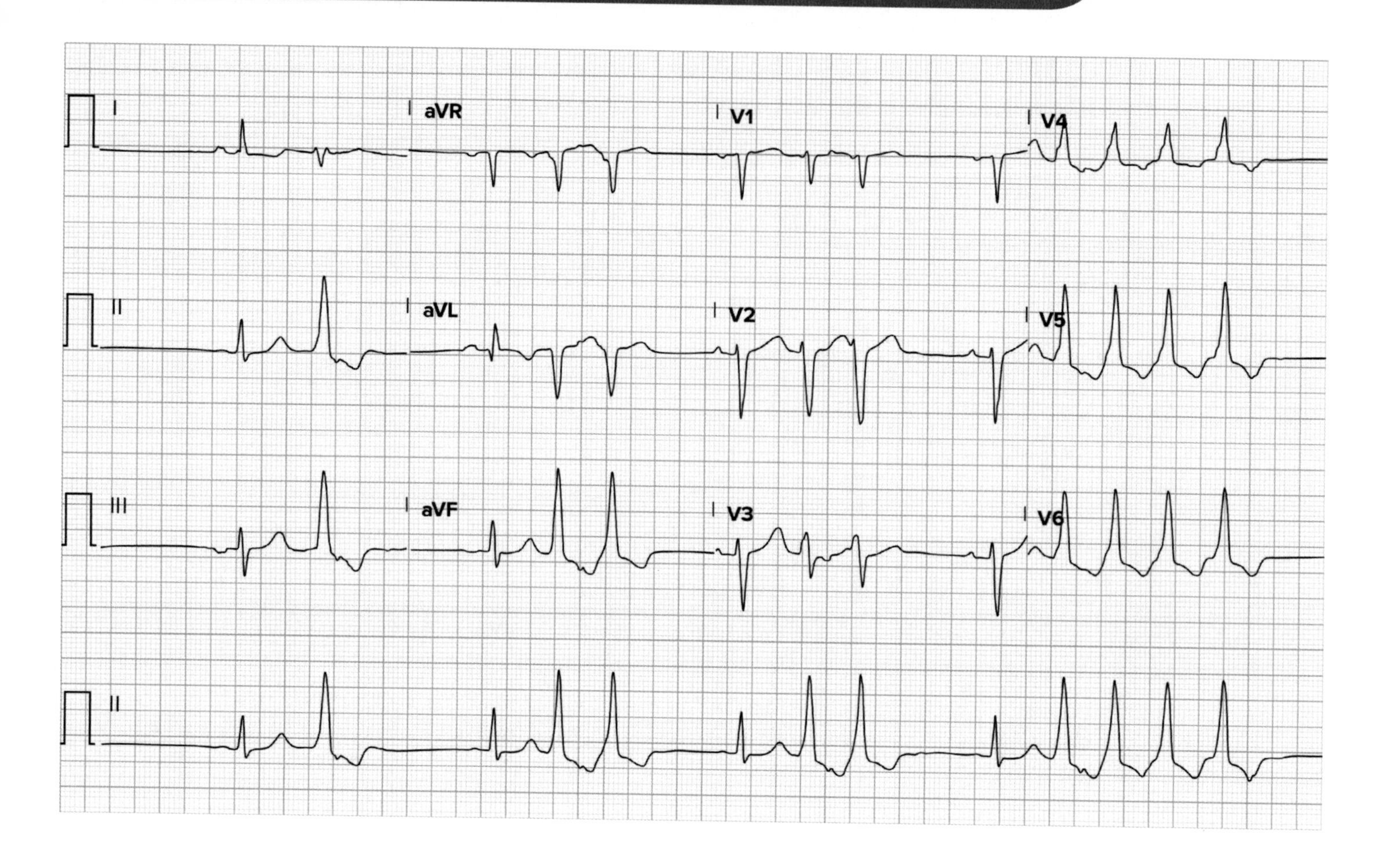

Case 7: Answer

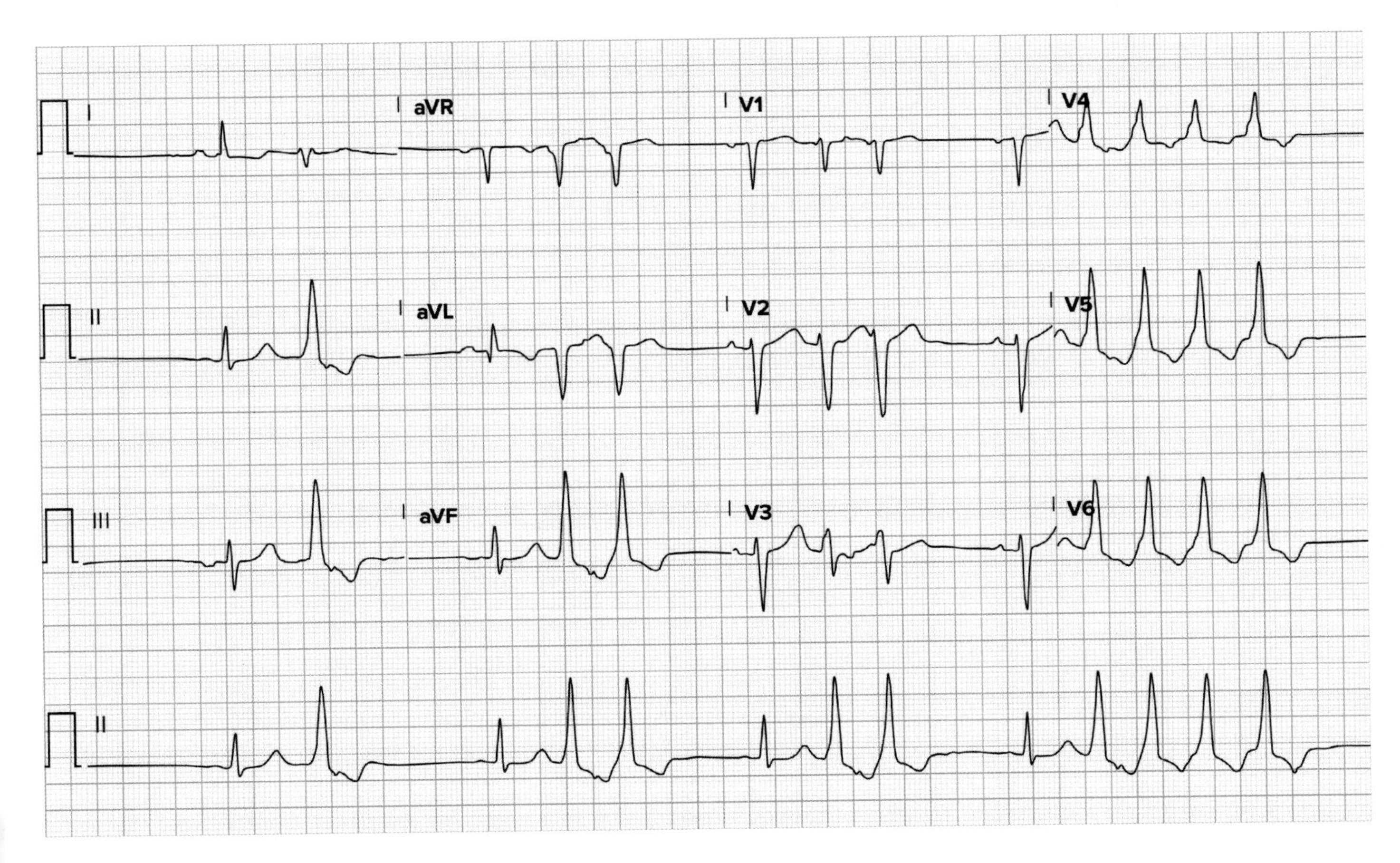

This ECG shows a sinus bradycardia with an irregular pattern of PVCs followed by a run of VT, normal axis, and left arm-left leg (LA-LL) lead reversal. This ECG would warrant hall of fame consideration if the 2nd PVC couplet was replaced by a PVC triplet.

Using the lead II rhythm strip ***(see Figure 1)***, the rhythm in this ECG is as follows:

- Sinus beat
- PVC with retrograde P-wave
- Sinus beat
- Unifocal PVC couplet (ie, 2 PVCs in a row with the same morphology)
- Sinus beat
- Unifocal PVC couplet (ie, 2 PVCs in a row with the same morphology)
- Sinus beat
- 4-beat run of VT

Figure 1.
The lead II rhythm strip shows frequent PVCs, a run of VT, and retrograde P-waves

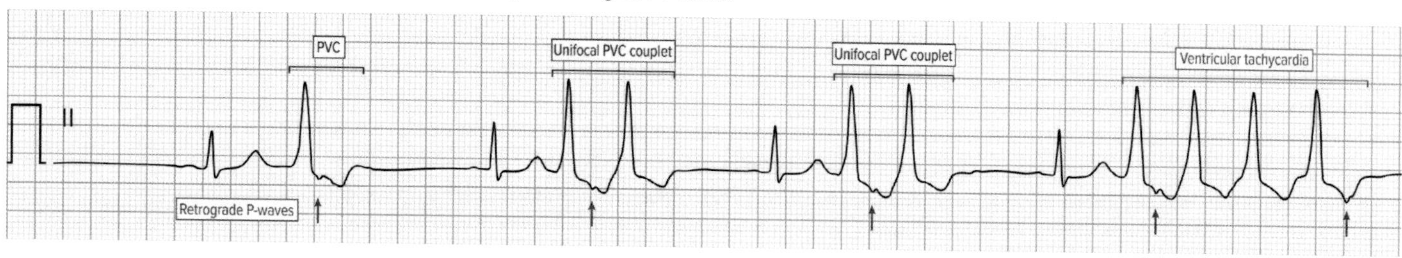

The retrograde P-waves are best visualized in leads V1-V3 where they clearly point in the opposite direction of the sinus P-waves, which is expected with retrograde P-waves. It is also worth noting that the 4-beat run off VT at the end of the ECG cannot be further differentiated into sustained or non-sustained without knowing whether there was any hemodynamic instability at that time (this patient remained hemodynamically stable so this was NSVT). Short runs of VT (ie, 3-5 PVCs) are often referred to as "bursts" or "salvos" of VT.

This ECG also shows LA-LL lead reversal. A notable finding in this ECG that should prompt concern for LA-LL lead reversal is the prominent P-wave in lead I when compared to lead II ***(see Figure 2)***. In general, the P-wave should be more prominent in lead II than lead I in normal sinus rhythm with correct lead placement.

Figure 2.
A more prominent P-wave in lead I than in lead II in the setting of normal sinus rhythm suggests LA-LL lead reversal

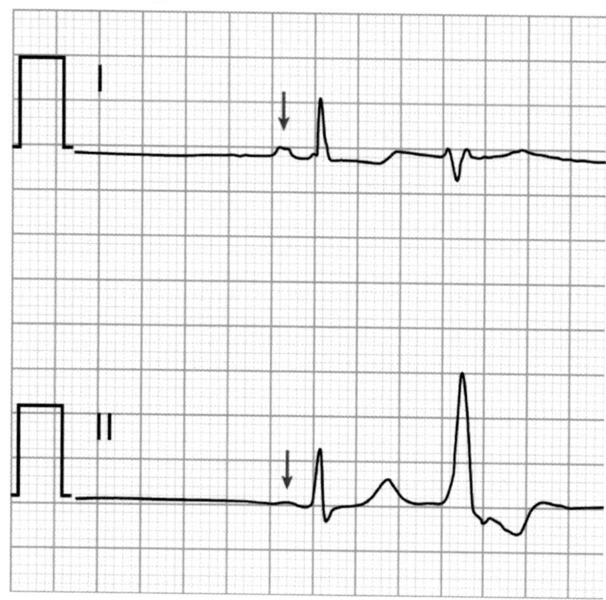

ECG findings seen with LA-LL lead reversal include:

- In comparison to normal P-QRS-T complexes (ie, normal sinus rhythm with normal lead placement), leads I and II "switch places," meaning that the normal findings in lead I are noted in lead II and vice versa
- In comparison to normal P-QRS-T complexes (ie, normal sinus rhythm with normal lead placement), leads aVL and aVF "switch places," so the normal findings in lead aVL are noted in lead aVF and vice versa
- Lead III is inverted, meaning that the P-QRS-T complexes are all oriented in the opposite direction from the normal P-QRS-T complexes (ie, normal sinus rhythm with normal lead placement)
- Lead aVR is unchanged

This patient had an unremarkable ED workup and was admitted to the cardiology service for telemetry and evaluation for AICD placement.

Monomorphic VT Learning Points

- ≥ 3 consecutive, regular, wide complex beats with rate > 120-130 bpm
- Non-sustained: < 30 sec duration with no hemodynamic instability
- Sustained: ≥ 30 sec duration OR causes hemodynamic instability

PVC Learning Points

- Wide-complex (≥120 msec) premature beat from a ventricular focus with no preceding P-wave
  - Unifocal: arising from a single ectopic focus, so each PVC is identical in any single lead
  - Multifocal: arising from ≥ 2 ectopic foci, so multiple PVC morphologies in any single lead
  - Usually followed by compensatory pause
- Patterns include:
  - Bigeminy: every other beat is a PVC
  - Trigeminy: every 3rd beat is a PVC
  - Quadrigeminy: every 4th beat is a PVC
  - Couplet: two consecutive PVCs
  - Triplet: three consecutive PVCs
- Clinical significance includes:
  - Right ventricular PVCs: LBBB-like morphology, not necessarily pathologic
  - Left ventricular PVCs: RBBB-like morphology, usually pathologic, more likely to precipitate ventricular fibrillation
  - R-on-T PVC: PVC falls on T-wave of normal beat and can precipitate ventricular fibrillation

Lead Reversal Summary

	I	II	III	aVR	aVL	aVF	V1-V6
LA-RA	Inverted	Switches with III	Switches with II	Switches with aVL	Switches with aVR	No change	No change
LA-LL	Switches with II	Switches with I	Inverted	No change	Switches with aVF	Switches with aVL	No change
LA-RL	Looks like II	Unchanged	Flatline	Looks like inverted II	Looks identical to aVF	Looks identical to aVL	No change
RA-LL	Switches with inverted III	Inverted	Switches with inverted I	Switches with aVF	No change	Switches with aVR	No change
RA-RL	Looks like inverted III	Flatline	Unchanged	Looks identical to aVF	Looks like inverted III	Looks identical to aVR	No change
LA-LL + RA-RL	Flatline	Looks like inverted III	Inverted	Looks identical to aVL	Looks identical to aVR	Looks like inverted III	No change
Dextrocardia	Inverted	Switches with III	Switches with II	Switches with aVL	Switches with aVR	No change	Dominant S-wave and poor R-wave progression

NOTE: *RL is a ground lead, so RL-LL reversal does not result in any significant changes*

Case 8: Presentation

An 89-year-old male with history of dual chamber permanent pacemaker placement presents with chest pain. What is your interpretation of his ECG?

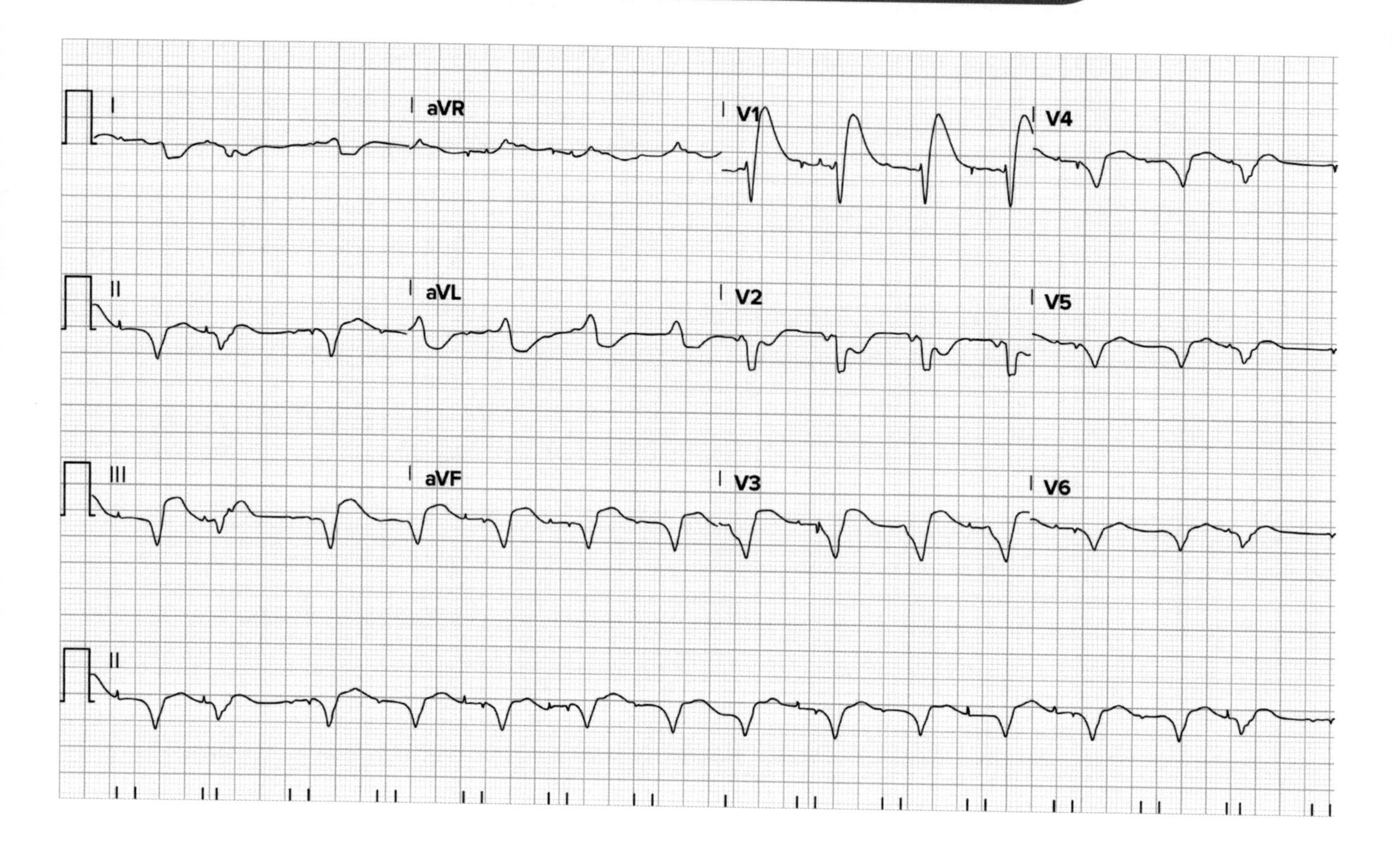

Case 8: Answer

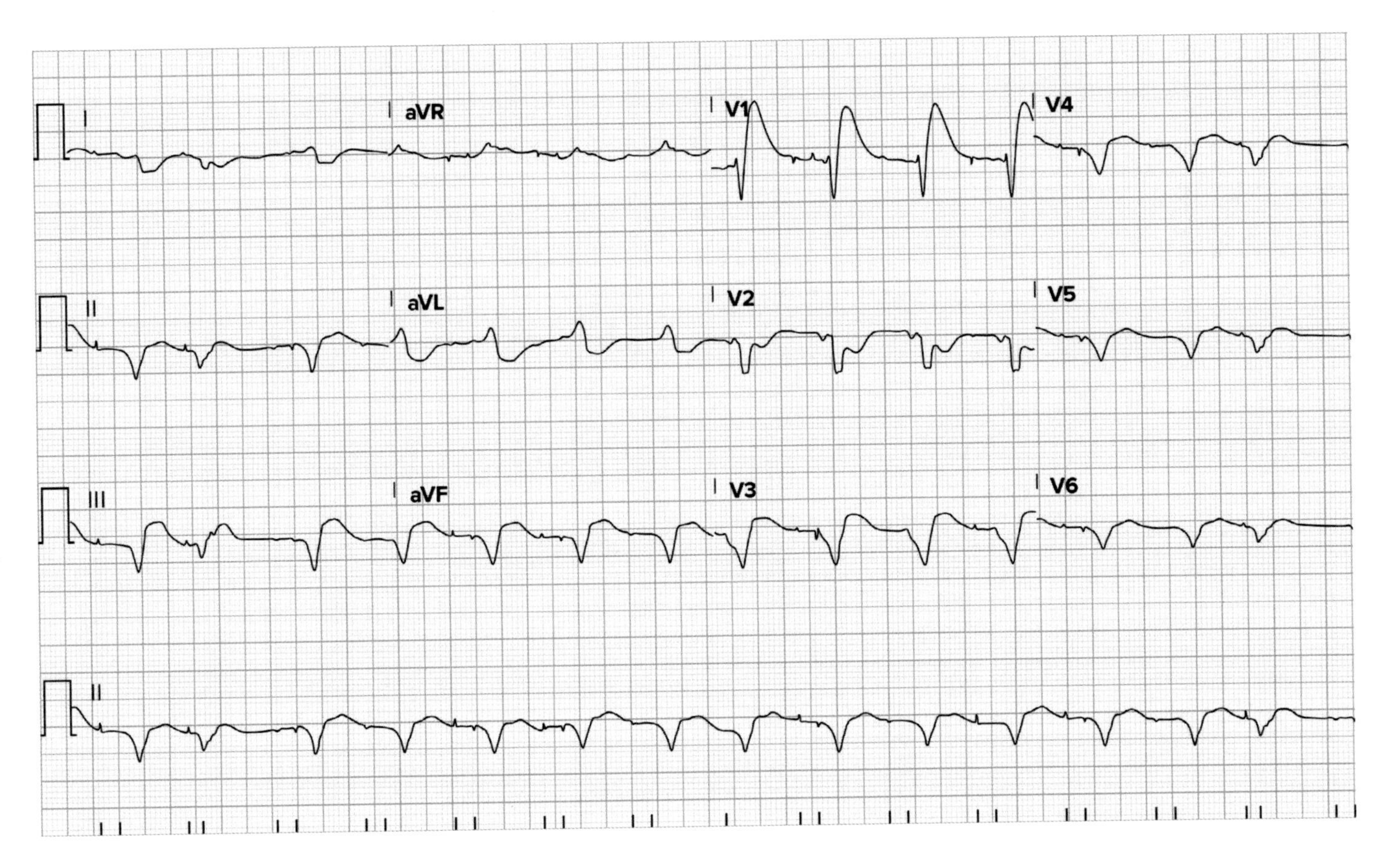

This ECG shows an AV-paced rhythm at 90 bpm, left axis deviation, prolonged QRS complex duration with LBBB-like morphology, discordant STE in lead V1, STD in lead V2, failure to capture, and intermittent failure to sense.

The fundamentals of right ventricular pacing include:

- Depolarization is initiated in the apex of the right ventricle
- Produces an abnormal but predictable pattern that mimics an intrinsic LBBB except for leads V-V6, which will almost always have negatively oriented QRS complexes with a ventricular-paced rhythm
  - These repolarization abnormalities confound the ECG's ability to detect an AMI and/or other findings suggestive of ACS

As with an intrinsic LBBB, the expected repolarization abnormalities in a paced rhythm follow the "rule of appropriate discordance" which describes the relationship between the direction of the QRS complex and its ST-segment. In other words, if the main vector of the QRS complex points up, there will be STD, and if the QRS complex points down, there will STE. These repolarization abnormalities confound the ECG's ability to detect an AMI and other ACS findings, so interpretation of the ECG in a presentation suggestive of ACS requires using the Sgarbossa criteria to diagnose an MI. It is important to note that a significant number of patients with an AMI and a ventricular-paced rhythm will not have any abnormalities, Sgarbossa or otherwise, on their ECG.

The Sgarbossa criteria are based on the underlying principle that concordance and excessive discordance in a LBBB are abnormal. The criteria assign a point value for any concordant STE ***(see Figures 1a and 1b)*** or excessively discordant STE ***(see Figure 1c)***. A score ≥ 3 is 98% specific for AMI, so the presence of criteria A or B are considered diagnostic of an AMI. Criterion C is only assigned 2 points, so the presence of just criterion C is not diagnostic of an AMI. However, in the setting of a right ventricular-paced rhythm, Sgarbossa criterion C was found to have 99% specificity for AMI.[1]

Figure 1a. Sgarbossa criterion A
Concordant STE ≥ 1 mm in ≥ 1 lead
(5 points = diagnostic of AMI)

Figure 1b. Sgarbossa criterion B
STD ≥ 1 mm in V1, V2, or V3
(3 points = diagnostic of AMI)

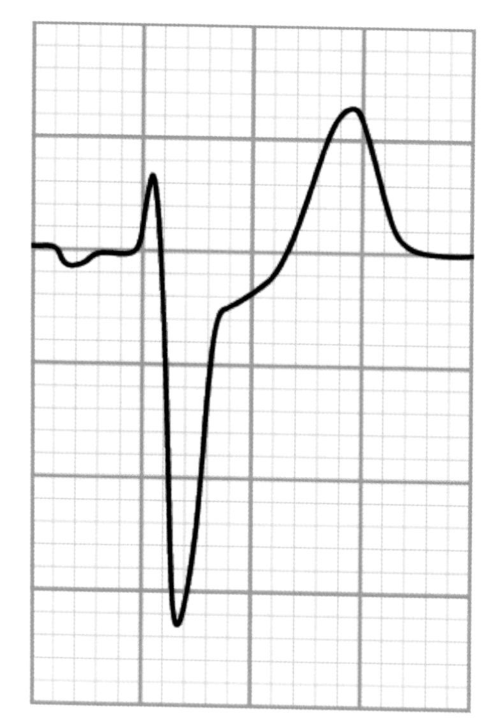

Figure 1c. Sgarbossa criterion C
Discordant STE ≥ 5 mm in ≥ 1 lead (99% specific for AMI in the setting of a right ventricular-paced rhythm)

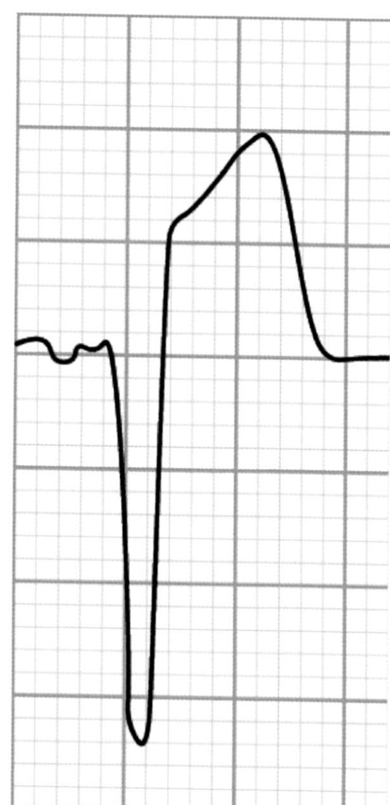

Figure 2. Modified Sgarbossa criterion C
STE/S ratio ≥ 0.25 in ≥ 1 lead (diagnostic of AMI but not mandated in current AHA/ACC STEMI guidelines)

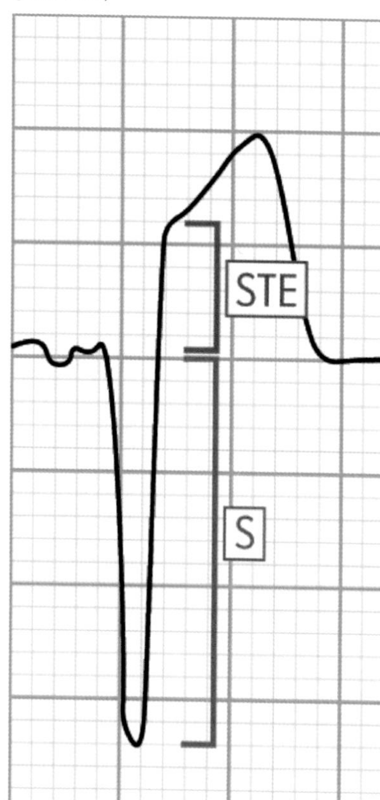

The Modified Sgarbossa criteria includes Sgarbossa criteria A and B with a variation of criterion C. Instead of using a fixed cutoff of 5 mm for discordant STE, it uses a ratio of the STE height to the S-wave depth ***(see Figure 2)***. A STE/S ratio ≥ 0.25 in ≥ 1 lead is considered diagnostic of an AMI. This means that more than 5 mm of STE is permissible if there is a large S-wave, and less than 5 mm of STE may be diagnostic if the accompanying S-wave is small. The Modified Sgarbossa criteria are not mandated in the current AHA/ACC STEMI guidelines, and at the time of publication, there are no published studies on the use of the Modified Sgarbossa criteria in ventricular-paced rhythms.

This ECG shows discordant STE in lead V1 and STD in lead V2 that meet Sgarbossa criteria. Identifying the J point in these lead V1 is difficult and best done by drawing a vertical line from lead V2 where the J point is more obvious ***(see Figure 3)***. The discordant STE ≥ 5 mm in lead V1 ***(see Figure 4)*** is not diagnostic of an AMI in the setting of a LBBB, but in the setting of a right ventricular-paced rhythm, this finding has a 99% specificity for AMI.[1] The STD ≥ 1 mm in lead V2 ***(see Figure 5)*** also meets Sgarbossa criterion B.

Figure 3.
Using the J point in lead V2, a vertical line can be extended up to help identify the J point in lead V1

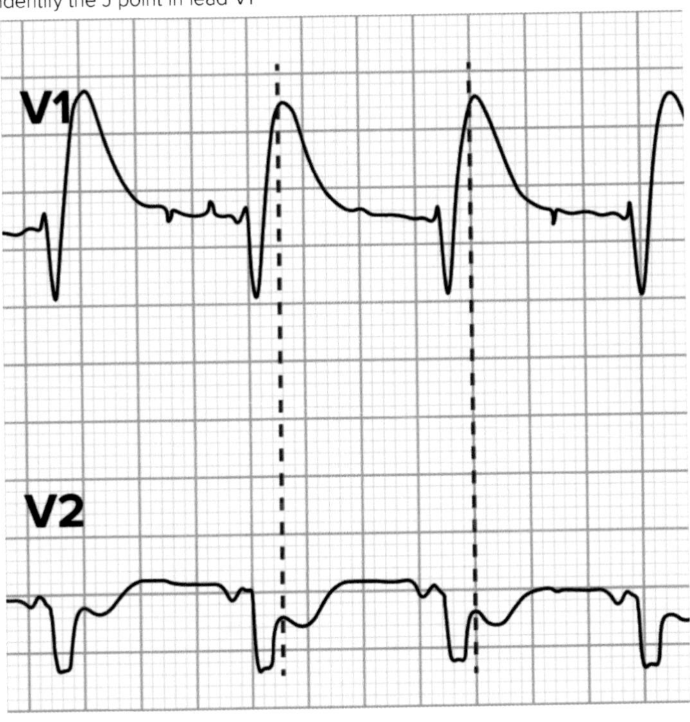

Figure 4.
Discordant STE ≥ 5 mm in lead V1 that meets Sgarbossa criterion C

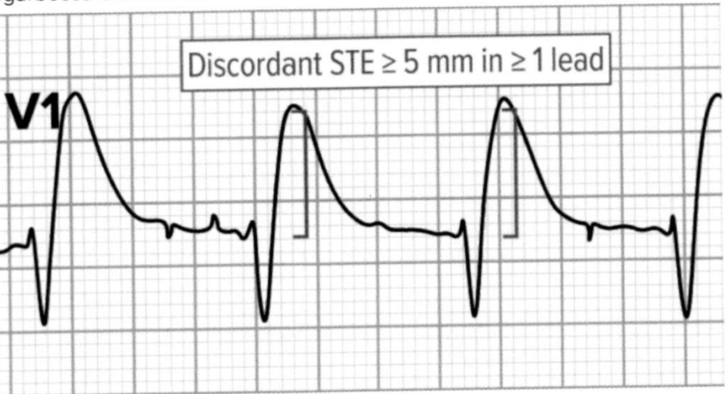

Figure 5.
STD ≥ 1 mm in lead V2 that meets Sgarbossa criterion B

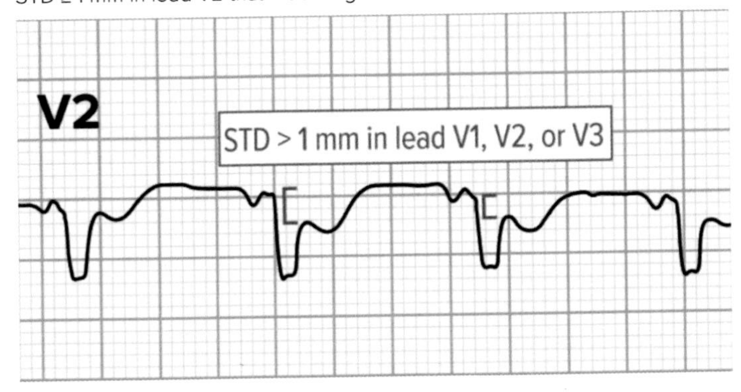

Failure to Sense
The defining feature of failure to sense is asynchronous pacing as the pacemaker fails to sense the native cardiac activity. This will frequently present as a pacer spike within a QRS complex, as seen on this ECG. The 2nd beat in the rhythm strip shows an atrial pacer spike followed by a PVC with a ventricular pacer spike that is within the QRS complex ***(see Figure 6)***. There may be a retrograde P-wave buried in the ascending limb of the PVC QRS complex which is only possible because the atrium was not depolarized by the atrial pacing **(see Failure to Capture)**, otherwise it would be refractory to any retrograde conduction. In a normally functioning pacemaker, the pacer spike seen in the middle of the QRS complex should have been inhibited by the pacer once it sensed the native ventricular depolarization.

Common causes of failure to sense include lead insulation break, new intrinsic bundle branch block, electrolyte abnormalities, and Class IC antiarrhythmics. Treatment is based on correcting the underlying etiology (eg, calcium for hyperkalemia).

Failure to Capture

The defining feature of failure to capture is the absence of depolarization after pacer spikes. The 3rd beat in the rhythm strip ***(see Figure 6)*** shows an atrial pacer spike with no visible P-wave on the ECG. This is seen in all leads including the leads that typically show atrial activity the best (ie, II, II, aVF, and V1) and is consistent with failure to capture. Note that this patient has a dual chamber pacemaker (ie, AV-paced) and the presence of failure to capture with the atria lead is far less concerning than if it were happening with the ventricular lead.

Common causes of failure to capture include electrode displacement, wire fracture, ischemia/infarct, and electrolyte abnormalities (especially hyperkalemia). Treatment is based on correcting the underlying etiology (eg, calcium for hyperkalemia).

Figure 6.

Failure to sense and failure to capture in the lead II rhythm strip

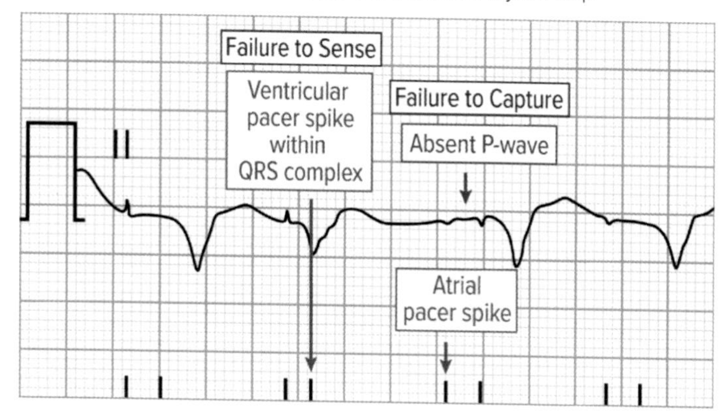

This patient went into cardiac arrest on the way to the cardiac catheterization lab and was not able to be resuscitated.

AMI in Right Ventricular-Paced Rhythms Learning Points

- In general, evaluate a paced ECG for ischemia as you would a LBBB, using Sgarbossa criteria
  - Discordant STE ≥ 5 mm: 99% specificity[1] (note that this study had no cases with STE > 1 mm)
  - Concordant STE ≥ 1 mm: 94% specificity[2]
  - At the time of publication, there are no published studies on the use of the Modified Sgarbossa criteria in ventricular-paced rhythms

Pacemaker Learning Points

- Pacer spikes are usually visible on the ECG, either at the bottom of the ECG and/or preceding the P-wave and/or QRS complex
  - Atrial pacing: spikes immediately precede P-waves
  - Ventricular pacing: spikes immediately precede QRS complexes
  - Dual chamber pacing: spikes immediately precede both P-waves and QRS complexes
  - Biventricular pacing: 2 spikes immediately precede QRS complexes
- Atrial pacing
  - Pacemaker lead usually implanted in the right atrial appendage
  - Results in P-waves with normal morphology
- Right ventricular pacing
  - Pacemaker lead usually implanted in the RV apex
  - Results in a LBBB pattern in the limb leads and anteroseptal precordial leads
  - The major difference between an intrinsic LBBB and a right ventricular-paced rhythm is that the QRS complex will almost always be negatively oriented in leads V5-V6 with a right ventricular-paced rhythm
- Biventricular pacing
  - Two pacemaker leads usually implanted in the RV apex and the surface of the posterior or lateral LV
  - Typically results in a narrower QRS complex than with right ventricular pacing
  - Dominant R-wave in lead V1 +/- V2 is common
- AICD will have a thick coil that differentiates it from a pacemaker

Failure to Sense Learning Points

- Pacemaker fails to sense native cardiac activity → asynchronous pacing ***(see figure below)***
  - Sensing refers to the pacer's ability to recognize native cardiac beats
- ECG shows pacer spikes before, after, or within P-waves and/or QRS complexes
- Causes include lead insulation break, new intrinsic bundle branch block, electrolyte abnormalities, and Class IC antidysrhythmics (eg, flecainide)

Failure to Capture Learning Points

- Delivery of pacing stimulus without subsequent myocardial depolarization ***(see figure below)***
- ECG shows absence of depolarization after pacer spikes
- Causes include functional (eg, electrode displacement, wire fracture) and pathologic (eg, electrolyte disturbances, AMI)

Failure to Pace Learning Points

- Paced stimulus is not generated when expected ***(see figure below)***
- ECG shows decreased or absent pacemaker function
- Causes include oversensing, lead fracture or insulation defect
  - Oversensing: pacing inhibited by non-cardiac activity (eg, skeletal muscle activity) inappropriately recognized as native cardiac activity

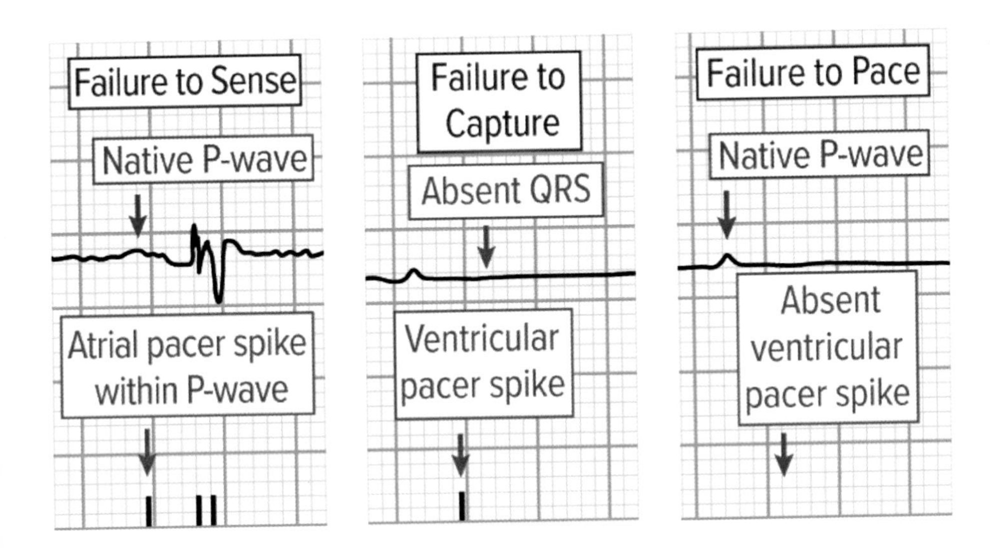

References

1. Maloy KR, Bhat R, Davis J, Reed K, Morrissey R. Sgarbossa Criteria Are Highly Specific for Acute Myocardial Infarction with Pacemakers. *West J Emerg Med.* 2010;11(4):354-357.
2. Sgarbossa EB, Pinski SL, Gates KB, Wagner GS, The GUSTO-1 Investigators. Early electrocardiographic diagnosis of acute myocardial infarction in the presence of ventricular paced rhythm. *J Am Coll Cardiol.* 1996;77(5):423-424.

Case 9: Presentation

A 63-year-old male presents due to an episode of chest pain with onset at rest that resolved a few hours prior to arrival. What is your interpretation of his ECG?

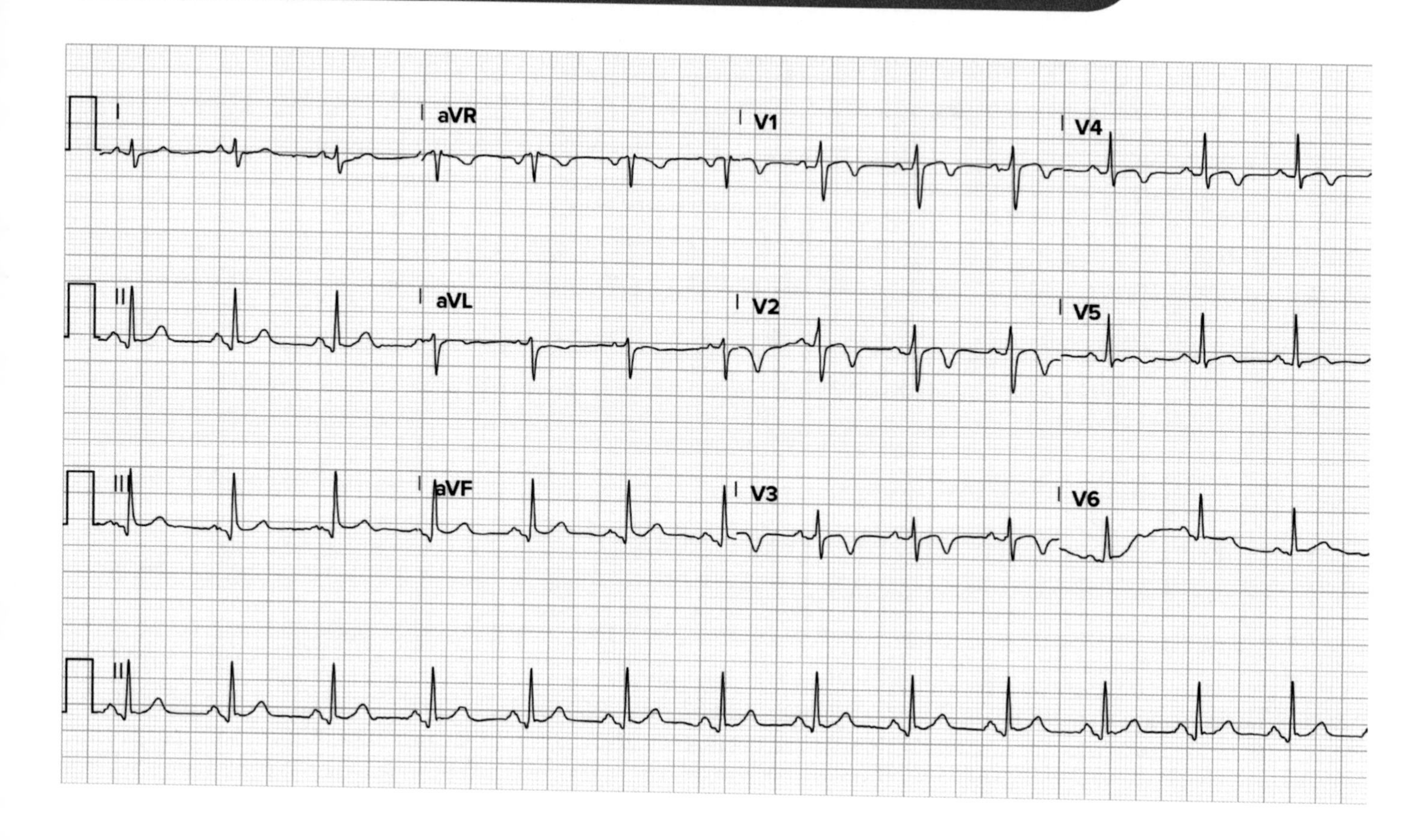

Case 9: Answer

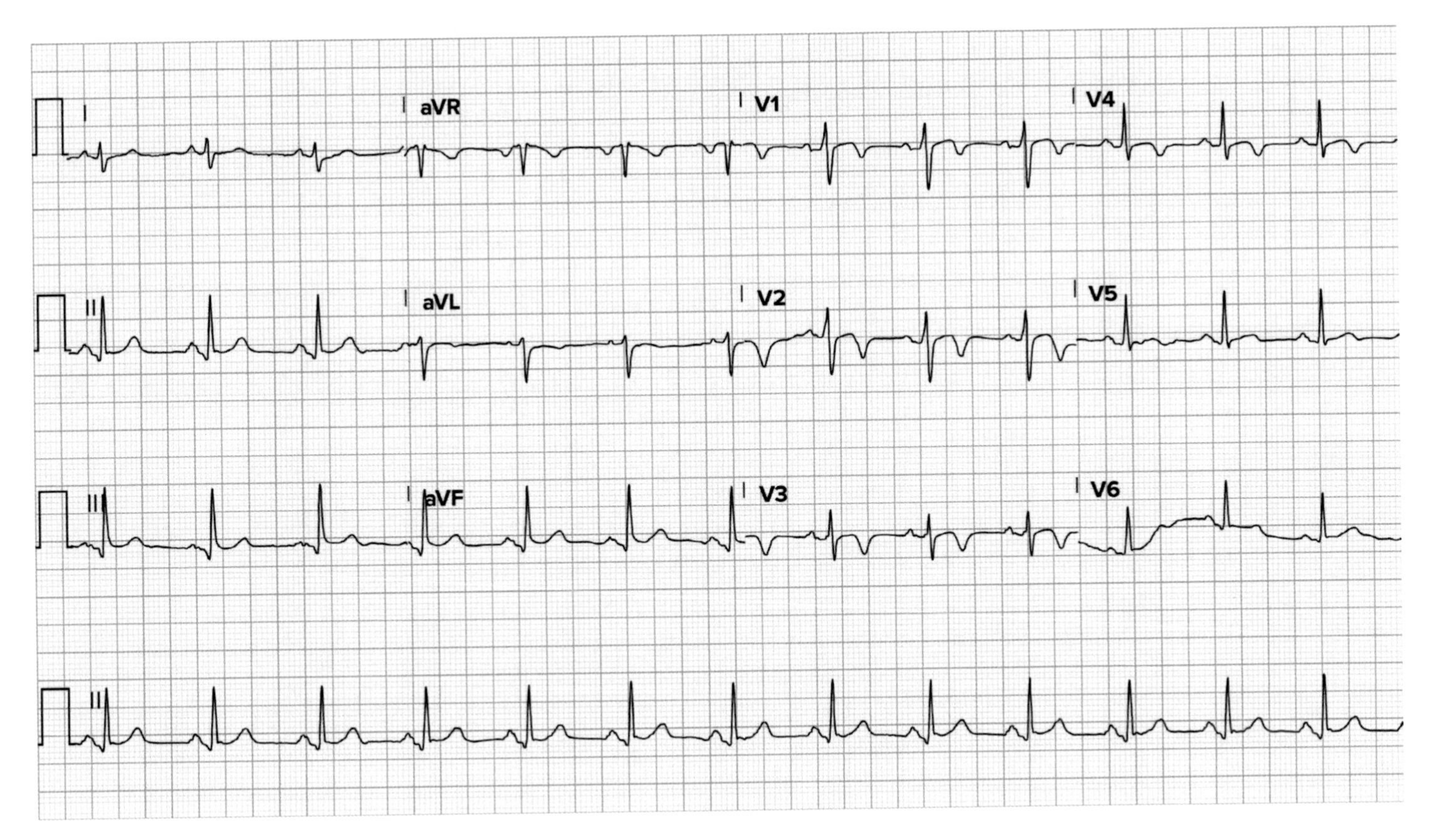

This ECG shows a normal sinus rhythm at 79 bpm, normal axis, normal QRS complex duration, and TWI in leads V1-V4. The J point in the inferior leads is isoelectric to the TP segment but appears to be elevated relative to the PR segment, but this is confounded by a down-sloping PR segment. There appears to be STD in beats 1 and 3 of lead I, but this is also confounded by a down sloping PR segment. There are also Q-waves in the inferior leads, but these are unlikely to be clinically significant as pathologic Q-waves are defined by have a duration ≥ 40 msec and ≥ amplitude ≥ 25-33% of accompanying R-wave height.

The morphology of the precordial TWI is typically seen in Wellens syndrome, also called "LAD coronary T-wave syndrome," which describes an abnormal T-wave pattern seen in a pain-free state with recent history of anginal symptoms. These characteristic ECG findings were first described in 1982 by Dr. Hein J.J. Wellens, a Dutch cardiologist, who found that 75% of patients with this syndrome developed an anterior MI within a few weeks of hospital admission if no intervention was performed.[1] The diagnostic criteria include:

- Biphasic (type A) or deeply inverted (type B, as seen in this example) T-waves in precordial leads, typically V2-V3 (***see Figures 1a and 1b***)
- Isoelectric or minimally elevated ST-segment (< 1 mm)
- No precordial Q-waves
- Preserved precordial R-wave progression
- Normal or minimally elevated troponins

Figure 1a.
Biphasic T-waves seen in Wellens type A
(from a different ECG)

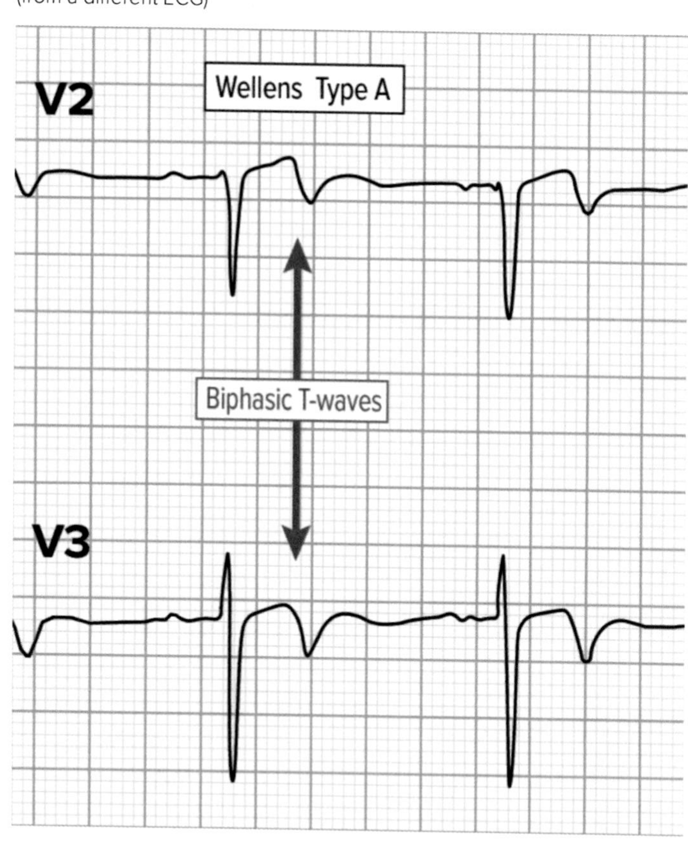

Figure 1b.
TWI seen in Wellens type B
(from case ECG)

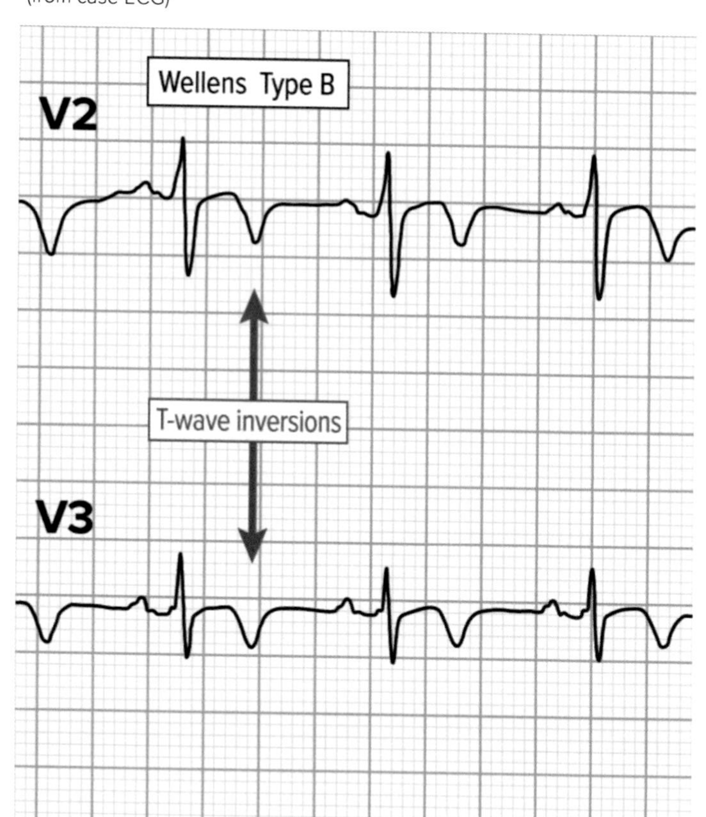

There is no universal definition for a preserved precordial R-wave progression, but common criteria include:

- R-wave > 2-4 mm in lead V3 or V4
- R-wave in lead V4 > lead V3 or lead V3 > lead V2
- R-wave in lead V3 ≥ 3 mm

This ECG pattern is concerning for a critical stenosis/lesion of the proximal LAD, and the T-wave abnormalities are thought to represent reperfusion after an ischemic event. Biphasic T-waves, also called Wellens type A, are an early finding, while deeply inverted T-waves, also called Wellens type B, are a later finding and more common (up to 75% of cases). Patients with these ECG findings in the appropriate clinical context have a high likelihood of developing an anterior MI within a short period of time[1] and warrant admission for cardiac catheterization. Coronary angiography is required to evaluate the need for early angioplasty or coronary bypass surgery, and provocative testing, especially exercise stress testing, should be avoided as it could precipitate an AMI or cardiac arrest.[2,3,4]

It is important to recognize that these ECG findings were originally described in patients in a pain-free state. In fact, it is not unusual to see these ECG changes persist from the painful presentation into the pain-free state as the ECG changes do not resolve until the LAD lesion is successfully managed with either PCI or CABG.

The term "Wellens waves" is sometimes used to describe these ECG findings in symptomatic patients. In these cases, the ECG changes are due to active ischemia. The term "pseudo-Wellens" is commonly used to describe these ECG findings when associated with causes other than LAD stenosis such as LVH, PE, hypertrophic cardiomyopathy, intracranial hemorrhage, and RBBB. In these cases, the ECG changes are due to repolarization abnormalities.

This patient was admitted for an urgent, but not emergent, cardiac catheterization. He was found to have a 99% occlusion of the proximal LAD which was successfully treated with a stent.

Wellens Syndrome Learning Points

- Wellens syndrome describes an abnormal T-wave pattern seen in the mid-precordial leads, typically V2-V3, in a pain-free state with recent history of anginal symptoms
  - Type A: biphasic T-wave, early finding
  - Type B: deeply inverted T-waves, later finding
- These findings represent critical stenosis of the proximal LAD and warrants admission for cardiac catheterization
  - Provocative testing should be avoided as it could precipitate an MI
- Associated with a high risk of an anterior MI if left untreated

Q-waves Learning Points

- Can be pathological or non-pathological (see table below)
- Pathologic Q-waves generally defined as ≥40 msec and/or ≥ 25-33% of accompanying R-wave height
- When due to an MI:
  - Occur in ≥ 2 contiguous leads that also have STE
  - Size correlates with volume of infarcted myocardium
  - Early appearance of Q-waves does not always indicate irreversible myocardial death, particularly with simultaneous STE and/or shorter period of ACS symptoms
  - Tall R-waves in leads V1 and V2 may represent Q-waves due to a posterior MI
- QS complex = single large negative deflection
  - Usually indicates significant irreversible myocardial loss when associated with ischemia
  - QS complex with STE and diminished T-wave should prompt evaluation for LV aneurysm
- Q-waves in leads V1 and V2 can be caused by misplacement of leads in the 2nd or 3rd intercostal spaces

Q-wave Causes	
Physiologic	Normal variant in leads V1, V2, III, and/or aVR
Structural	LVH RVH HCM
Conduction	LBBB Pre-excitation rhythms
Myocardial	Infarct Cardiomyopathy Myocarditis Infiltrative disease

References

1. de Zwaan C, Bär FW, Wellens HJ. Characteristic electrocardiographic pattern indicating a critical stenosis high in left anterior descending coronary artery in patients admitted because of impending myocardial infarction. *Am Heart J.* 1982;103(4 Pt 2):730-736.
2. de Zwann C, FW Bar, JH Janssen, et al. Angiographic and clinical characteristics of patients with unstable angina showing an ECG pattern indicating critical narrowing of the proximal LAD coronary artery. *Am Heart J.* 1989;117(3):657-665.
3. Rhinehardt J, Brady WJ, Perron AD, Mattu A. Electrocardiographic manifestations of Wellens syndrome. Am J Emerg Med. 2002;20(7):638-643.
4. Patel K, Alattar F, Koneru J, Shamoon F. ST-Elevation Myocardial Infarction after Pharmacologic Persantine Stress Test in a Patient with Wellens Syndrome. *Case Rep Emerg Med.* v2014; 2014:PMC4006572.

Case 10: Presentation

A 70-year-old female presents with exertional dyspnea. What is your interpretation of her ECG?

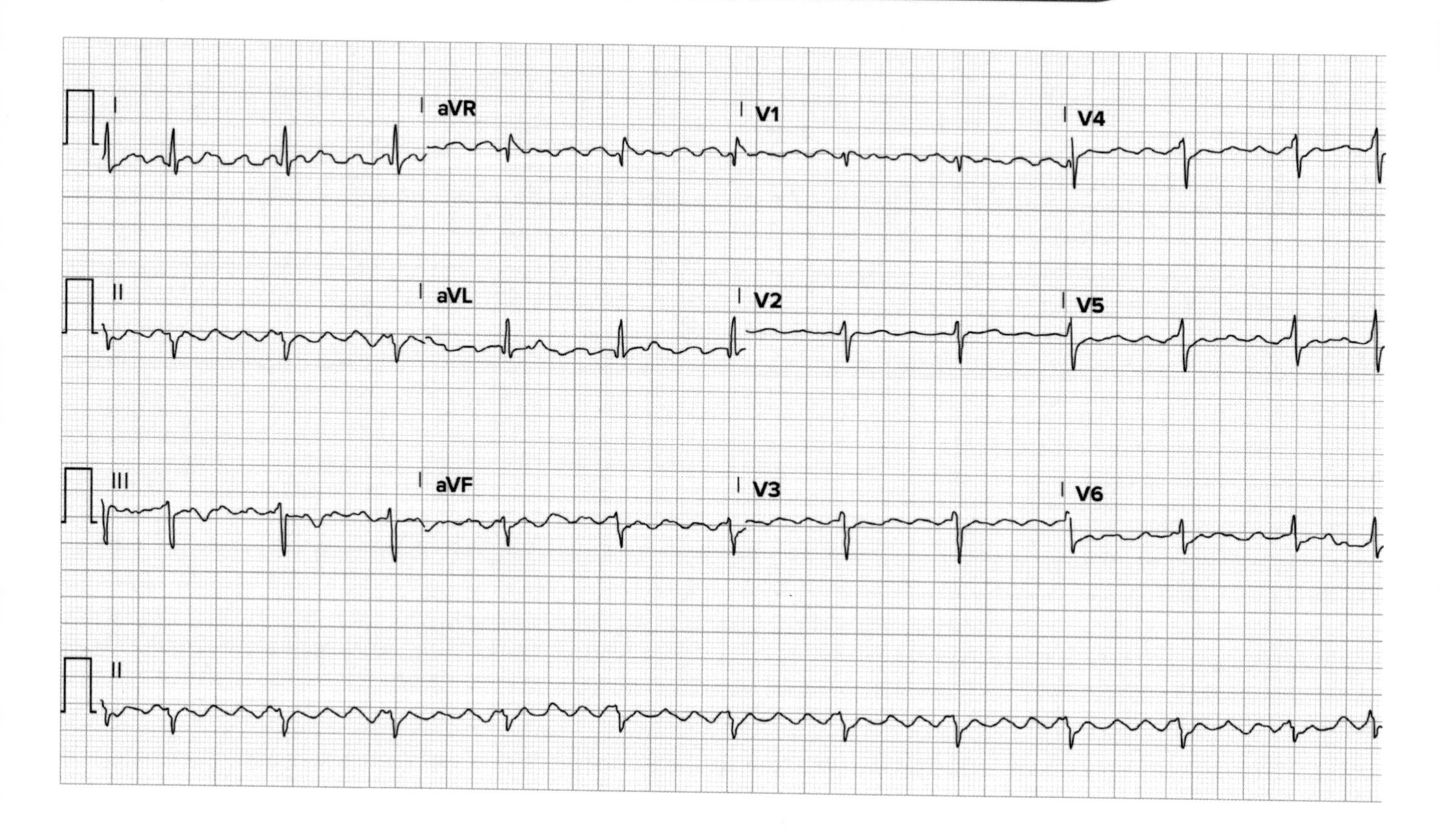

Case 10: Answer

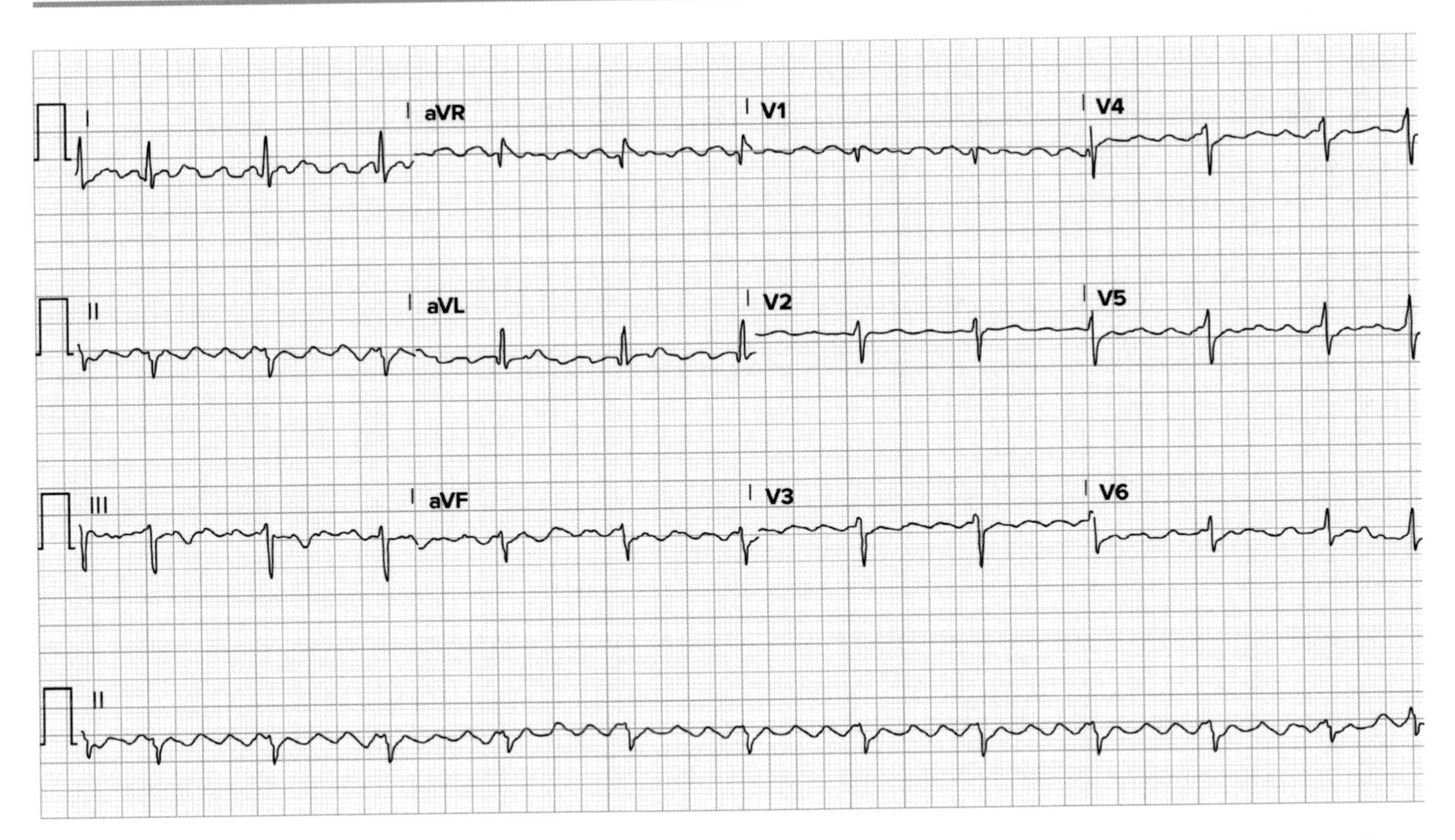

This ECG shows atrial flutter with variable block and an average ventricular rate of 68 bpm, left axis deviation, and a left anterior fascicular block.

This ECG shows flutter waves, also called F-waves, best seen in the inferior leads, that are diagnostic of atrial flutter. Atrial flutter is typically due to a right atrial re-entry circuit around the tricuspid ring. It is classified as a macro-reentry tachycardia because it revolves around a large obstacle, the right atrium, as opposed to a small obstacle like the AV node. This ECG shows atrial flutter with both 4:1 and 3:1 conduction ***(see Figures 1a and 1b).***

Figure 1a.
Atrial flutter with 4:1 conduction seen here in the initial portion of the lead II rhythm strip

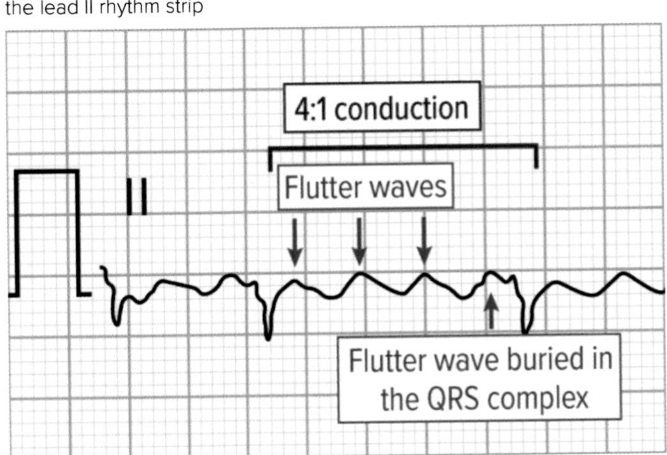

Figure 1b.
Atrial flutter with 3:1 conduction is seen at the end of the lead II rhythm strip (the last and 2nd to last QRS complexes are shown here)

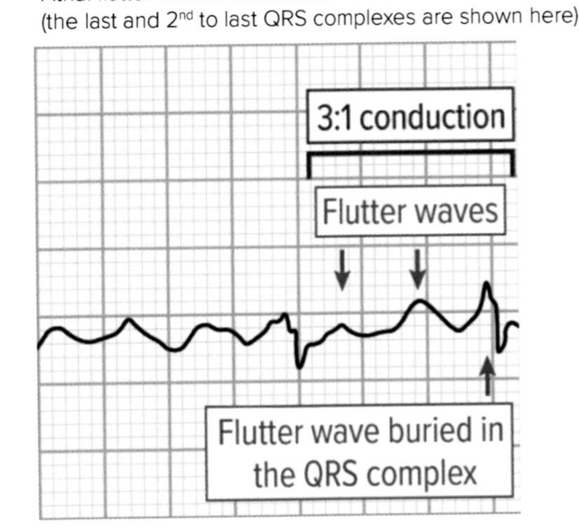

The flutter waves have a consistent FF interval of 220 msec which equates to ~272 bpm. The majority of the ECG shows 4:1 conduction with an RR interval of 880 msec which is exactly 4 times the FF interval of 220 msec ***(see Figure 2).***

Figure 2.
The initial portion of the lead II rhythm strip shows an atrial rate exactly four times the ventricular rate, consistent with atrial flutter with 4:1 conduction

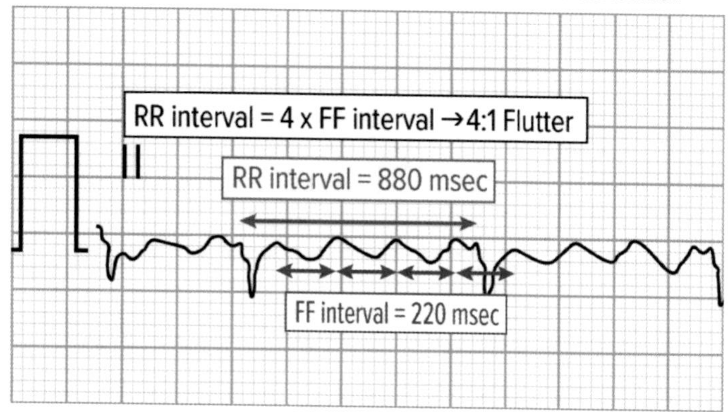

The presence of a LAFB in this ECG is not clinically important but is worth reviewing for the times when it can be. Any time there is a RBBB with an axis deviation there may be a concurrent fascicular block. A new RBBB + fascicular block + 1st/2nd AV block is concerning for an incomplete trifascicular block, and when seen in the setting of syncope can warrant admission for cardiac monitoring. Patients with trifascicular blocks can have transient episodes of 3rd degree AV block and require pacemaker placement.

The characteristic findings in a LAFB include ***(see Figure 3)***:

- Left axis deviation between -45° and -90°
- qR complex in lead aVL +/- lead I
- rS complex in leads II, III, and aVF
- Prolonged R-wave peak time ≥ 45 msec in lead aVL
- QRS complex duration < 120 msec in the absence of a concurrent conduction delay

Figure 3.
Findings in this ECG consistent with a left anterior fascicular block include qR complexes in leads I and aVL (red box), rS complexes in leads II, III, and aVF (purple box), and left axis deviation (green arrow)

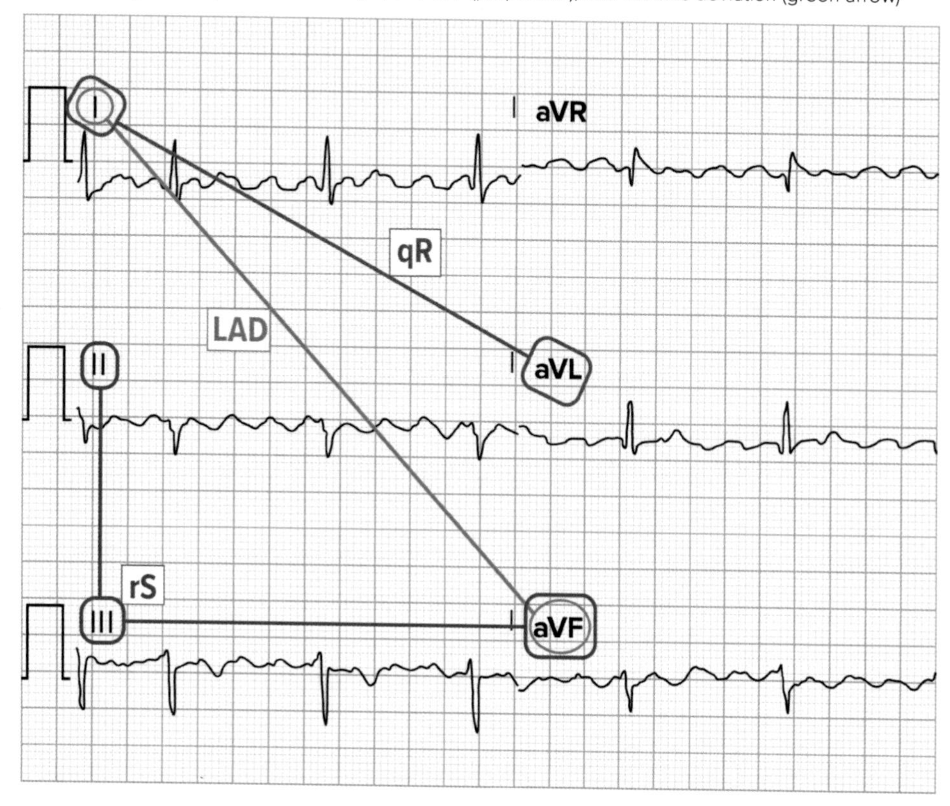

This patient had a history of atrial flutter and was on chronic oral anticoagulation. She was admitted to the internal medicine service for pneumonia and a new oxygen requirement.

Atrial Flutter Learning Points

- Due to a re-entrant circuit in the right atrium
- Stereotypical sawtooth pattern of P-waves seen best in the inferior leads
  - Absence of isoelectric baseline (eg, TP segment) in lead II
- Atrial rate is 250-350 bpm and typically fixed over time
  - Ventricular rate is a fraction of atrial rate (ie, for an atrial rate of 300 bpm, 2:1 conduction produces a ventricular rate of 150 bpm, 3:1 conduction produces a ventricular rate of 100 bmp, 4:1 conduction produces a ventricular rate of 75 bpm, etc.)
- Consider atrial flutter when ventricular rate is consistently around 150 bpm
- Vagal maneuvers or adenosine will slow ventricular rate but have no effect on flutter waves

Fascicular Blocks Learning Points

- Complete trifascicular block
  - 3rd degree AV block + RBBB + LAFB or LPFB
  - Always gets admitted for pacemaker placement
- Incomplete trifascicular block
  - 1st or 2nd degree AV block + RBBB + LAFB or LPFB, or RBBB + alternating LAFB/LPFB on successive ECGs
  - Syncope + incomplete trifascicular block = usually requires admission for cardiac monitoring for transient 3rd degree AV block and evaluation for pacemaker placement

Case 11: Presentation

An 82-year-old male presents with near syncope. What is your interpretation of his ECG?

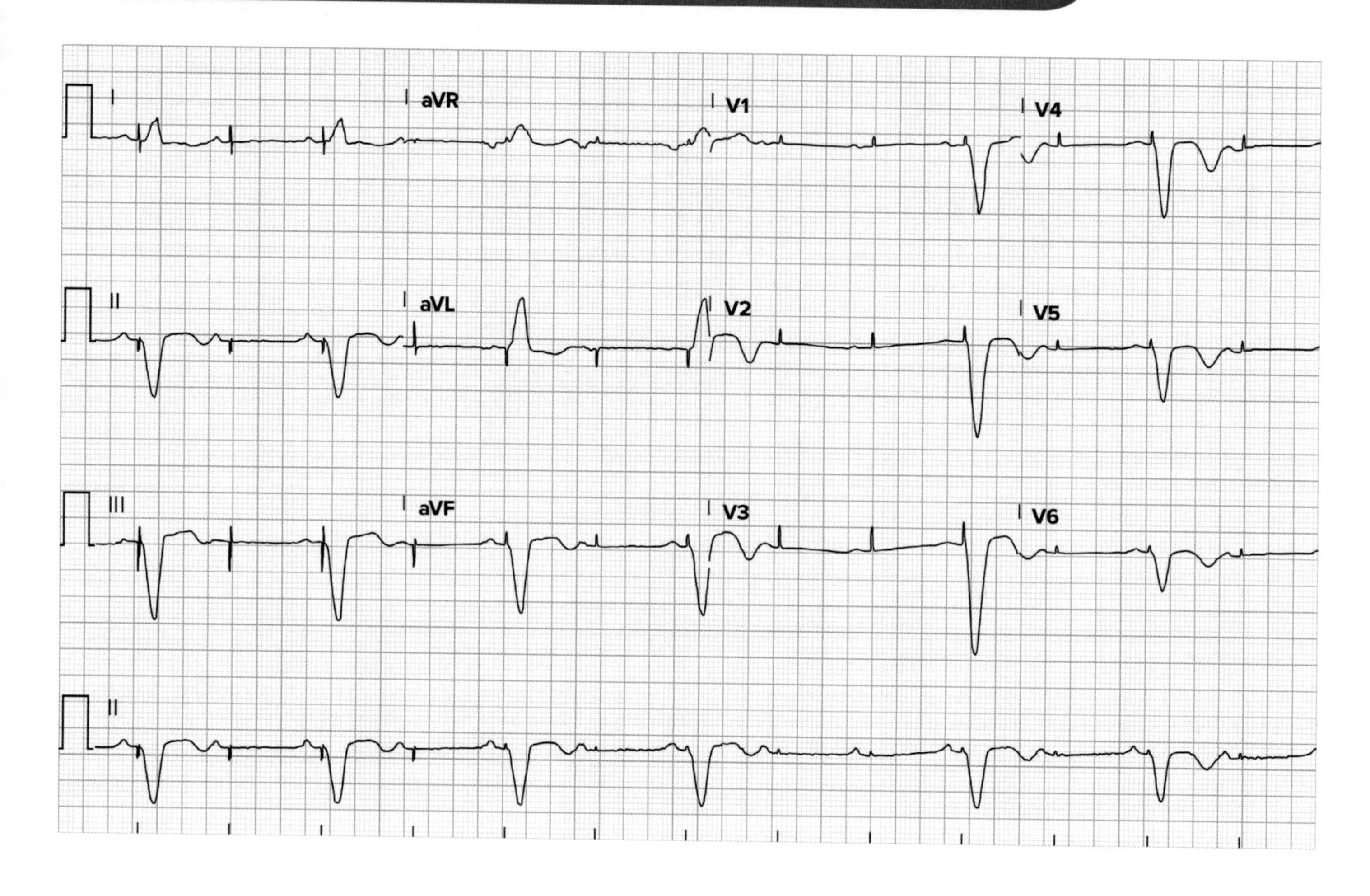

Case 11: Answer

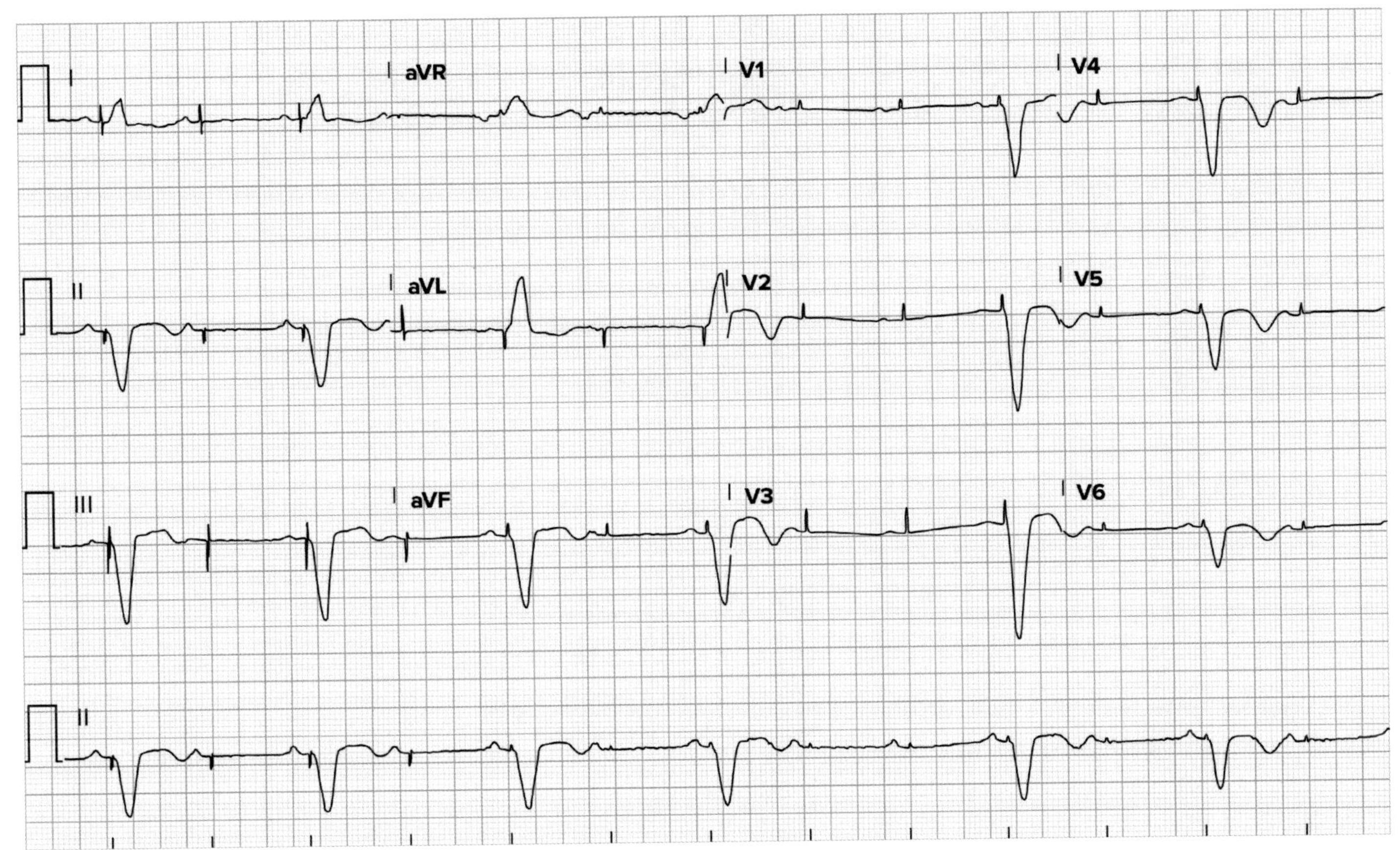

This ECG shows an atrial-sensed, ventricular-paced rhythm with an average ventricular rate of 36 bpm and frequent failure to capture ***(see Figure 1)***, left axis deviation, and prolonged QRS complex duration with a LBBB-like morphology. Note that the QRS complex in lead V6 is negatively oriented which is normal for right ventricular pacing.

Figure 1.
The lead II rhythm strip shows an atrial-sensed, ventricular-paced rhythm (green boxes) with frequent failure to capture (red boxes)

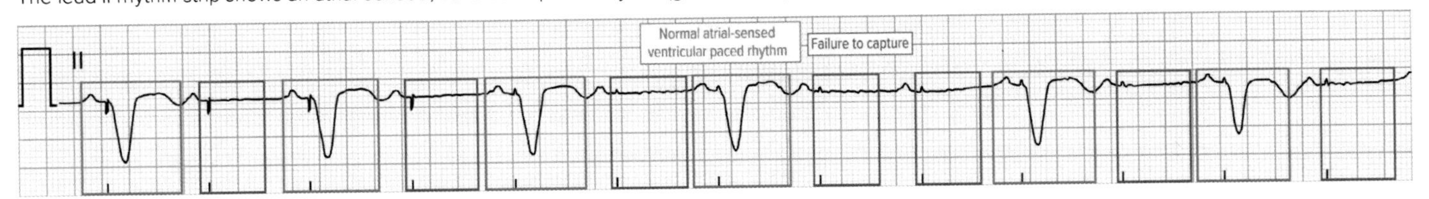

The P-QRS-T complexes associated with the 1st, 3rd, 5th, 7th, 10th, and 12th pacer spikes show a normal atrial-sensed ventricular-paced rhythm. There is a native P-wave that is sensed by the pacemaker which then triggers a paced ventricular beat ***(see Figure 2)***.

The 2nd, 4th, 6th, 8th, 9th, 11th, and 13th pacer spikes show failure to capture. The defining feature of failure to capture is the absence of depolarization after a pacer spike ***(see Figure 3)***. Common causes of failure to capture include electrode displacement, wire fracture, ischemia/infarct, and electrolyte abnormalities (especially hyperkalemia). Treatment is based on correcting the underlying etiology (eg, calcium for hyperkalemia).

Figure 2.
The initial P-QRS-T complex of the lead II rhythm strip shows an atral-sensed, ventricular-paced rhythm

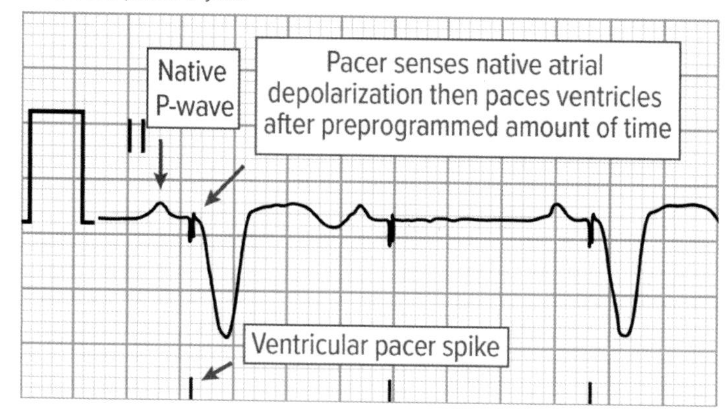

Figure 3.
The 2nd P-wave of the lead II rhythm strip is sensed by the pacemaker which then triggers a pacer spike. The absence of subsequent ventricular depolarization is called failure to capture.

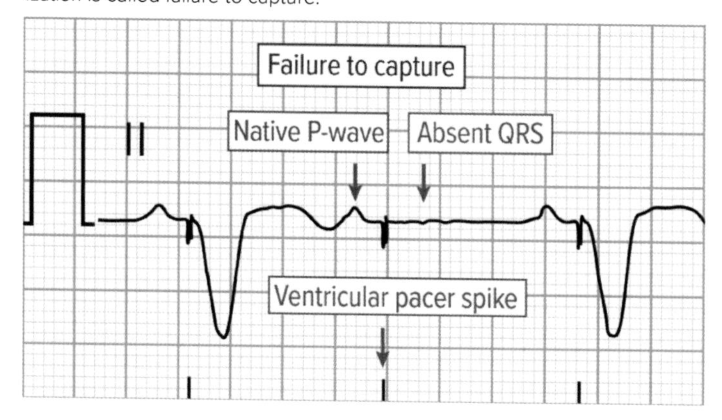

Pacemaker Learning Points

- Pacer spikes are usually visible on the ECG, either at the bottom of the ECG and/or preceding the P-wave and/or QRS complex
  - Atrial pacing: spikes immediately precede P-waves
  - Ventricular pacing: spikes immediately precede QRS complexes
  - Dual chamber pacing: spikes immediately precede both P-waves and QRS complexes
  - Biventricular pacing: 2 spikes immediately precede QRS complexes
- Atrial pacing
  - Pacemaker lead usually implanted in the right atrial appendage
  - Results in P-waves with normal morphology
- Right ventricular pacing
  - Pacemaker lead usually implanted in the RV apex
  - Results in a LBBB pattern in the limb leads and anteroseptal precordial leads
  - The major difference between an intrinsic LBBB and a right ventricular-paced rhythm is that the QRS complex will almost always be negatively oriented in leads V5-V6 with a right ventricular-paced rhythm
- Biventricular pacing
  - Two pacemaker leads usually implanted in the RV apex and the surface of the posterior or lateral LV
  - Typically results in a narrower QRS complex than with right ventricular pacing
  - Dominant R-wave in lead V1 +/- V2 is common
- AICD will have a thick coil that differentiates it from a pacemaker

Failure to Sense Learning Points

- Pacemaker fails to sense native cardiac activity → asynchronous pacing ***(see figure below)***
  - Sensing refers to the pacer's ability to recognize native cardiac beats
- ECG shows pacer spikes before, after, or within P-waves and/or QRS complexes
- Causes include lead insulation break, new intrinsic bundle branch block, electrolyte abnormalities, and Class IC antidysrhythmics (eg, flecainide)

Failure to Capture Learning Points

- Delivery of pacing stimulus without subsequent myocardial depolarization ***(see figure below)***
  ECG shows absence of depolarization after pacer spikes
- Causes include functional (eg, electrode displacement, wire fracture) and pathologic (eg, electrolyte disturbances, AMI)

Failure to Pace Learning Points

- Paced stimulus is not generated when expected ***(see figure below)***
- ECG shows decreased or absent pacemaker function
- Causes include oversensing, lead fracture or insulation defect
  - Oversensing: pacing inhibited by non-cardiac activity (eg, skeletal muscle activity) inappropriately recognized as native cardiac activity

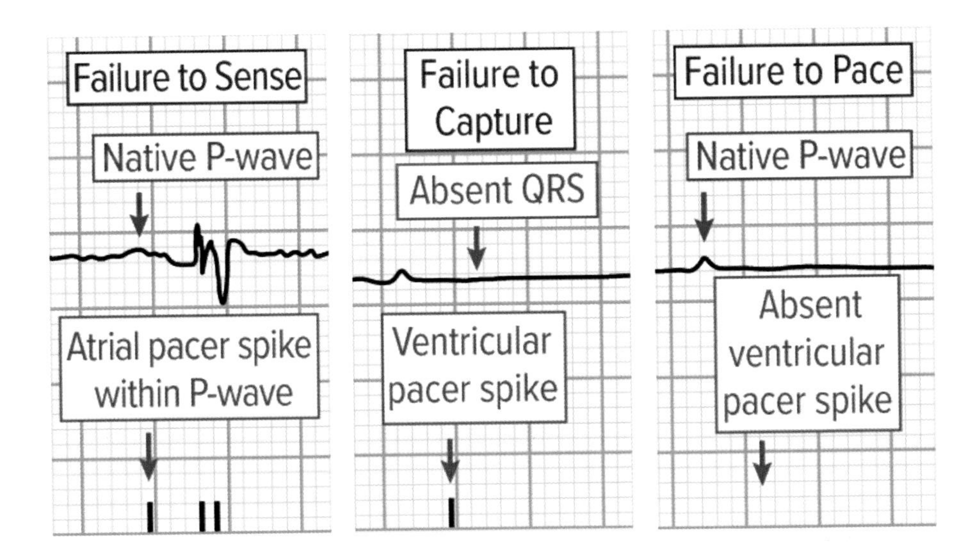

Case 12: Presentation

This is the preop ECG of a 79-year-old female being admitted for a hip fracture. What is your interpretation of her ECG?

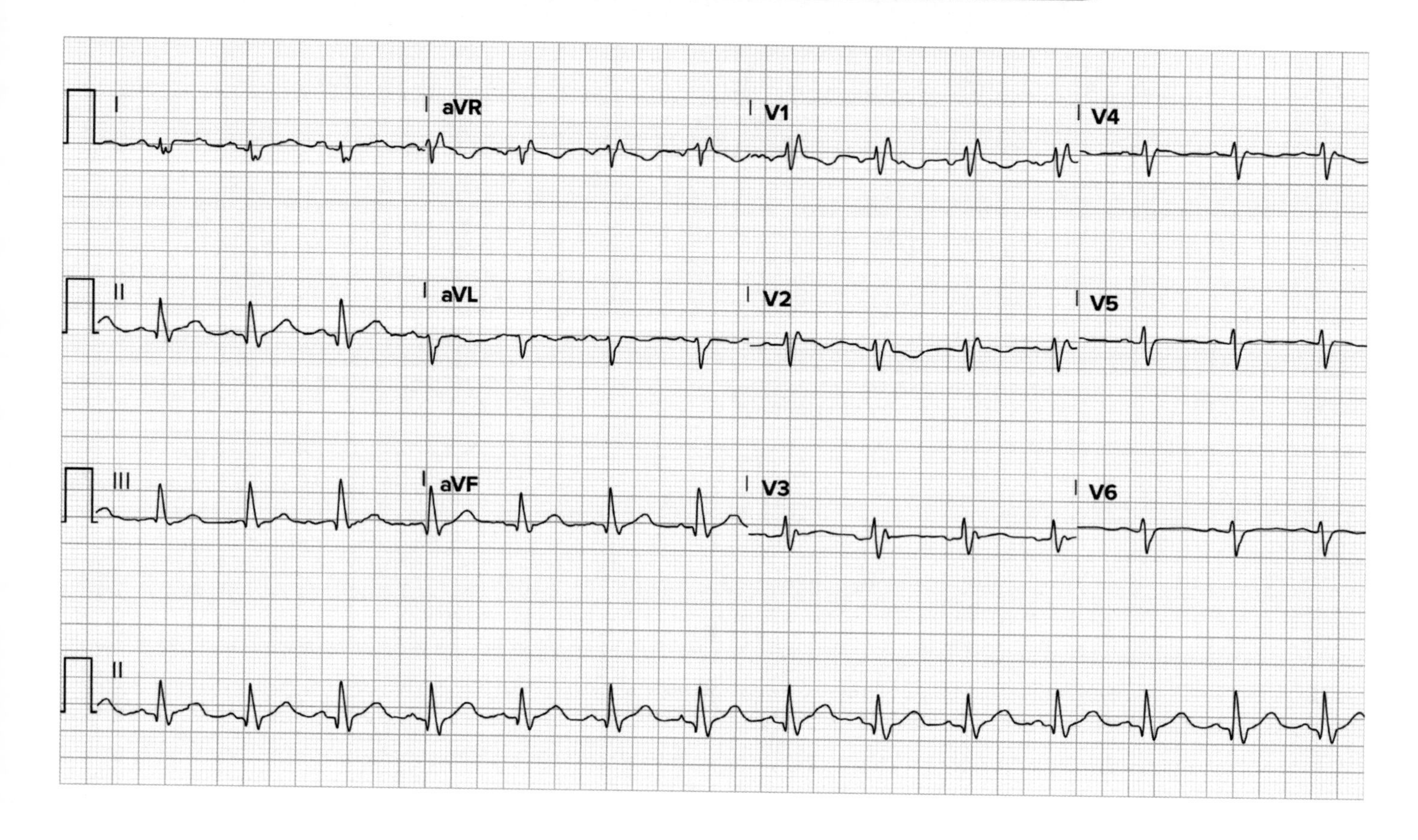

Case 12: Answer

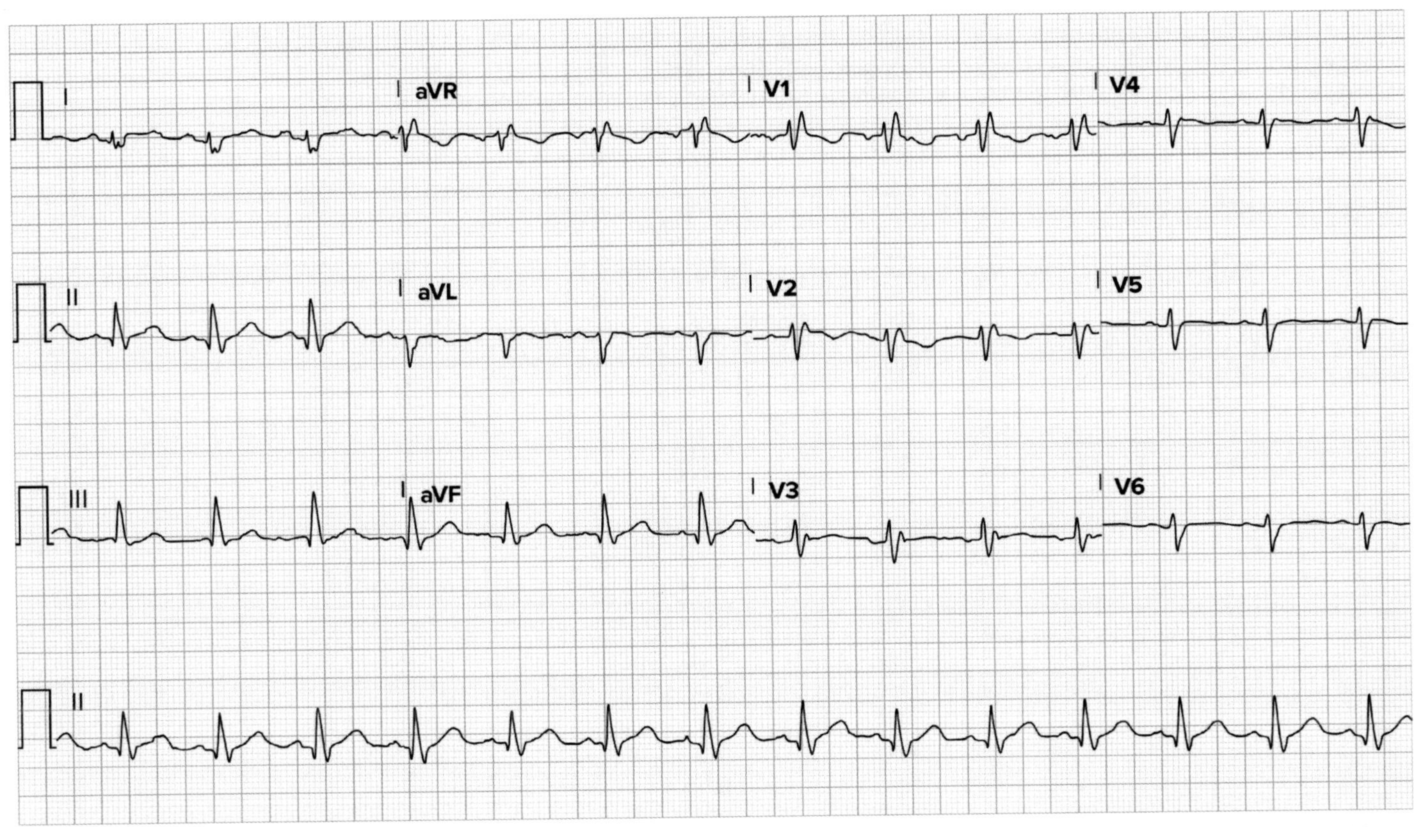

This ECG shows left arm-left leg (LA-LL) lead reversal. A notable finding in this ECG that should prompt concern for LA-LL lead reversal is the prominent P-wave in lead I when compared to lead II. In general, the P-wave should be more prominent in lead II than lead I in normal sinus rhythm with correct lead placement. **Figure 1** shows a repeat ECG with correct lead placement.

Figure 1.
Repeat ECG with correct lead placement

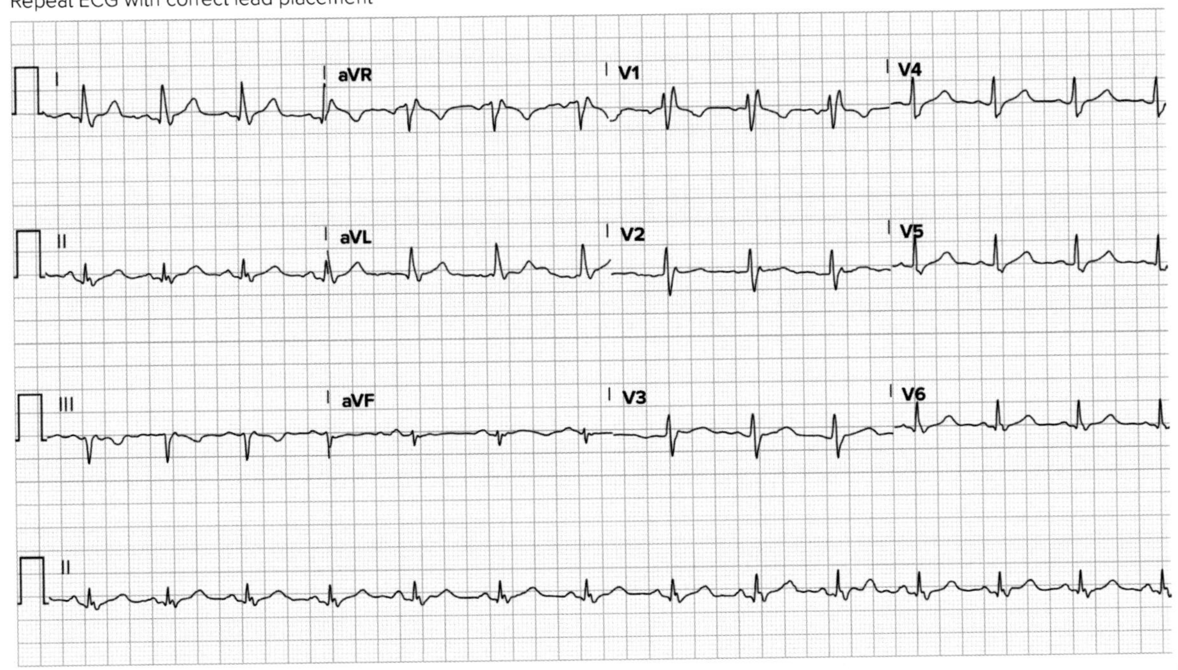

ECG findings seen with LA-LL lead reversal include ***(see Figure 2)***:

1. In comparison to normal P-QRS-T complexes (ie, normal sinus rhythm with normal lead placement), leads I and II "switch places," meaning that the normal findings in lead I are noted in lead II and vice versa
2. In comparison to normal P-QRS-T complexes (ie, normal sinus rhythm with normal lead placement), leads aVL and aVF "switch places," so the normal findings in lead aVL are noted in lead aVF and vice versa
3. Lead III is inverted, meaning that the P-QRS-T complexes are all oriented in the opposite direction from the normal P-QRS-T complexes (ie, normal sinus rhythm with normal lead placement)
4. Lead aVR is unchanged

Figure 2.
Comparison of the limb leads from the case ECG with LA-RA lead reversal with the repeat ECG with correct lead placement

2a. LA-LL lead reversal (case ECG)

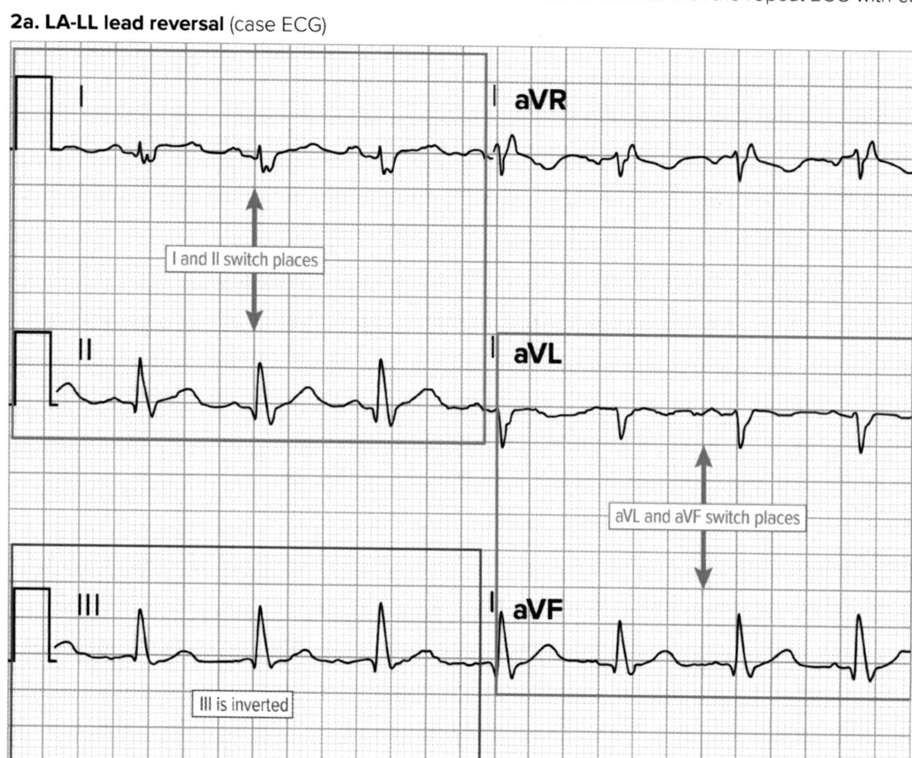

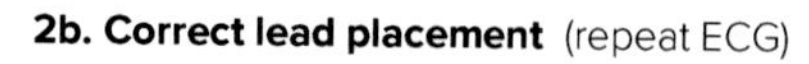
2b. Correct lead placement (repeat ECG)

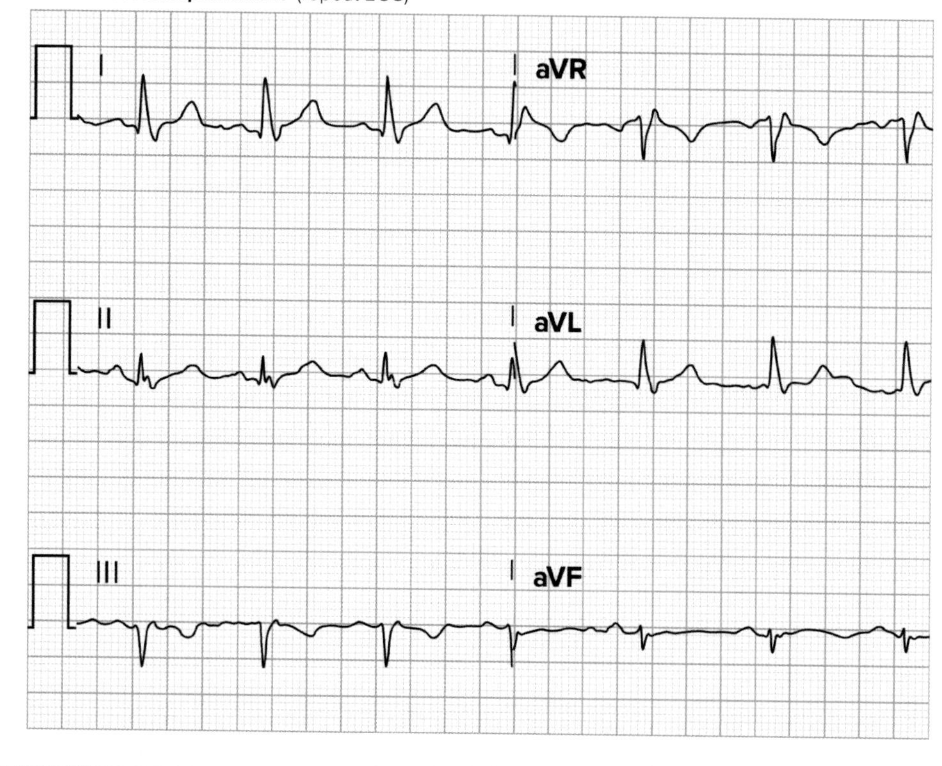

Lead Reversal Summary							
	I	II	III	aVR	aVL	aVF	V1-V6
LA-RA	Inverted	Switches with III	Switches with II	Switches with aVL	Switches with aVR	No change	No change
LA-LL	Switches with II	Switches with I	Inverted	No change	Switches with aVF	Switches with aVL	No change
LA-RL	Looks like II	Unchanged	Flatline	Looks like inverted II	Looks identical to aVF	Looks identical to aVL	No change
RA-LL	Switches with inverted III	Inverted	Switches with inverted I	Switches with aVF	No change	Switches with aVR	No change
RA-RL	Looks like inverted III	Flatline	Unchanged	Looks identical to aVF	Looks like inverted III	Looks identical to aVR	No change
LA-LL + RA-RL	Flatline	Looks like inverted III	Inverted	Looks identical to aVL	Looks identical to aVR	Looks like inverted III	No change
Dextrocardia	Inverted	Switches with III	Switches with II	Switches with aVL	Switches with aVR	No change	Dominant S-wave and poor R-wave progression

NOTE: *RL is a ground lead, so RL-LL reversal does not result in any significant changes*

Case 13: Presentation

An 81-year-old female with history of congestive heart failure and permanent cardiac pacemaker placement presents with shortness of breath. What is your interpretation of her ECG?

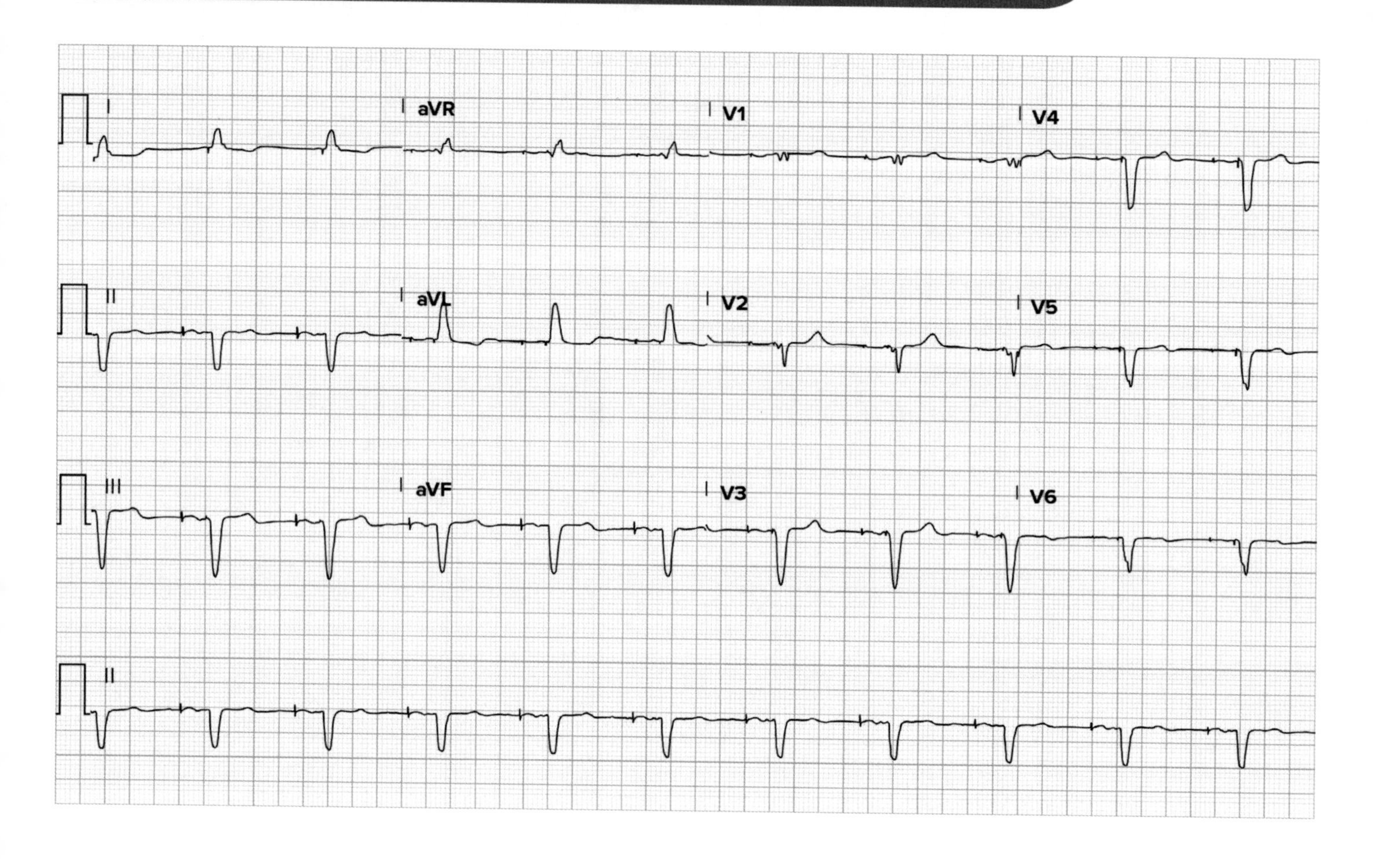

Case 13: Answer

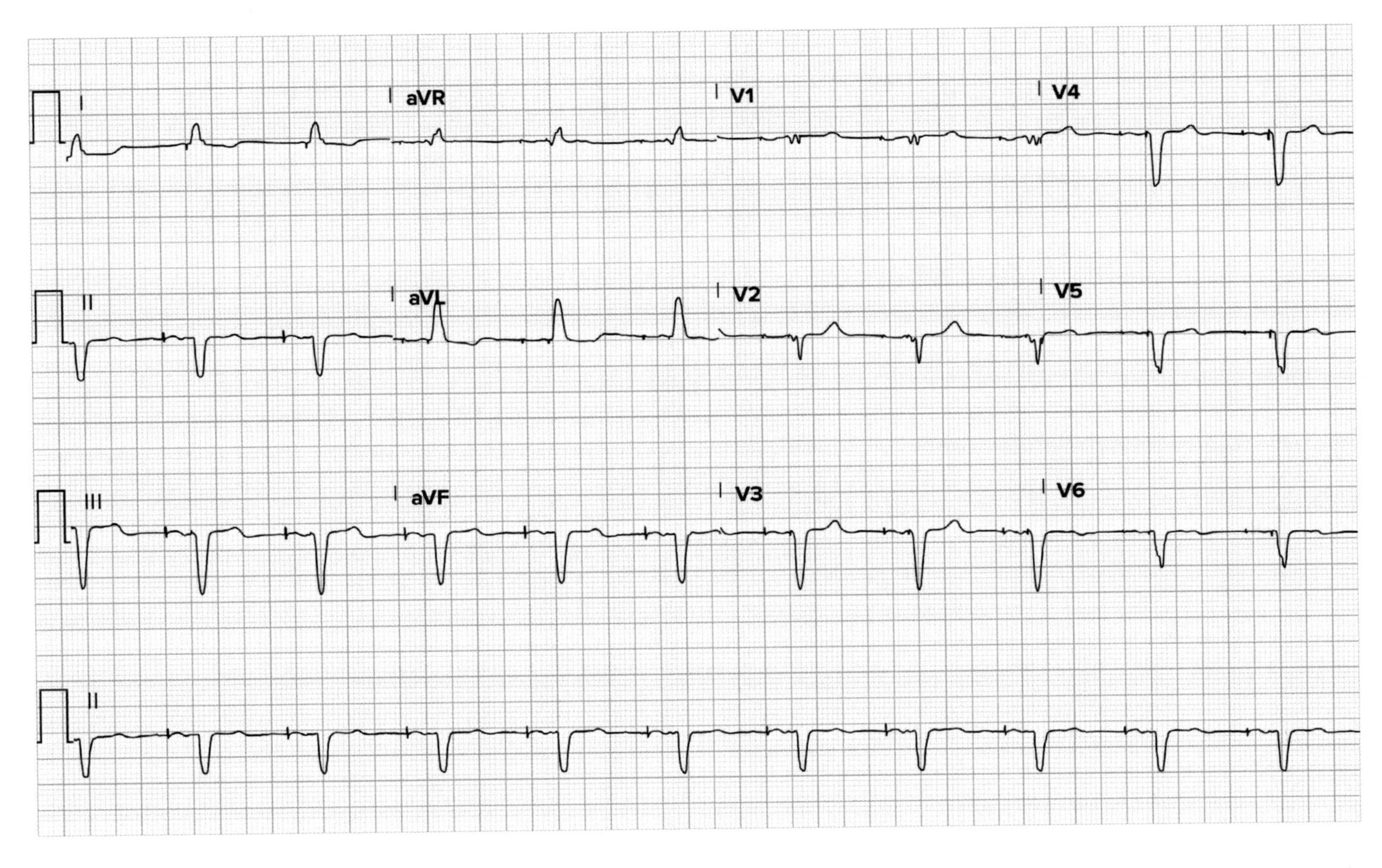

This ECG shows a dual chamber paced rhythm (also called A-V sequential pacing) at 82 bpm, left axis deviation, normal QTc interval, and prolonged QRS complex duration at 130 msec with a LBBB-like morphology. Note that the QRS complex in lead V6 is negatively oriented which is normal for right ventricular pacing.

Dual chamber pacing, also called A-V sequential pacing, involves pacing of both the right atria and right ventricle. There is one atrial lead and one ventricular lead:

- The right atrial lead paces the right atrial appendage
- The RV lead paces the RV apex

The atrial lead is programmed to sense for native atrial activity and act accordingly:

- The pacemaker senses native atrial activity, waits a programmed amount of time, then paces the ventricles (ie, atrial-sensed, ventricular-paced rhythm)
- The pacemaker paces the atria if no native atrial activity is detected during a programmed amount of time, waits another programmed amount of time, then paces the ventricles (ie, A-V sequential pacing)

With A-V sequential pacing, the ECG will show 2 pacer spikes: one preceding the P-wave and one preceding the QRS complex ***(see Figure 1)***. When compared to right ventricular pacing, the advantage of the atrial pacing is that it allows for coordination of the atrial kick in order to maximize cardiac output.

Figure 1.
Lead III shows normal A-V sequential pacing with 2 pacer spikes, one preceding the P-wave and one preceding the QRS complex

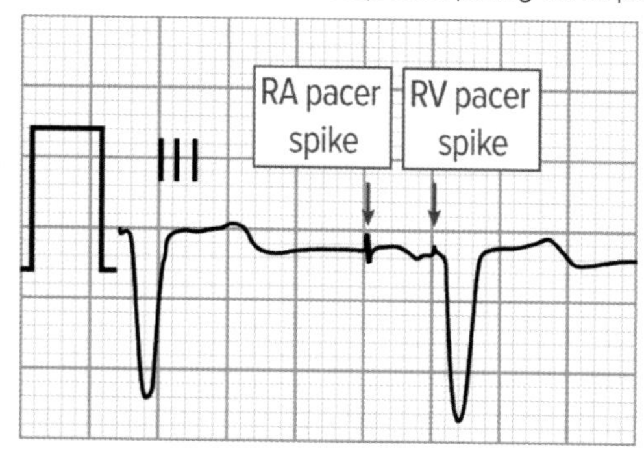

In an atrial-sensed ventricular-paced rhythm ***(see Figure 2)***, the pacemaker senses the patient's native atrial depolarization (ie, P-wave) and triggers ventricular depolarization after a programmed amount of time. The ECG will show a pacer spike preceding the QRS complexes but not the native P-waves ***(see Figure 3)***.

Figure 2.
Normal atrial-sensed, ventricular-paced rhythm (from a different ECG)

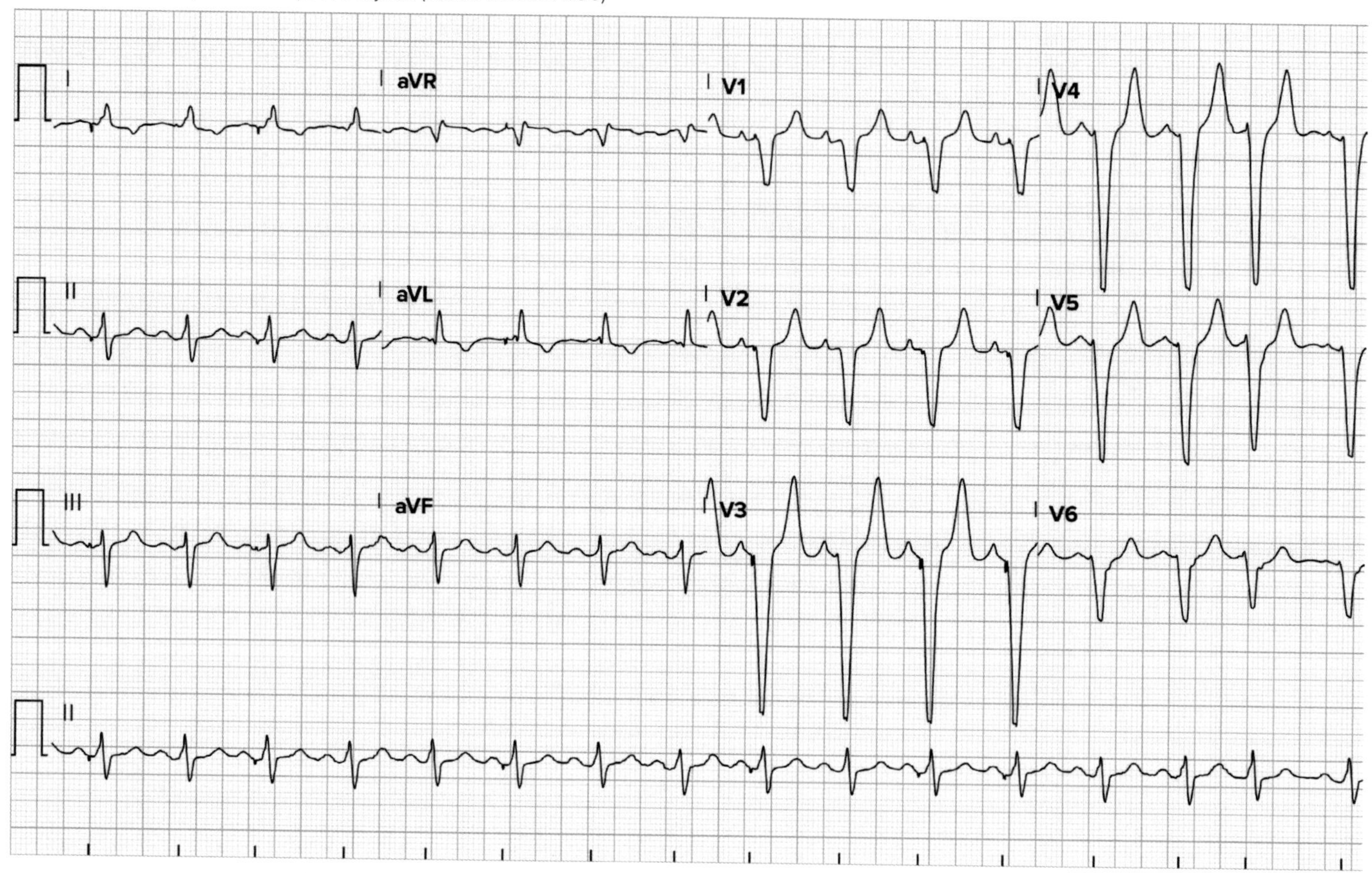

Figure 3.
Lead V1 from Figure 2 shows a normal atrial-sensed, ventricular-paced rhythm

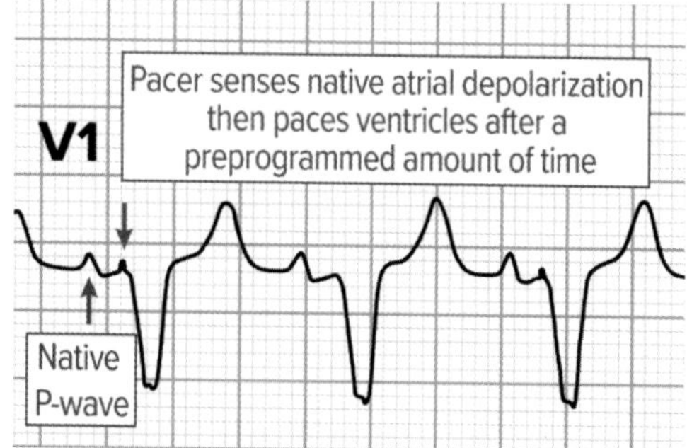

Pacing of the ventricles from the RV apex leads to a LBBB-like morphology. The major difference between an intrinsic LBBB and the LBBB-like morphology seen in a paced rhythm is that the QRS complex will almost always be negatively oriented in leads V5-V6 with a paced rhythm.

This patient's ECG was unchanged from prior, and her ED workup was consistent with a CHF exacerbation. She was admitted to the Cardiology service for diuresis.

Pacemaker Learning Points

- Pacer spikes are usually visible on the ECG, either at the bottom of the ECG and/or preceding the P-wave and/or QRS complex
  - Atrial pacing: spikes immediately precede P-waves
  - Ventricular pacing: spikes immediately precede QRS complexes
  - Dual chamber pacing: spikes immediately precede both P-waves and QRS complexes
  - Biventricular pacing: 2 spikes immediately precede QRS complexes
- Atrial pacing
  - Pacemaker lead usually implanted in the right atrial appendage
  - Results in P-waves with normal morphology
- Right ventricular pacing
  - Pacemaker lead usually implanted in the RV apex
  - Results in a LBBB pattern in the limb leads and anteroseptal precordial leads
  - The major difference between an intrinsic LBBB and a right ventricular-paced rhythm is that the QRS complex will almost always be negatively oriented in leads V5-V6 with a right ventricular-paced rhythm
- Biventricular pacing
  - Two pacemaker leads usually implanted in the RV apex and the surface of the posterior or lateral LV
  - Typically results in a narrower QRS complex than with right ventricular pacing
  - Dominant R-wave in lead V1 +/- V2 is common
- AICD will have a thick coil that differentiates it from a pacemaker

Case 14: Presentation

A 54-year-old male presents after collapsing at work. During transport to the emergency department, he lost pulses and was defibrillated once by EMS for ventricular fibrillation with return of spontaneous circulation. What is your interpretation of his pre-arrest ECG?

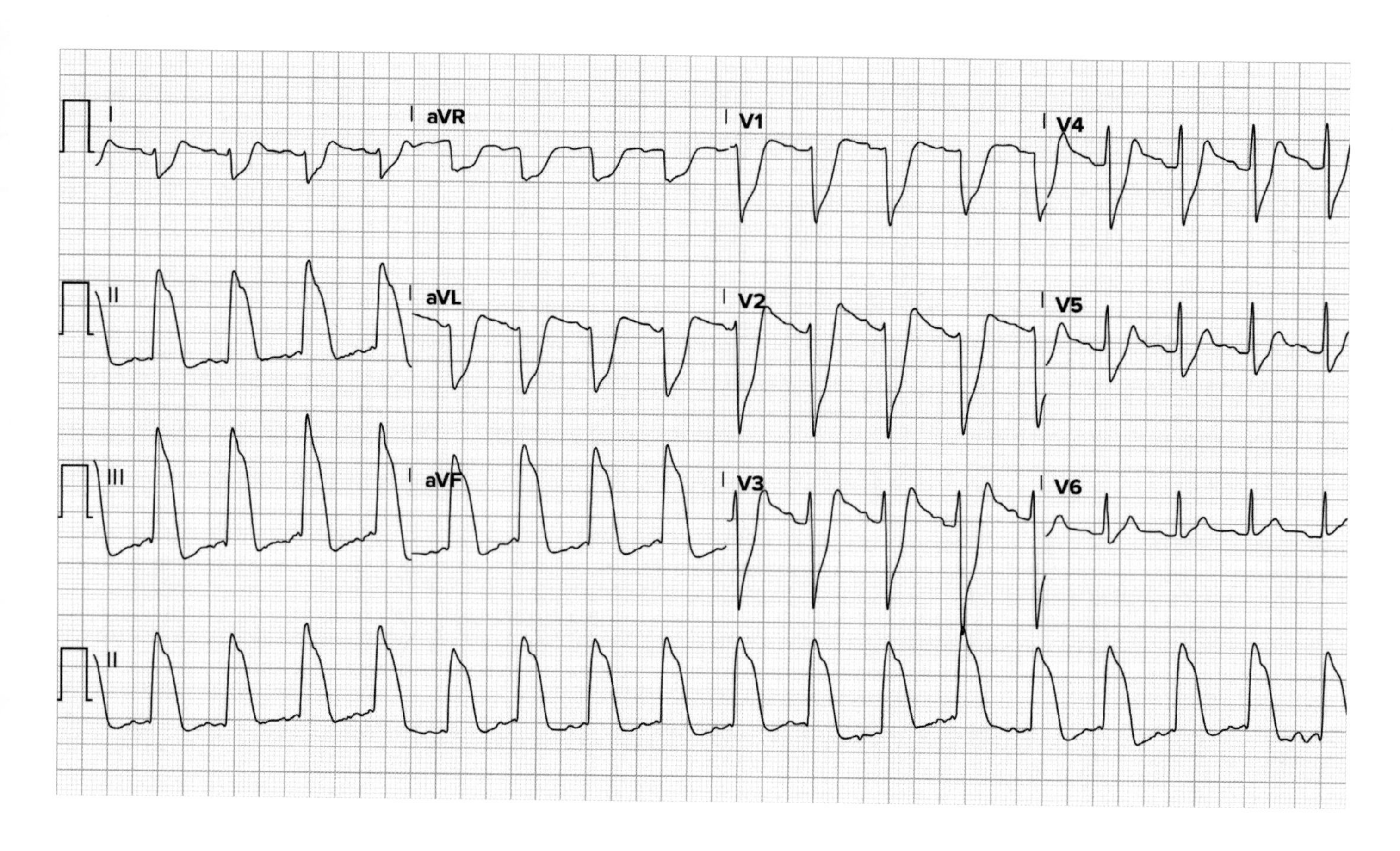

Case 14: Answer

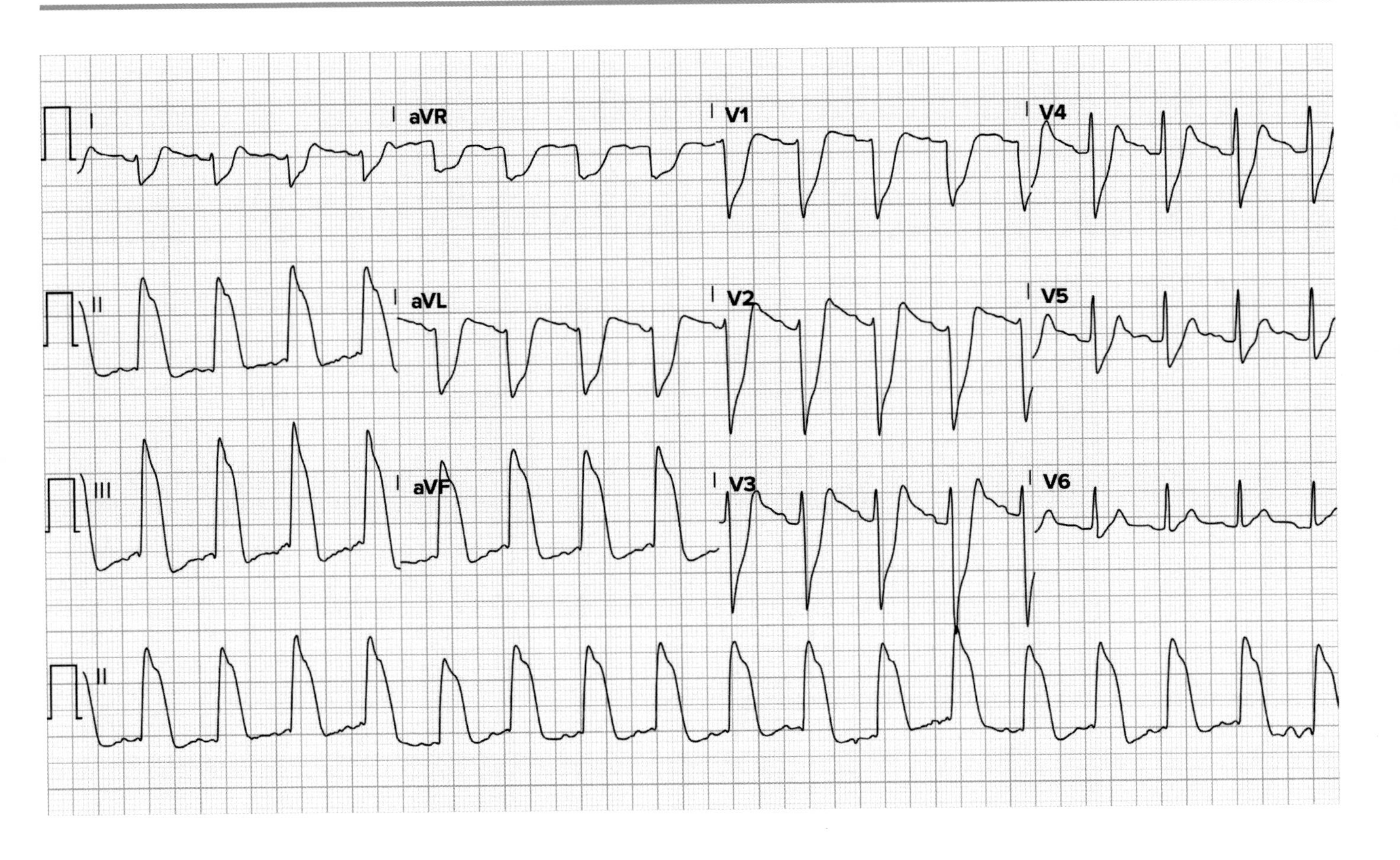

This ECG shows sinus tachycardia at approximately 102 bpm, right axis deviation, prolonged QRS complex duration of 120 msec, STE in leads II, III, aVF, and STD in leads I, aVL, aVR, and V1-V6.

The QRS-T complexes in the inferior leads are called "Shark Fins" and are due to a massive AMI. These complexes are a fusion of a widened QRS complex with an elevated ST segment and hyperacute T wave. The presence of hyperacute T-waves with this patten suggests an early STEMI in most instances. Patients presenting with this ECG pattern have a very high risk for rapid decompensation and cardiac arrest.

The key to interpreting this ECG is identifying the J point which is best seen in lead V6 and can be used to find the J point in the leads above and below it ***(see Figure 1).***

Figure 1.
The J point in lead V6 can be used to find the J point in the leads above and below

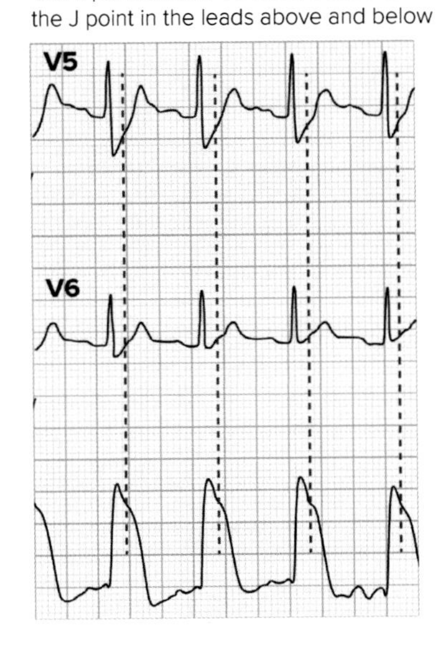

The lead II rhythm strip can be used to identify the J point in the other leads and it becomes clear that the QRS complex duration is only 120 msec and the other 85 msec is STE/STD ***(see Figures 2 and 3).*** The inferior lead STE with STD in the lateral leads is consistent with an inferior MI and the STD in leads V1-V3 suggest posterior extension.

Figure 2.
Identification of the QRS complex duration, J point, and STE in lead II

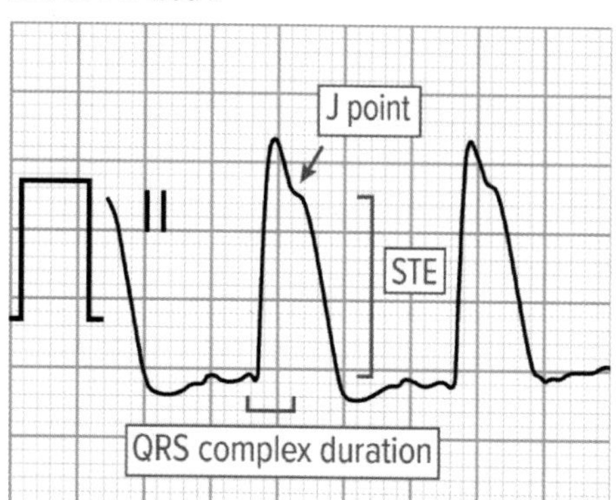

Figure 3.
Identification of the QRS complex duration, J point, T-wave, and STD in lead I

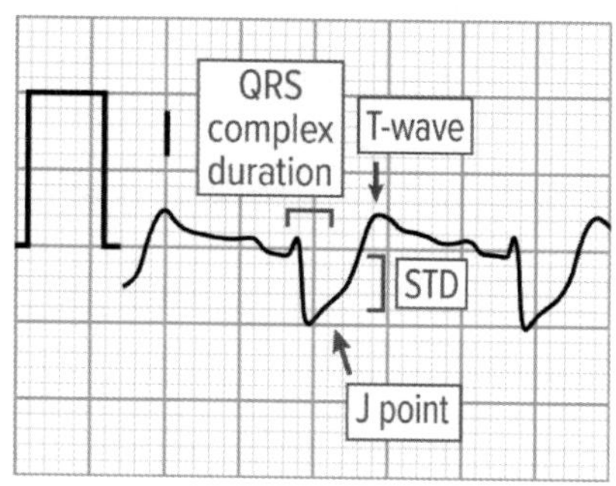

Although the QRS complex duration is not as prolonged as it appears, there is value in the mental exercise of considering the differential diagnosis for a very prolonged QRS complex duration. The differential diagnosis for a QRS complex duration > 200 msec includes hyperkalemia, sodium channel blocker toxicity, and VT. With respect to this patient's ECG:

- The presence of non-dissociated P-waves rules out VT, and the rate would be very slow for VT, which is typically > 120-130 bpm
- Although there is a positive QRS complex in lead II and right axis deviation, both of which are seen with sodium channel blocker toxicity, there is no dominant R-wave or R/S ratio > 0.7 in lead aVR which would be expected with a sodium channel blocker toxicity
- Treating presumptively for hyperkalemia with calcium would be a reasonable initial step in management in conjunction with either point-of-care or traditional laboratory-based testing for serum potassium

This patient went to the catheterization laboratory and had a 100% RCA occlusion successfully treated with a stent. He was discharged 5 days later after placement of an internal cardiac defibrillator.

"Shark Fin" Learning Points

- Very wide QRS-T complex with significant ST-segment elevation
    - ST-segment is typically convex
    - T-wave becomes indistinguishable from ST-segment making it difficult to determine STE
- Consistent with a massive AMI
    - Associated with a very high risk for rapid decompensation and cardiac arrest

STEMI Learning Points

- STEMI is defined by new, or presumed new, STE at the J point in ≥ 2 anatomically contiguous leads in the absence of LVH by voltage pattern, LBBB, or ventricular-paced rhythm
  - ≥ 2.5 mm in men < 40 years old and ≥ 2 mm in men ≥ 40 years old in leads V2-V3 (or an increase of ≥ 1 mm when compared to baseline ECG)
  - ≥ 1.5 mm in women in leads V2-V3 (or an increase of ≥ 1 mm when compared to baseline ECG)
  - ≥ 1 mm in all other leads
- ST-segment is measured from the isoelectric baseline, typically the TP segment (see below)
- Reciprocal STD are not required for the diagnosis of STEMI, but their presence does increase the likelihood of the diagnosis of STEMI
  - Reciprocal STD are only present in 70% of anterior MI[1]
- Posterior MI
  - Consider whenever there is STD in leads V1-V4
  - STE ≥ 0.5 mm in posterior leads V7, V8 or V9 is diagnostic- does not require 2 contiguous leads
- Right ventricular MI
  - Consider with any inferior MI (RV MI is seen in approximately 1/3 of inferior MI)
  - STE in right precordial leads V3R and V4R ≥ 0.5 mm (≥ 1 mm for men ≤ 30 years old)
  - STE in right precordial lead V4R > 1 mm is most predictive of RV MI
  - STE in right precordial lead V4R > STE in leads V1-V3 = highly specific for RV MI
- Significant STE that does not meet the traditional distribution (ie, ≥ 2 anatomically contiguous leads) in a presentation concerning for ACS may still represent coronary artery occlusion and warrant consideration for emergent coronary reperfusion

How to Measure STE per most recent 2018 AHA Guidelines[2]

- The J point is the junction between QRS termination and ST-segment onset and is used to determine the magnitude of the ST-segment shift
- **In patients with a stable baseline, the TP segment (isoelectric interval) is a more accurate method to assess the magnitude of ST-segment shift** ***(see Figure 4)***, and in distinguishing pericarditis from acute myocardial ischemia
- QRS onset should be used if TP segment does not have a stable baseline ***(see Figure 5)***
- Measurement should be made from the top of the ECG line tracing

Figure 4.
Measure STE from the TP segment if the TP segment is isoelectric (ie, horizontal)

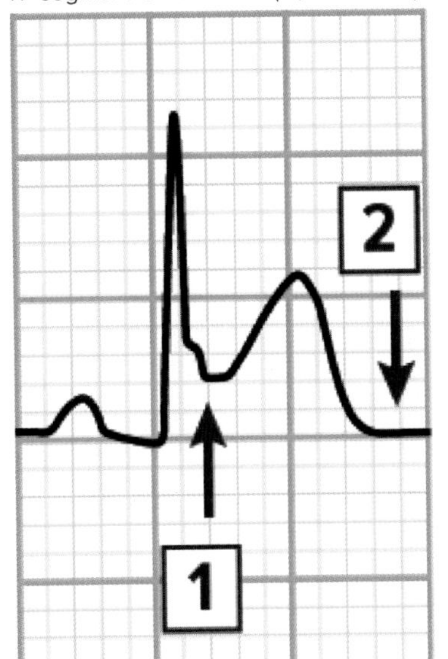

Arrow 1: onset of the ST-segment (ie, J point)
Arrow 2: TP segment

Figure 5.
Measure STE from onset of the QRS complex if the TP segment is not isoelectric (ie, not horizontal)

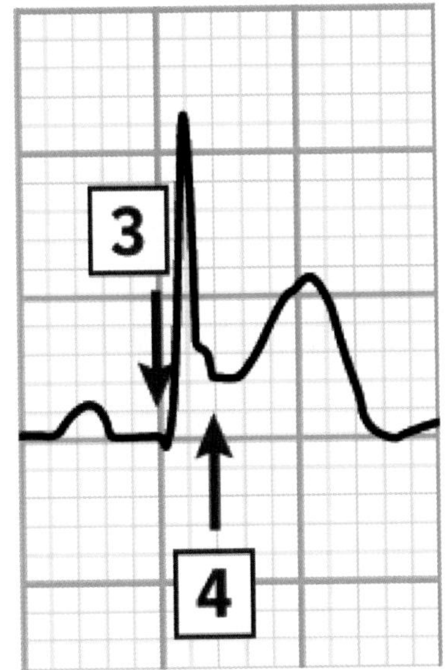

Arrow 3: initial onset of the Q-wave
Arrow 4: onset of the ST-segment (ie, J point)

References

1. Knilans T, Surawicz B. Chou's Electrocardiography in Clinical Practice. Philadelphia, PA: Elsevier. 2020.
2. Thygesen K, Alpert JS, Jaffe AS, et al. 2018 ESC/ACC/AHA/WHF Expert Consensus Document: Fourth Universal Definition of Myocardial Infarction (2018). *Circulation.* 2018;138:e618-e651.

Case 15: Presentation

A 17-year-old male with no known past medical history presents after a syncopal episode. What is your interpretation of his ECG?

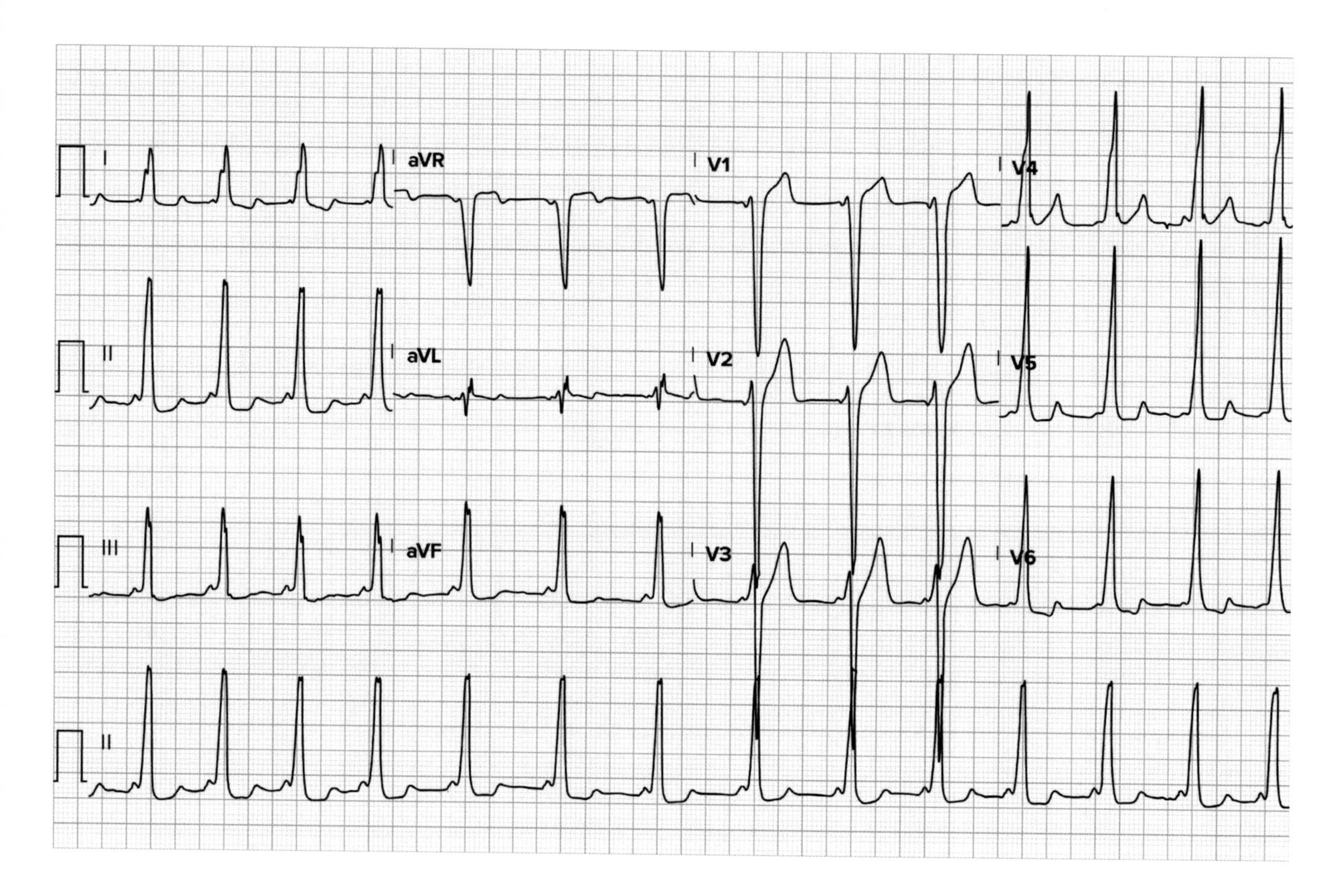

Case 15: Answer

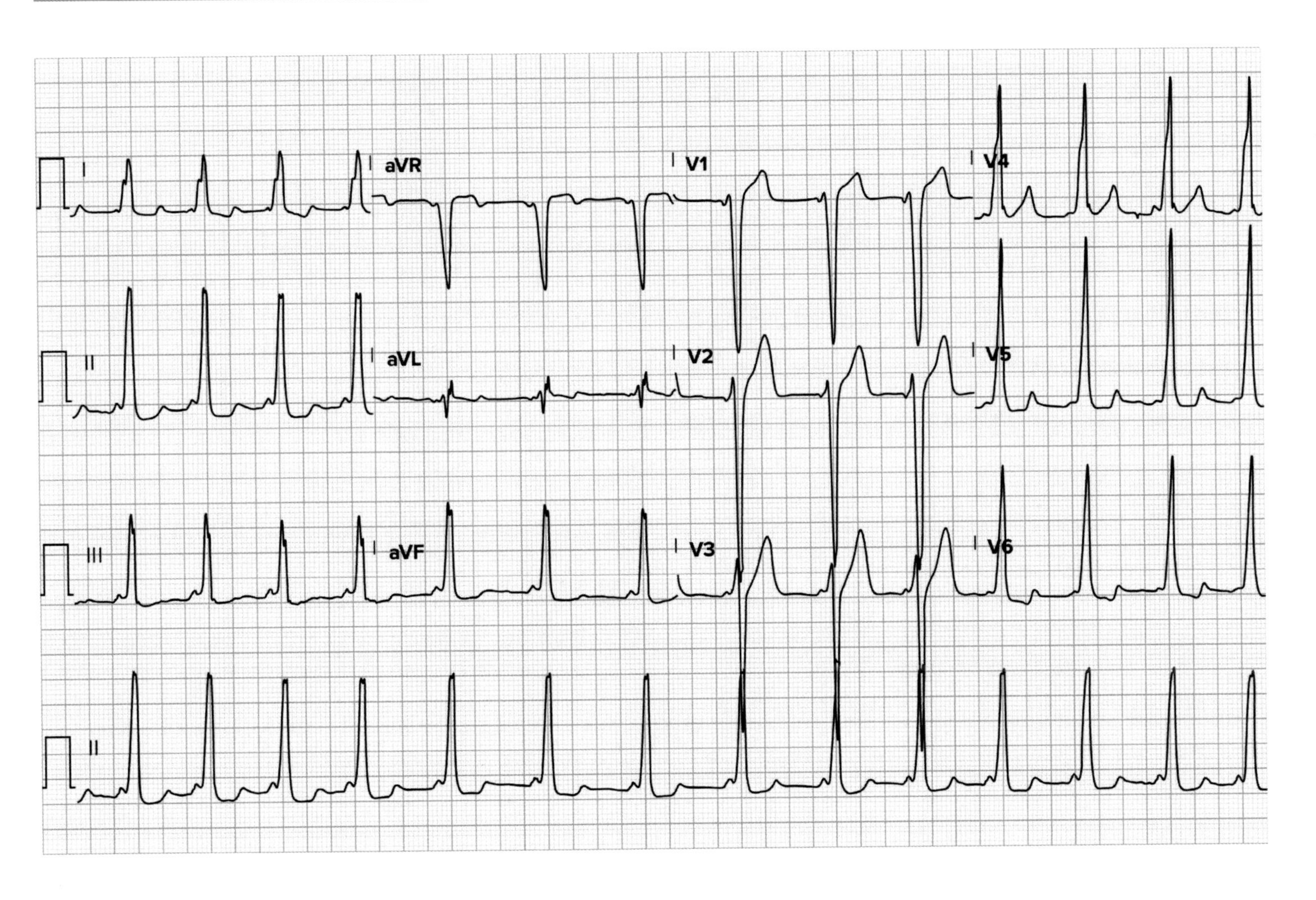

This ECG shows normal sinus rhythm with a ventricular rate of 82 bpm, normal axis, shortened PR interval, prolonged QRS complex duration ~130 msec, and delta waves, best seen in leads I and V4-V6, consistent with pre-excitation and WPW syndrome. There are ST-segment changes that mimic a LBBB or the LVH with strain pattern.

In patients with WPW, ECG findings seen in sinus rhythm include:

- Shortened PR interval (< 120 msec)
- Delta wave: slurring of initial portion of the QRS complex that interrupts the P-wave or arises immediately after its termination
- QRS complex duration prolonged, usually > 110 msec
- Secondary ST and T-wave changes

Wolff-Parkinson-White syndrome is a congenital pre-excitation syndrome due to an abnormal conduction pathway between the atria and the ventricle, called the accessory pathway (AP). Conduction from the atria to the ventricles can occur via both the AV node and AP, but conduction via the AP is typically faster than the AV node due to its shorter refractory period. The early ventricular depolarization via the AP, called ventricular pre-excitation, subsequently fuses with the depolarization caused by conduction via the AV node to create the characteristic delta wave ***(see Figure 1)***.

Figure 1.
Lead V4 shows delta waves and short PR intervals consistent with WPW in sinus rhythm

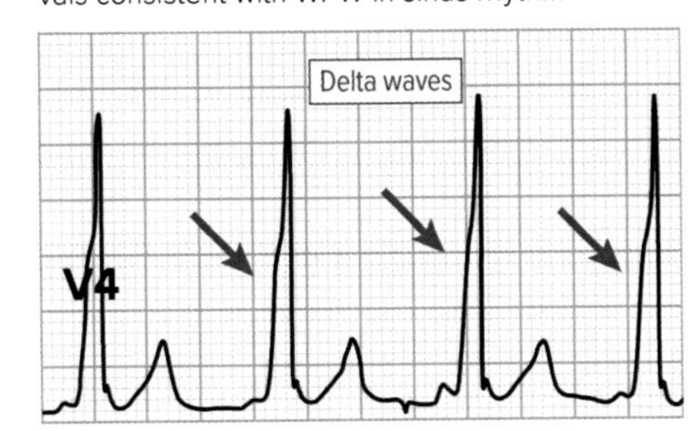

The PR interval represents the time it takes for an impulse to propagate from the atria through the AV node and His-Purkinje system until the ventricles begin to depolarize. It is measured from the beginning of the P-wave to the beginning of the QRS complex and a normal value in adults is 120-200 msec.

The differential diagnosis for a short PR interval includes:

- Pre-excitation syndromes
- Ectopic atrial rhythms originating near AV node
- Junctional rhythms with retrograde P-waves

In WPW, the short PR interval and often prolonged QRS complex duration are due to the presence of a delta wave, and not due to conduction abnormalities in the AV node and/or His-Purkinje system. This is important because patients with WPW can have baseline ECGs (ie, in normal sinus rhythm) without delta waves that will show a normal PR interval and normal QRS complex duration.

Patients with WPW will often have ST-segment and T-wave abnormalities on their baseline ECGs (ie, in normal sinus rhythm). Most often, the ST-segment deviation and T-wave will point opposite to the main vector of the QRS complex ***(see Figure 2).*** These findings can mimic the changes seen with a LBBB ***(see Figure 3)*** or LVH with strain pattern ***(see Figure 4).***

Figure 2.
ST-segment and T-wave abnormalities seen with WPW in normal sinus rhythm (case ECG)

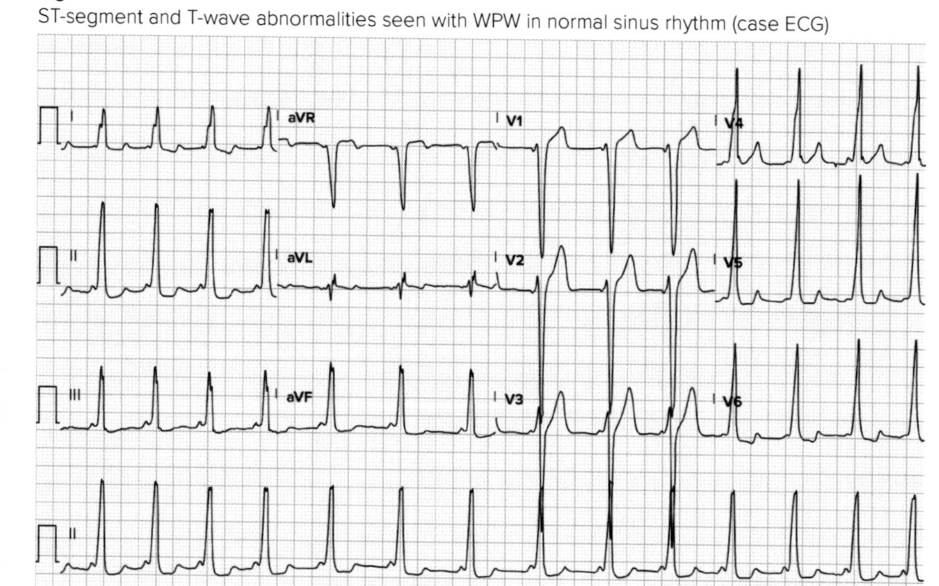

Figure 3.
ST-segment and T-wave abnormalities seen with a LBBB (ECG from a different patient)

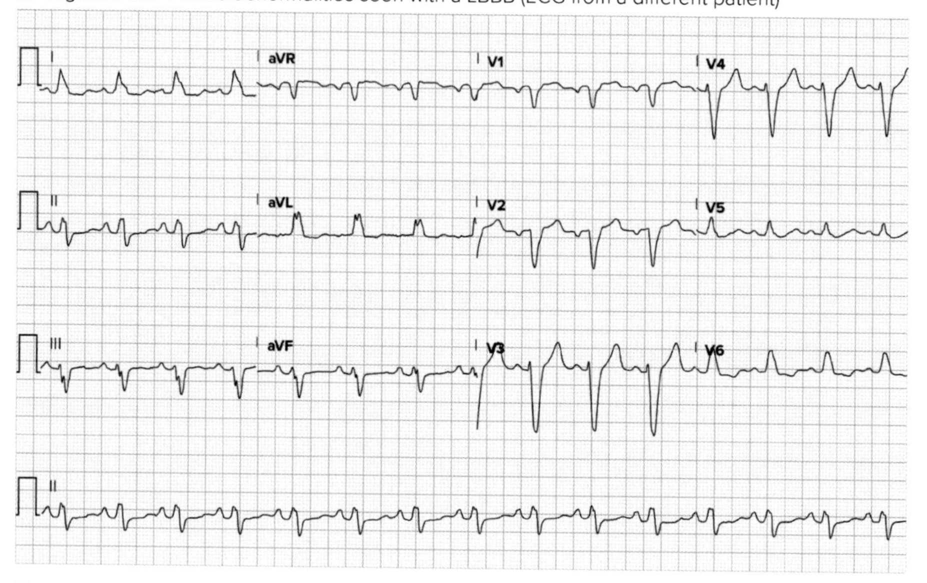

Figure 4.
ST-segment and T-wave abnormalities seen with LVH with strain pattern (ECG from a different patient)

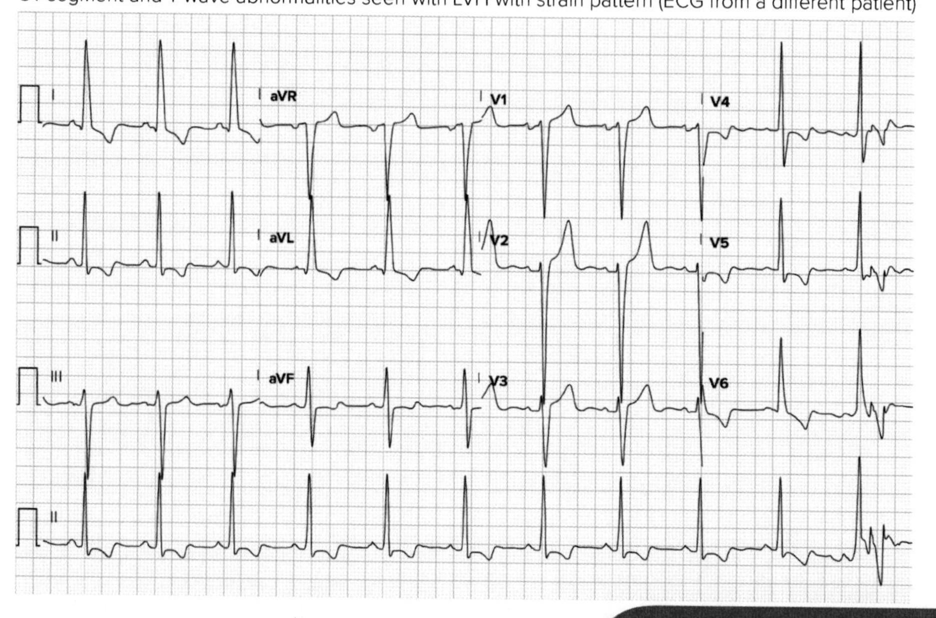

There are multiple dysrhythmias that are seen in patients with WPW syndrome. Anterograde conduction via the AV node is called orthodromic conduction and will result in a narrow QRS complex (ie, duration < 110 msec) in the absences of a rate-related or fixed conduction delay or electrolyte abnormality. Anterograde conduction via the AP will result in a prolonged QRS complex duration and is called antidromic conduction. Tachydysrhythmias associated with WPW include:

- WPW with orthodromic AVRT
  - Rapid, regular narrow complex tachycardia
  - Treat like AVNRT (PSVT)
- WPW with antidromic AVRT
  - Rapid, regular wide complex tachycardia
  - Can look like monomorphic VT
  - Treat like VT
- WPW with atrial fibrillation
  - Rapid, irregularly irregular wide complex tachycardia with beat-to-beat variation in QRS morphologies
  - Avoid AV nodal blocking agents (eg, adenosine, beta- and calcium channel blockers, amiodarone)

This patient had an unremarkable ED work-up and was admitted to the cardiology service. He was diagnosed with WPW and discharged home on oral flecainide.

WPW Learning Points

- Congenital condition involving abnormal conduction pathway between atria and ventricle
  - Most common dysrhythmia is orthodromic AVRT
- ECG findings seen in sinus rhythm include:
  - Shortened PR interval (< 120 msec)
  - Delta wave: slurring of initial portion of the QRS complex
  - QRS complex duration prolonged, usually > 110 msec
  - Secondary ST-segment and T-wave changes
  - Patients with WPW can have baseline ECGs (ie, in normal sinus rhythm) with a normal PR interval, normal QRS complex duration, and/or without delta waves
- Regular rhythm tachycardias in WPW can be narrow (orthodromic conduction via AV node) or wide (antidromic conduction via accessory pathway)
  - WPW with orthodromic AVRT (most common dysrhythmia): regular NCT, treat like AVNRT (PSVT)
  - WPW with antidromic AVRT: regular WCT, treat like monomorphic VT
- WPW with atrial fibrillation
  - Rapid, irregularly irregular wide complex tachycardia with beat-to-beat variation in QRS complex morphologies
  - Treatment includes electrical cardioversion (for stable or unstable patients) and IV procainamide or ibutilide for stable patients (avoid AV nodal blocking medications)
- In wide-complex atrial fibrillation, ventricular rates > 220-240 bpm suggest anterograde conduction via an accessory pathway

References

1. January CT, Wann LS, Alpert JS, et al. 2014 AHA/ACC/ HRS guideline for the management of patients with atrial fibrillation: a report of the American College of Cardiology/American Heart Association Task Force on Practice Guidelines and the Heart Rhythm Society. J Am Coll Cardiol. 2014;64:e1–76

Case 16: Presentation

A 51-year-old male with no past medical history presents after a syncopal episode. What is your interpretation of his ECG? A prior ECG is below for comparison.

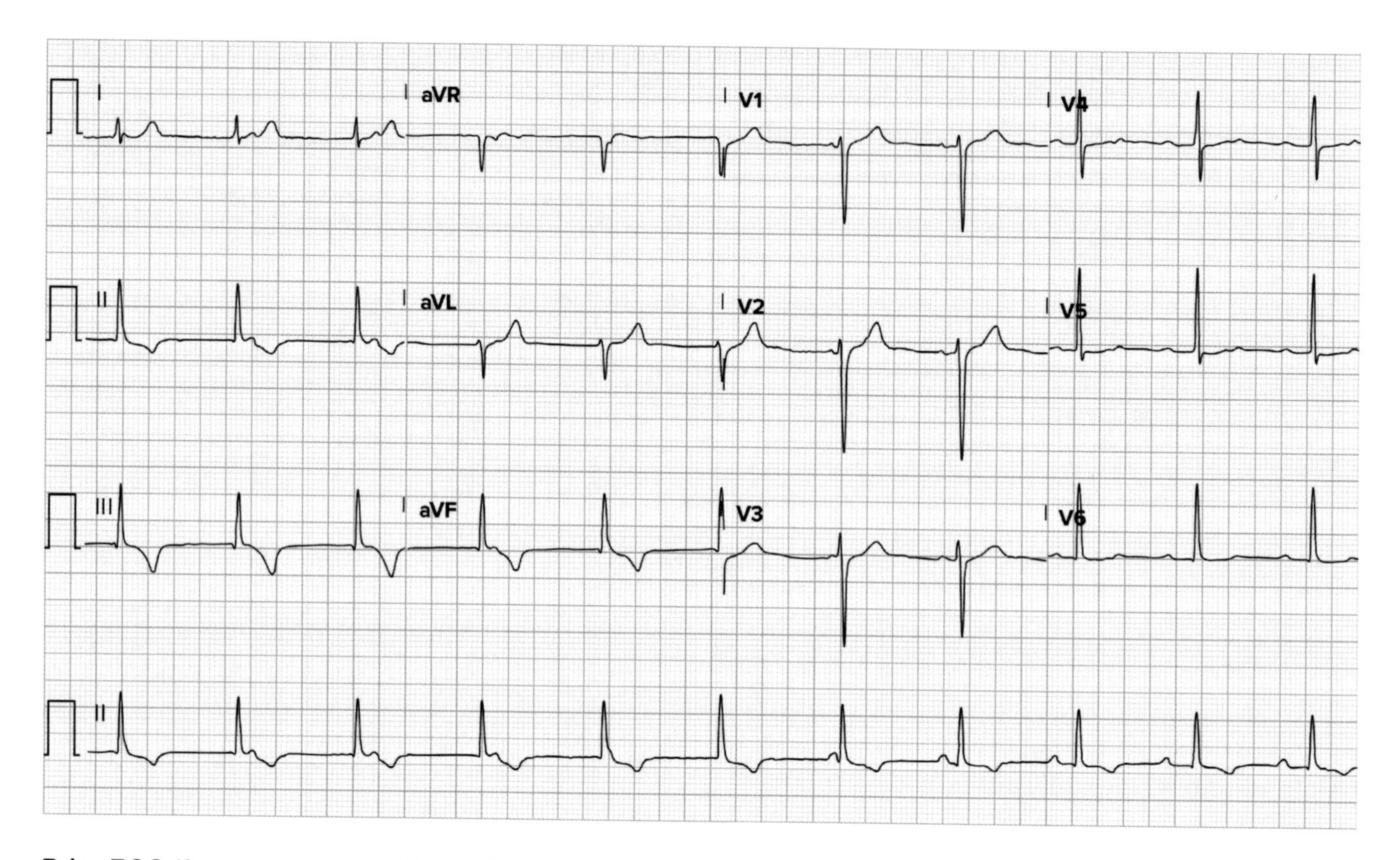

Prior ECG (from several months ago)

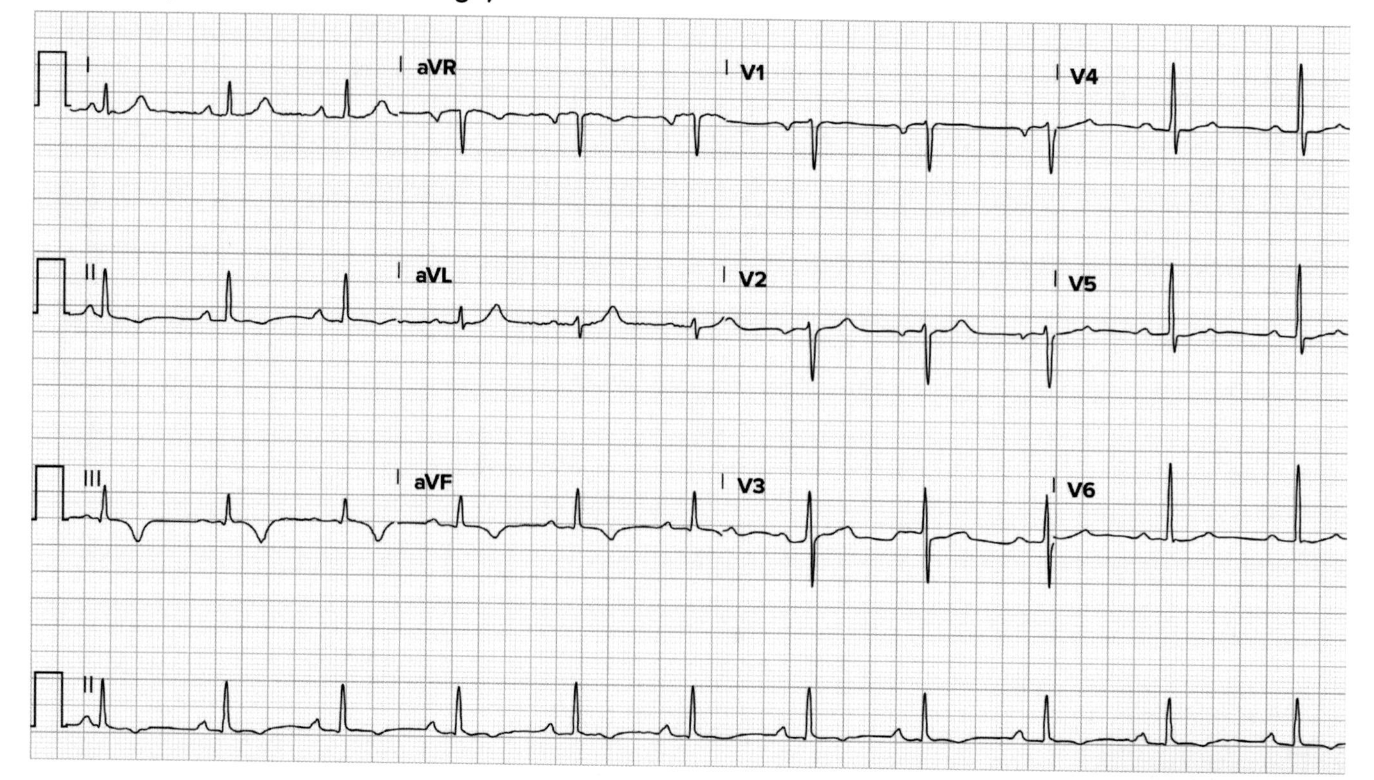

Case 16: Answer

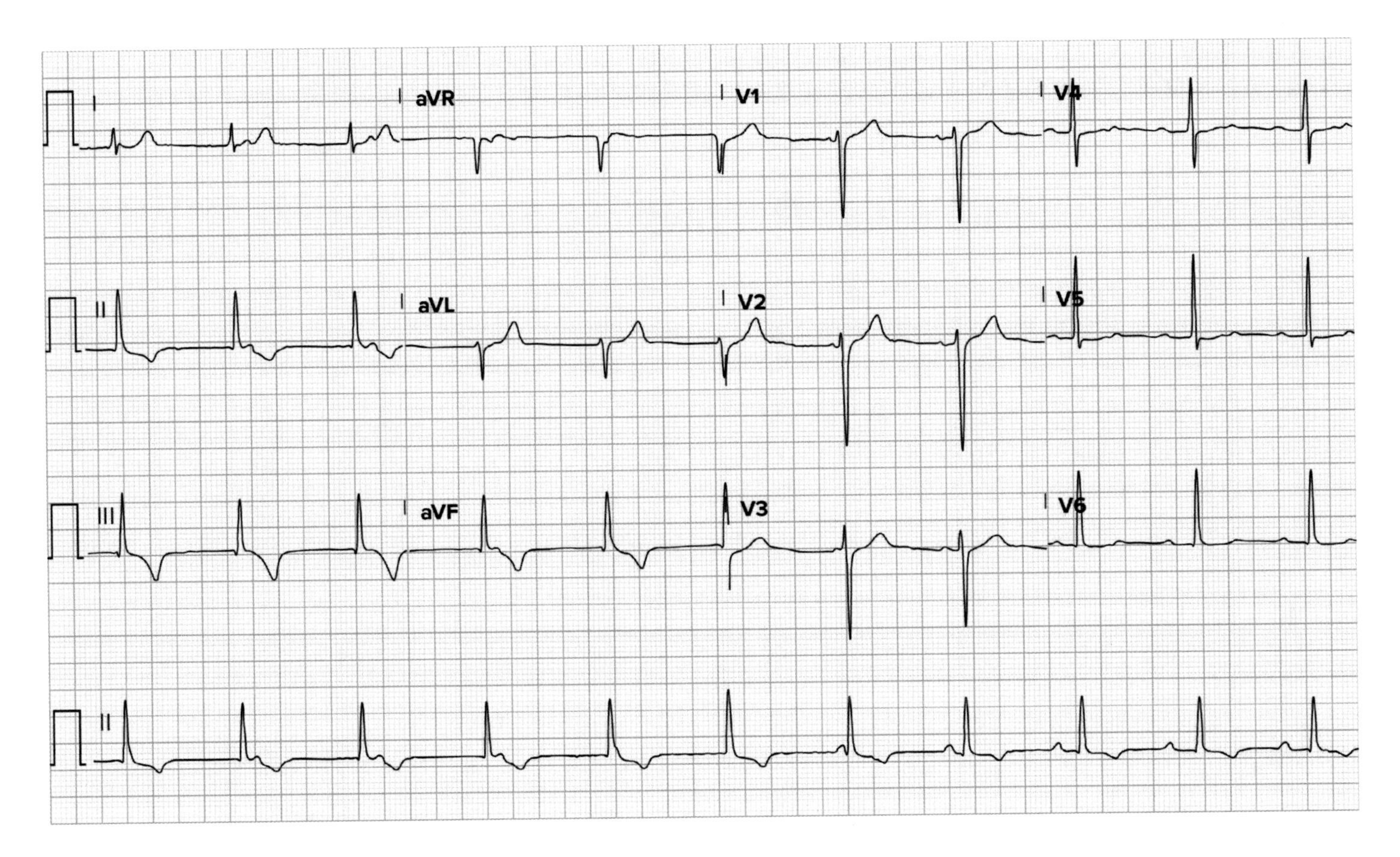

Prior ECG (from several months ago)

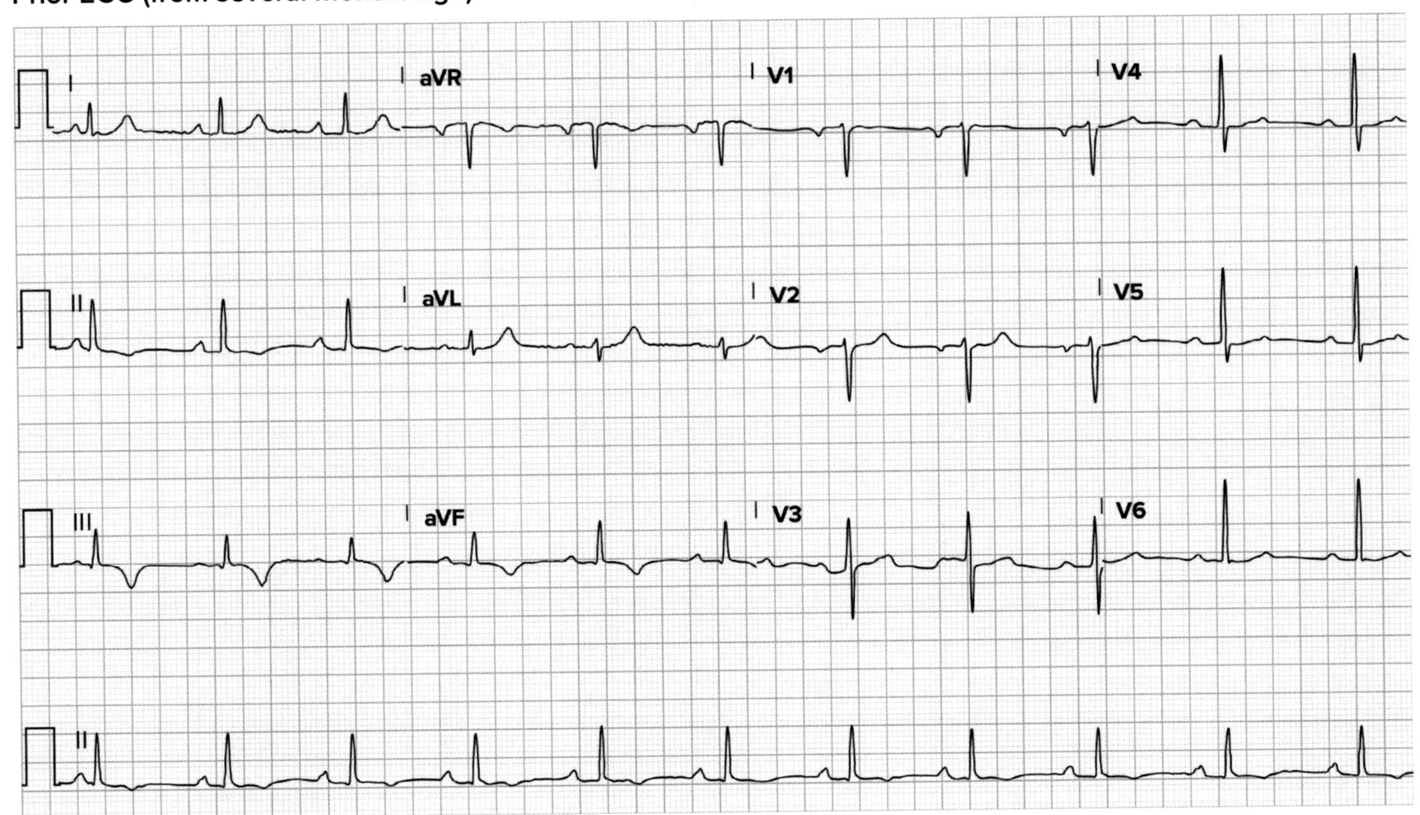

This ECG shows an accelerated junctional rhythm at 65 bpm with AV dissociation, TWI in leads II, III, and aVF unchanged from prior, and a new upright T-wave in lead V1 when compared to prior. Note that the P-wave in lead V1 in the prior ECG is entirely negative which suggests that it was placed above the 4th intercostal space. This inappropriate lead placement will typically produce a negatively oriented T-wave so the new upright T-wave in lead V1 seen on the initial EG may be due to better lead placement.

The key finding in this ECG is the AV dissociation in the absence of a 3rd degree, or complete, AV block. It is important to differentiate a 3rd degree AV block from AV dissociation. A 3rd degree AV block describes the absence of conduction from the atria to the ventricles via the AV node. AV dissociation describes when the atria and ventricles operate independently of each other. A 3rd degree AV block will always have AV dissociation, but there can be AV dissociation without a 3rd degree AV block. Examples of this include ventricular tachycardia, decreased SA node automaticity such that a junctional or ventricular site takes over pacing, or if there is increased automaticity in a junctional or ventricular site that is faster than the SA node. In these cases, the AV node functions normally, but the impulses from the SA node are blocked by the retrograde conduction from the faster junctional or ventricular pacing.

Isorhythmic AV dissociation describes when the atrial and ventricular rates are the same or very similar. In these cases, it is impossible to tell whether there is a 3rd degree AV block unless there is a P-QRS-T complex with a PR interval that would be reasonable to see with normal conduction. In other words, identifying a 3rd degree AV block requires the presence of a P-wave that should conduct under normal circumstances but doesn't.

This ECG begins with isorhythmic AV dissociation ***(see Figure 1)*** with atrial and ventricular rates that are very similar although not exactly identical. The P-waves occur after the QRS complexes so it impossible to tell if the AV node is blocked. The P-waves are upright in leads I, II, and aVF which is consistent with sinus P-waves and not retrograde P-waves.

Figure 1.
The initial portion of the ECG (seen here in the lead II rhythm strip) shows isorhythmic AV dissociation with very similar atrial and ventricular rates

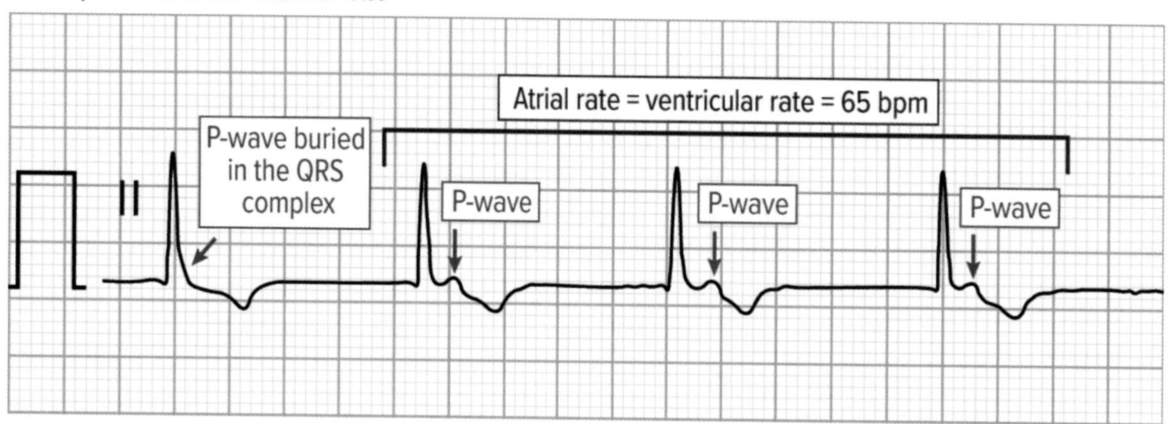

The next portion of this ECG shows an increasing atrial rate while the ventricular rate, paced by the junction, remains constant ***(see Figure 2).*** This is not uncommon as the sinus rate is more influenced by sympathetic/parasympathetic stimulation than junctional or ventricular-paced rates.

Figure 2.
The middle portion of the ECG (seen here in the lead II rhythm strip) shows an increasing atrial rate with a constant ventricular rate

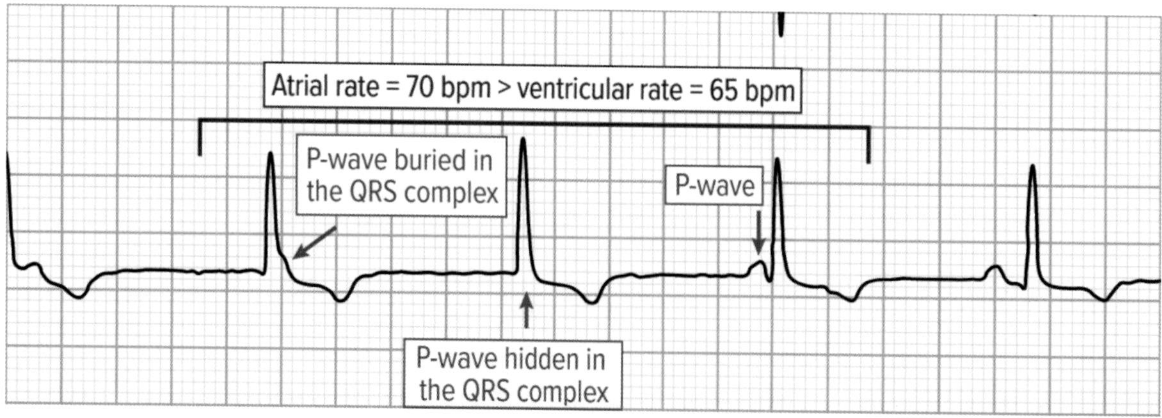

The final portion of the ECG shows P-waves preceding the QRS complexes with consistent PR intervals and an increase in the ventricular rate to match the sinus rate ***(see Figure 3).*** This proves that there is AV conduction and eliminates a 3rd degree AV block as a cause of the AV dissociation. In this ECG, the AV dissociation was due to increased automaticity of a junctional pacing site which should typically only take over pacing when the sinus rate falls below 60 bpm.

Figure 3.
The last portion of the ECG (seen here in the lead II rhythm strip) shows a sinus rhythm with the atrial and ventricular rates exactly equal and constant PR intervals

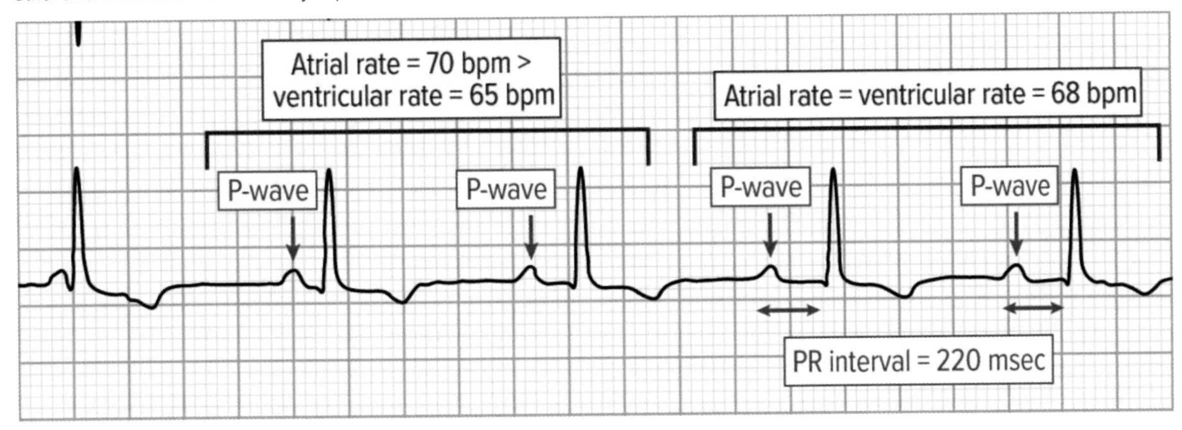

This patient had an unremarkable workup in the ED and was admitted to the cardiology service. Further evaluation for the etiology of his syncope was unrevealing and the patient was discharged with an ambulatory cardiac monitor.

AV dissociation Learning Points

- Independent atrial and ventricular pacing
  - Ventricular pacing can be from a junctional or ventricular pacing site
  - Isorhythmic AV dissociation describes when the atrial and ventricular rates are the same or very similar
- Etiologies include:
  - 3rd degree AV block
  - Ventricular tachycardia
  - Decreased sinus rate that allows for a junctional or ventricular site to take over pacing
  - Increased junctional or ventricular pacing rate that is faster than the sinus rate

Junctional Rhythm Learning Points

- Ectopic focus from AV node or proximal Purkinje system
  - Also called AV junctional rhythm, nodal rhythm, nodal escape rhythm, junctional escape rhythm, AV nodal rhythm
- ECG shows ventricular rate of 40-60 bpm with normal QRS complex duration unless concurrent conduction abnormality (eg, bundle branch block)
- May have retrograde P-waves that precede (with PR interval < 120 msec) or follow QRS complex, typically best seen in the inferior leads
- Variations include:
  - Junctional Bradycardia: ventricular rate < 40 bpm
  - Accelerated Junctional Rhythm: ventricular rate 61–100 bpm
  - Junctional Tachycardia: ventricular rate > 100 bpm

Case 17: Presentation

A 74-year-old female with history of atrial fibrillation and pacemaker placement for sick sinus syndrome presents with altered mental status in the setting of a recent viral GI illness. What is your interpretation of her ECG?

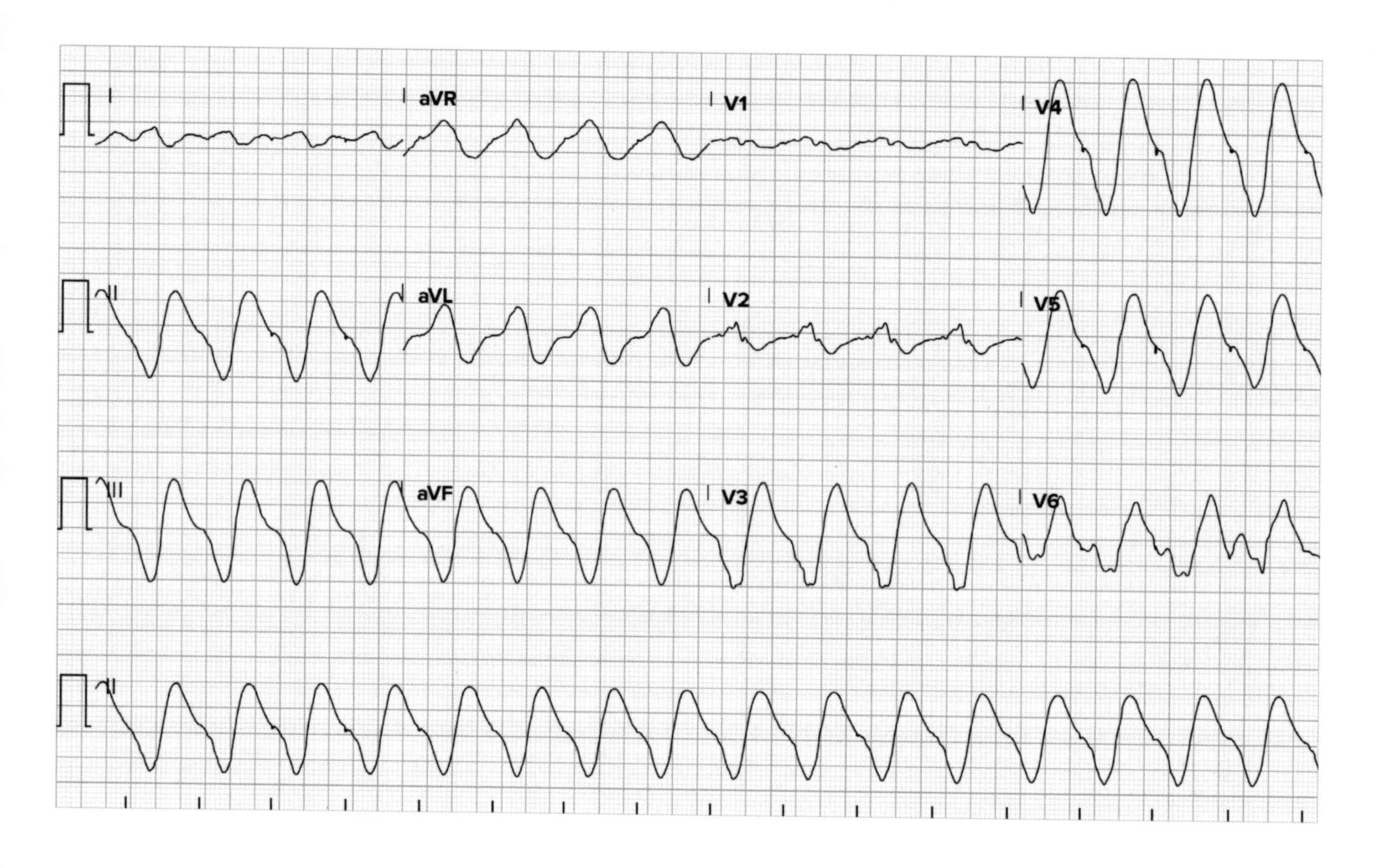

Case 17: Answer

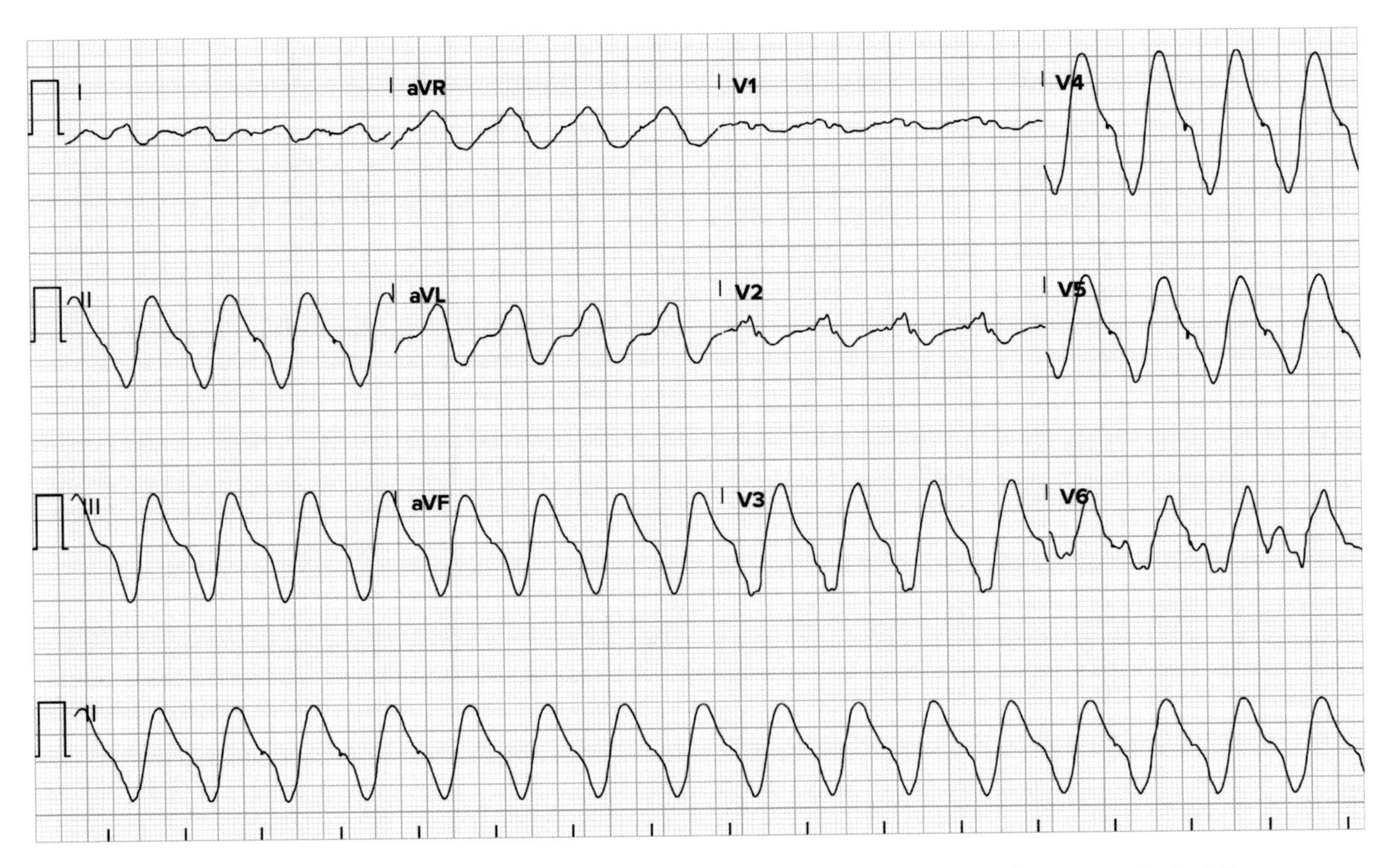

This ECG shows a ventricular-paced rhythm at 100 bpm with no visible P-waves, northwest/extreme axis deviation, prolonged QRS complex duration of ~280 msec, and a sinusoidal QRS-T complex morphology. Lead V2 has the appearance of a RBBB ***(see Figure 1)***. The pacer spikes are best seen preceding the QRS complexes in leads V4-V5.

Figure 1.
The rSR' morphology of the QRS complexes in lead V2 are consistent with a RBBB

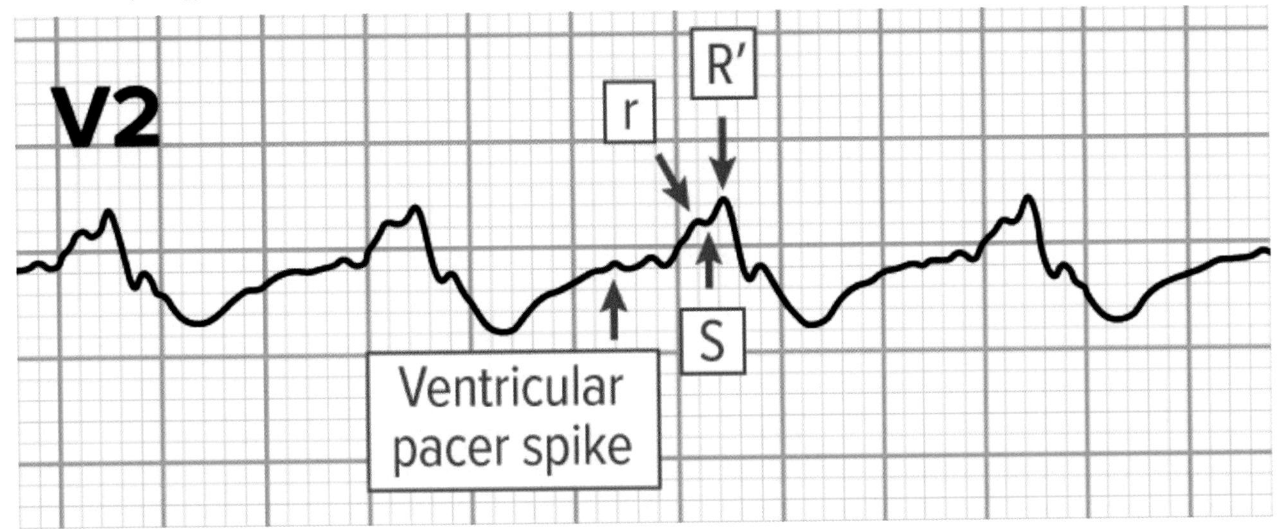

The differential diagnosis for a regular paced rhythm with QRS complexes this wide includes a paced rhythm with hyperkalemia, a paced rhythm with sodium channel blocker toxicity, and pacemaker-mediated tachycardia. The findings in this ECG that support those diagnoses include:

- The sinusoidal QRS-T complex morphology can be seen with hyperkalemia
- The terminal R-wave > 3 mm in lead aVR can be seen with sodium channel blocker toxicity
- The presence of pacer spikes that precede each QRS complex ***(see Figure 2)*** with a constant rate of 100 bpm and no visible P-waves can be seen with pacemaker-mediated tachycardia

Figure 2.
The lead II rhythm strip shows pacer spikes preceding each QRS complex

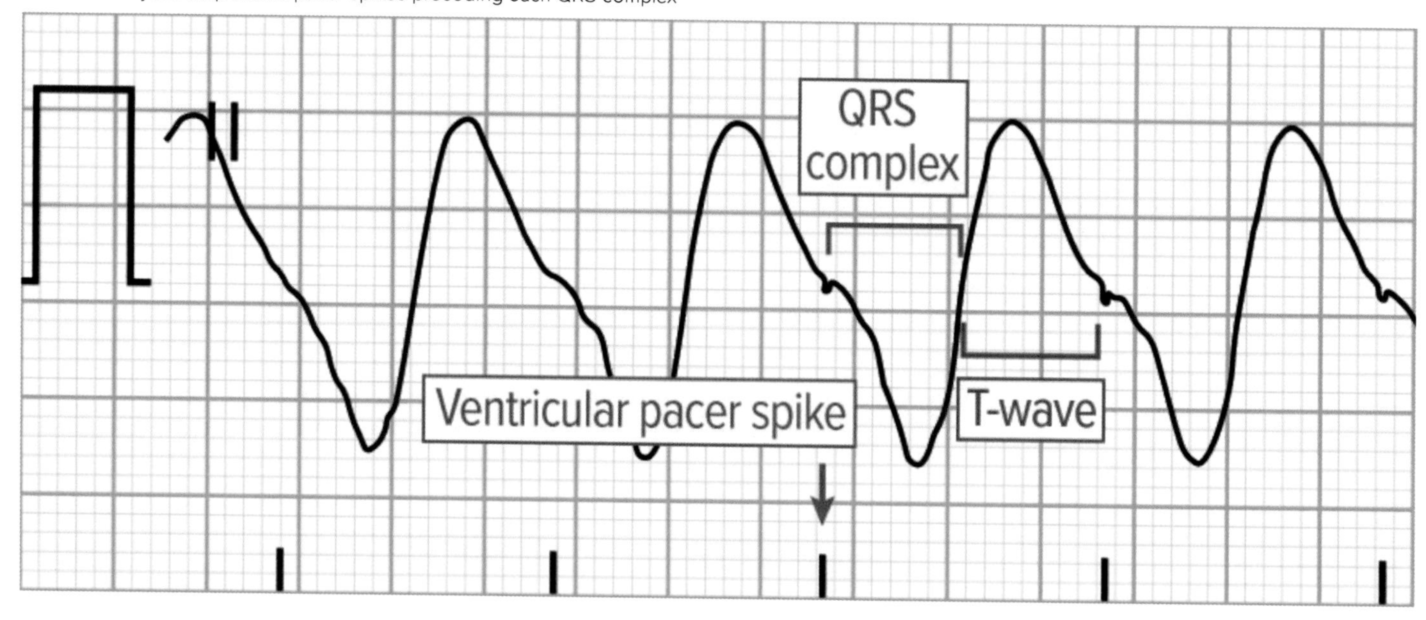

This patient was treated with IV calcium for presumptive hyperkalemia with no change in the ECG. Further history revealed the patient was on flecainide, a class 1C sodium-channel blocker. Notable lab findings included a normal potassium level, elevated lactate of 12.1 mmol/L, elevated BUN (the suspected cause of the patient's altered mental status), and elevated creatinine (thought to be caused by dehydration from the gastrointestinal illness). Overdrive pacing was attempted by cardiology, which resulted in rapid ventricular tachycardia, requiring cardioversion. The etiology of the prolonged QRS complex duration is thought to be a combination of the lactic acidosis and flecainide toxicity (acting via its sodium channel blocking effects) secondary to acute renal failure.

Sodium Channel Blocker Toxicity Learning Points

- ECG triad of prolonged QRS complex duration, prolonged QTc interval, and right axis deviation
- ECG features include:
  - Tachycardia
  - Right axis deviation
  - R/S ratio > 0.7 in lead aVR
  - QRS complex duration > 100 msec
  - Prolonged QTc interval
  - Terminal R-wave in lead aVR > 3 mm
- Tachycardia is common
  - Due to competing muscarinic or sympathomimetic effects
  - Bradycardia is typically a sign of severe toxicity
- QRS complex duration > 100 msec is associated with toxicity
  - Mortality increases as QRS duration increases
  - Treat with sodium bicarbonate
- Sodium channel blocking drugs include:
  - Anesthetics: bupivacaine
  - Anticonvulsants: carbamazepine
  - Antidepressants: bupropion, mirtazapine, venlafaxine
  - Antiarrhythmics: Class IA (procainamide), IC (flecainide), and II (propranolol)
  - Antihistamines: diphenhydramine
  - Antimalarial drugs: chloroquine, hydroxychloroquine, quinine
  - Cocaine
  - Phenothiazines: prochlorperazine, chlorpromazine
  - Tricyclic antidepressants: amitriptyline, nortriptyline

NOTES:

Case 18: Presentation

This is the preop ECG of an 82-year-old male being admitted for a hip fracture.
What is your interpretation of her ECG

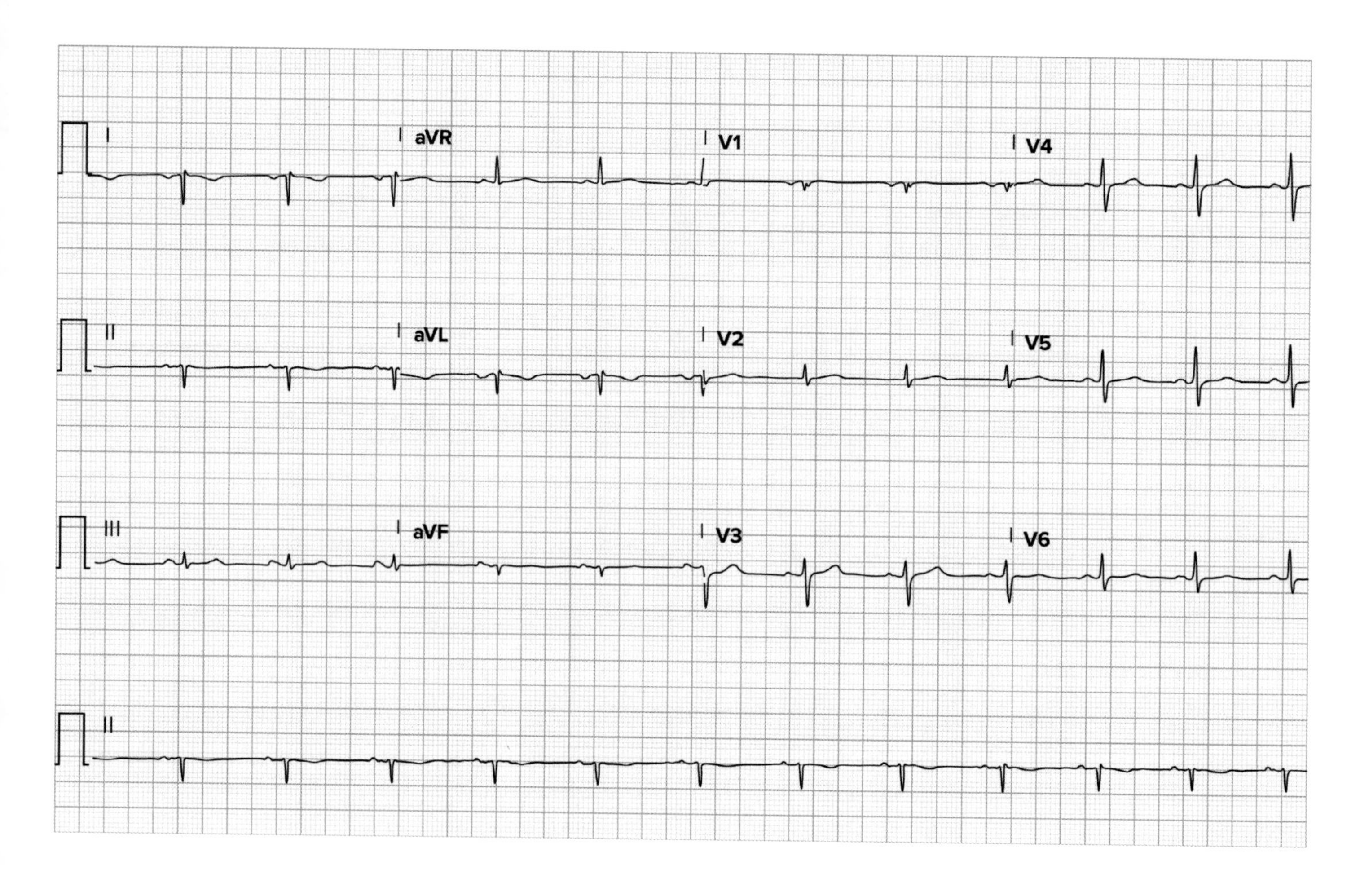

Case 18: Answer

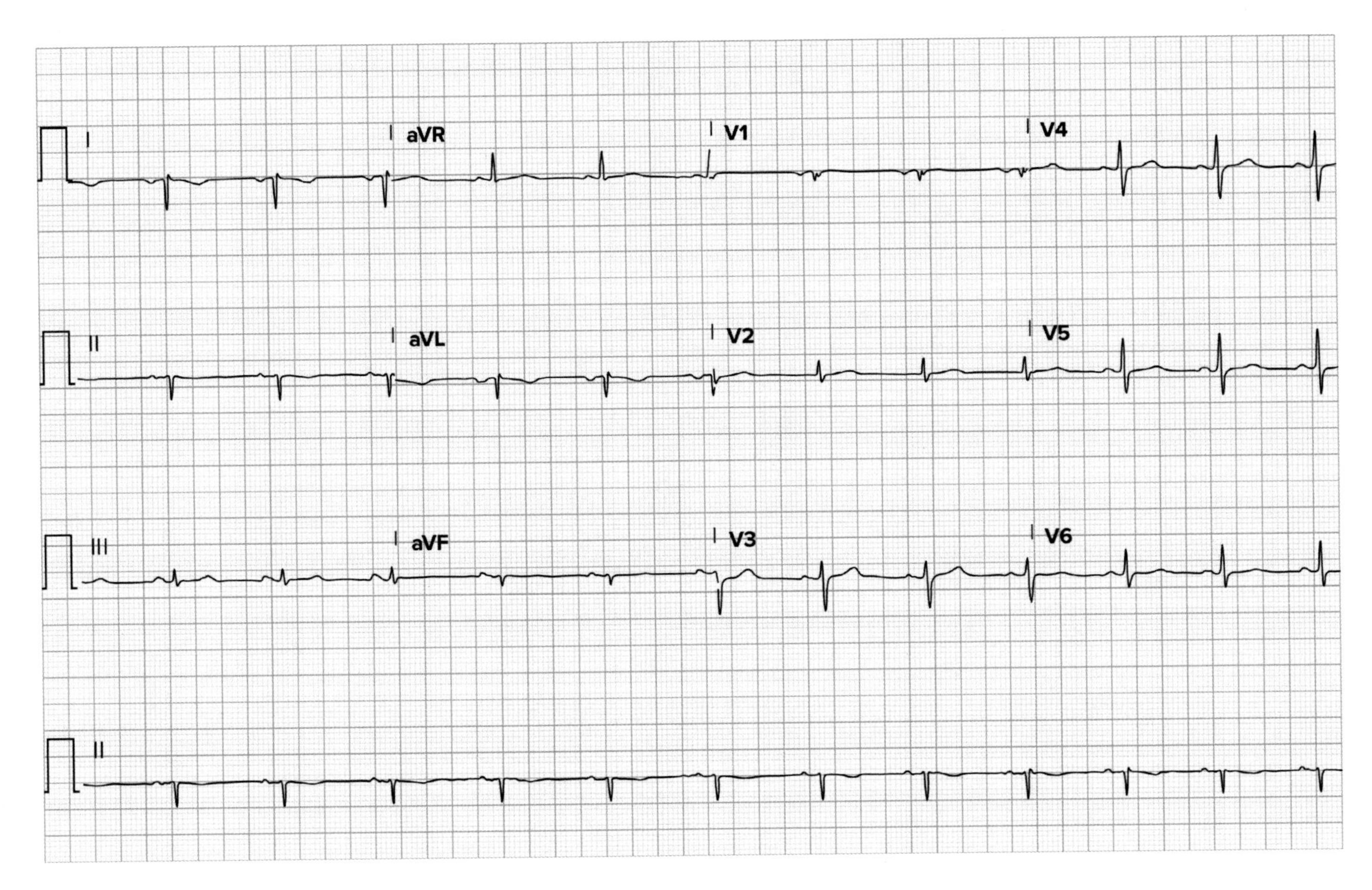

This ECG shows left arm-right arm (LA-RA) lead reversal. An easy way to scan for LA-RA lead reversal is to compare leads I and V6, which should appear similarly with normal lead placement since they both look at the heart from the same direction. In this case, the QRS complexes are negatively oriented in lead I and positively oriented in lead V6, suggesting that "the view" of lead I is coming from the wrong side of the body, which is what would happen if the arm leads were reversed. Another clue is that the QRS complex in lead aVR is predominantly upright which is very atypical and should prompt evaluation for lead reversal. ***Figure 1*** shows a repeat ECG with correct lead placement.

Figure 1.
Repeat ECG with correct lead placement

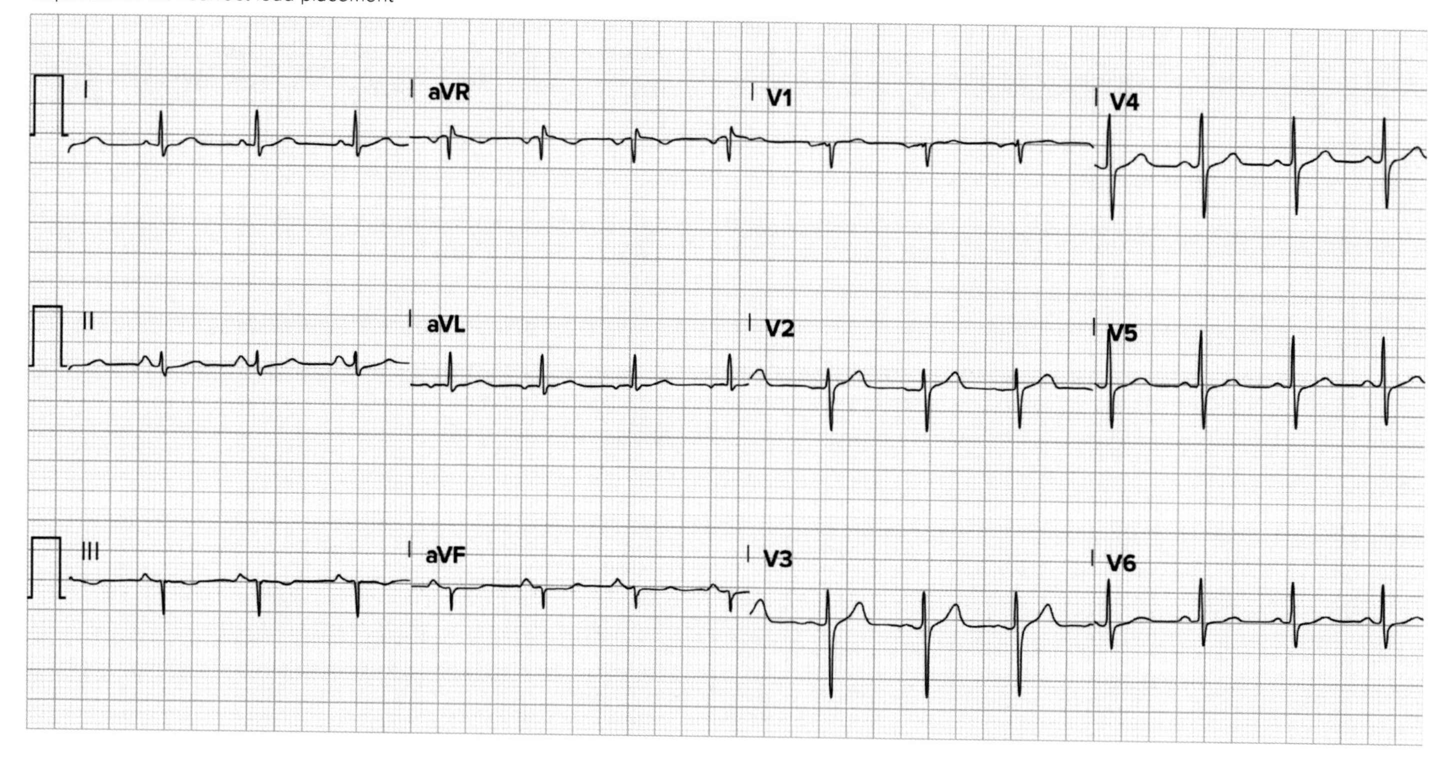

ECG findings seen with LA-RA lead reversal include ***(see Figure 2)***:

1. Lead I is inverted, indicating that P-QRS-T complexes are all oriented in the opposite direction from the normal P-QRS-T complexes (ie, normal sinus rhythm with normal lead placement)
2. In comparison to normal P-QRS-T complexes (ie, normal sinus rhythm with normal lead placement), leads II and III "switch places," so the normal findings in lead II are noted in lead III and vice versa
3. In comparison to normal P-QRS-T complexes (ie, normal sinus rhythm with normal lead placement), leads aVR and aVL "switch places," so the normal findings in lead aVR are noted in lead aVL and vice versa
4. Lead aVF is unchanged

Figure 2.
Comparison of the limb leads from the case ECG with LA-RA lead reversal with the repeat ECG with correct lead placement

2a. LA-RA lead reversal (case ECG)

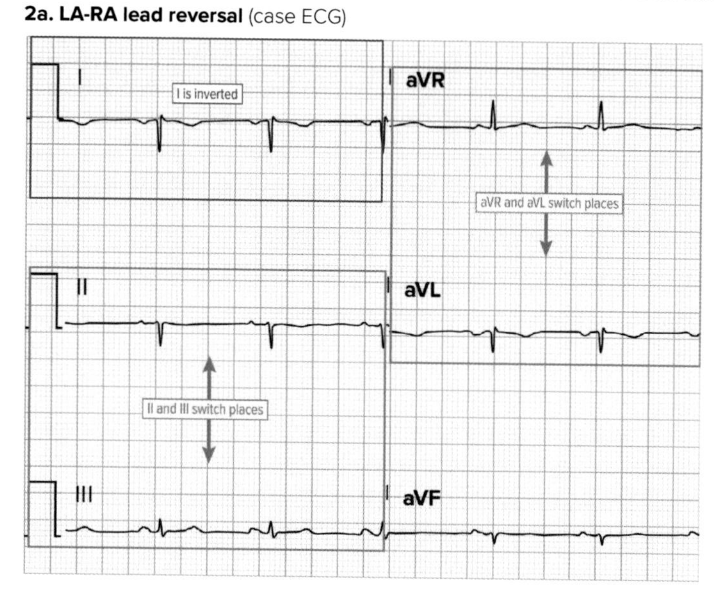

2b. Correct lead placement (repeat ECG)

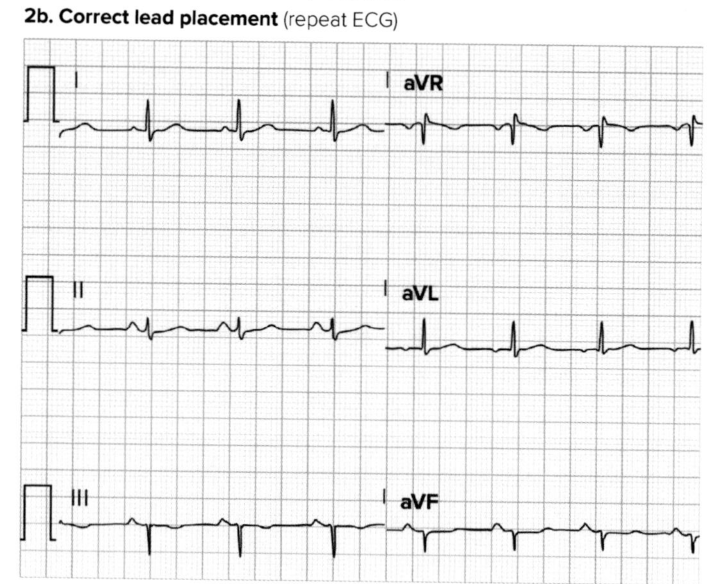

Lead Reversal Summary							
	I	II	III	aVR	aVL	aVF	V1-V6
LA-RA	Inverted	Switches with III	Switches with II	Switches with aVL	Switches with aVR	No change	No change
LA-LL	Switches with II	Switches with I	Inverted	No change	Switches with aVF	Switches with aVL	No change
LA-RL	Looks like II	Unchanged	Flatline	Looks like inverted II	Looks identical to aVF	Looks identical to aVL	No change
RA-LL	Switches with inverted III	Inverted	Switches with inverted I	Switches with aVF	No change	Switches with aVR	No change
RA-RL	Looks like inverted III	Flatline	Unchanged	Looks identical to aVF	Looks like inverted III	Looks identical to aVR	No change
LA-LL + RA-RL	Flatline	Looks like inverted III	Inverted	Looks identical to aVL	Looks identical to aVR	Looks like inverted III	No change
Dextrocardia	Inverted	Switches with III	Switches with II	Switches with aVL	Switches with aVR	No change	Dominant S-wave and poor R-wave progression

NOTE: *RL is a ground lead, so RL-LL reversal does not result in any significant changes*

Case 19: Presentation

A 7-week-old male is brought in by parents due to an episode of cyanosis. What is your interpretation of his ECG?

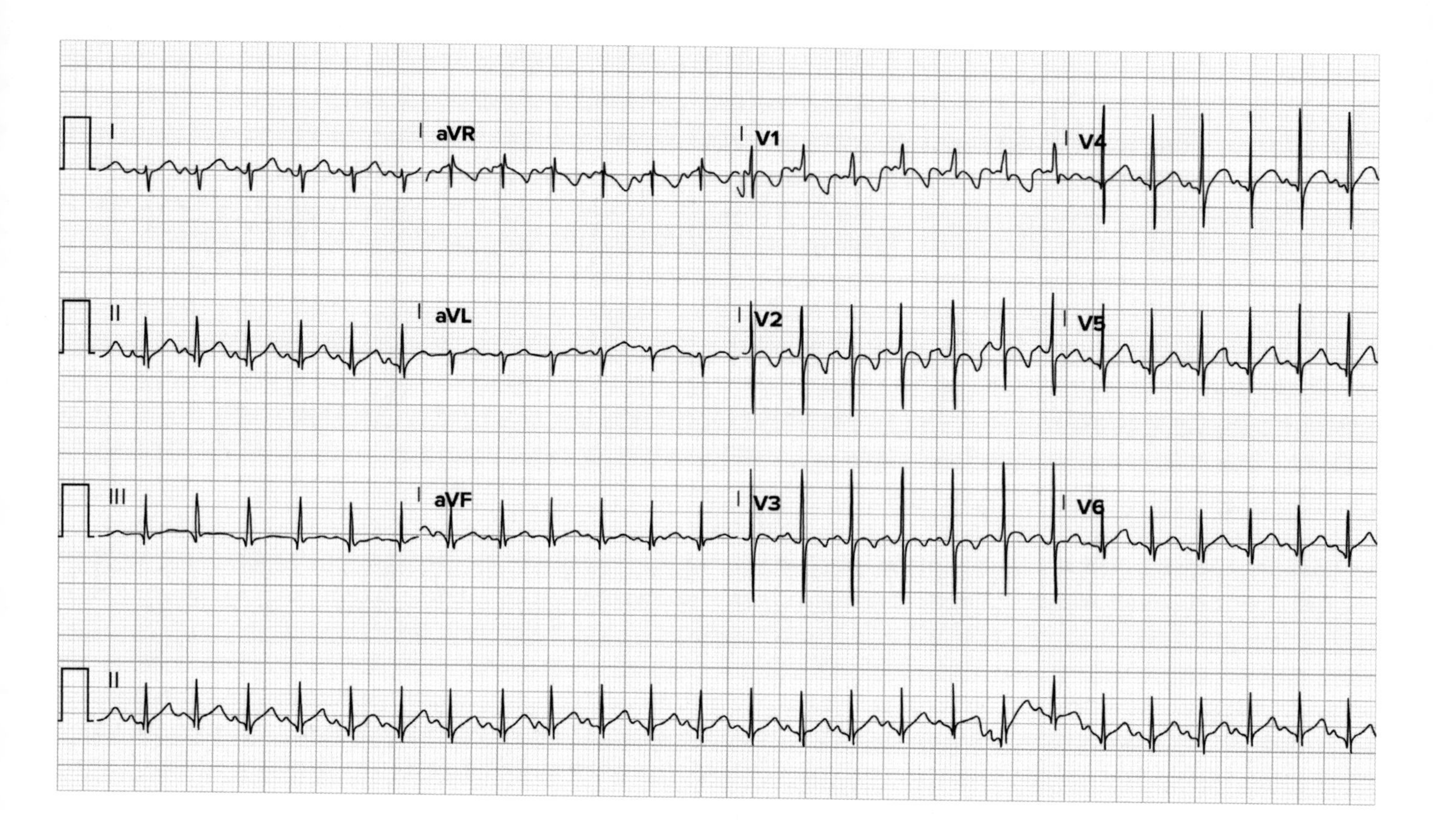

Case 19: Answer

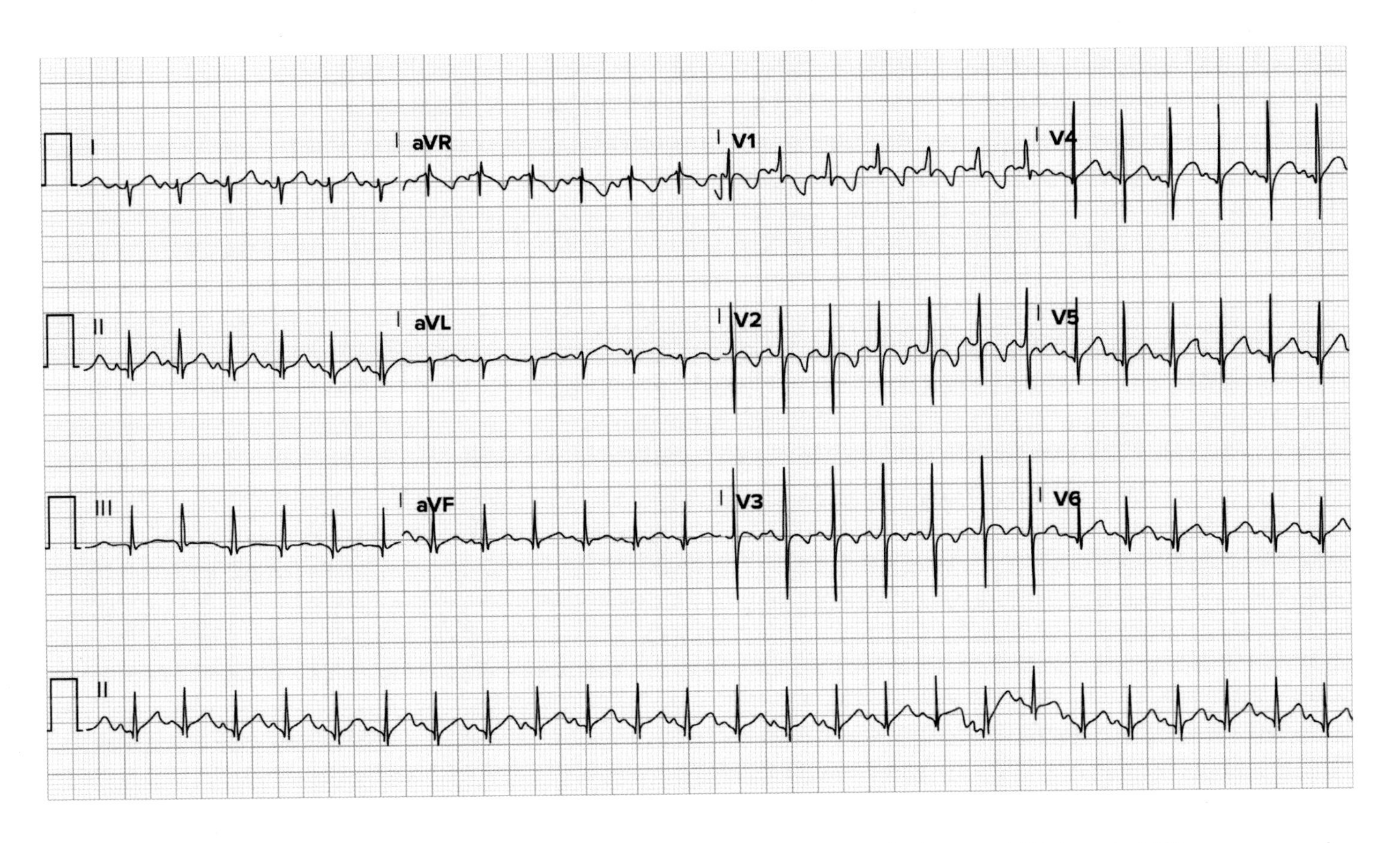

This ECG shows sinus tachycardia with a ventricular rate of 150 bpm, right axis deviation, a PR interval of 110 msec, normal QRS duration and QTc interval, tall R-waves and TWI in leads V1-V3, and deep S-waves in leads I, aVL, and V4-V5. This constellation of findings mimics RVH but is normal in this age group.

The challenge in interpreting pediatric ECGs is the age- and size-related changes in the normal healthy patient, which vary from adults. Heart rate, intervals, QRS complex axis and morphology, and T-waves all change with age and should be referenced to normal values for that age group (see table in Learning Points below).

The QRS complex axis and morphology changes are most pronounced in the first year of life. These findings are mainly due to the increased mass of the right ventricle and position of the heart relative to that of an adult. In a newborn, the right ventricle will be larger than the left. By 6 months of age, the relative sizes of the ventricles will mimic that of an adult, but the ECG will still differ from that of an adult due to the differences in the position of the heart in the body. In a newborn, these ECG changes include prominent R-waves (and often S-waves) in the right precordial leads and prominent S-waves (and often small R-waves) in the left precordial leads. By 6 months of age, these ECG changes include increased amplitude in mid-precordial leads and decreased amplitude in lateral precordial leads. Right axis deviation is often seen during the first year of life.

T-waves are typically inverted in leads V1-V3 after the first week of life, during which time lead V1 can show an upright T-wave. These changes are often seen in children up to 8 years of age and are called persistent juvenile T-waves if they persist into adulthood. Upright T-waves in leads V1-V3 in children younger than age 8 is uncommon and should prompt evaluation for RVH and the underlying pathologic etiology.

Measurement of the QT interval is important when evaluating for congenital or acquired long QT syndrome, typically in the setting as the cause of syncope. Unlike other intervals, the QT interval does not vary much with age after 6 months of life. QT interval measurement should be measured in the lead with the longest QT interval, and calculation of the of the QTc interval should use the Bazett formula (QTc = QT / √RR interval). In general, after 6 months of age, a normal QTc is < 440 msec, 440-460 msec is borderline, and > 460 msec is abnormal.

It is useful to compare the ECG in this case to that of an adult with RVH ***(see Figure 1)***. Common findings in the adult with RVH would include right axis deviation, increased R-wave amplitude with STD and TWI in leads III, aVR, and V1-V3, increased S-wave depth in leads I, aVL and V4-V6, and increased QRS complex and QT interval duration. These repolarization abnormalities can mimic the appearance of a posterolateral MI. Comparison with prior ECGs and obtaining serial ECGs can help differentiate between the two.

Figure 1.
ECG of an adult with RVH

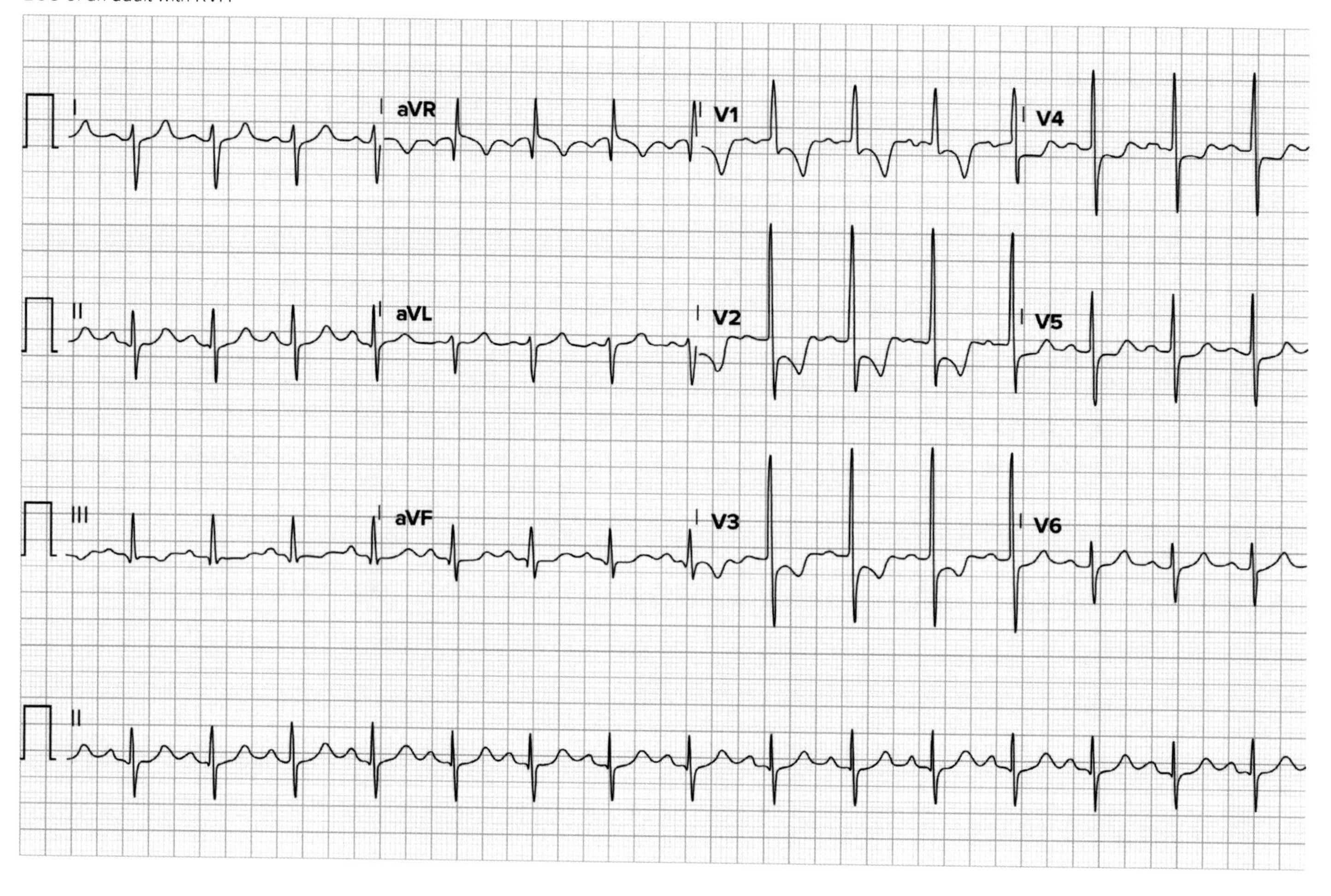

This patient was admitted for further workup of a Brief Resolved Unexplained Event (formerly called an Apparent Life-Threatening Event or ALTE).

Pediatric ECG Learning Points

- Normal values vary by age
- P-waves
  - Similar to adults, typically upright in leads I, II, III, and aVF
  - P-wave duration varies by age
- PR interval
  - Lower limit is 70-90 msec (depending on age) which can confound ability to diagnose ventricular preexcitation (ie, WPW)
  - Upper limit varies by age
- QRS complex
  - Newborns: prominent R-wave s (and often S-waves) in the right precordial leads and prominent S-waves (and often small R-waves) in the left precordial leads
  - 6-month-olds: increased amplitude in mid-precordial leads and decreased amplitude in lateral precordial leads
  - Right axis deviation often seen in infants under 1 year old
- QRS duration
  - Shorter: 30-80 msec for infants and 50-100 msec for adolescents
  - Important because ventricular dysrhythmias can be seen with narrow appearing QRS complexes

- Q-waves
  - Normal in inferior and lateral precordial leads
  - Usually < 20 msec long but can have large amplitude
  - Presence in leads I and aVL in infants is often pathologic
  - Presence in right precordial leads is always pathologic
- ST-segment
  - Can be difficult to determine STE due to lack of a stable isoelectric baseline
  - STE in precordial leads is seen most often in adolescent males
- T-waves
  - Typically negative in leads V1-V3 in children up to 8 years of age
  - Upright T-waves in leads V1-V3 in children < 8 years of age should prompt evaluation for RVH
  - T-wave in lead V1 is often upright in the first week of life
- QT interval
  - QTc calculated with Bazett formula: QTc = QT / √RR interval
  - After 6 months of age, normal is < 440 msec and > 460 msec is abnormal

Age	HR (bpm)	QRS axis (degrees)	PR interval (msec)	QRS interval (msec)	R-wave in V1 (mm)	S-wave in V1 (mm)	R-wave in V6 (mm)	S-wave in V6 (mm)
1st week	90-160	60-180	80-150	30-80	5-26	0-23	0-12	0-10
1-3 weeks	100-180	45-160	80-150	30-80	3-21	0-16	2-16	0-10
1-2 months	120-180	30-135	80-150	30-80	3-18	0-15	5-21	0-10
3-5 months	105-185	0-135	80-150	30-80	3-20	0-15	6-22	0-10
6-11 months	110-170	0-135	70-160	30-80	2-18	0.5-20	6-23	0-7
1-2 years	90-165	0-110	80-160	30-80	2-18	0.5-21	6-23	0-7
3-4 years	70-140	0-110	90-170	40-80	1-18	0.5-21	4-24	0-5
5-7 years	65-140	0-110	90-170	40-80	0.5-14	0.5-24	4-26	0-4
8-11 years	60-130	(-)15-110	90-170	40-80	0-14	0.5-25	4-25	0-4
12-15 years	65-130	(-)15-110	90-180	40-80	0-14	0.5-21	4-25	0-4
≥ 16 years	50-120	(-)15-110	120-200	50-100	0-14	0.5-22	4-21	0-4

RVH Learning Points

- ECG is only suggestive of anatomic RVH; echocardiography is the superior diagnostic modality for this anatomic abnormality
  - No criteria are recommended for use exclusive of other validated criteria
  - Diagnosis of RVH in the presence of a RBBB should be made with caution as it may impact the accuracy of the ECG criteria for RVH
- Common ECG findings include:
  - STD and TWI in leads III, aVR, and V1-V3
  - Increased R-wave amplitude in leads III, aVR, and V1-V3
  - Increased S-wave depth in leads I, aVL and V4-V6
  - Right axis deviation
  - Increased QRS complex and QT interval duration
- Repolarization abnormalities can mimic the appearance of a posterolateral MI

Case 20: Presentation

A 77-year-old female presents with substernal chest pain, intermittent all day and now constant for past 20 minutes. What is your interpretation of her ECG?

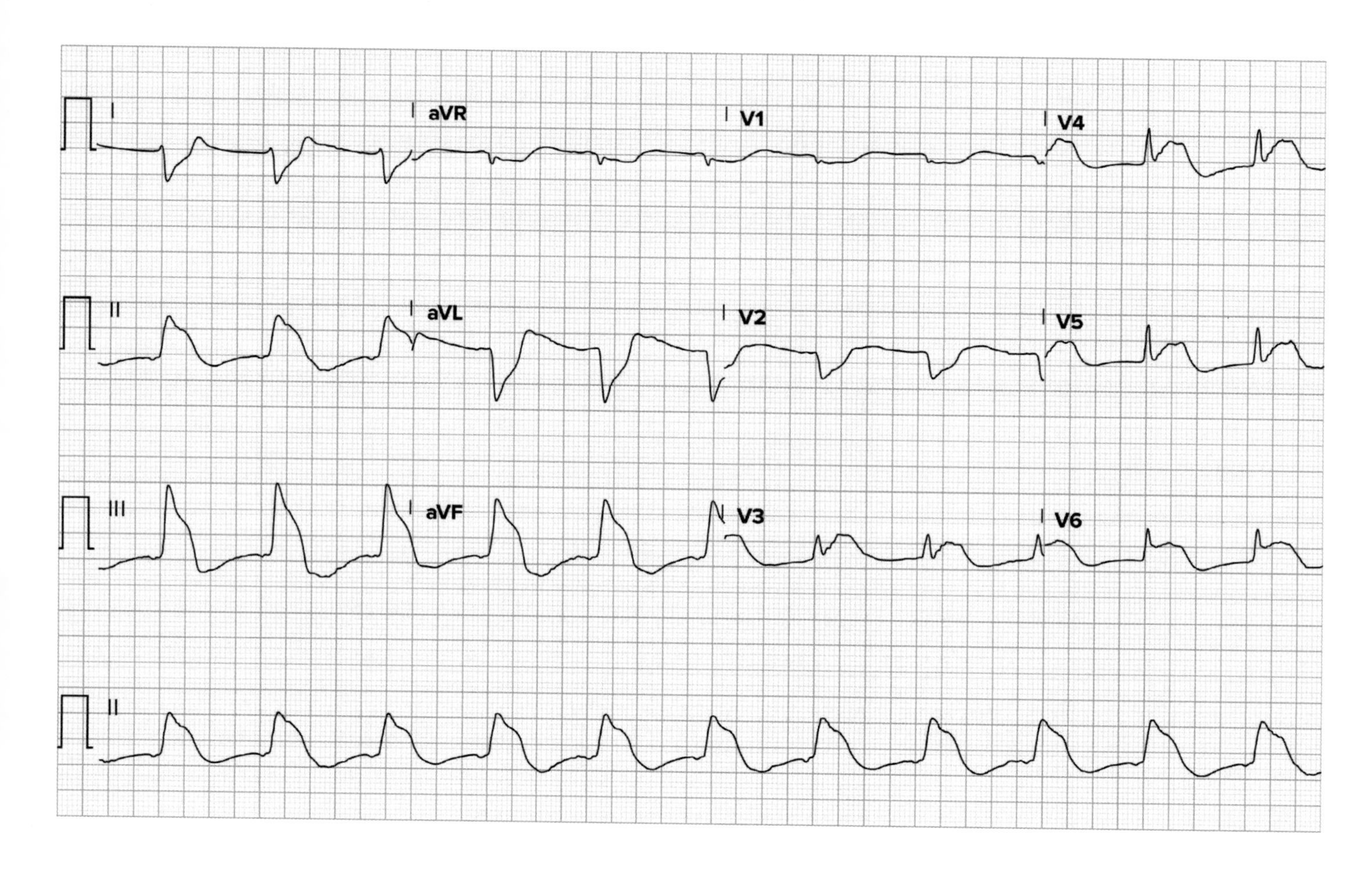

Case 20: Answer

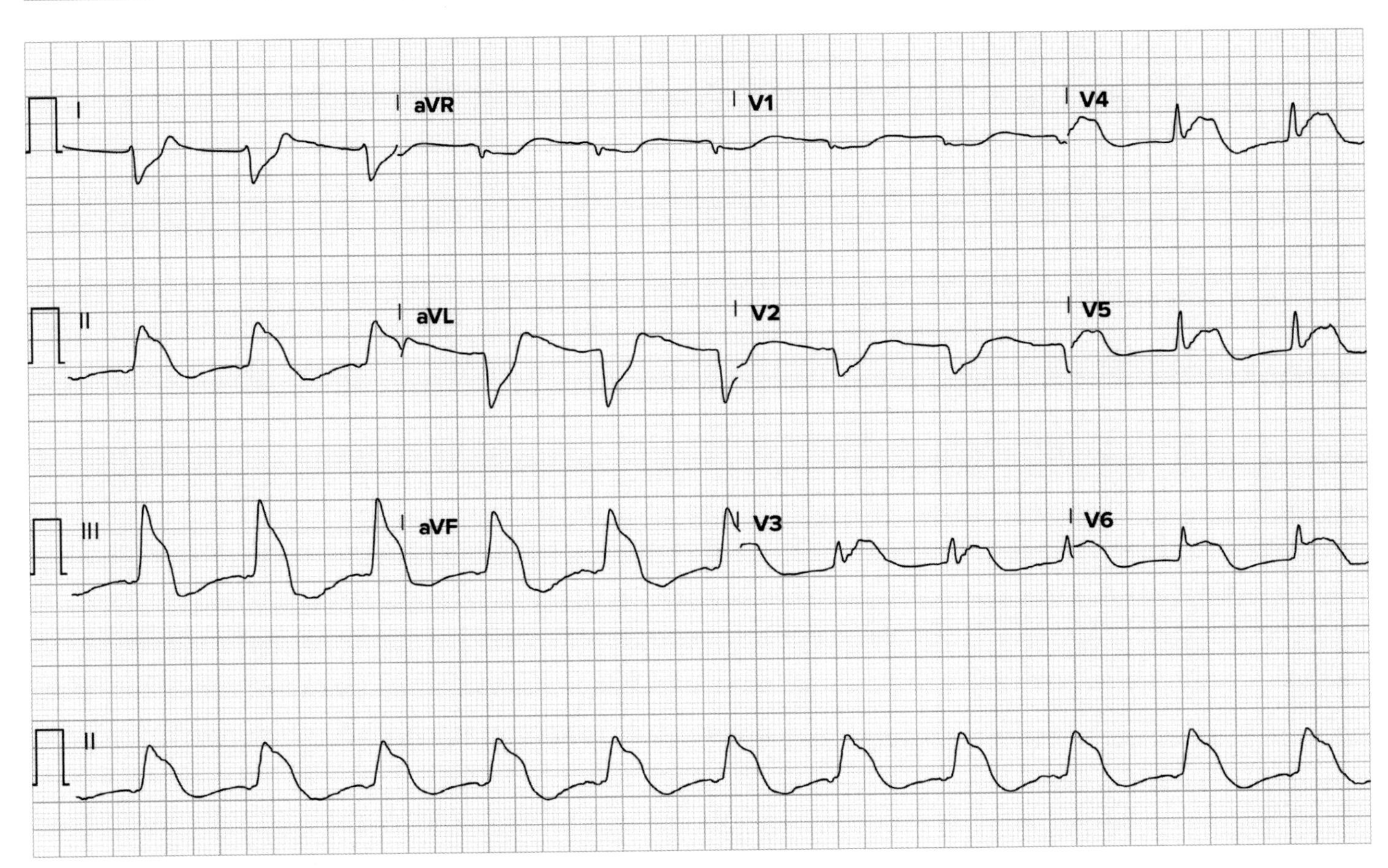

This ECG shows an accelerated junctional rhythm with a ventricular rate of 68 bpm, retrograde P-waves with a short PR interval, right axis deviation, prolonged QRS complex duration of 120 msec, STE in leads II, III, aVF, and V3-V6, and STD in leads I, aVL, aVR, and V1-V2.

The QRS-T complexes in the inferior leads are called "Shark Fins" and are due to a massive AMI. These complexes are a fusion of a widened QRS complex with an elevated ST segment and hyperacute T-wave. The presence of hyperacute T-waves with this patten suggests an early AMI in most instances. Patients presenting with this ECG pattern have a very high risk for rapid decompensation and cardiac arrest.

The key to interpreting this ECG is identifying the J point. The QRS complex duration in the limb leads appears very prolonged, but is actually only 120 msec. The other ~140 msec is the ST-segment and T-wave ***(see Figures 1 and 2)***.

Figure 1.
Identification of the P-wave, QRS complex duration, J point, and STE in lead II

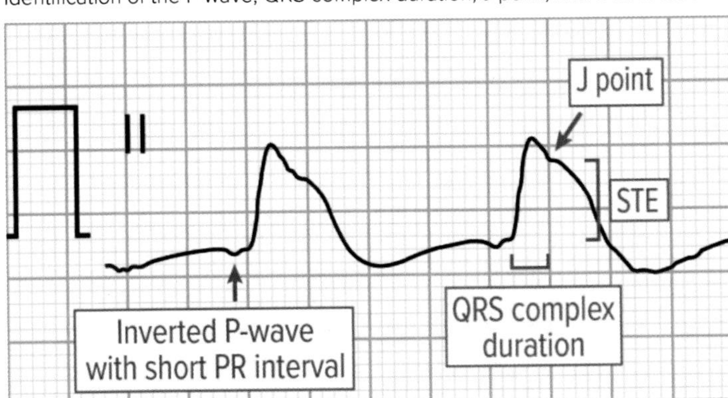

Although the QRS complex duration is not as prolonged as it appears, there is value in the mental exercise of considering the differential diagnosis for a very prolonged QRS complex duration. The differential diagnosis for a QRS complex duration > 200 msec includes hyperkalemia, sodium channel blocker toxicity, and VT. With respect to this patient's ECG:

- The presence of non-dissociated P-waves and ventricular rate < 120-130 bpm rules out VT
- Although there is a positive QRS complex in lead II and right axis deviation, both of which are seen with sodium channel blocker toxicity, there is no dominant R-wave or R/S ratio > 0.7 in lead aVR which would be expected with a sodium channel blocker toxicity
- Treating presumptively for hyperkalemia with calcium would be a reasonable initial step in management in conjunction with either point-of-care or traditional laboratory-based testing for serum potassium

Figure 2.
Identification of the QRS complex duration, J point, T-wave, and STD in lead I

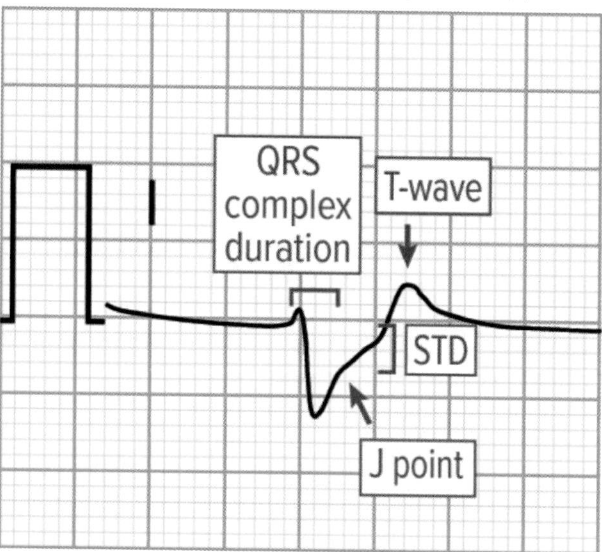

This ECG also shows a shortened PR interval ***(see Figure 1)***. The differential diagnosis for a short PR interval includes:

- Pre-excitation rhythms
- Ectopic atrial rhythms originating near the AV node
- Junctional rhythms with retrograde P-waves

The presence of inverted P-waves in leads II and aVF, which are normally upright in sinus rhythm, suggests they are retrograde and due to a junctional rhythm. This diagnosis is confounded by the absence of visible P-waves in other leads, but the distinction between a junctional rhythm and ectopic atrial rhythm is not clinically important given that the patient is having an MI.

This patient was taken to the cardiac catheterization laboratory and had a 100% RCA occlusion treated with a stent.

"Shark Fin" Learning Points

- Very wide QRS-T complex with significant ST-segment elevation
  - ST-segment is typically convex
  - T-wave becomes indistinguishable from ST-segment making it difficult to determine STE
- Consistent with a massive AMI
  - Associated with a very high risk for rapid decompensation and cardiac arrest

STEMI Learning Points

- STEMI is defined by new, or presumed new, STE at the J point in ≥ 2 anatomically contiguous leads in the absence of LVH by voltage pattern, LBBB, or ventricular-paced rhythm
  - ≥ 2.5 mm in men < 40 years old and ≥ 2 mm in men ≥ 40 years old in leads V2-V3 (or an increase of ≥ 1 mm when compared to baseline ECG)
  - ≥ 1.5 mm in women in leads V2-V3 (or an increase of ≥ 1 mm when compared to baseline ECG)
  - ≥ 1 mm in all other leads
- ST-segment is measured from the isoelectric baseline, typically the TP segment (see below)
- Reciprocal STD are not required for the diagnosis of STEMI, but their presence does increase the likelihood of the diagnosis of STEMI
  - Reciprocal STD are only present in 70% of anterior MI[1]
- Posterior MI
  - Consider whenever there is STD in leads V1-V4
  - STE ≥ 0.5 mm in posterior leads V7, V8 or V9 is diagnostic- does not require 2 contiguous leads

- Right ventricular MI
  - Consider with any inferior MI (RV MI is seen in approximately 1/3 of inferior MI)
  - STE in right precordial leads V3R and V4R ≥ 0.5 mm (≥ 1 mm for men ≤ 30 years old)
  - STE in right precordial lead V4R > 1 mm is most predictive of RV MI
  - STE in right precordial lead V4R > STE in leads V1-V3 = highly specific for RV MI
- Significant STE that does not meet the traditional distribution (ie, ≥ 2 anatomically contiguous leads) in a presentation concerning for ACS may still represent coronary artery occlusion and warrant consideration for emergent coronary reperfusion

How to Measure STE per most recent 2018 AHA Guidelines[2]

- The J point is the junction between QRS termination and ST-segment onset and is used to determine the magnitude of the ST-segment shift
- **In patients with a stable baseline, the TP segment (isoelectric interval) is a more accurate method to assess the magnitude of ST-segment shift** ***(see Figure 3)***, and in distinguishing pericarditis from acute myocardial ischemia
- QRS onset should be used if TP segment does not have a stable baseline ***(see Figure 4)***
- Measurement should be made from the top of the ECG line tracing

Figure 3.
Measure STE from the TP segment if the TP segment is isoelectric (ie, horizontal)

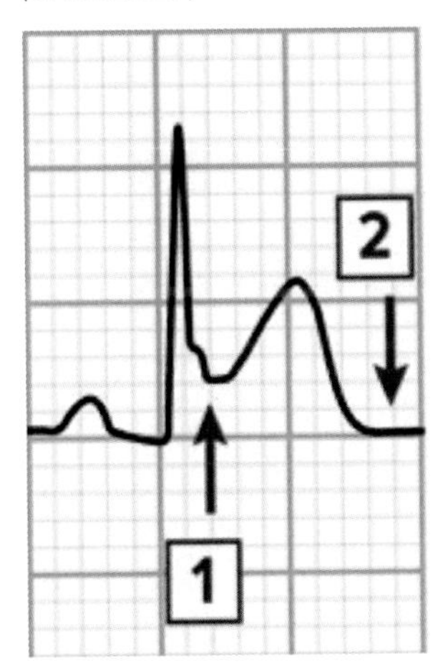

Arrow 1: onset of the ST-segment (ie, J point)
Arrow 2: TP segment

Figure 4.
Measure STE from onset of the QRS complex if the TP segment is not isoelectric (ie, not horizontal)

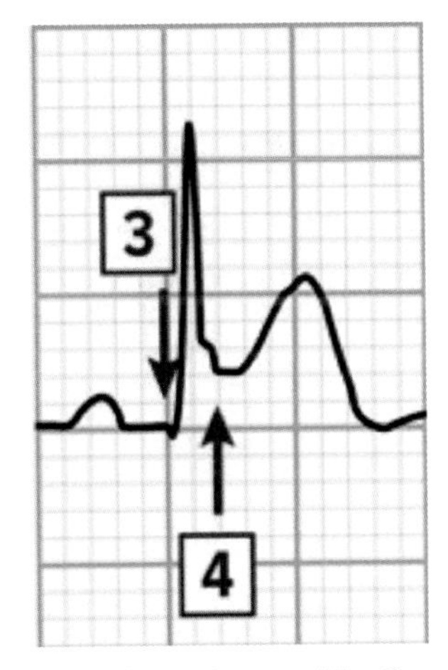

Arrow 3: initial onset of the Q-wave
Arrow 4: onset of the ST-segment (ie, J point)

Junctional Rhythm Learning Points

- Ectopic focus from AV node or proximal Purkinje system
  - Also called AV junctional rhythm, nodal rhythm, nodal escape rhythm, junctional escape rhythm, AV nodal rhythm
- ECG shows ventricular rate of 40-60 bpm with normal QRS complex duration unless concurrent conduction abnormality (eg, bundle branch block)
- May have retrograde P-waves that precede (with PR interval < 120 msec) or follow QRS complex, typically best seen in the inferior leads
- Variations include:
  - Junctional Bradycardia: ventricular rate < 40 bpm
  - Accelerated Junctional Rhythm: ventricular rate 61–100 bpm
  - Junctional Tachycardia: ventricular rate > 100 bpm

References

1. Knilans T, Surawicz B. Chou's Electrocardiography in Clinical Practice. Philadelphia, PA: Elsevier. 2020.
2. Thygesen K, Alpert JS, Jaffe AS, et al. 2018 ESC/ACC/AHA/WHF Expert Consensus Document: Fourth Universal Definition of Myocardial Infarction (2018). Circulation. 2018;138:e618-e651.

Case 21: Presentation

An 83-year-old female presents with exertional near syncope.
What is your interpretation of her ECG?

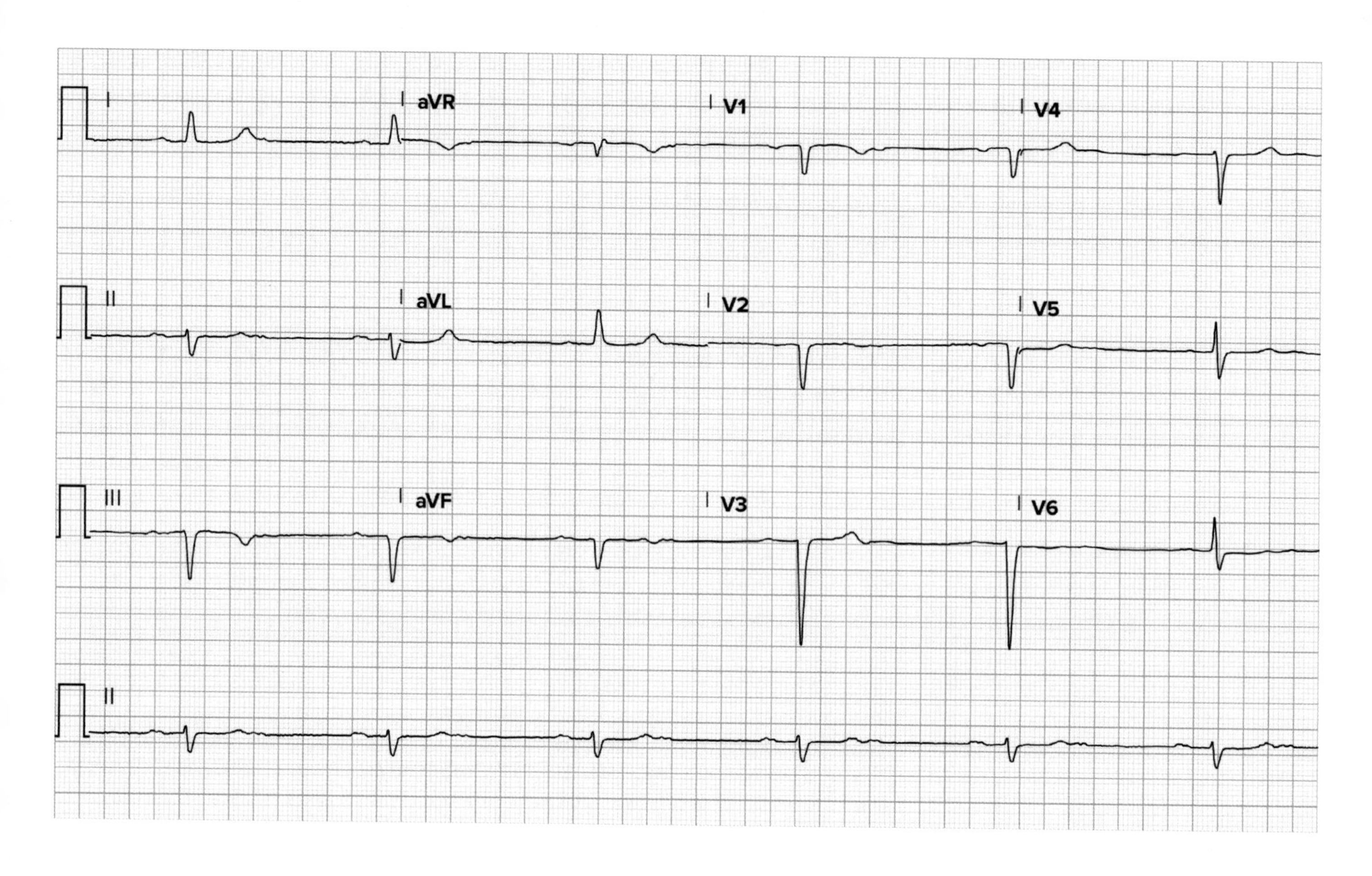

Case 21: Answer

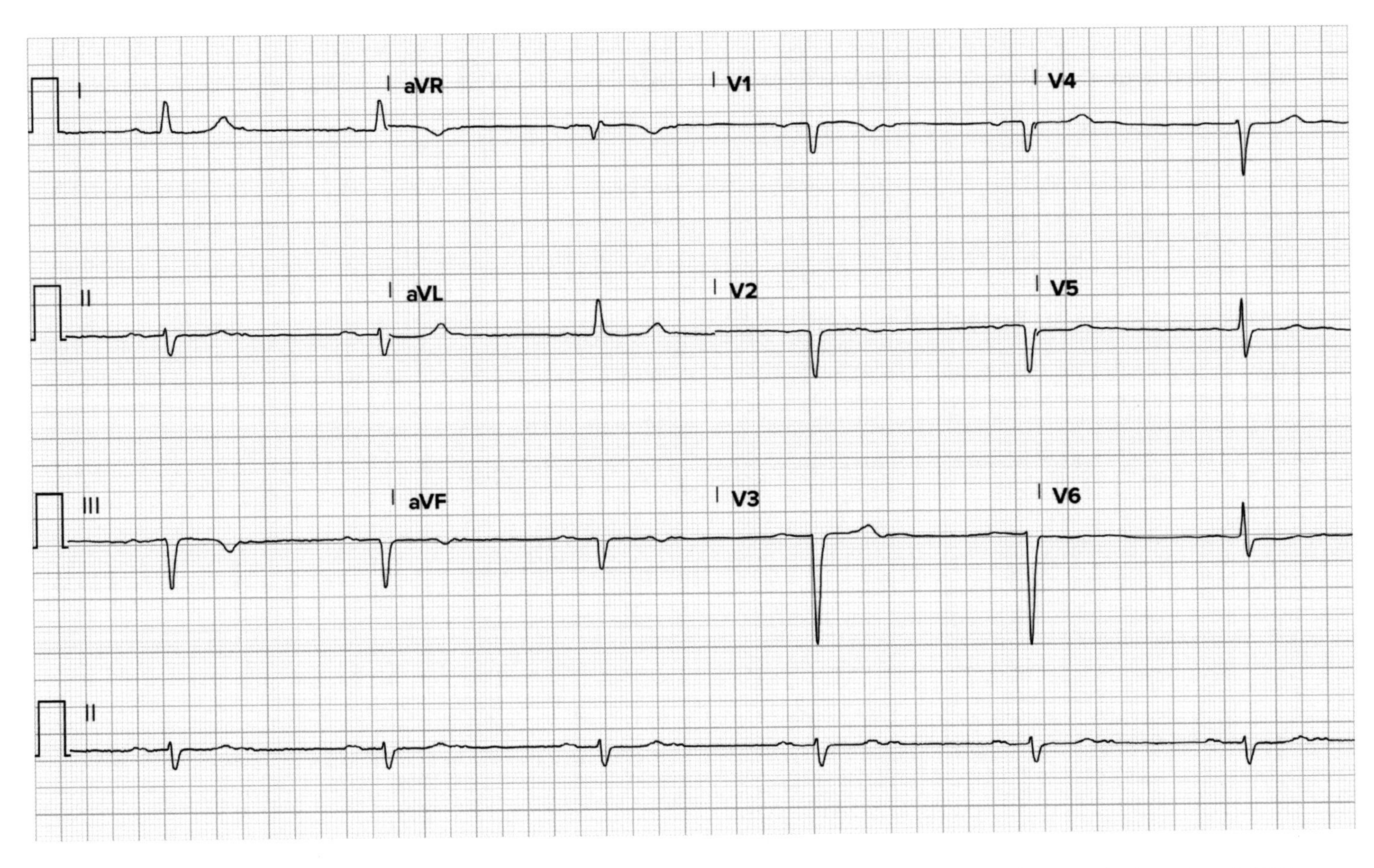

This ECG shows a 2nd degree AV block with 2:1 AV conduction, an atrial rate of ~72 bpm, and a ventricular rate of ~36 bpm. A leftward axis is present due to the presence of an old inferior wall infarction as evidenced by Q-waves in leads III and aVF. There are also Q-waves in leads V1-V2, consistent with a prior septal wall anterior infarction. The QRS complex duration is prolonged at ~115 msec with a non-specific intraventricular conduction delay.

The differential diagnosis for a regular narrow complex rhythm with bradycardic ventricular rates includes:

- Sinus bradycardia
- Junctional rhythm
- Junctional bradycardia
- Atrial flutter with block (rate controlled)
- Atrial tachycardia with block (rate controlled)
- 2:1 AV block
- High-grade AV block (eg, 3:1, 4:1, etc.)
- 3rd degree AV block with junctional escape rhythm
- 3rd degree sinoatrial block with junctional escape rhythm

When interpreting an ECG with subtle findings, it can be helpful to increase the gain. This will be reflected in the calibration signal box on the left side of the ECG. This box represents the calibration of the recording speed (x-axis) and voltage (y-axis) of the ECG. Time is represented by the width of the rectangle and is set for 0.2 sec. Voltage is represented by the height and is set for 10 mV (except for Nigel Tufnel's, which goes up to 11). Standard calibration is 25 mm/sec (ie, one small box = 0.04 sec) and 10 mm/mV (ie, one small box = 0.1 mV). When the gain (ie, amplitude) is increased 2x, the height of the calibration box will become twice as tall, so now 20 mm = 1 mV (ie, one small box = 0.05 mV). ***Figure 1*** shows lead II of this ECG with standard calibration and ***Figure 2*** shows the same P-QRS-T complex with the amplitude increased 2x.

The 2nd degree AV block seen in this ECG is subtle and it is more apparent when the amplitude is increased 2x ***(see Figure 3)***. Note that the calibration box on the left-hand side of the page is now 20 mm, twice as tall as the original ECG.

Figure 1.
The calibration signal box from the lead II rhythm strip denotes the recording speed (x-axis) and voltage (y-axis) of the ECG

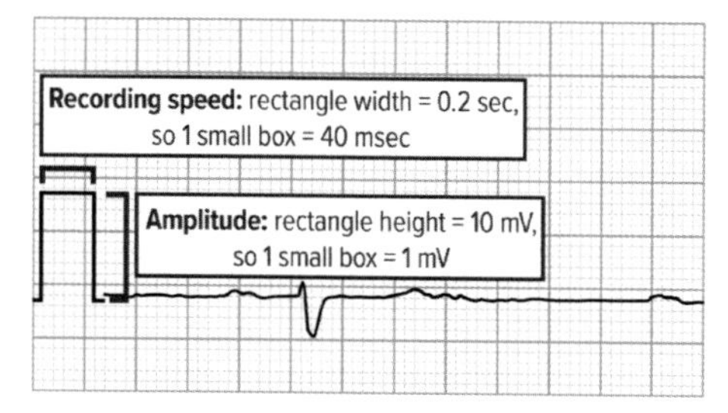

Figure 2.
The calibration signal box from the lead II rhythm strip from Figure 3 when the amplitude is increased 2x (note the amplitude is twice as high as in Figure 1)

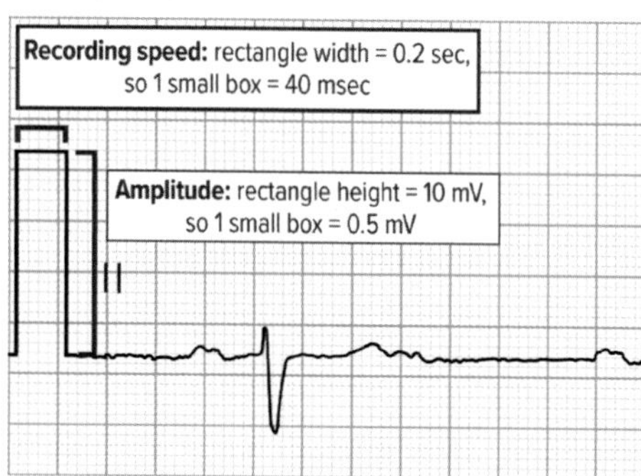

Figure 3.
The initial ECG with the gain increased 2x (note that calibration signal box is now twice as tall)

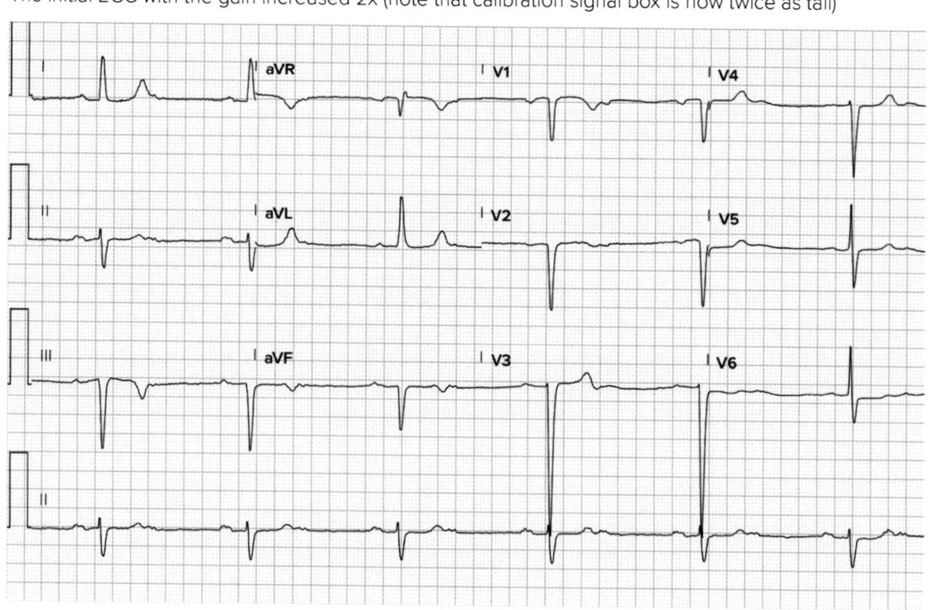

A closer look at the rhythm strip shows non-conducted P-waves after every QRS complex ***(see Figure 4)*** that march out regularly at exactly twice the ventricular rate ***(see Figure 5)***.

Figure 4.
The lead II rhythm strip from Figure 3 shows every other P-wave is non-conducted

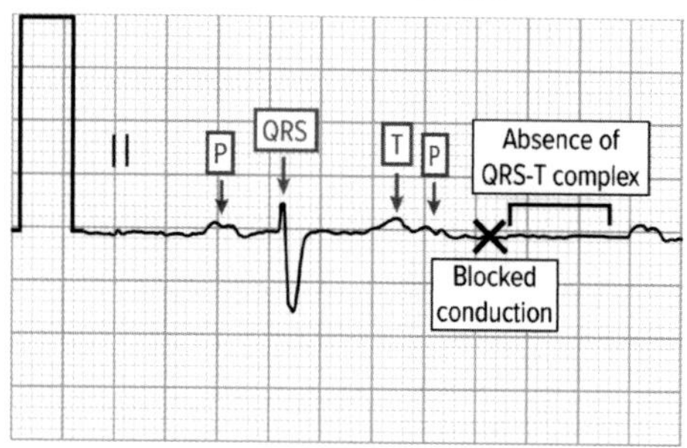

Figure 5.
The lead II rhythm strip from Figure 3 shows P-waves that march out at a rate that is exactly twice the ventricular rate

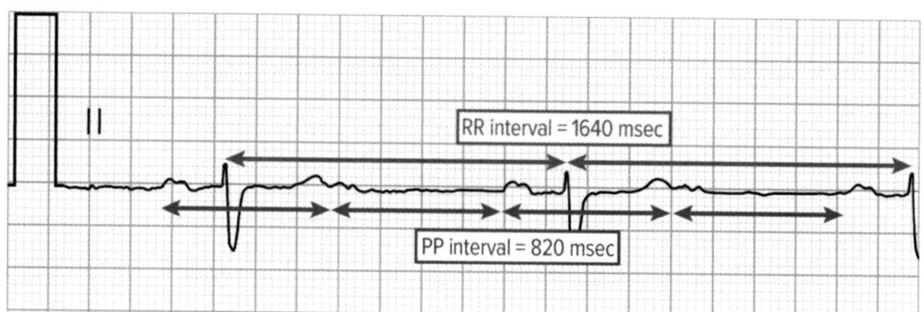

In a 2:1 AV block, there are no sequential conducting P-waves to compare PR intervals, so it is often impossible to determine if the underlying pathology is a Mobitz type I or Mobitz type II. Note that while a wide QRS complex suggests an underlying Mobitz type II, a narrow QRS complex is not specific for an underlying Mobitz type I. Although a 2:1 AV block can be encountered in situations simply involving increased vagal tone, it is always appropriate to assume the higher risk Mobitz type II until proven otherwise.

This patient was admitted to the cardiology service and eventually required placement of a permanent pacemaker.

2nd degree AV Block with 2:1 Conduction Learning Points

- 2nd degree AV block with 2:1 conduction will show blocked conduction of every other P-wave
- It is not always possible to determine if the underlying block is a Mobitz type I or type II, so assume the higher risk Mobitz type II conduction

Mobitz type I AV Block Learning Points

- Progressively increasing PR interval and decreasing RR interval until a non-conducted P-wave occurs (ie, P-wave without accompanying QRS complex)
  - PR interval immediately after non-conducted P-wave is shorter than PR interval preceding non-conducted P-wave
  - RR interval that includes non-conducted P-wave < twice the PP interval
- Can be normal variant and usually does not produce hemodynamic compromise
  - Typically associated with excess vagal tone and therefore usually responds to atropine when acute treatment is needed
  - Can lead to a more advanced AV block if associated with a pathologic etiology
  - Can be seen with inferior MI

Mobitz type II AV Block Learning Points

- Constant PR interval in conducted beats
  - Described as ratio of P-waves to QRS complexes
  - Typically an infranodal block resulting in a prolonged QRS complex duration
  - RR interval that includes non-conducted P-wave = twice the PP interval
- Never a normal variant and frequently produces hemodynamic compromise
  - High risk of progressing to a 3rd degree AV block
  - Atropine is unlikely to lead to clinical improvement and may lead to a high-grade AV block

Case 22: Presentation

A 76-year-old female presents to the emergency department with exertional dyspnea and chest tightness that is now persistent while at rest. Notable vital signs include an oxygen saturation of 85%. What is your interpretation of her ECG?

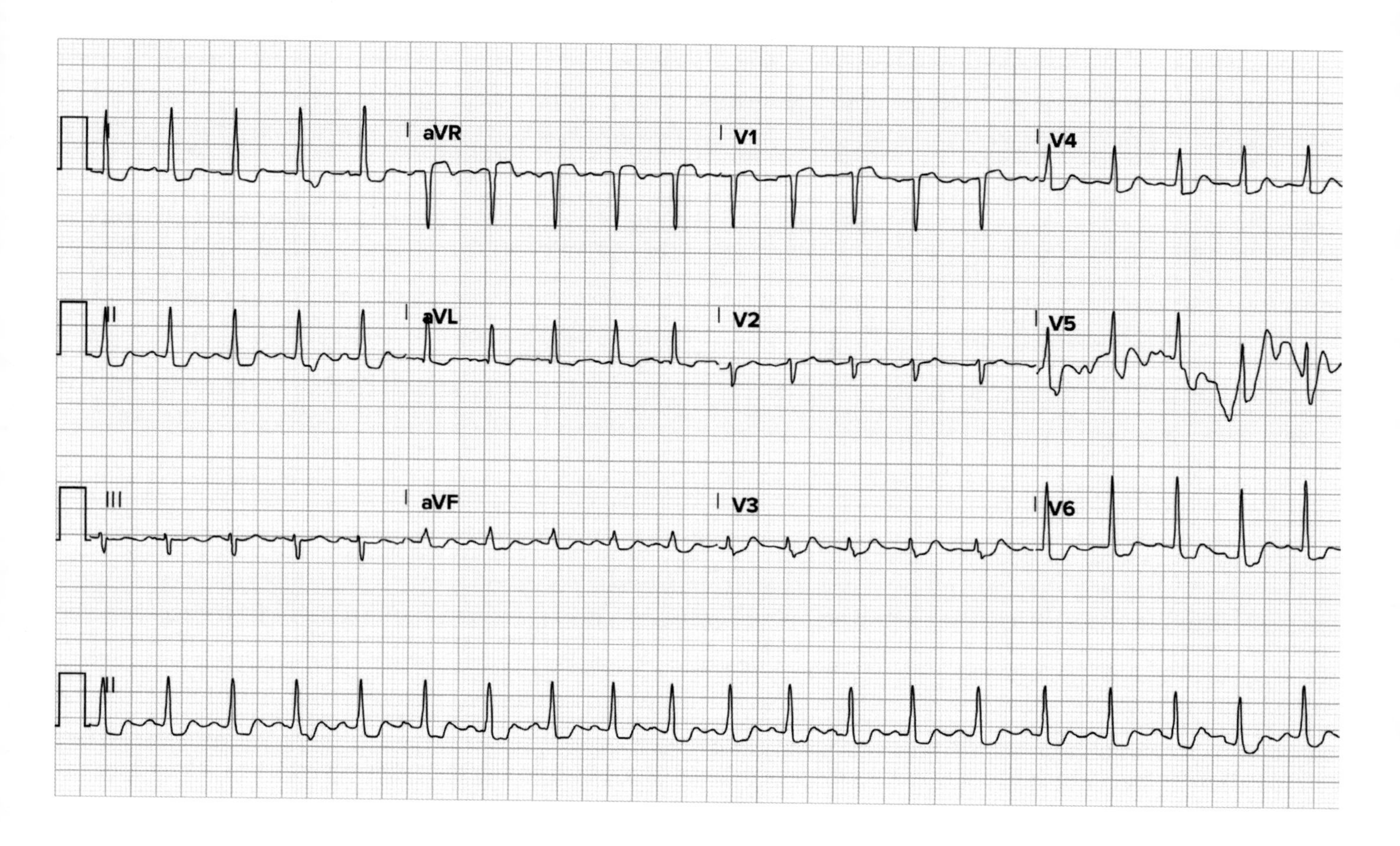

Case 22: Answer

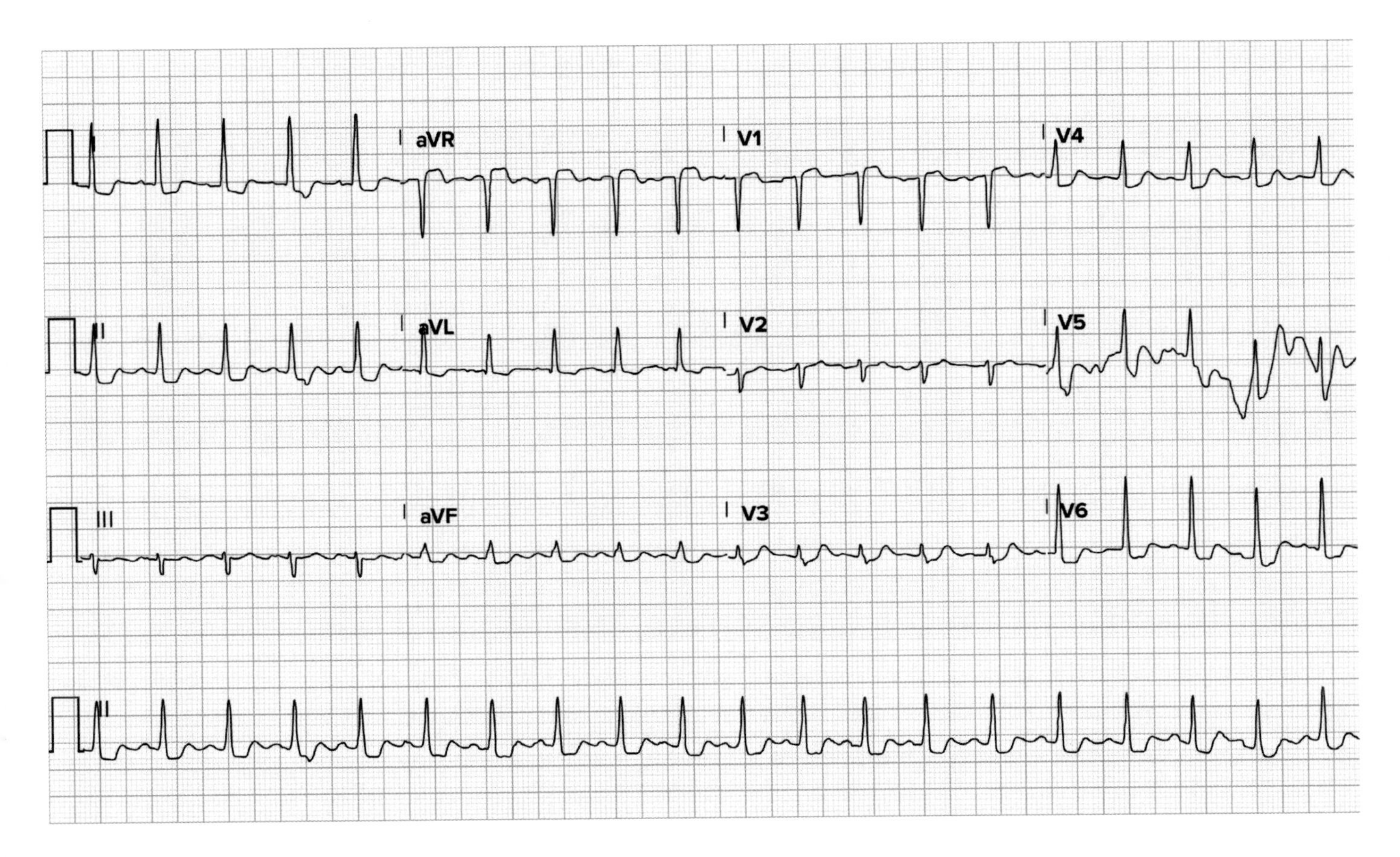

This ECG shows sinus tachycardia with a ventricular rate of 120 bpm, normal axis, normal intervals, STE in leads aVR and V1, and STD in leads I, aVL, II, aVF, V3-V4, V6, and presumably lead V5 which is obscured by artifact.

The differential diagnosis for the pattern of STE in lead aVR +/- lead V1 with diffuse STD includes both ACS and non-ACS etiologies:

ACS causes[1]	Non-ACS causes[2]
• LMCA insufficiency (can see STE aVR > V1)	• Acute and/or severe anemia
• Prox LAD insufficiency (can see STE V1 > aVR)	• Aortic dissection
• Triple vessel disease	• LBBB and ventricular-paced rhythms
• Global cardiac ischemia	• LVH with strain pattern
• Prinzmetal angina	• Pulmonary embolism
	• ROSC s/p epinephrine or defibrillation
	• Severe hypokalemia or hyperkalemia
	• Sodium channel blockade
	• Supraventricular tachycardia (especially with rapid rates)

Although the pattern of STE in lead aVR +/- lead V1 with diffuse STD is discussed in the cardiology literature, its clinical significance is not without some controversy. This is likely due to the broad differential diagnosis associated with this pattern that includes both ACS and non-ACS causes. The 2018 Fourth Universal Definition of MI states "ST-segment depression ≥ 1 mm in 6 or more leads, which may be associated with ST-segment elevation in leads aVR and/or V1 and hemodynamic compromise, is suggestive of multivessel disease or left main disease" but does not provide specific management recommendations.

Treatment should be guided by the underlying etiology, and it is imperative to consider both ACS and non-ACS causes. For patients suspected of having an ACS cause, this ECG pattern is highly suggestive of LMCA insufficiency, proximal LAD insufficiency, or triple vessel disease. So, while this pattern does not meet "traditional" STEMI criteria, it can represent high-risk ACS, including possible acute coronary occlusion, in the correct clinical context, and immediate angiography should be considered. Whether this is done by emergent cardiology consultation or activation of the cardiac catheterization lab depends on local practice preferences.

This patient's ED workup was notable for pulmonary edema seen on chest radiograph and a hemoglobin of 6.0 g/dL, down from 12.2 g/dL a week prior. In this case, the severe acute blood loss anemia led to subendocardial ischemia and acute decompensated heart failure which led to pulmonary edema and hypoxia. The patient received a blood transfusion and judicious diuresis, and after correcting the underlying problem, her ECG normalized as expected with non-ACS causes of this ECG pattern.

The diagnostic reasoning involved in this case illustrates how failing to consider the non-ACS causes of this ECG pattern can lead to patient harm. This patient's history and vital sign abnormalities, including tachycardia and hypoxia, was concerning for PE, and sending the patient to the catheterization laboratory would have been an inappropriate disposition if the patient had a PE. As well, PE became the presumptive diagnosis without consideration of the other possible non-ACS causes, so much so that we considered starting heparin immediately after the ECG was obtained which would have likely worsened the patient's condition. This type of cognitive bias is called anchoring and is especially relevant to this ECG pattern given its prevalence in both ACS and non-ACS presentations.

Lead aVR Learning Points

- Lead aVR views the right upper portion of the heart including the basal part of the septum
- STE in lead aVR +/- V1 with diffuse STD ≥ 1 mm in ≥ 6 leads can be due to ACS or non-ACS etiologies; therefore, always consider the clinical context when considering the differential diagnosis
- In ACS presentations, this pattern is highly suggestive of LMCA obstruction, proximal LAD obstruction, and triple vessel disease, and immediate angiography should be considered[3]
- In non-ACS causes, the ECG changes should resolve with treatment of non-ACS cause
- Anterior or inferior MI with STE > 1 mm in lead aVR are associated with an increased 30-day mortality[4]

References

1. Thygesen K, Alpert JS, Jaffe AS, et al. 2018 ESC/ACC/AHA/WHF Expert Consensus Document: Fourth Universal Definition of Myocardial Infarction (2018). Circulation. 2018;138:e618-e651.
2. Mattu A. ECG Weekly.
3. Writing Committee, et al. 2013 ACCF/AHA Guideline for the Management of ST-Elevation Myocardial Infarction: A Report of the American College of Cardiology Foundation/American Heart Association Task Force on Practice Guidelines. Circulation. 2013;127:e362-e425.
4. Wong CK, Gao W, Stewart RA, Benatar J, French JK, Aylward PE,White HD; HERO-2 Investigators. aVR ST elevation: an important but neglected sign in ST elevation acute myocardial infarction. Eur Heart J. 2010;31:1845–1853.

Case 23: Presentation

A 32-year-old male with recent history of tricuspid valve replacement and postoperative 3rd degree AV block requiring transvenous pacing (TVP) has the TVP turned off to determine if a permanent pacemaker is needed. What is your interpretation of his ECG?

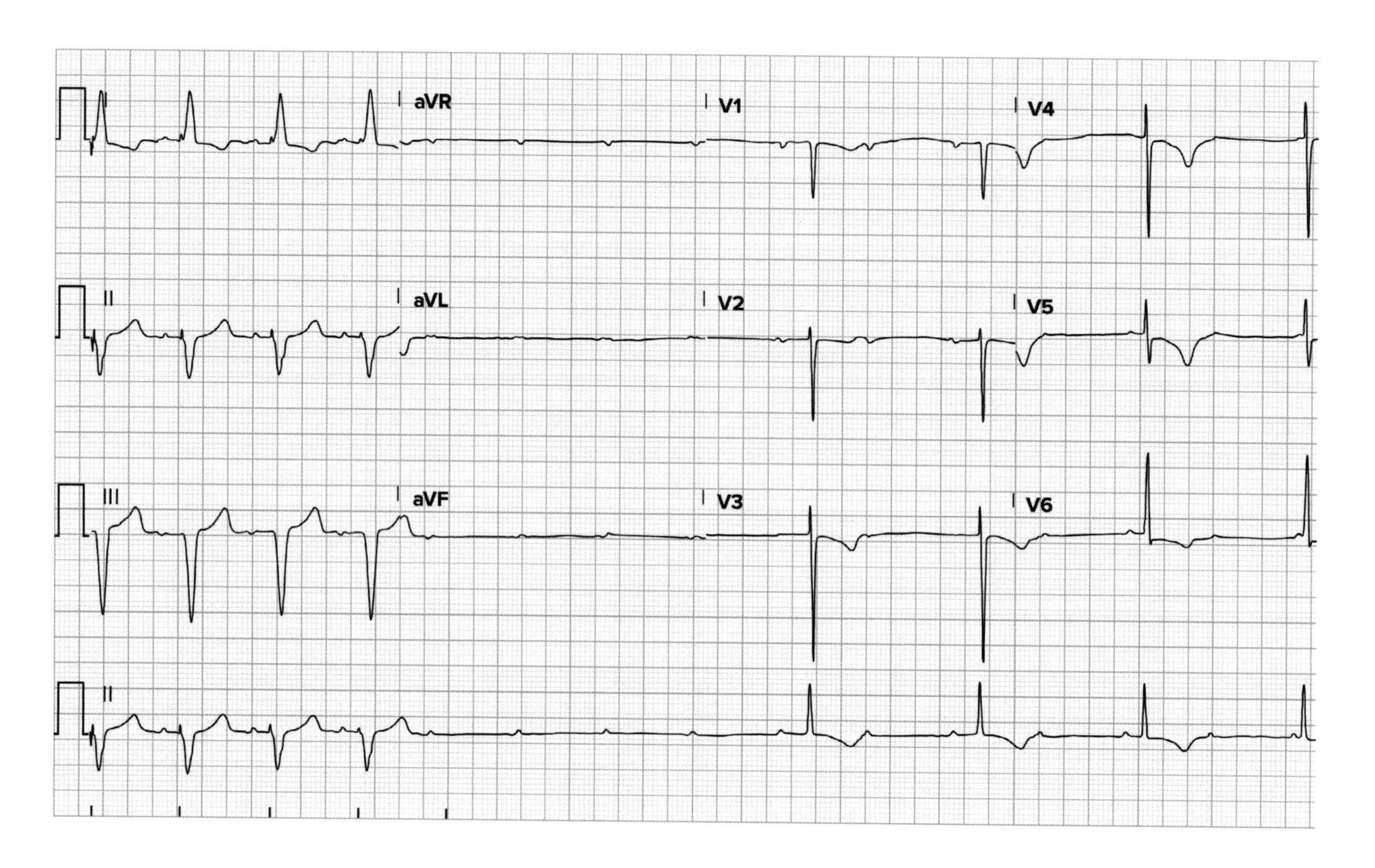

Case 23: Answer

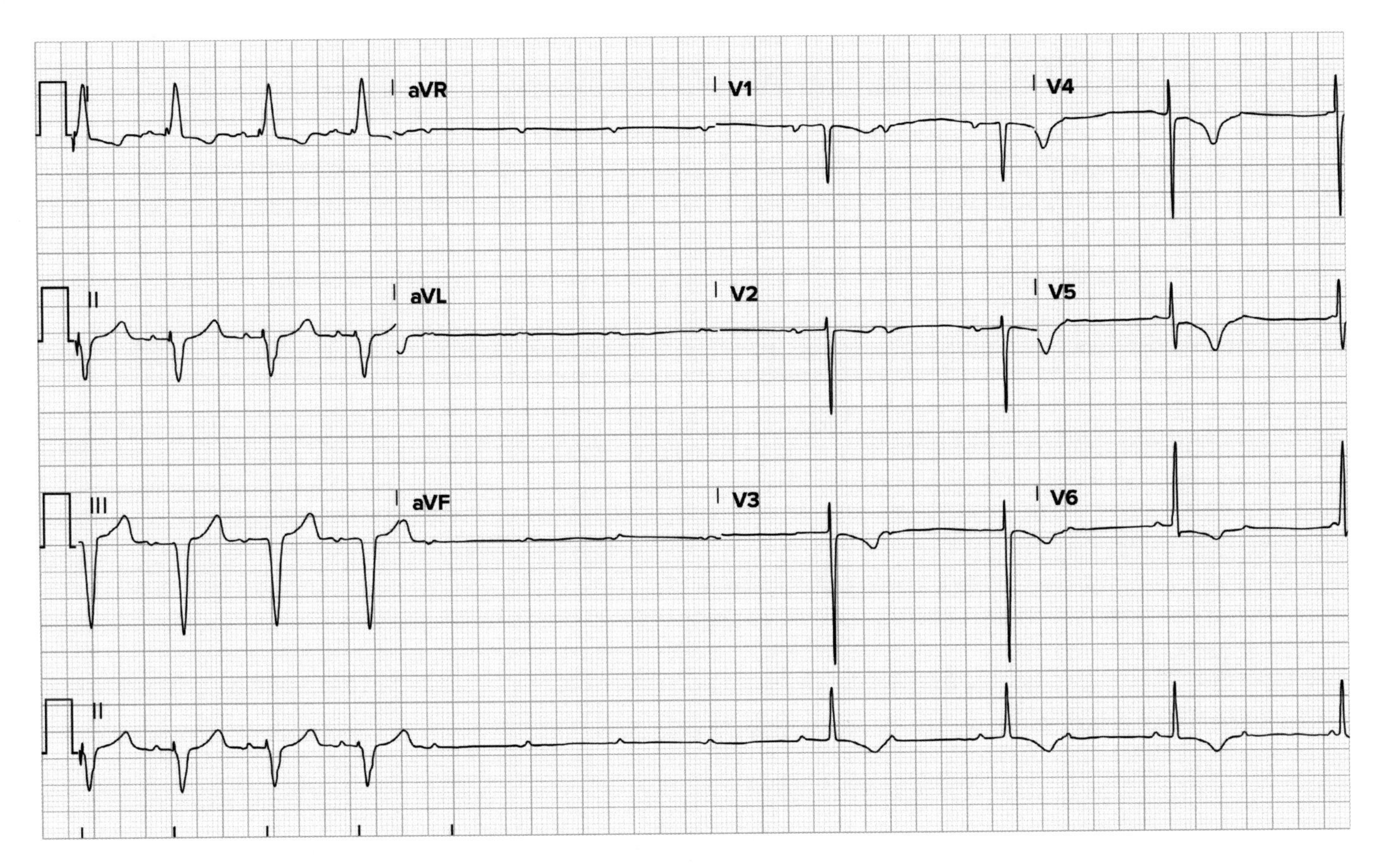

This ECG shows three distinct rhythms that are best described individually.

The initial section of this ECG shows an atrial-sensed, ventricular-paced rhythm with an average ventricular rate of 88 bpm ***(see Figure 1).*** There is a native P-wave that is sensed by the pacemaker which then triggers a paced ventricular beat. This is a normal functioning atrial-sensed ventricular pacemaker. The QRS complexes have a LBBB-like morphology which is expected with right ventricular pacing. The middle section of this ECG shows four P-waves with no associated QRS-T complexes ***(see Figure 2)***. The first P-wave is followed by a pacer spike with no ventricular depolarization which is called failure to capture. The defining feature of failure to capture is the absence of depolarization after pacer spikes. Common causes of failure to capture include electrode displacement, wire fracture, ischemia/infarct, and electrolyte abnormalities (especially hyperkalemia). Treatment is based on correcting the underlying etiology (eg, calcium for hyperkalemia).

The remaining P-waves are not followed by any pacer spikes or QRS complexes ***(see Figure 2)*** which is called failure to pace. The defining feature of failure to pace is when a pacer spike is expected but not generated. The common causes include oversensing, lead fracture, or insulation defect. Oversensing describes when non-cardiac activity (eg, skeletal muscle activity) is inappropriately recognized as native cardiac activity and subsequently inhibits pacing.

Figure 1.
The initial section of this ECG shows a normal atrial-sensed, ventricular-paced rhythm

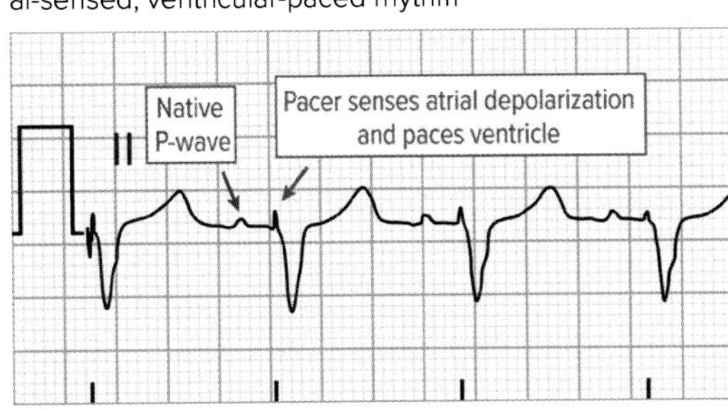

Figure 2.
The middle section of this ECG shows failure to capture (pacer spike with no subsequent depolarization) followed by failure to pace (pacer spike is expected but absent)

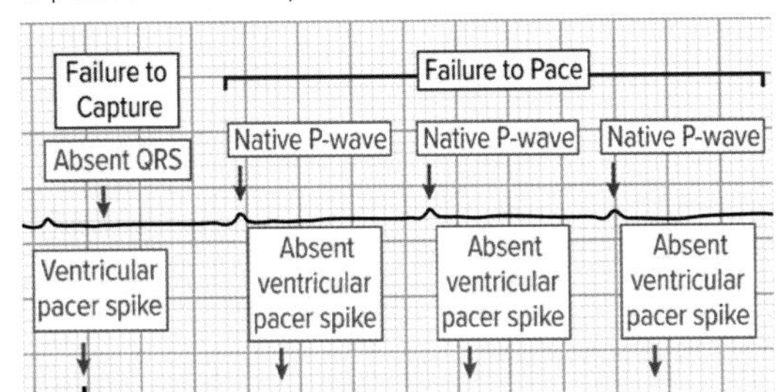

The final section of this ECG shows a regular narrow complex bradycardia with a ventricular rate of 45 bpm and an atrial rate of 88 bpm, consistent with AV dissociation and a 3rd degree AV block with a junctional escape rhythm.

The differential diagnosis for a regular narrow complex rhythm with bradycardic ventricular rates includes:

- Sinus bradycardia
- Junctional rhythm
- Junctional bradycardia
- Atrial flutter with block (rate controlled)
- Atrial tachycardia with block (rate controlled)
- 2:1 AV block
- High-grade AV block (eg, 3:1, 4:1, etc.)
- 3rd degree AV block with junctional escape rhythm
- 3rd degree sinoatrial block with junctional escape rhythm

The QRS complex duration is narrow (ie, < 110 msec) which is consistent with a junctional escape rhythm. The PP and RR intervals are close to a 2:1 ratio but the PR intervals for the P-waves that immediately precede a QRS complex get progressively shorter which is consistent with AV dissociation ***(see Figure 3)***. Leads V4-V6 show TWI and STD suggestive of the strain pattern seen with LVH, but it impossible to state this definitively based on this ECG alone.

Figure 3.
The final section of this ECG shows a 3rd degree AV block with a junctional escape rhythm

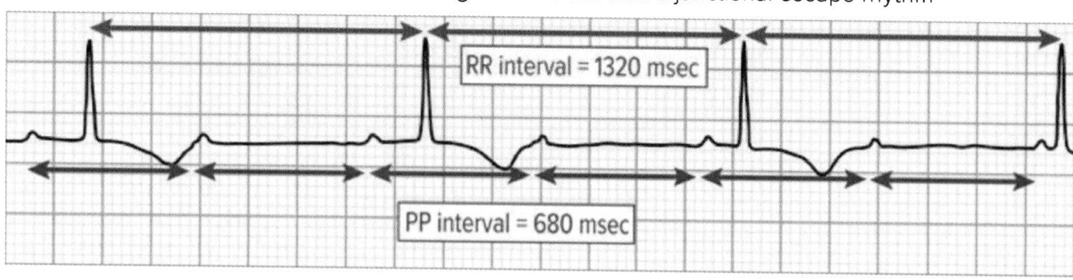

This patient had a permanent pacemaker placed due to the persistent 3rd degree AV block.

Pacemaker Learning Points

- Pacer spikes are usually visible on the ECG, either at the bottom of the ECG and/or preceding the P-wave and/or QRS complex
  - Atrial pacing: spikes immediately precede P-waves
  - Ventricular pacing: spikes immediately precede QRS complexes
  - Dual chamber pacing: spikes immediately precede both P-waves and QRS complexes
  - Biventricular pacing: 2 spikes immediately precede QRS complexes
- Atrial pacing
  - Pacemaker lead usually implanted in the right atrial appendage
  - Results in P-waves with normal morphology
- Right ventricular pacing
  - Pacemaker lead usually implanted in the RV apex
  - Results in a LBBB pattern in the limb leads and anteroseptal precordial leads
  - The major difference between an intrinsic LBBB and a right ventricular-paced rhythm is that the QRS complex will almost always be negatively oriented in leads V5-V6 with a right ventricular-paced rhythm
- Biventricular pacing
  - Two pacemaker leads usually implanted in the RV apex and the surface of the posterior or lateral LV
  - Typically results in a narrower QRS complex than with right ventricular pacing
  - Dominant R-wave in lead V1 +/- V2 is common
- AICD will have a thick coil that differentiates it from a pacemaker

Failure to Sense Learning Points

- Pacemaker fails to sense native cardiac activity → asynchronous pacing ***(see figure below)***
  - Sensing refers to the pacer's ability to recognize native cardiac beats
- ECG shows pacer spikes before, after, or within P-waves and/or QRS complexes
- Causes include lead insulation break, new intrinsic bundle branch block, electrolyte abnormalities, and Class IC antidysrhythmics (eg, flecainide)

Failure to Capture Learning Points

- Delivery of pacing stimulus without subsequent myocardial depolarization ***(see figure below)***
- ECG shows absence of depolarization after pacer spikes
- Causes include functional (eg, electrode displacement, wire fracture) and pathologic (eg, electrolyte disturbances, AMI)

Failure to Pace Learning Points

- Paced stimulus is not generated when expected ***(see figure below)***
- ECG shows decreased or absent pacemaker function
- Causes include oversensing, lead fracture or insulation defect
  - Oversensing: pacing inhibited by non-cardiac activity (eg, skeletal muscle activity) inappropriately recognized as native cardiac activity

3rd Degree AV Block Learning Points

- A 3rd degree AV block, or complete heart block, is defined by the absence of conduction through the AV node leading to complete AV dissociation
  - P-waves "march out" (ie, constant PP interval) and do not conduct to produce a QRS complex
  - PR intervals are variable
  - Atrial rate > ventricular rate
  - Ventricular rhythm is usually junctional or ventricular escape rhythm
- All patients require admission and evaluation for pacemaker placement

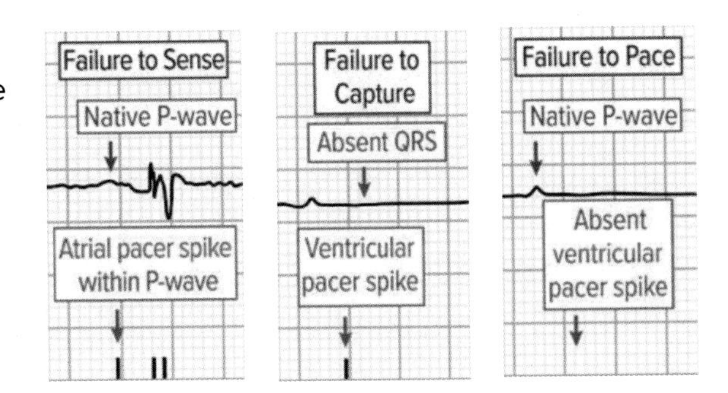

Junctional Rhythm Learning Points

- Ectopic focus from AV node or proximal Purkinje system
  - Also called AV junctional rhythm, nodal rhythm, nodal escape rhythm, junctional escape rhythm, AV nodal rhythm
- ECG shows ventricular rate of 40-60 bpm with normal QRS complex duration unless concurrent conduction abnormality (eg, bundle branch block)
- May have retrograde P-waves that precede (with PR interval < 120 msec) or follow QRS complex, typically best seen in the inferior leads
- Variations include:
  - Junctional Bradycardia: ventricular rate < 40 bpm
  - Accelerated Junctional Rhythm: ventricular rate 61–100 bpm
  - Junctional Tachycardia: ventricular rate > 100 bpm

Case 24: Presentation

A 61-year-old female presents with chest pain. A prior ECG from one year ago was normal. What is your interpretation of her ECG?

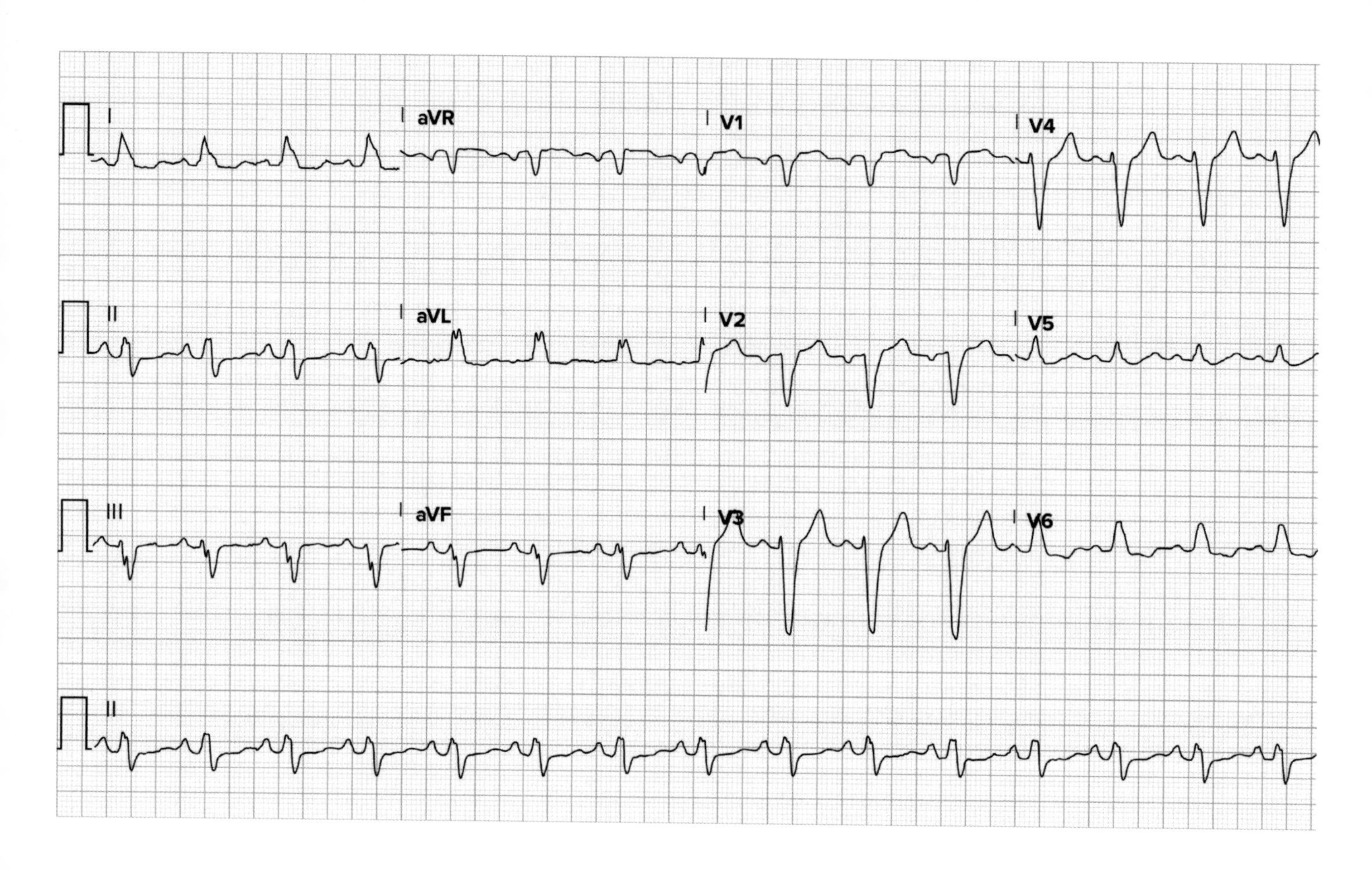

Case 24: Answer

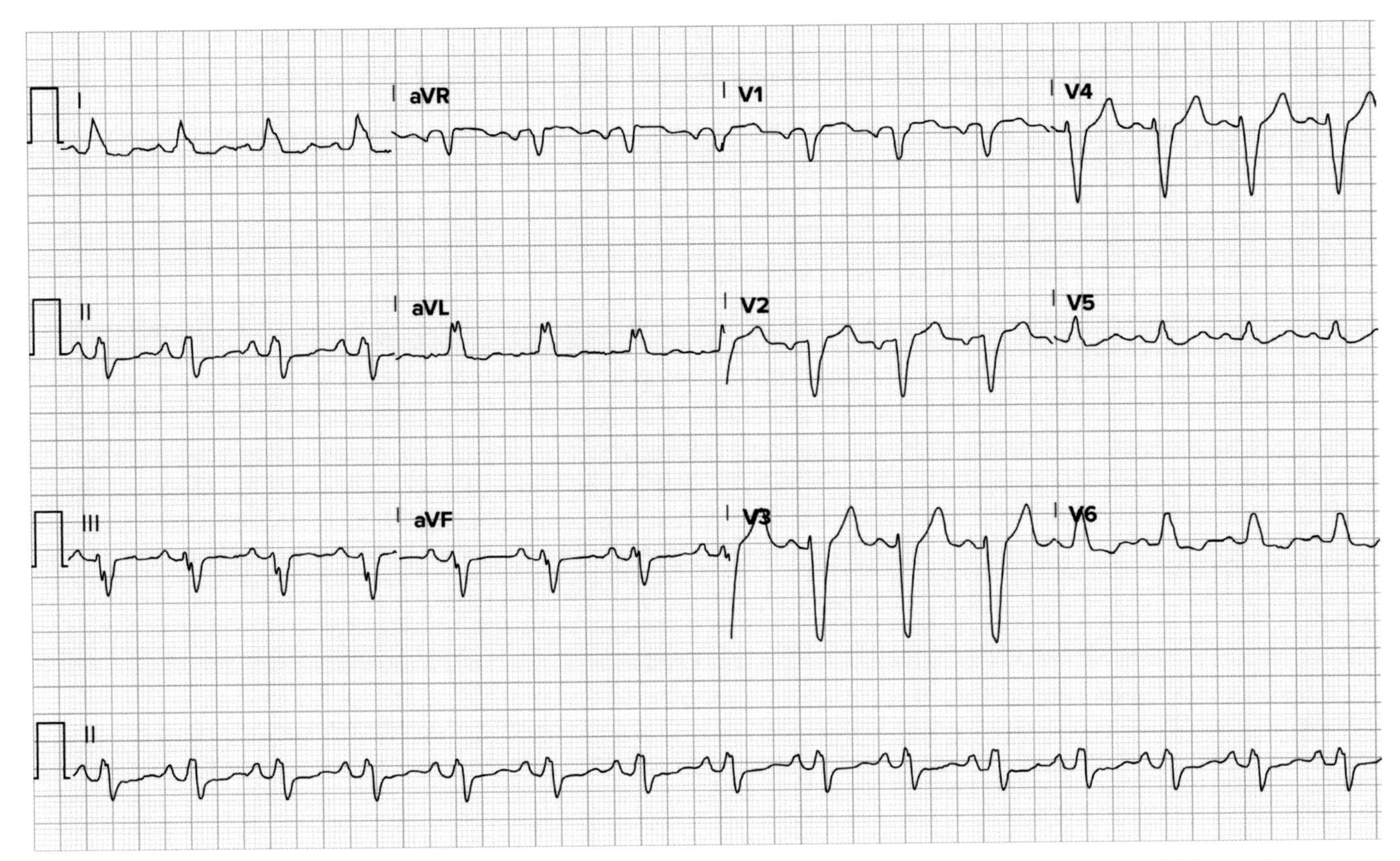

This ECG shows a normal sinus rhythm with a ventricular rate of 90 bpm, left axis deviation, prolonged QRS complex duration with a LBBB, and a prolonged QTc interval.

The characteristic findings in a LBBB include:

- QRS complex duration ≥ 120 msec
- Dominant S-wave in leads V1, V2, and frequently V3 ***(see Figure 1)***
- Broad and notched or slurred R-wave in leads I, aVL, V5, and V6 ***(see Figures 2 and 3)***
- Absent Q-waves in leads I, V5, and V6 (can see small Q-wave in lead aVL)
- R-wave peak time > 60 msec in leads V5 and V6 but normal in leads V1-V3 ***(see Figure 3)***
- Axis usually normal or leftward
- ST segments follow the "Rule of Appropriate Discordance"
  - ST-segment deviation in the opposite direction from the QRS complex ***(see Figures 1, 2, and 3)***

Figure 1.
Lead V1 shows a dominant S-wave and appropriate discordance, consistent with a LBBB

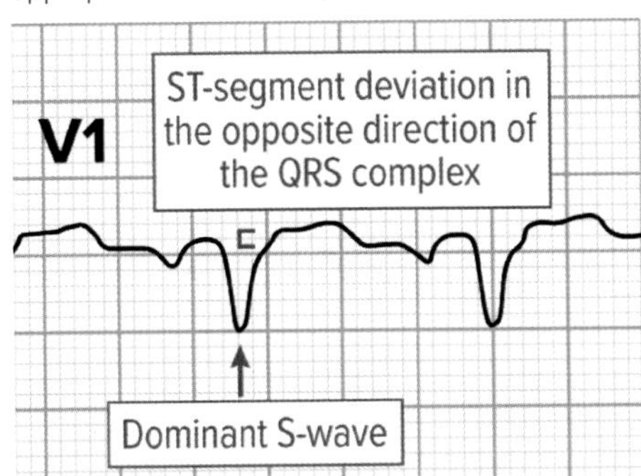

Figure 2.
Lead shows a broad notched R-wave and appropriate discordance, consistent with a LBBB

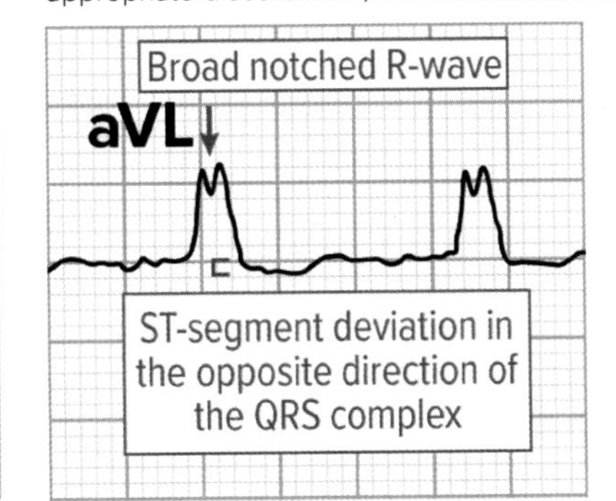

A defining feature of a LBBB is the "rule of appropriate discordance" which describes the relationship between the direction of the QRS complex and its ST-segment. In other words, if the main vector of the QRS complex points up, there will be STD, and if the main vector of the QRS complex points down, there will STE. These repolarization abnormalities confound the ECG's ability to detect AMI and other ACS findings, so interpretation of the ECG with a LBBB in a presentation suggestive of ACS requires using the Sgarbossa criteria to diagnose an MI.

The Sgarbossa criteria are based on the underlying principle that concordance and excessive discordance in a LBBB are abnormal. The criteria assign a point value for any concordant STE ***(see Figures 4a and 4b)*** or excessively discordant STE ***(see Figure 4c)***. A score ≥ 3 is 98% specific for AMI, so the presence of criterion A or B are considered diagnostic of an AMI. Criterion C is only assigned 2 points, so the presence of just criterion C is not diagnostic of an AMI.

Figure 3.
Lead V6 shows a broad slurred R-wave, R-wave peak time > 60 msec, and appropriate discordance, consistent with a LBBB

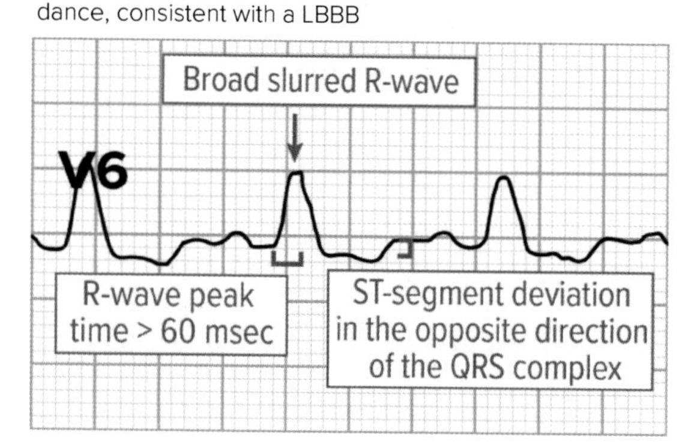

Figure 4a.
Sgarbossa criterion A: concordant STE ≥ 1 mm in ≥ 1 lead (5 points = diagnostic of AMI)

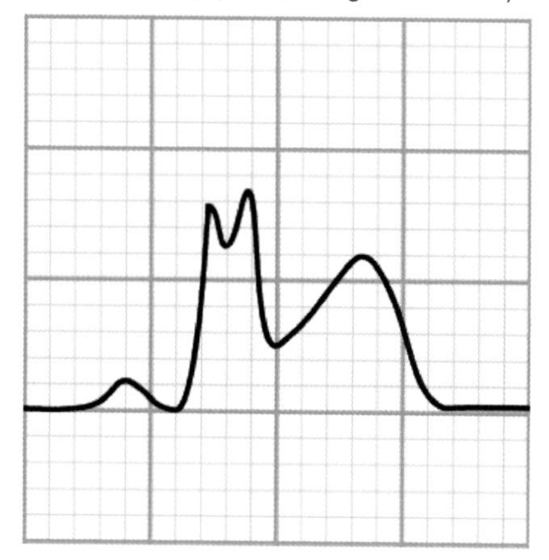

Figure 4b.
Sgarbossa criterion B: STD ≥ 1 mm in leads V1 or V2 or V3 (3 points = diagnostic of AMI)

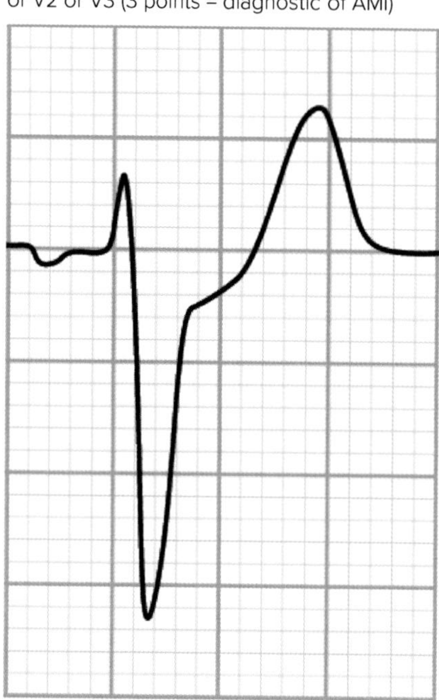

Figure 4c.
Sgarbossa criterion C: discordant STE ≥ 5 mm in ≥ 1 lead (2 points = not diagnostic of AMI)

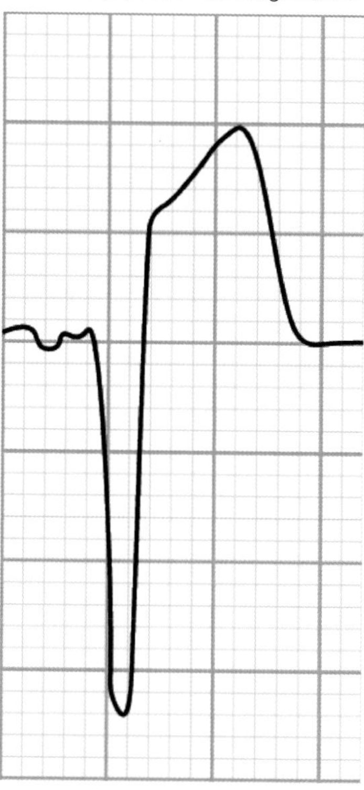

The Modified Sgarbossa criteria includes Sgarbossa criteria A and B with a variation of criterion C. Instead of using a fixed cutoff of 5 mm for discordant STE, it uses a ratio of the STE height to the S-wave depth **(see *Figure 5*)**. A STE/S ratio ≥ 0.25 in ≥ 1 lead is considered diagnostic of an AMI. This means that more than 5 mm of STE is permissible if there is a large S-wave, and less than 5 mm of STE may be diagnostic if the accompanying S-wave is small. The Modified Sgarbossa criteria are not mandated in the current AHA/ACC STEMI guidelines.

This patient had an unremarkable ED workup and was admitted to the cardiology service for further ACS risk stratification.

LBBB Learning Points

- Ventricular depolarization from right to left (opposite of normal)
- ST segments follow the "Rule of Appropriate Discordance"
  - ST-segment deviation in the opposite direction from the QRS complex
- Confounds ECG's ability to detect AMI and other ACS findings
  - If ACS suspected, must use the Sgarbossa criteria to diagnose an AMI
  - A presumed new LBBB in itself is no longer considered a STEMI equivalent, but is a high risk finding in ACS, so if an AMI is suspected, urgent reperfusion therapy should be considered

Sgarbossa Criteria Learning Points

- Used to evaluate for STEMI in the presence of LBBB
- Based on "Rule of Appropriate Discordance"
  - In the absence of AMI, LBBB will have ST-segment deviation in the opposite direction from the QRS complex
  - Concordance and excessive discordance in LBBB are abnormal
- Concordant STE ≥ 1 mm in ≥ 1 lead or STD ≥ 1 mm in lead V1, V2, or V3 is considered diagnostic of AMI
- Modified Sgarbossa criteria
  - For discordant STE, a ratio of STE to S-wave depth ≥ 0.25 in ≥ 1 lead is considered diagnostic of AMI
  - Not mandated in current AHA/ACC STEMI guidelines

Figure 5.
Modified Sgarbossa criterion C- STE/S ratio ≥ 0.25 in ≥ 1 lead (diagnostic of AMI but not mandated in current AHA/ACC STEMI guidelines)

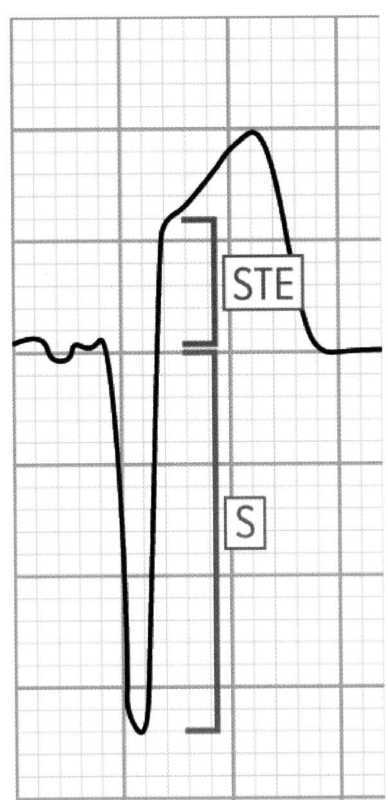

Case 25: Presentation

A 23-year-old male presents with SOB, hemoptysis, and chest pain. Notable vital signs include a respiratory rate of 26 and an oxygen saturation of 89%. What is your interpretation of his ECG?

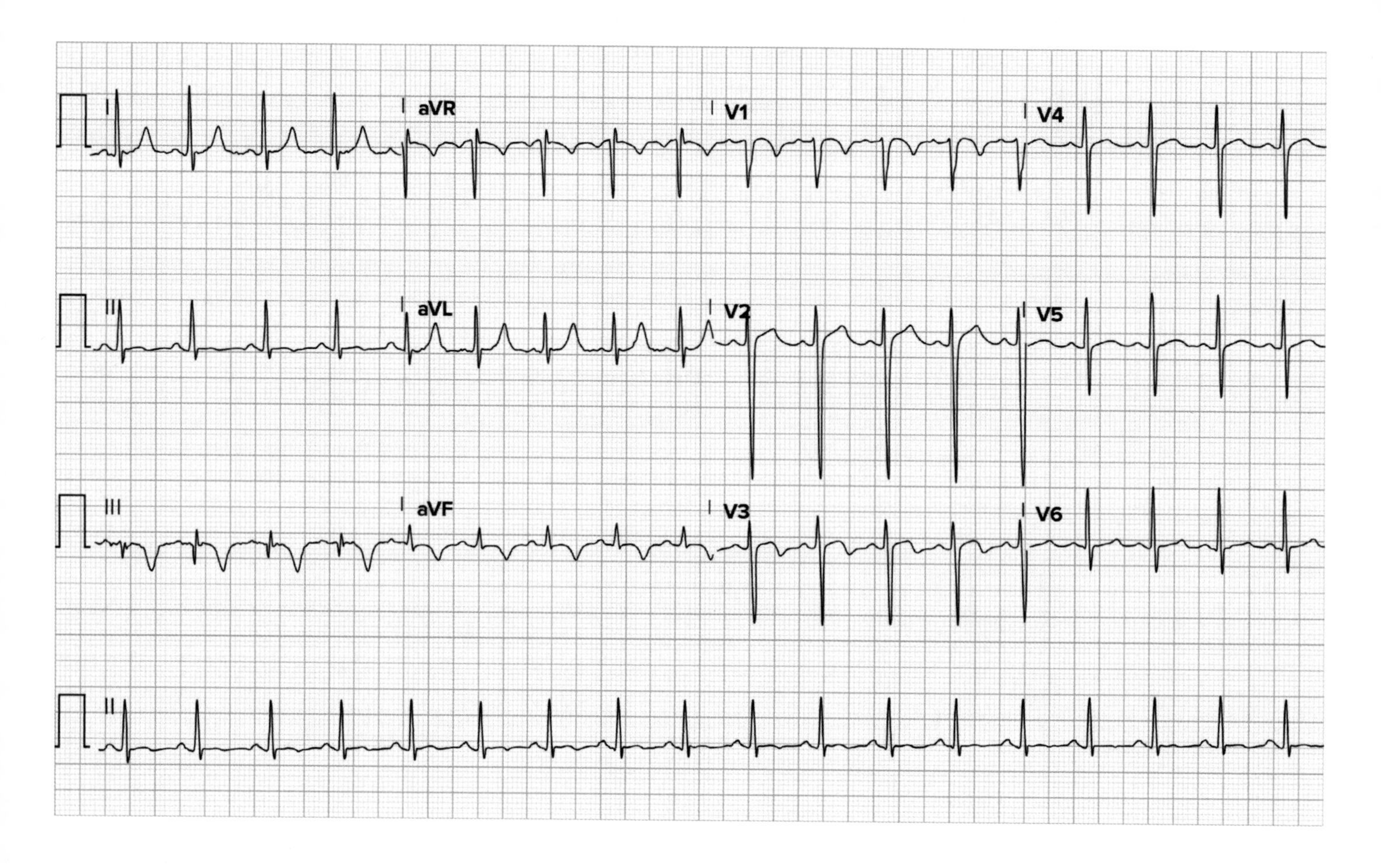

Case 25: Answer

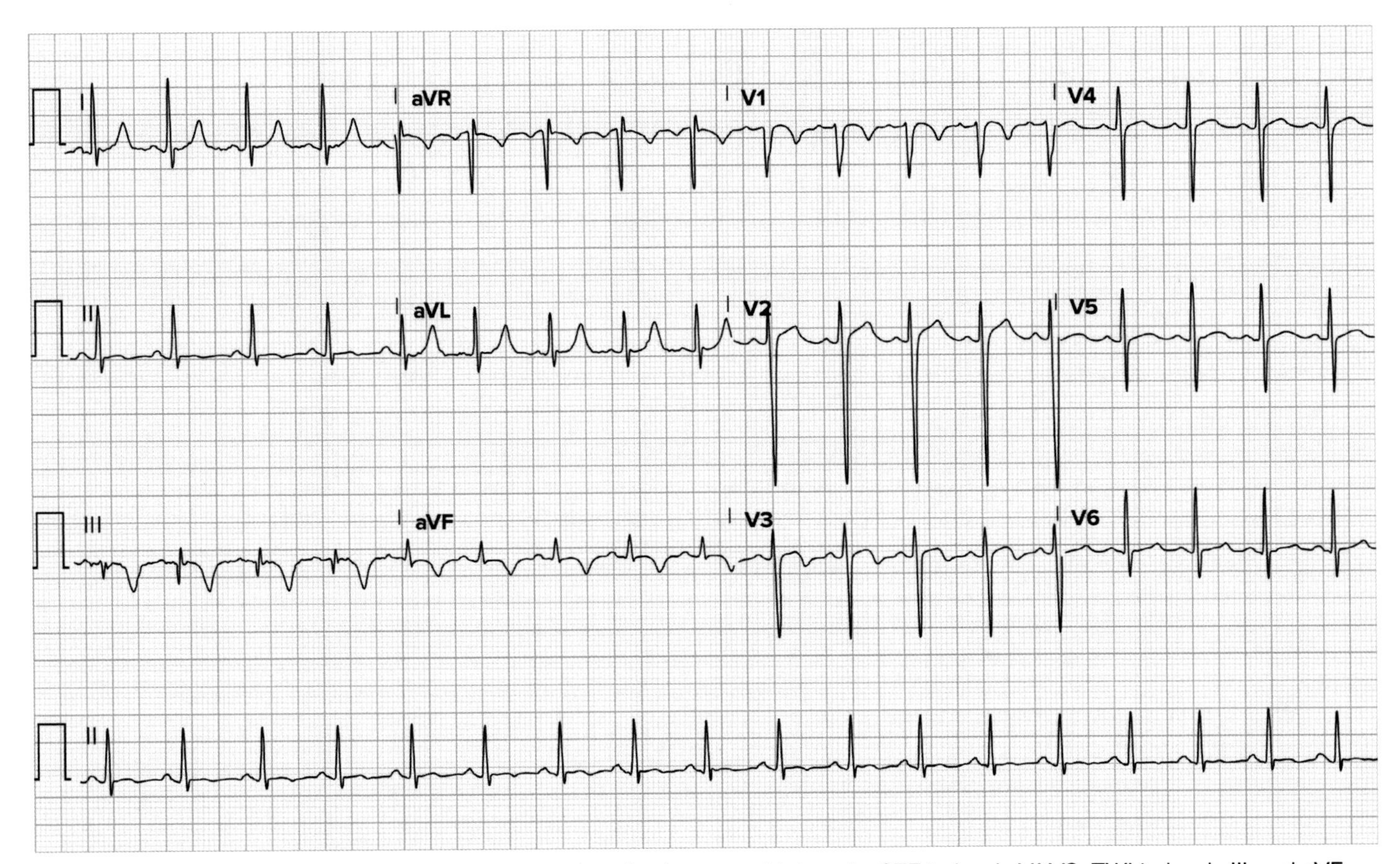

This ECG shows a sinus tachycardia at 110 bpm, normal axis, normal intervals, STE in leads V1-V3, TWI in leads III and aVF, and a biphasic T-wave in lead V3.

The differential diagnosis for TWI includes:	The differential diagnosis for STE includes[1]:
• Acute ischemia (early reciprocal changes)	• Acute myocardial infarction
• Bundle branch blocks	• Acute myocarditis
• CNS injury	• Acute pericarditis
• Digitalis effect	• Benign early repolarization
• Intra-abdominal disorders	• Brugada syndrome
• Juvenile T-wave pattern	• Bundle branch blocks
• LVH	• Cardiomyopathy
• Metabolic abnormalities	• CNS injury
• Pericarditis	• Coronary vasospasm
• Pre-excitation syndromes	• Hypercalcemia
• Pulmonary embolism	• Hyperkalemia
• Toxicologic abnormalities	• Hypothermia
• Ventricular rhythms (paced or intrinsic) or ectopy	• Left ventricular aneurysm
	• Left ventricular hypertrophy
	• Non-ACS myocardial injury
	• Pre-excitation Syndromes
	• Post-electrical cardioversion
	• Spiked Helmet Sign
	• Ventricular rhythms (paced or intrinsic) or ectopy

Although this patient's ECG shows STE in leads V1-V3, his history and vital sign abnormalities are concerning for a pulmonary embolism (PE). It is important to always consider the non-ACS causes of STE in the context of a patient's history and exam as sending a patient with a PE to the cath lab is not ideal.

The ECG findings in PE (see Learning Points below) are varied and neither sensitive nor specific. This ECG has multiple findings that can be seen with PE:

1. Sinus tachycardia (the most common ECG rhythm abnormality)
2. TWI in the inferior leads
3. STE in lead V1
4. Large S-wave in leads I and aVL
5. R/S transition point shift towards lead V6

Figure 1.
A right-sided ECG shows Qr pattern in leads V5R-V6R

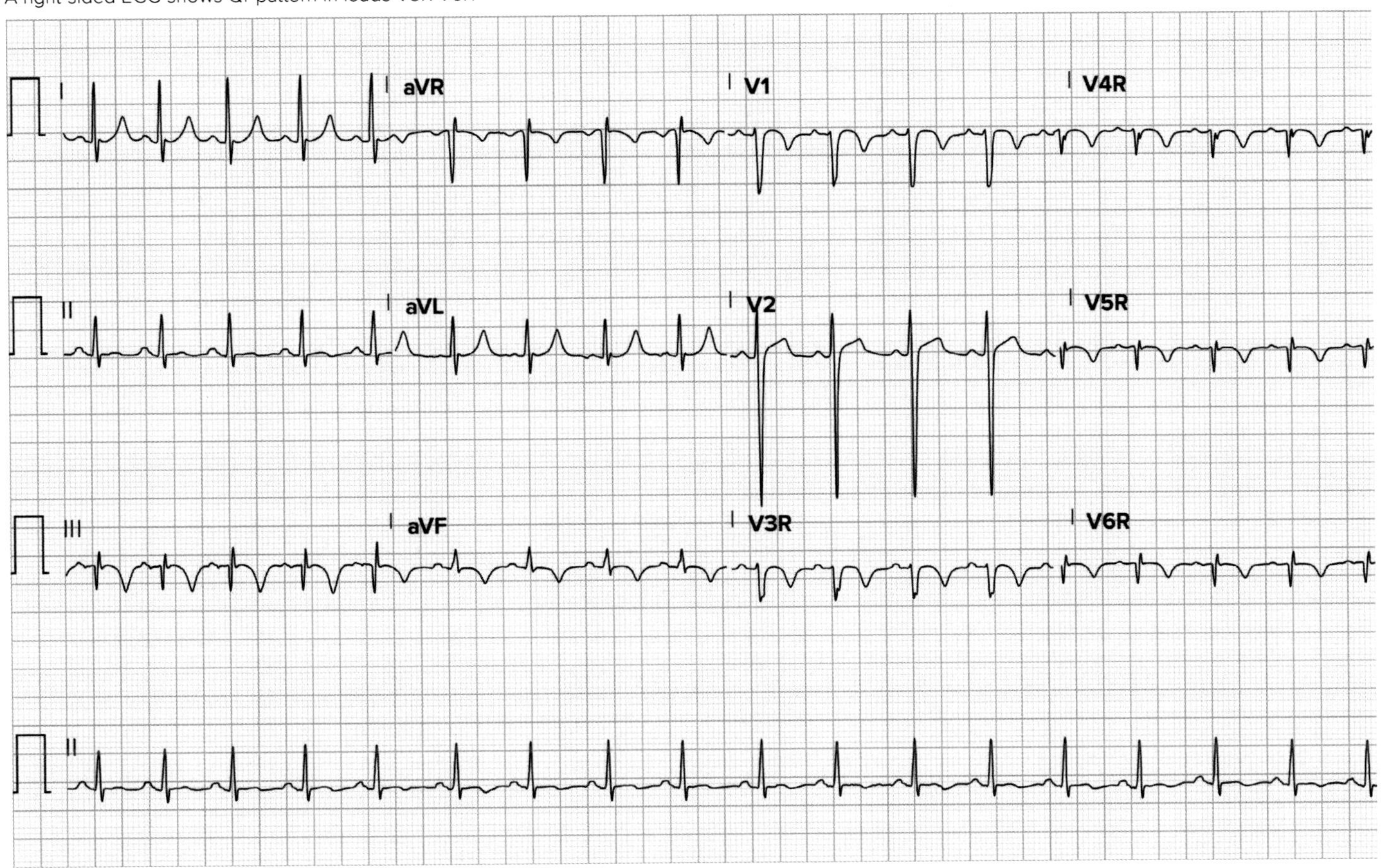

A right-sided ECG was obtained, mostly for academic purposes, and showed a Qr pattern in leads V5R-V6R (***see Figure 1***).

This patient was started on heparin after a bedside echo showed right heart strain. A subsequent CTA showed a saddle PE, and labs showed an elevated troponin and BNP. The patient's hypoxia corrected with a non-rebreather and BiPAP was avoided due to concern that it could lead to decreased venous return in the setting of preload dependence. The patient was admitted to the ICU and did not require catheter directed thrombolysis or thrombectomy.

ECG in PE Learning Points

- ECG is neither sensitive nor specific for PE
  - No single ECG criterion is diagnostic- ECG can only suggest diagnosis
  - Most common ECG rhythm is sinus
  - Most common ECG abnormality is T-wave abnormalities
  - Most common ECG rhythm abnormality is sinus tachycardia
- ECG findings in PE include:
  - Non-specific ST-segment/T-wave changes +/- sinus tachycardia
  - TWI in leads V1-V4 +/- inferior leads (highly specific)
  - STE in lead V1 or aVR
  - Small Q-wave with prominent R-wave in lead V1
  - Large S-wave in lead I and/or aVL
  - RBBB (complete or incomplete)
  - Right axis deviation
  - R/S transition point shift towards lead V6
  - STE, Qr, or Qs pattern in leads V4R- V6R
  - S1Q3T3: poor sensitivity/specificity (found in ~10% of PE patients and ~10% of patients with RV strain unrelated to PE)

References

1. 1. Mattu A. ECG Weekly.

Case 26: Presentation

A 78-year-old female presents with intermittent near syncope.
What is your interpretation of her ECG?

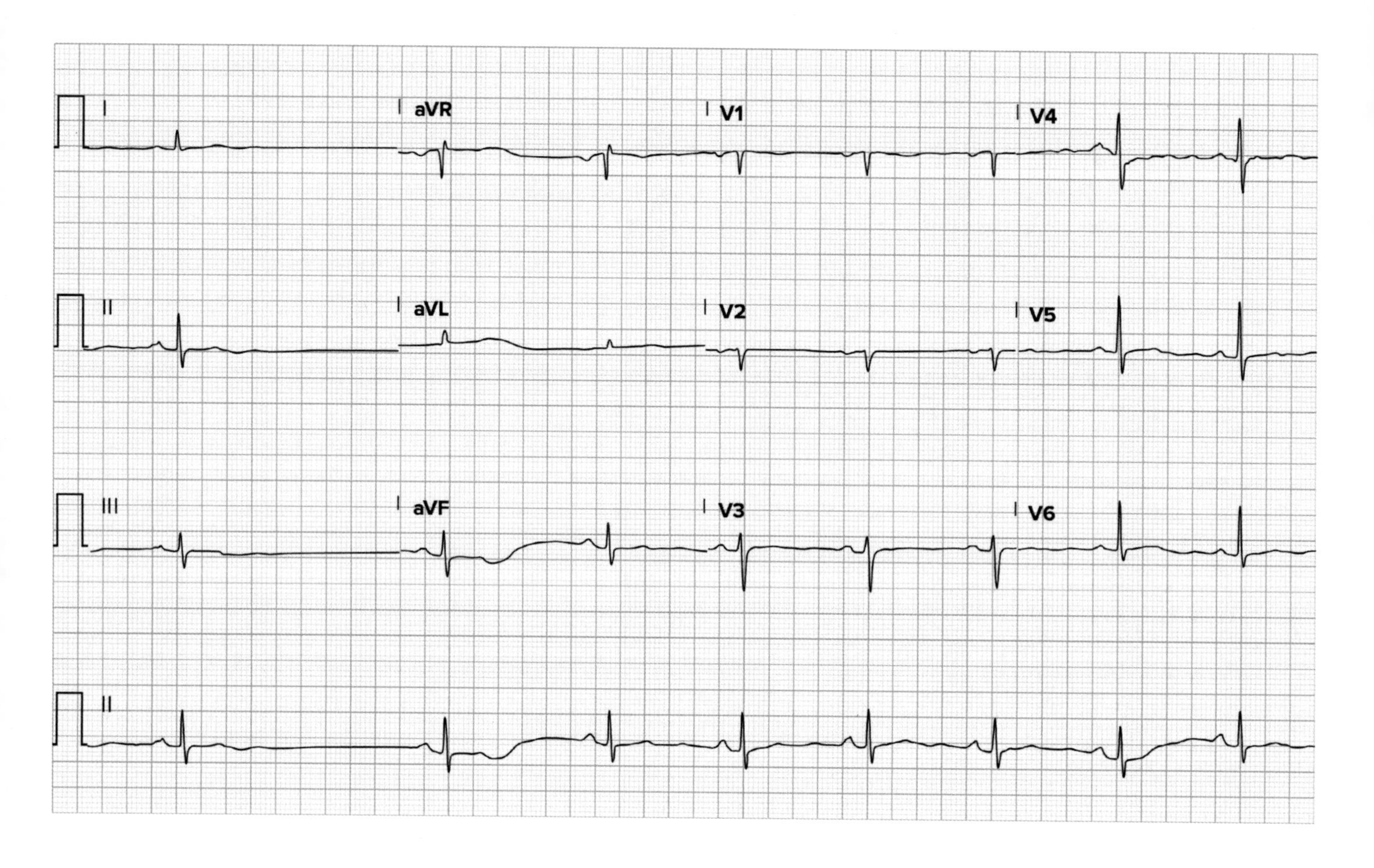

Case 26: Answer

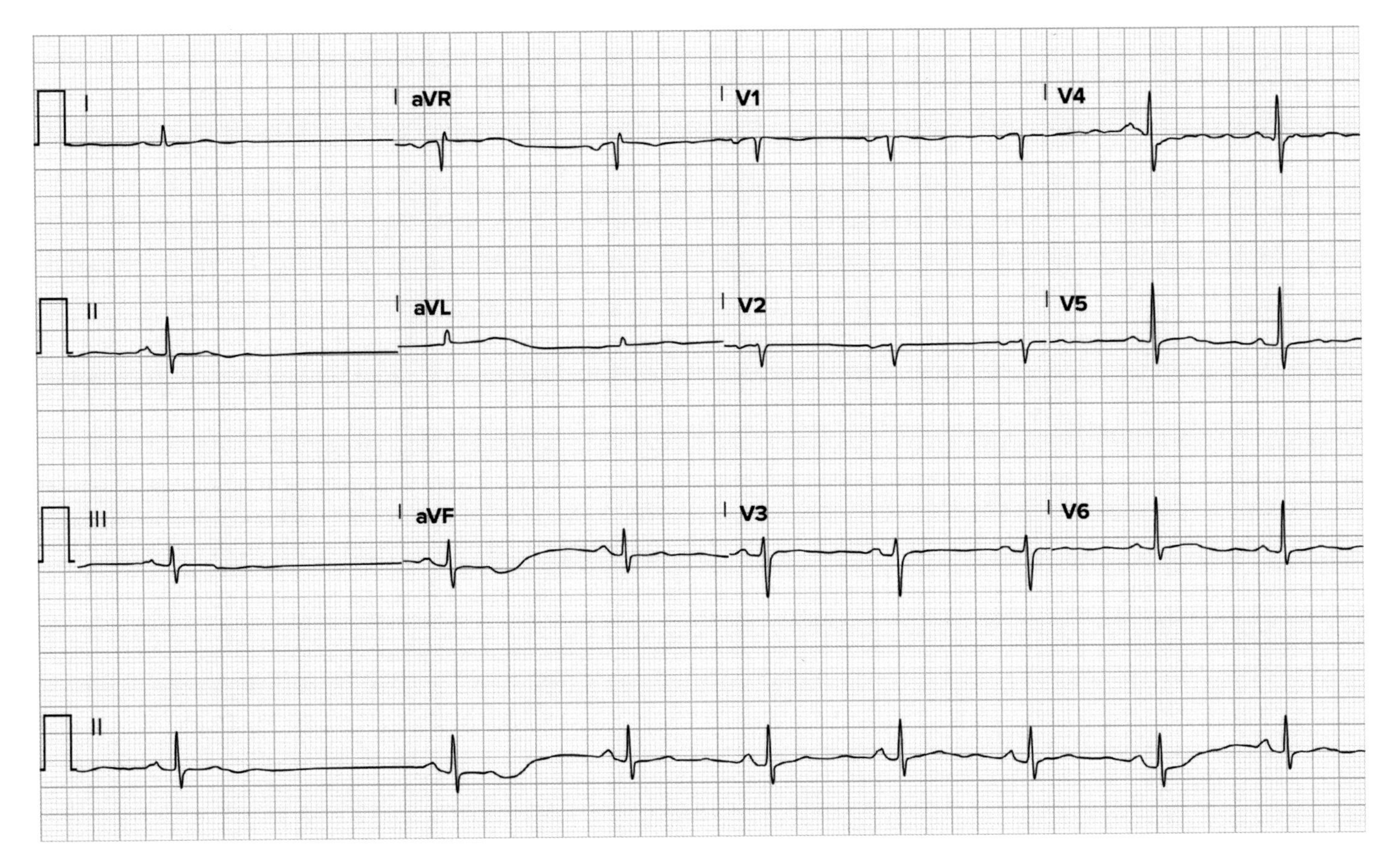

This ECG shows a sinus pause followed by a bradycardic sinus arrhythmia with an average ventricular rate of 48 bpm, normal intervals, normal axis, and diffuse T-wave flattening.

The differential diagnosis for an irregular narrow complex rhythm with bradycardic ventricular rates includes:

- Atrial fibrillation (rate controlled)
- Atrial flutter with variable block (rate controlled)
- Atrial tachycardia with variable block (rate controlled)
- Wandering atrial pacemaker
- 2nd degree AV block Mobitz types I and II
- Variable high-grade AV block (eg, 3:1, 4:1, etc.)
- 2nd degree sinoatrial block
- Sinus arrhythmia
- Sinus bradycardia, junctional rhythm, or junctional bradycardia with irregular pattern of PAC, PJC, and/or PVC
- Sinus bradycardia, junctional rhythm, or junctional bradycardia with regular patterns of PAC, PJC, and/or PVC (bigeminy, trigeminy, etc.)

ECG findings to look for in syncope patients include:

- Ischemia/infarct
- Severe bradycardia or tachycardia
- Conduction abnormalities (eg, AV blocks)
- Low voltage +/- electrical alternans
- Syncope syndromes:
  - ARVD/ARVC
  - Brugada
  - HCM
  - QT syndromes (long and short)
  - WPW

This ECG starts with a sinus pause ***(see Figure 1)*** which is the absence of sinus node depolarization for > 2 seconds, although some criteria set this cutoff at 3 seconds. This can be caused by increased parasympathetic activity or impairment of all pacemaker cells (including those in the atria, His bundle, and Purkinje systems). The effect of the autonomic nervous system is greatest in the SA node and least in the Purkinje system, so more distal pacing sites will usurp pacing responsibilities when more proximal sites are suppressed from increased parasympathetic activity.

The other cause of an absent P-QRS-T sequence is a sinoatrial block. This is defined as the failure of an impulse to emerge from the SA node. It is often difficult to distinguish between a sinus pause and a SA block, but a SA block should show a mathematical relationship between the longer and short cycle lengths (ie, the PP interval of the longer interval should be twice the PP interval of the shorter PP interval).

Figure 1.
The lead II rhythm strip shows a sinus pause followed by variable RR intervals consistent with a sinus arrhythmia

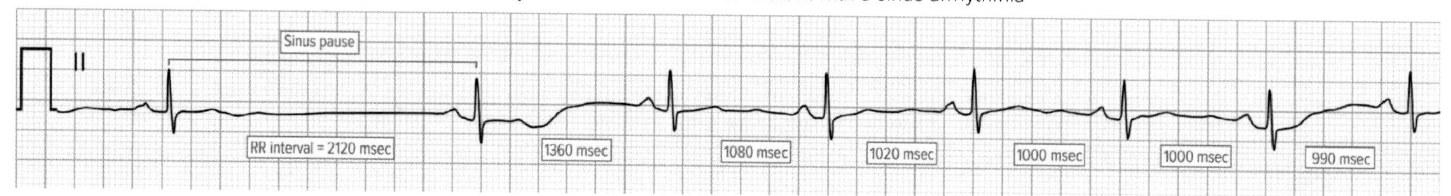

This ECG also shows a sinus arrhythmia. There is no universally accepted definition for sinus arrhythmia, but commons criteria include variation in sequential RR intervals > 10% or 120 msec. The most common cause of heart rate variation is respiratory inspiration leading to decreased vagal tone and subsequent increased heart rate. This ECG shows a sinus arrhythmia with beats 2 and 3 where the difference in the RR interval is both > 10% and 120 msec. This is followed by a steady increase in the heart rate which is commonly seen following episodes of increased parasympathetic activity.

Sick sinus syndrome, also called sinoatrial disease or sinus node dysfunction, describes a series of abnormalities that include sinus node dysfunction, escape pacemaker dysfunction, and AV node conduction dysfunction. The term "sick sinus syndrome" is often used interchangeably with tachy-brady syndrome, but it is really an umbrella term that includes multiple other ECG abnormalities (see table below).

This patient had an unremarkable ED workup and was admitted to the cardiology service. She had multiple episodes of sinus pauses on telemetry which prompted placement of a permanent pacemaker.

Sick Sinus Syndrome Learning Points

- Describes a series of abnormalities that includes sinus node dysfunction, escape pacemaker dysfunction, and AV node conduction dysfunction[1]
- Diagnosis requires both ECG abnormalities (see table below) and symptoms

Sinus bradycardia	Sinus rate < 50 bpm
Ectopic atrial bradycardia	Atrial depolarization attributable to an atrial pacemaker other than the sinus node with a rate < 50 bpm
Sinoatrial exit block	Evidence that blocked conduction between the sinus node and adjacent atrial tissue is present. Multiple electrocardiographic manifestations including "group beating" of atrial depolarization and sinus pauses
Sinus pause	Sinus node depolarizes >3 s after the last atrial depolarization
Sinus node arrest	No evidence of sinus node depolarization
Tachycardia-bradycardia ("tachy-brady") syndrome	Sinus bradycardia, ectopic atrial bradycardia, or sinus pause alternating with periods of abnormal atrial tachycardia, atrial flutter, or atrial fibrillation. The tachycardia may be associated with suppression of sinus node automaticity and a sinus pause of variable duration when the tachycardia terminates
Chronotropic incompetence	Broadly defined as the inability of the heart to increase its rate commensurate with increased activity or demand, in many studies translates to failure to attain 80% of expected heart rate reserve during exercise
Isorhythmic dissociation	Atrial depolarization (from either SA node or ectopic atrial site) is slower than ventricular depolarization (from an AV nodal, His bundle, or ventricular site)

References

1. Kusumoto FM, Schoenfeld MH, Barrett C, et al. 2018 ACC/AHA/HRS guideline on the evaluation and management of patients with bradycardia and cardiac conduction delay: executive summary: a report of the American College of Cardiology/American Heart Association Task Force on Clinical Practice Guidelines and the Heart Rhythm Society. Circulation. 2019;140:e333–e381.

Case 27: Presentation

A 70-year-old female with history of congestive heart failure with EF of 15-20% and paroxysmal atrial fibrillation on anticoagulation presents with palpitations and lightheadedness.
What is your interpretation of her ECG?

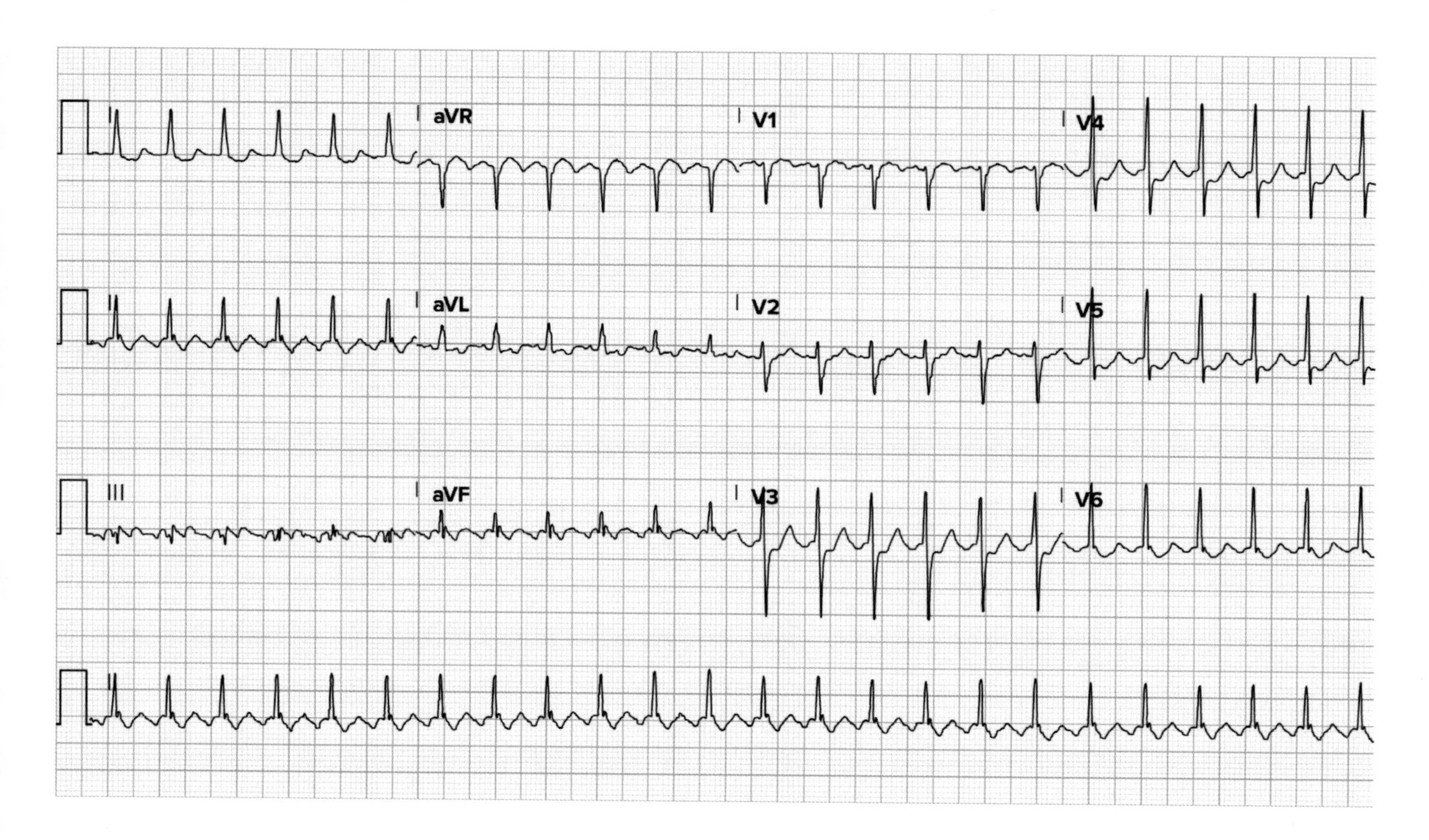

Case 27: Answer

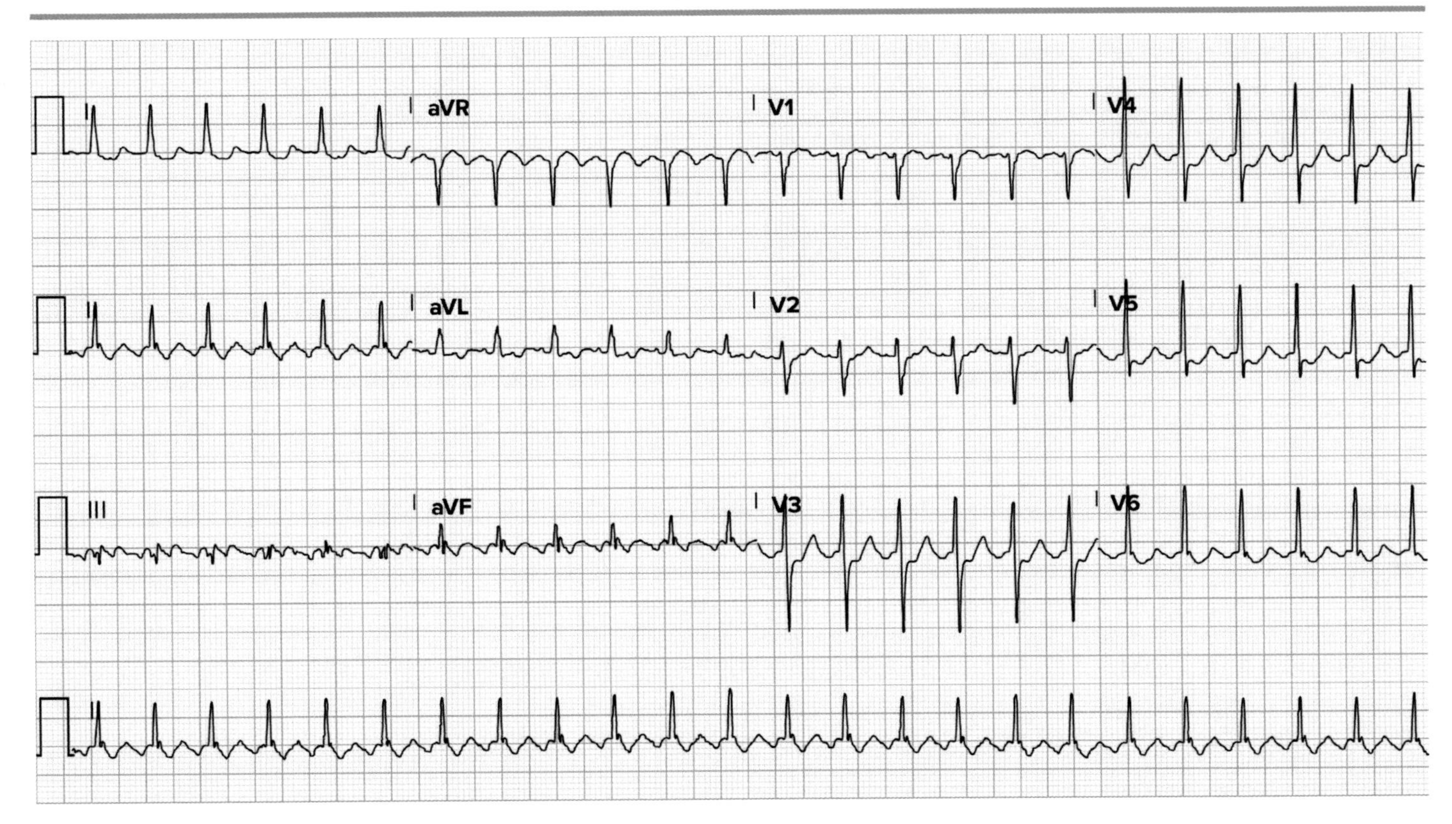

This ECG shows a regular narrow-complex tachycardia with a ventricular rate of 143 bpm, flutter waves best seen in leads II, III, and aVF, normal axis, STE in leads aVR and V1, and STD in leads I, aVL, and V2-V6.

The differential diagnosis for a regular narrow-complex tachycardia includes:

- Atrial flutter
- Atrial tachycardia
- AV nodal reentrant tachycardia
- AVRT (ie, WPW) with orthodromic conduction
- Junctional Tachycardia
- Narrow complex VT
- Sinus tachycardia

The presence of flutter waves, also called F-waves, that are best seen in the inferior leads, is diagnostic of atrial flutter, but it is always important to go through the differential diagnosis to rule out other possible NCT. The absence of P-waves rules out atrial tachycardia and sinus tachycardia. The QRS complex duration is ~90 msec, so narrow complex VT is unlikely. The rate is too fast for a junctional tachycardia. If not for the flutter waves, this could be AVNRT or orthodromic AVRT (ie, anterograde conduction via the AV node with retrograde conduction via the AP).

Atrial flutter is typically due to a right atrial re-entry circuit around the tricuspid ring. It is classified as a macro-reentry tachycardia because it revolves around a large obstacle, the right atrium, as opposed to a small obstacle like the AV node. One of the distinguishing features of atrial flutter is an atrial rate that typically fixed over time. The ventricular rate will be a whole number ratio of the atrial rate ***(see Figure 1)*** and named accordingly ***(see Figure 2)***. Treatment with AV nodal blockade (eg, vagal maneuvers, adenosine, etc.) will affect the ventricular rate but not the atrial rate and can be used diagnostically to differentiate between flutter and other NCTs.

Figure 1.
The lead II rhythm strip shows a flutter rate (210 msec) is exactly twice the ventricular rate (420 msec), consistent with atrial flutter with 2:1 conduction

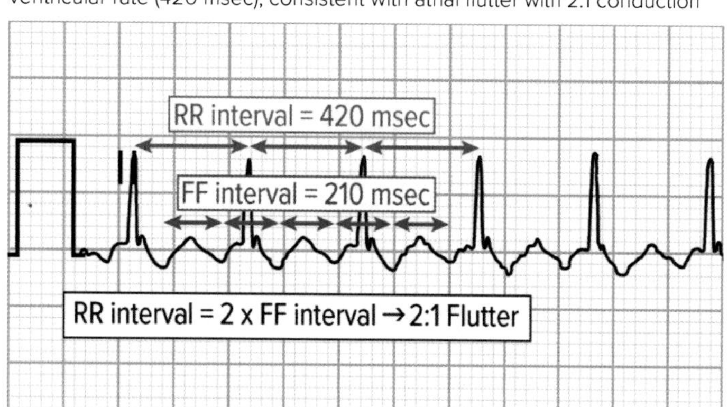

Figure 2.
The lead II rhythm strip shows 2 flutter waves per QRS complex consistent with atrial flutter with 2:1 conduction

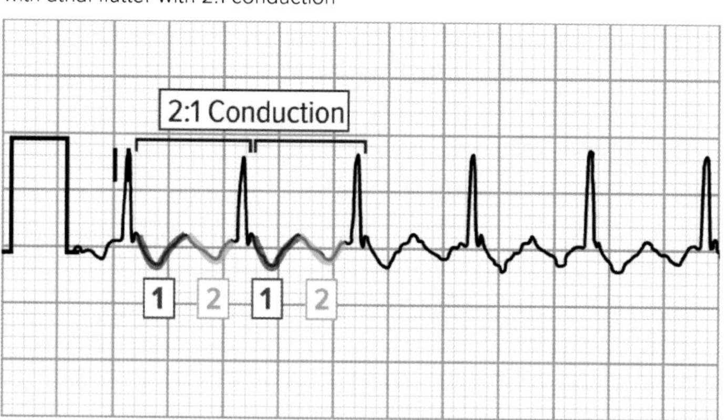

The ECG also shows STE in lead aVR +/- lead V1 with diffuse STD. The differential diagnosis for this pattern includes both ACS and non-ACS etiologies:

ACS causes[1]	Non-ACS causes[2]
• LMCA insufficiency (can see STE aVR > V1)	• Acute and/or severe anemia
• Prox LAD insufficiency (can see STE V1 > aVR)	• Aortic dissection
• Triple vessel disease	• LBBB and ventricular-paced rhythms
• Global cardiac ischemia	• LVH with strain pattern
• Prinzmetal angina	• Pulmonary embolism
	• ROSC s/p epinephrine or defibrillation
	• Severe hypokalemia or hyperkalemia
	• Sodium channel blockade
	• Supraventricular tachycardia (especially with rapid rates)

Although the pattern of STE in lead aVR +/- lead V1 with diffuse STD is discussed in the cardiology literature, its clinical significance is not without some controversy. This is likely due to the broad differential diagnosis associated with this pattern that includes both ACS and non-ACS causes. The 2018 Fourth Universal Definition of MI states "ST-segment depression ≥ 1 mm in 6 or more leads, which may be associated with ST segment elevation in leads aVR and/or V1 and hemodynamic compromise, is suggestive of multivessel disease or left main disease" but does not provide specific management recommendations.

Treatment should be guided by the underlying etiology, and it is imperative to consider both ACS and non-ACS causes. For patients suspected of having an ACS cause, this ECG pattern is highly suggestive of LMCA insufficiency, proximal LAD insufficiency, or triple vessel disease. So, while this pattern does not meet "traditional" STEMI criteria, it can represent high-risk ACS, including possible acute coronary occlusion, in the correct clinical context, and immediate angiography should be considered. Whether this is done by emergent cardiology consultation or activation of the cardiac catheterization lab depends on local practice preferences.

In this case, the pattern of STE in lead aVR +/- lead V1 with diffuse STD is likely due to the abnormal conduction associated with the supraventricular tachycardia. The ECG changes alone do not constitute a "failed stress test" and the decision to evaluate for ischemia that caused, or was caused by, the tachydysrhythmia should be a clinical one.

This patient's history of heart failure with a severely reduced EF played a significant role in determining treatment. Her workup was notable for a chest X-ray showing pulmonary edema consistent with a CHF exacerbation likely secondary to the tachycardia induced decrease in cardiac output (recall that CO = SV x HR). The initial ventricular rate of 143 bpm did not allow for adequate filling time which reduces the already poor baseline stroke volume. Slowing the rate down should improve the SV but ultimately this contribution is limited by the patient's poor baseline EF. It only makes sense to rate control this patient if the increase in SV improves the CO more than the decreased HR worsens the CO. Another important consideration is that patients with very low EF are often dependent on the atrial kick to maximize their CO. This patient was electrically cardioverted back to sinus rhythm and admitted to the cardiology service.

Atrial Flutter Learning Points

- Due to a re-entrant circuit in the right atrium
- Stereotypical sawtooth pattern of P-waves seen best in the inferior leads
  - Absence of isoelectric baseline (eg, TP segment) in lead II
- Atrial rate is 250-350 bpm and typically fixed over time
  - Ventricular rate is a fraction of atrial rate (ie, for an atrial rate of 300 bpm, 2:1 conduction produces a ventricular rate of 150 bpm, 3:1 conduction produces a ventricular rate of 100 bmp, 4:1 conduction produces a ventricular rate of 75 bpm, etc.)
- Consider atrial flutter when ventricular rate is consistently around 150 bpm
- Vagal maneuvers or adenosine will slow ventricular rate but have no effect on flutter waves

Lead aVR Learning Points

- Lead aVR views the right upper portion of the heart including the basal part of the septum
- STE in lead aVR +/- V1 with diffuse STD ≥ 1 mm in ≥ 6 leads can be due to ACS or non-ACS etiologies; therefore, always consider the clinical context when considering the differential diagnosis
- In ACS presentations, this pattern is highly suggestive of LMCA obstruction, proximal LAD obstruction, and triple vessel disease, and immediate angiography should be considered[3]
- In non-ACS causes, the ECG changes should resolve with treatment of non-ACS cause
- Anterior or inferior MI with STE > 1 mm in lead aVR are associated with an increased 30-day mortality[4]

References

1. Thygesen K, Alpert JS, Jaffe AS, et al. 2018 ESC/ACC/AHA/WHF Expert Consensus Document: Fourth Universal Definition of Myocardial Infarction (2018). Circulation. 2018;138:e618-e651.
2. Mattu A. ECG Weekly.
3. Writing Committee, et al. 2013 ACCF/AHA Guideline for the Management of ST-Elevation Myocardial Infarction: A Report of the American College of Cardiology Foundation/American Heart Association Task Force on Practice Guidelines. Circulation. 2013;127:e362-e425.
4. Wong CK, Gao W, Stewart RA, Benatar J, French JK, Aylward PE,White HD; HERO-2 Investigators. aVR ST elevation: an important but neglected sign in ST elevation acute myocardial infarction. Eur Heart J. 2010;31:1845–1853.

Case 28: Presentation

A 62-year-old male presents to the emergency department with severe substernal chest pain. What is your interpretation of his ECG?

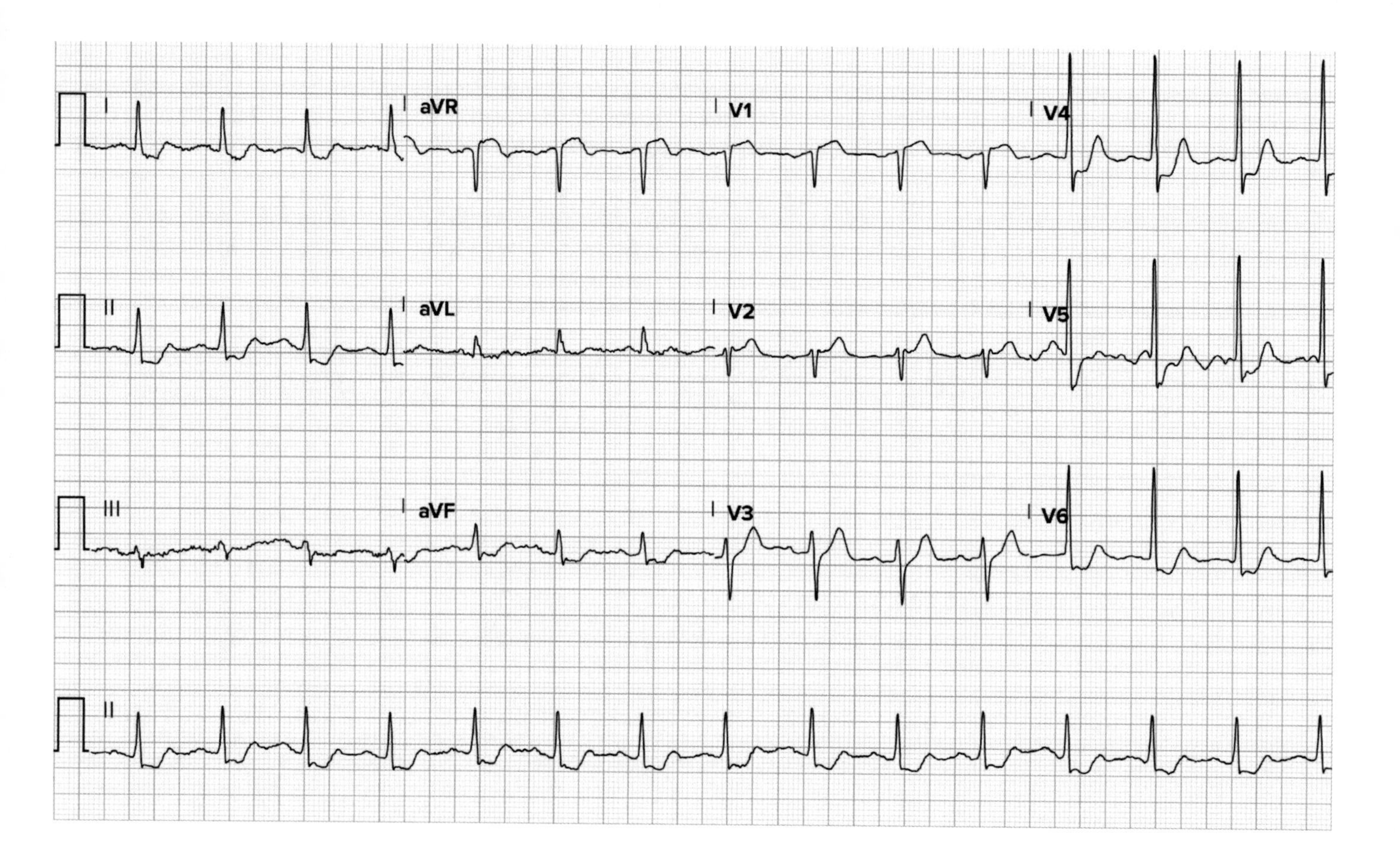

Case 28: Answer

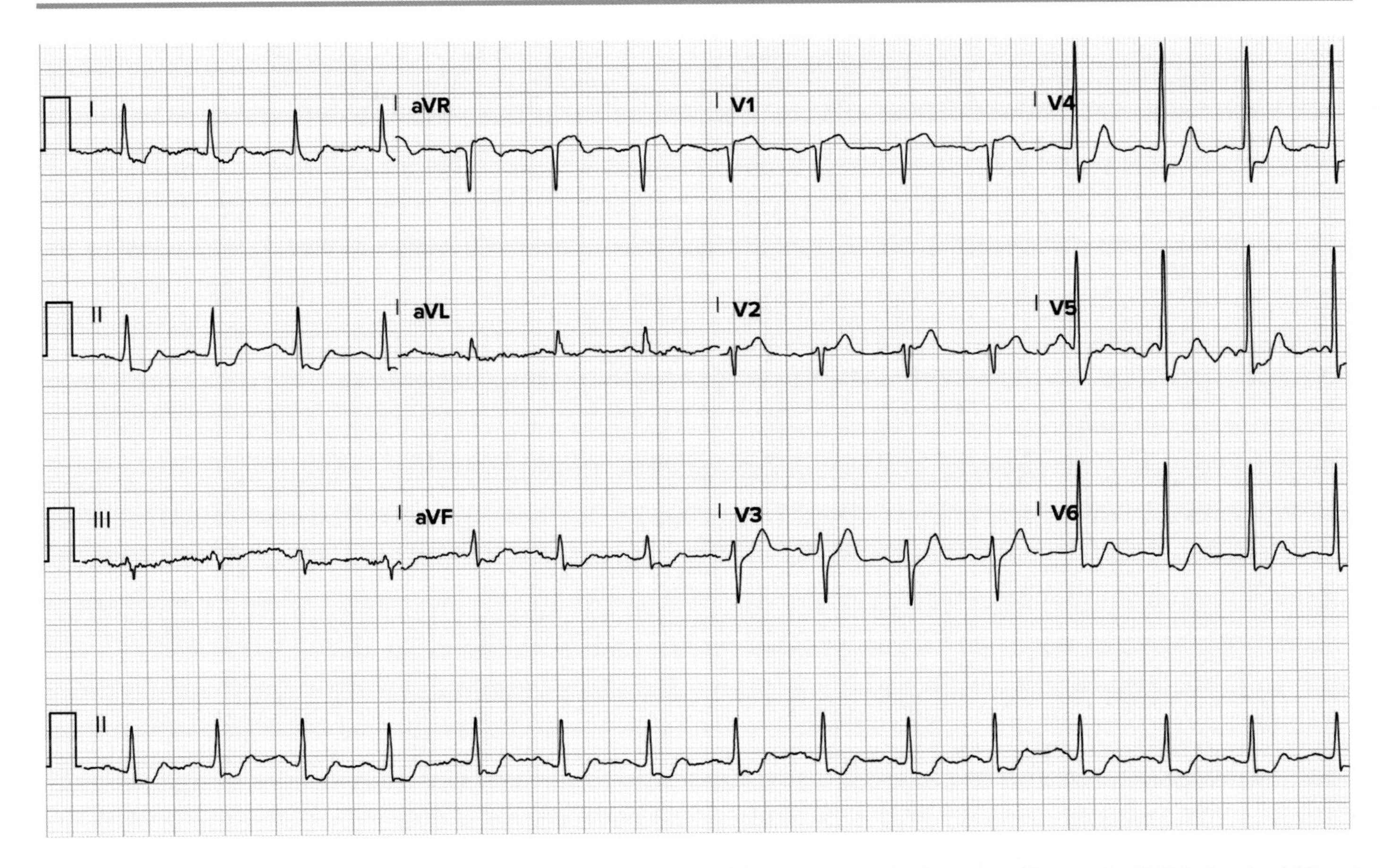

This ECG shows a normal sinus rhythm with a ventricular rate of 89 bpm, normal axis, normal intervals, STE in leads aVR and V1, and STD in leads I, II, III, aVF, and V3-V6.

The differential diagnosis for the pattern of STE in lead aVR +/- lead V1 with diffuse STD includes both ACS and non-ACS etiologies:

ACS causes[1]	Non-ACS causes[2]
• LMCA insufficiency (can see STE aVR > V1)	• Acute and/or severe anemia
• Prox LAD insufficiency (can see STE V1 > aVR)	• Aortic dissection
• Triple vessel disease	• LBBB and ventricular-paced rhythms
• Global cardiac ischemia	• LVH with strain pattern
• Prinzmetal angina	• Pulmonary embolism
	• ROSC s/p epinephrine or defibrillation
	• Severe hypokalemia or hyperkalemia
	• Sodium channel blockade
	• Supraventricular tachycardia (especially with rapid rates)

Although the pattern of STE in lead aVR +/- lead V1 with diffuse STD is discussed in the cardiology literature, its clinical significance is not without some controversy. This is likely due to the broad differential diagnosis associated with this pattern that includes both ACS and non-ACS causes. The 2018 Fourth Universal Definition of MI states "ST-segment depression ≥ 1 mm in 6 or more leads, which may be associated with ST-segment elevation in leads aVR and/or V1 and hemodynamic compromise, is suggestive of multivessel disease or left main disease" but does not provide specific management recommendations.

Treatment should be guided by the underlying etiology, and it is imperative to consider both ACS and non-ACS causes. For patients suspected of having an ACS cause, this ECG pattern is highly suggestive of LMCA insufficiency, proximal LAD insufficiency, or triple vessel disease. So, while this pattern does not meet "traditional" STEMI criteria, it can represent high-risk ACS, including possible acute coronary occlusion, in the correct clinical context, and immediate angiography should be considered. Whether this is done by emergent cardiology consultation or activation of the cardiac catheterization lab depends on local practice preferences.

This patient had resolution of his symptoms after nitroglycerin and a repeat ECG showed resolution of the abnormalities seen on his presenting ECG. The case was discussed with cardiology and he was taken urgently (ie, within 2 hours) to the catheterization laboratory. The patient's initial ECG showed STE in leads aVR > V1 which suggests the LMCA as the culprit artery, but the cardiac catheterization showed a 90% mid-LAD lesion.

Lead aVR Learning Points

- Lead aVR views the right upper portion of the heart including the basal part of the septum
- STE in lead aVR +/- V1 with diffuse STD ≥ 1 mm in ≥ 6 leads can be due to ACS or non-ACS etiologies; therefore, always consider the clinical context when considering the differential diagnosis
- In ACS presentations, this pattern is highly suggestive of LMCA obstruction, proximal LAD obstruction, and triple vessel disease, and immediate angiography should be considered[3]
- In non-ACS causes, the ECG changes should resolve with treatment of non-ACS cause
- Anterior or inferior MI with STE > 1 mm in lead aVR are associated with an increased 30-day mortality[4]

References

1. Thygesen K, Alpert JS, Jaffe AS, et al. 2018 ESC/ACC/AHA/WHF Expert Consensus Document: Fourth Universal Definition of Myocardial Infarction (2018). Circulation. 2018;138:e618-e651.
2. Mattu A. ECG Weekly.
3. Writing Committee, et al. 2013 ACCF/AHA Guideline for the Management of ST-Elevation Myocardial Infarction: A Report of the American College of Cardiology Foundation/American Heart Association Task Force on Practice Guidelines. Circulation. 2013;127:e362-e425.
4. Wong CK, Gao W, Stewart RA, Benatar J, French JK, Aylward PE,White HD; HERO-2 Investigators. aVR ST elevation: an important but neglected sign in ST elevation acute myocardial infarction. Eur Heart J. 2010;31:1845–1853.

NOTES:

Case 29: Presentation

A 64-year-old female with history of atrial fibrillation presents with chest pain. What is your interpretation of her ECG?

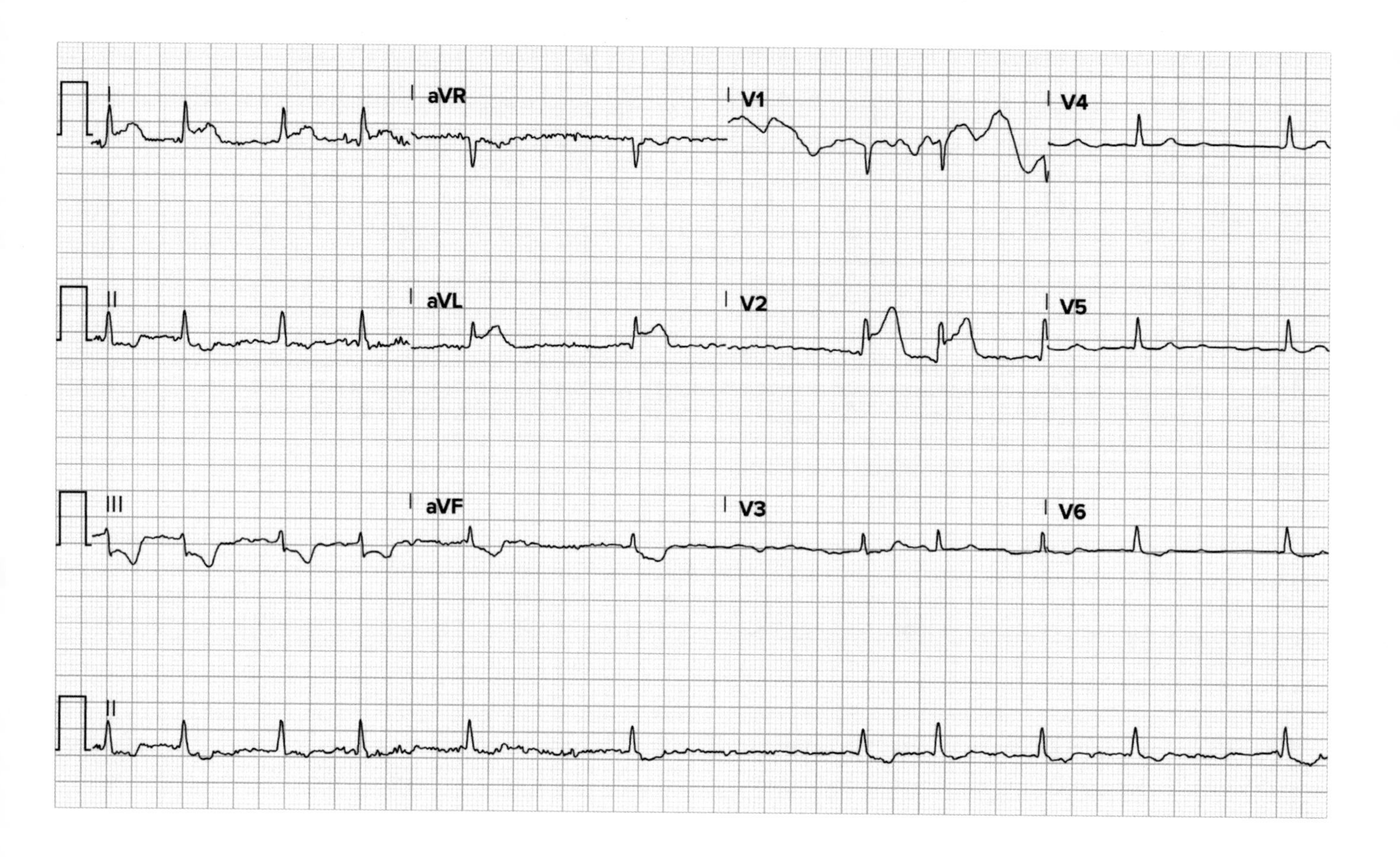

Case 29: Answer

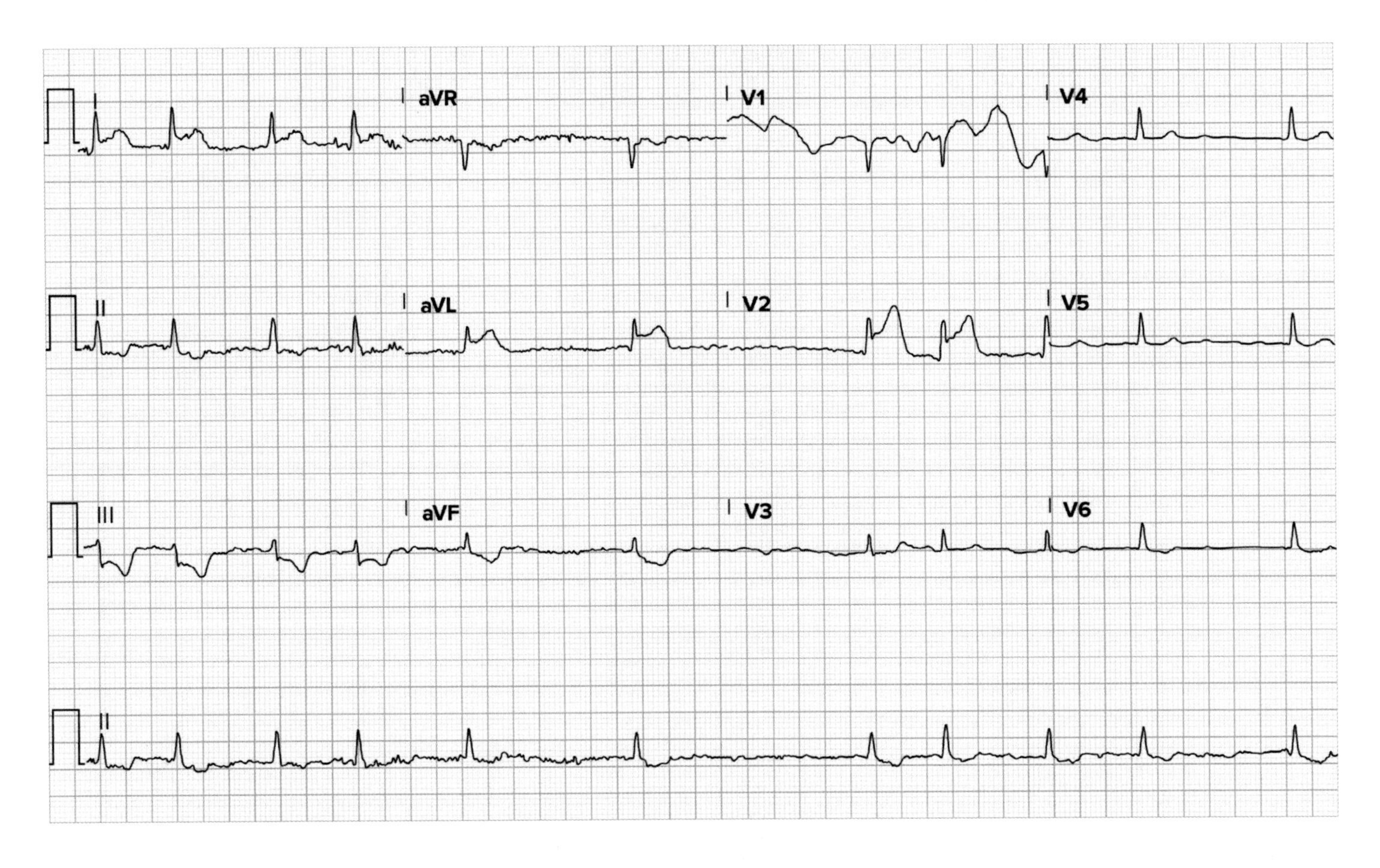

This ECG shows atrial fibrillation with an average ventricular rate of 77 bpm, normal axis, normal QRS complex and QTc interval durations, STE in leads I, aVL, and V2, STD with TWI in leads II, III, and aVF, and artifact in lead V1 that confounds the interpretation of ST-T changes in this lead.

This pattern of STE and STD in this ECG is consistent with a high lateral MI. The culprit artery is typically the 1st diagonal branch of the LAD. This pattern is sometimes called the South African Flag sign because the leads that show STE (leads I, aVL, and V2) and STD (lead III) fit into the central green coloration of the South African flag ***(see Figure 1)***. Note that there will usually be STD in lead aVF as well.

Figure 1.
The South African Flag sign: the leads that show STE (leads I, aVL, and V2) and STD (lead III) fit into the central green coloration of the South African flag

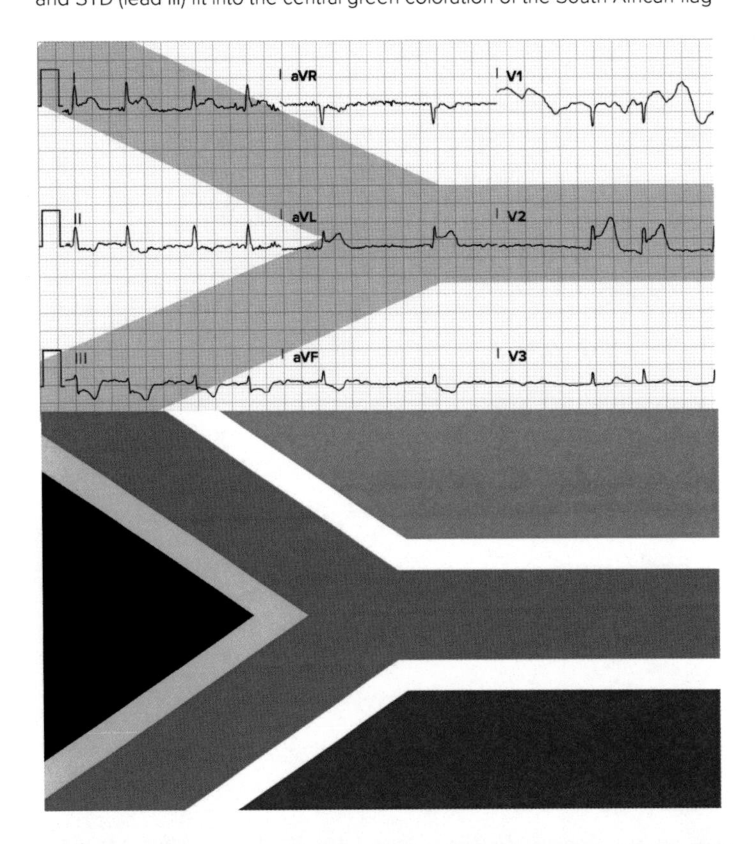

While this ECG meets STEMI criteria in leads I and aVL, occlusions of the 1st diagonal often result in minimal STE in lead I. In these cases, it is important to recognize that STE in leads aVL and V2 with STD in lead III is consistent with an occlusion of the 1st diagonal even though it does not meet traditional STEMI criteria since lead V2 is not considered contiguous with lead aVL. It is important to note that significant STE that does not meet the traditional distribution (ie, ≥ 2 anatomically contiguous leads) may still represent acute coronary artery occlusion and warrant consideration for emergent coronary reperfusion.

This patient was taken to the cardiac catheterization laboratory where a 100% occlusion of the 1st diagonal branch of the LAD (also denoted as D1) was successfully treated with a stent.

STEMI Learning Points

- STEMI is defined by new, or presumed new, STE at the J point in ≥ 2 anatomically contiguous leads in the absence of
- LVH by voltage pattern, LBBB, or ventricular-paced rhythm
  - ≥ 2.5 mm in men < 40 years old and ≥ 2 mm in men ≥ 40 years old in leads V2-V3 (or an increase of ≥ 1 mm when compared to baseline ECG)
  - ≥ 1.5 mm in women in leads V2-V3 (or an increase of ≥ 1 mm when compared to baseline ECG)
  - ≥ 1 mm in all other leads
- ST-segment is measured from the isoelectric baseline, typically the TP segment (see below)
- Reciprocal STD are not required for the diagnosis of STEMI, but their presence does increase the likelihood of the diagnosis of STEMI
  - Reciprocal STD are only present in 70% of anterior MI1
- Posterior MI
  - Consider whenever there is STD in leads V1-V4
  - STE ≥ 0.5 mm in posterior leads V7, V8 or V9 is diagnostic- does not require 2 contiguous leads
- Right ventricular MI
  - Consider with any inferior MI (RV MI is seen in approximately 1/3 of inferior MI)
  - STE in right precordial leads V3R and V4R ≥ 0.5 mm (≥ 1 mm for men ≤ 30 years old)
  - STE in right precordial lead V4R > 1 mm is most predictive of RV MI
  - STE in right precordial lead V4R > STE in leads V1-V3 = highly specific for RV MI
- Significant STE that does not meet the traditional distribution (ie, ≥ 2 anatomically contiguous leads) in a presentation concerning for ACS may still represent coronary artery occlusion and warrant consideration for emergent coronary reperfusion

How to Measure STE per most recent 2018 AHA Guidelines[2]

- The J point is the junction between QRS termination and ST-segment onset and is used to determine the magnitude of the ST-segment shift
- **In patients with a stable baseline, the TP segment (isoelectric interval) is a more accurate method to assess the magnitude of ST-segment shift *(see Figure 2)***, and in distinguishing pericarditis from acute myocardial ischemia
- QRS onset should be used if TP segment does not have a stable baseline ***(see Figure 3)***
- Measurement should be made from the top of the ECG line tracing

Figure 2.
Measure STE from the TP segment if the TP segment is isoelectric (ie, horizontal)

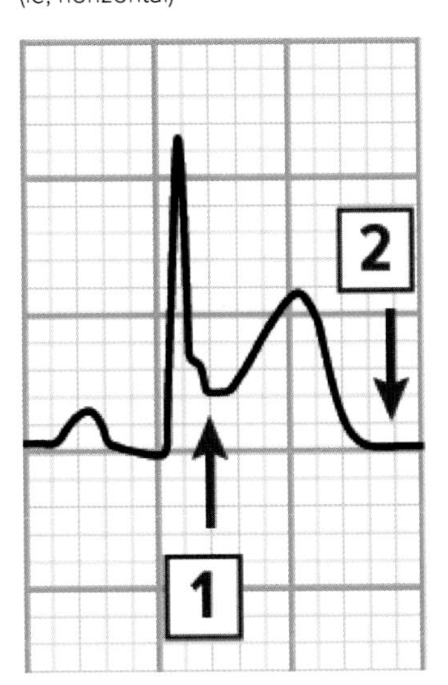

Arrow 1: onset of the ST-segment (ie, J point)
Arrow 2: TP segment

Figure 3.
Measure STE from onset of the QRS complex if the TP segment is not isoelectric (ie, not horizontal)

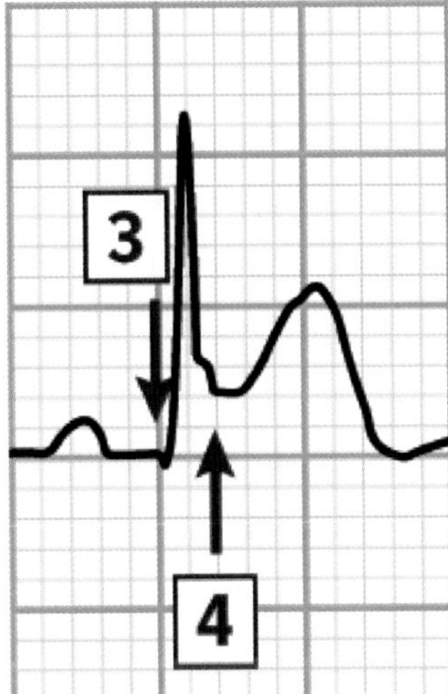

Arrow 3: initial onset of the Q-wave
Arrow 4: onset of the ST-segment (ie, J point)

References

1. 1. Knilans T, Surawicz B. Chou's Electrocardiography in Clinical Practice. Philadelphia, PA: Elsevier. 2020.
2. 2. Thygesen K, Alpert JS, Jaffe AS, et al. 2018 ESC/ACC/AHA/WHF Expert Consensus Document: Fourth Universal Definition of Myocardial Infarction (2018). Circulation. 2018;138:e618-e651.

Case 30: Presentation

A 19-year-old female with no past medical history presents after a syncopal episode at work.
She denies any prodromal symptoms or similar episodes in the past.
What is your interpretation of her ECG

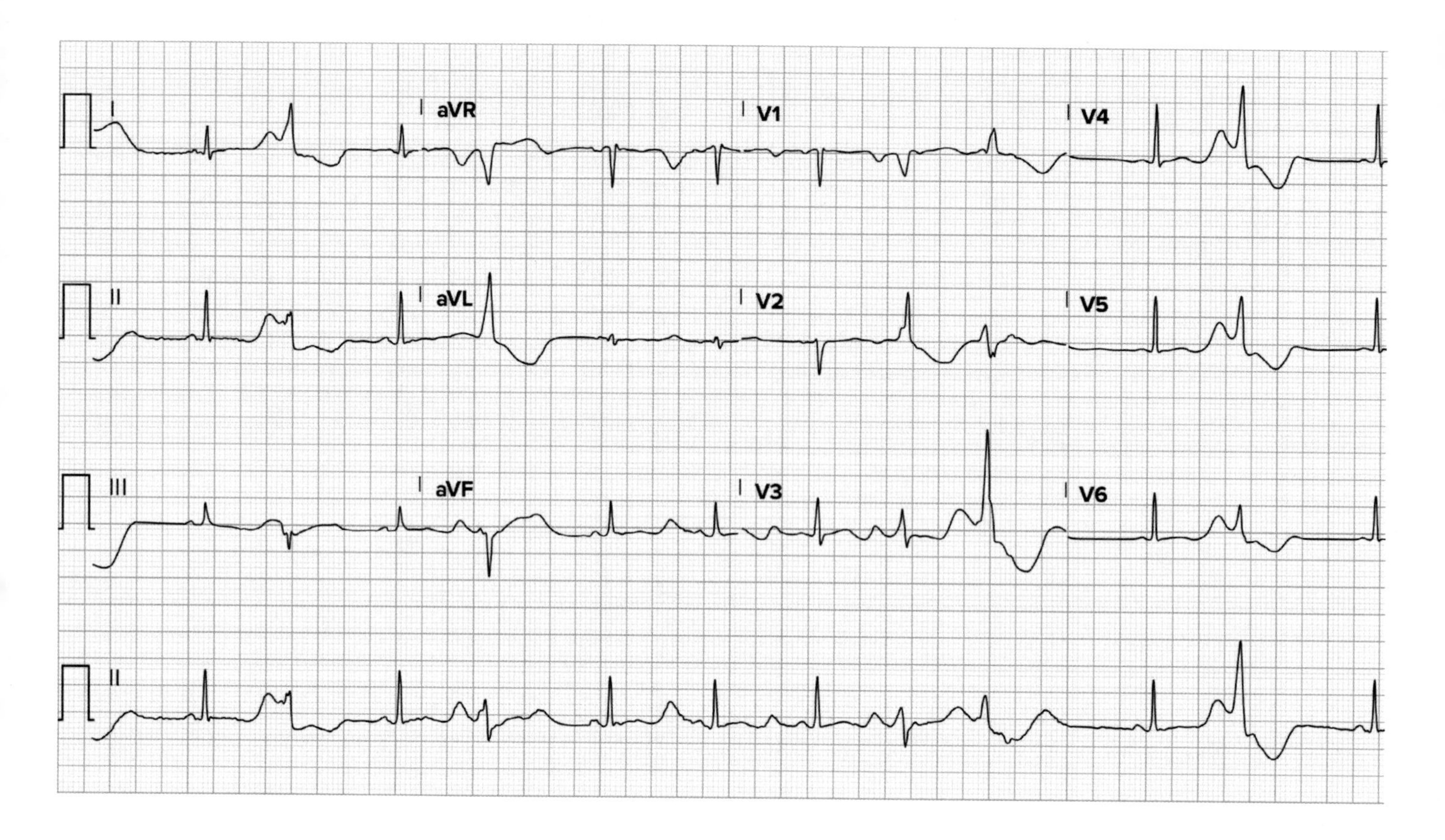

Case 30: Answer

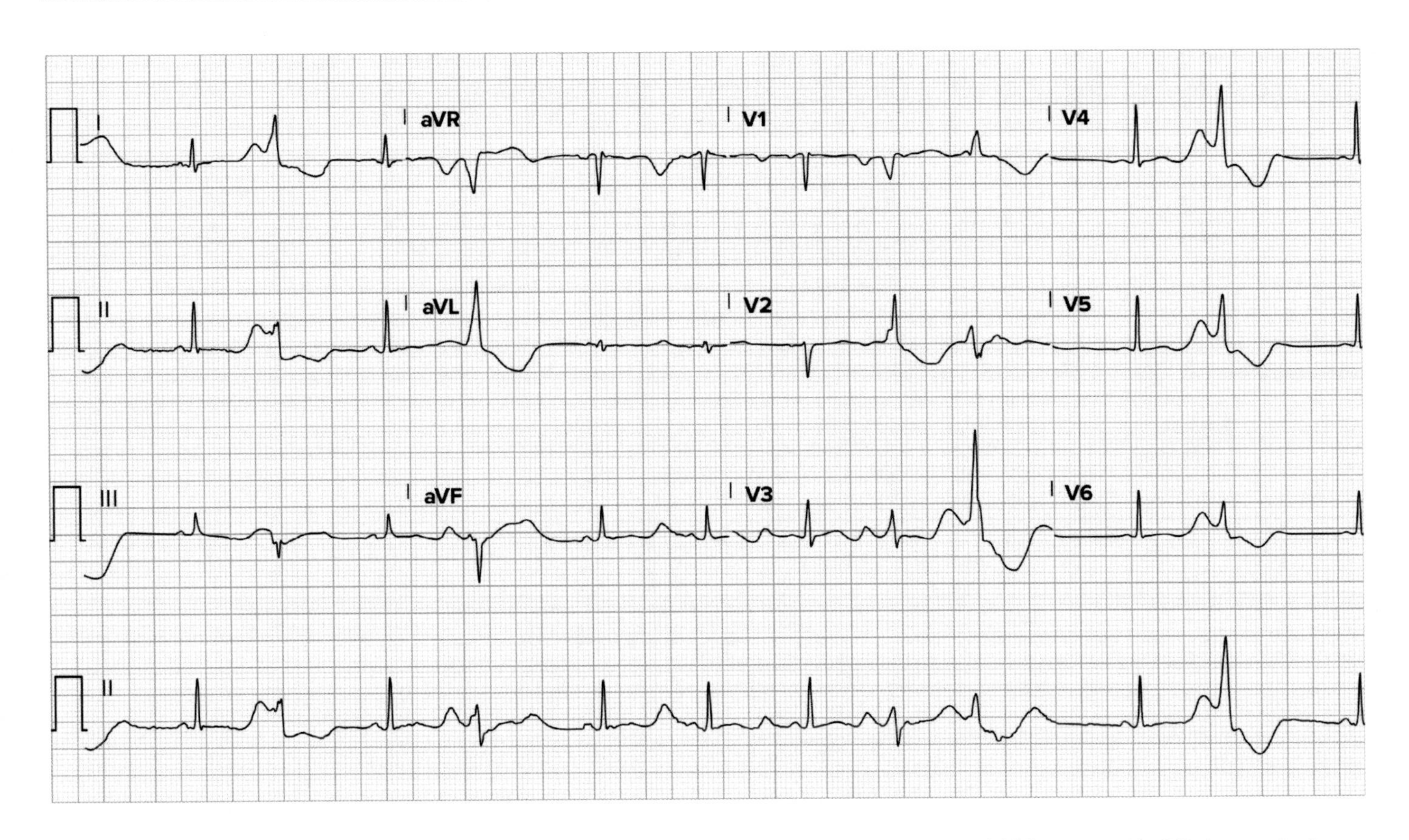

This ECG shows a normal sinus rhythm at 73 bpm, normal axis, prolonged QT interval of 600 msec with QTc interval of 623-662 msec (depending on which formula is used), and frequent multifocal PVCs including a multifocal PVC couplet.

ECG findings to look for in syncope patients include:

- Ischemia/infarct
- Severe bradycardia or tachycardia
- Conduction abnormalities (eg, AV blocks)
- Low voltage +/- electrical alternans
- Syncope syndromes:
  - ARVD/ARVC
  - Brugada
  - HCM
  - QT syndromes (long and short)
  - WPW

The differential diagnosis for a prolonged QTc interval includes:

- Cardiac ischemia
- Elevated intracranial pressure
- Hypocalcemia
- Hypokalemia
- Hypomagnesemia
- Hypothermia
- Long QT syndrome
- Medications

The most significant abnormality in this ECG is the prolonged QTc interval. Per the 2009 AHA/ACCF/HRS guidelines[1], the QT interval should be measured in the lead with longest QT (typically lead V2 or V3) and cutoffs for adults are ≥ 460 msec for women and ≥ 450 msec for men. There is no consensus recommendation for which formula should be used to calculate the QTc interval.

Long QT Syndrome (LQTS) can be congenital or acquired and the increased QTc interval increases the risk of torsades de pointes (TdP). TdP is a type of polymorphic ventricular tachycardia associated with a prolonged QTc interval on baseline ECG. It is triggered when a PVC occurs at the same time as the T-wave associated with the previous QRS complex (called "R-on-T phenomenon"). One of the key differences in the two types of LQTS is the treatment. Magnesium and electrical overdrive pacing can be used for both, but chemical overdrive pacing, typically with isoproterenol, should only be used for acquired LQTS. Congenital LQTS is considered "adrenergic dependent" and patients will often be on beta-blockers for dysrhythmia prevention, so the use of a beta agonist like isoproterenol is contraindicated.

This ECG also shows multiple PVCs, including multiform couplets and some with R-on-T phenomenon ***(see Figure 1).*** Premature beats, which include PACs, PJCs, and PVCs, are generally defined as QRS complexes that occur earlier than expected due to either altered impulse formation or altered impulse conduction. The nomenclature for PVCs is discussed below in the Learning Points.

Figure 1.
The lead II rhythm strip shows a prolonged QT interval, R-on-T PVCs, and a multifocal PVC couplet

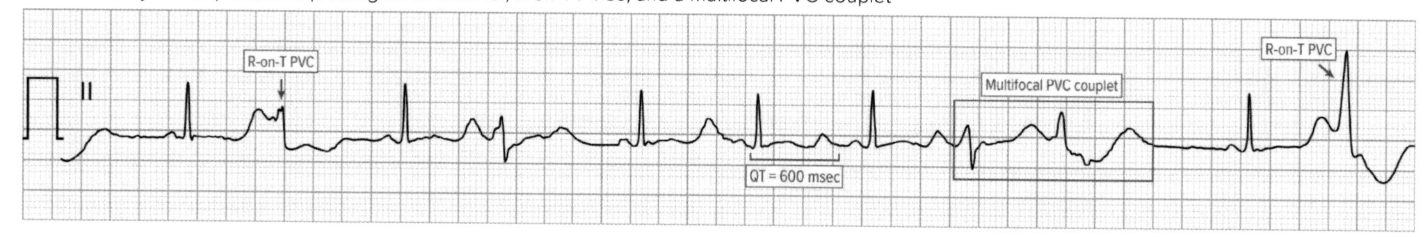

This patient was not on any medications and had an unremarkable ED workup. A repeat ECG was obtained ***(see Figure 2),*** which showed worsening ectopy and impending TdP. The patient was admitted to the cardiology service for AICD placement.

Figure 2.
Repeat ECG showing worsening ectopy

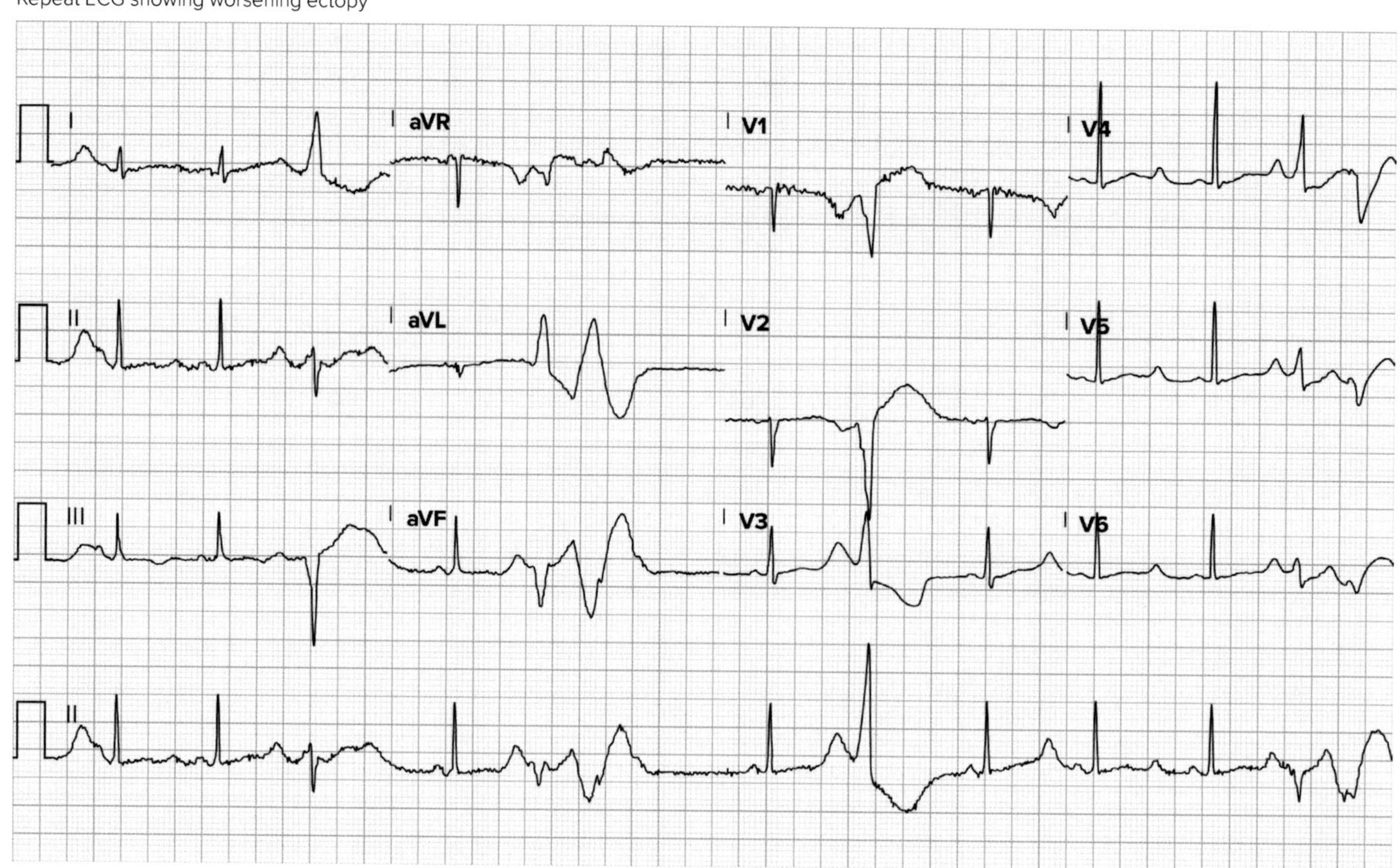

An important pattern that is associated with a prolonged QTc interval is T-wave alternans (not seen in this case). T-wave alternans is the beat-to-beat alternation of the duration, morphology, and/or polarity of the T-wave ***(see Figure 3)*** not related to alternans of other components of the ECG (ie, QRS complex alternans). It is a marker of myocardial electrical instability and impending ventricular dysrhythmia. T-wave alternans is frequently associated with a long QTc interval that is caused by electrolyte abnormalities (eg, hypokalemia, hypocalcemia), treatment with quinidine, and congenital LQTS.[2]

When seen with a long QTc interval, T-wave alternans is considered a precursor to torsades de pointes. It can also be seen in the absence of a long QTc interval, often with myocardial ischemia and both ischemic and non-ischemic cardiomyopathies, in which cases it often precedes ventricular tachycardia and/or ventricular fibrillation.

Figure 3.
Beat-to-beat alteration in the morphology of the T-waves, consistent with T-wave alternans (not from case ECG)

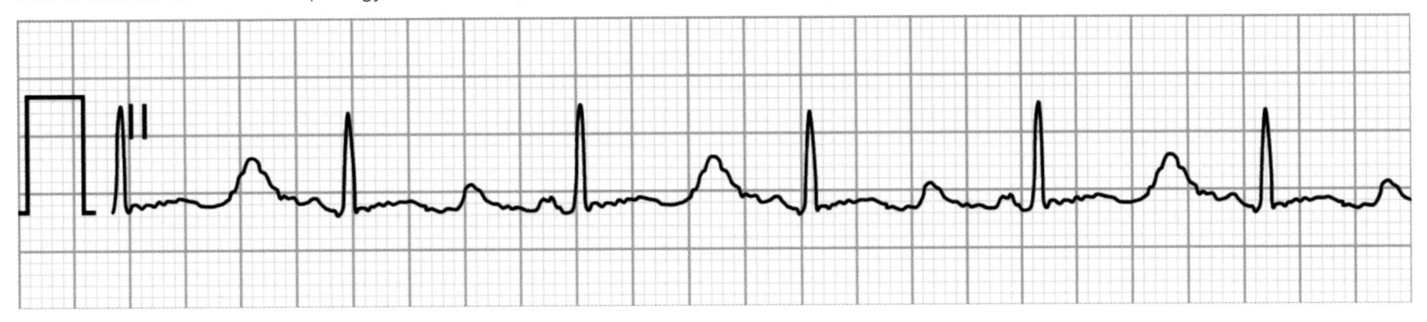

Long QT Syndrome Learning Points

- Congenital or acquired
  - Common acquired etiologies include electrolyte abnormalities (hypokalemia, hypomagnesemia, hypocalcemia), medications, hypothermia, ischemia, elevated ICP
- Prolonged QTc interval is defined as ≥ 460 msec for women and ≥ 450 msec for men
  - QT interval should be measured in the lead with the longest QT interval, usually lead V2 or V3
  - If U-waves superimposed on T-waves are present, measure QT interval in a lead without U-waves, usually lead aVR or aVL
  - Validate computer generated QTc interval with visual inspection of serial ECGs
- Increased risk for torsades typically occurs with QTc > 500 msec
  - AICD is recommended if no reversible cause is found
  - Presence of T-wave alternans = increased risk for ventricular dysrhythmias

PVC Learning Points

- Wide-complex (≥120 msec) premature beat from a ventricular focus with no preceding P-wave
  - Unifocal: arising from a single ectopic focus, so each PVC is identical in any single lead
  - Multifocal: arising from ≥ 2 ectopic foci, so multiple PVC morphologies in any single lead
  - Usually followed by compensatory pause
- Patterns include:
  - Bigeminy: every other beat is a PVC
  - Trigeminy: every 3rd beat is a PVC
  - Quadrigeminy: every 4th beat is a PVC
  - Couplet: two consecutive PVCs
  - Triplet: three consecutive PVCs
- Clinical significance includes:
  - Right ventricular PVCs: LBBB-like morphology, not necessarily pathologic
  - Left ventricular PVCs: RBBB-like morphology, usually pathologic, more likely to precipitate ventricular fibrillation
  - R-on-T PVC: PVC falls on T-wave of normal beat and can precipitate ventricular fibrillation

References

1. Rautaharju PM, Surawicz B, Gettes LS. AHA/ACCF/HRS recommendations for the standardization and interpretation of the electrocardiogram, part IV: the ST segment, T and U waves, and the QT interval: a scientific statement from the American Heart Association Electrocardiography and Arrhythmias Committee, Council on Clinical Cardiology; the American College of Cardiology Foundation; and the Heart Rhythm Society. Circulation. 2009;119:e241– e250.
2. Knilans T, Surawicz B. Chou's Electrocardiography in Clinical Practice. Philadelphia, PA: Elsevier. 2020.

Case 31: Presentation

A 65-year-old male with known DVT on warfarin with recent subtherapeutic INR presents with SOB and chest pain. Notable vital signs include a respiratory rate of 24 and an oxygen saturation of 83%. What is your interpretation of his ECG?

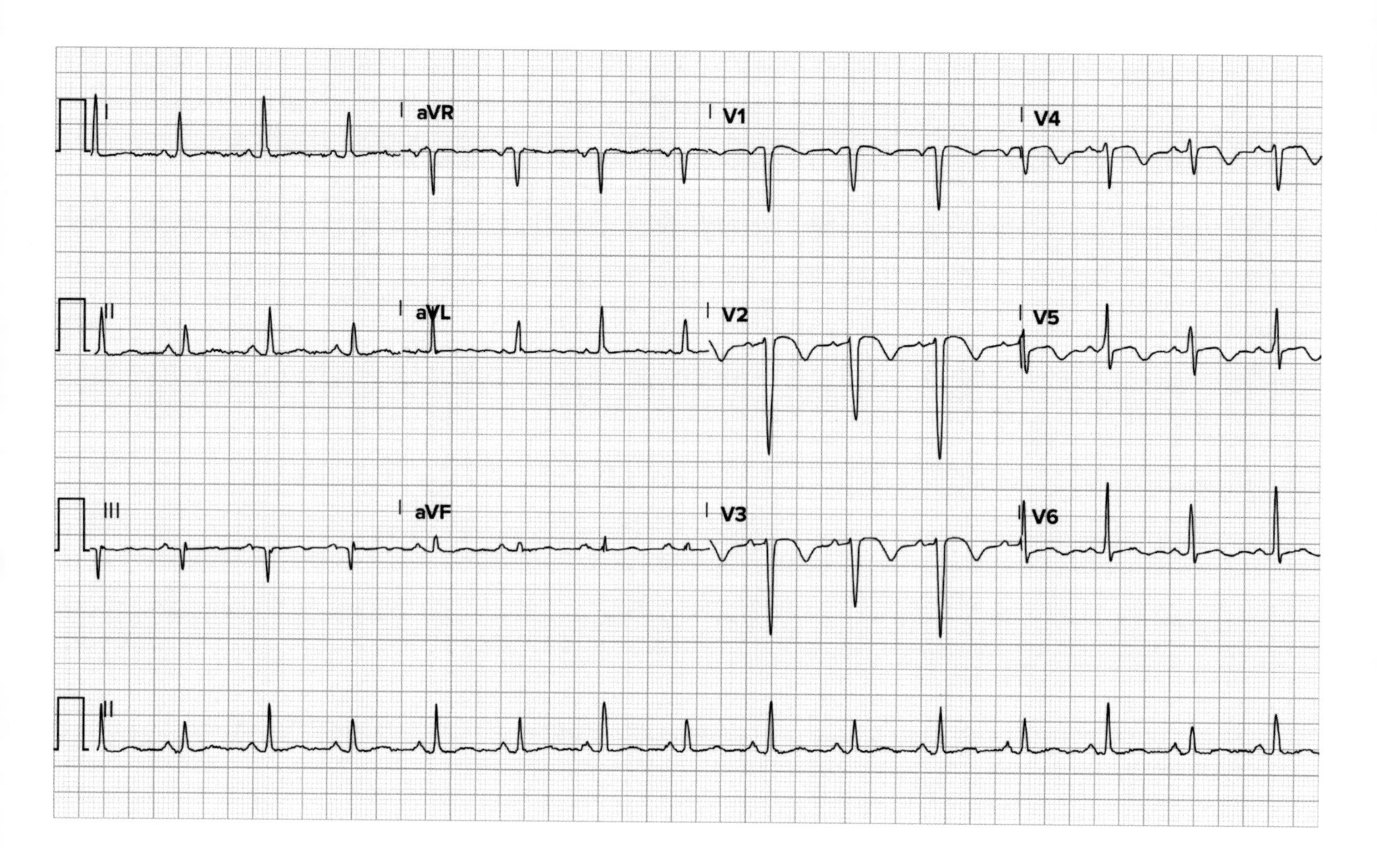

Case 31: Answer

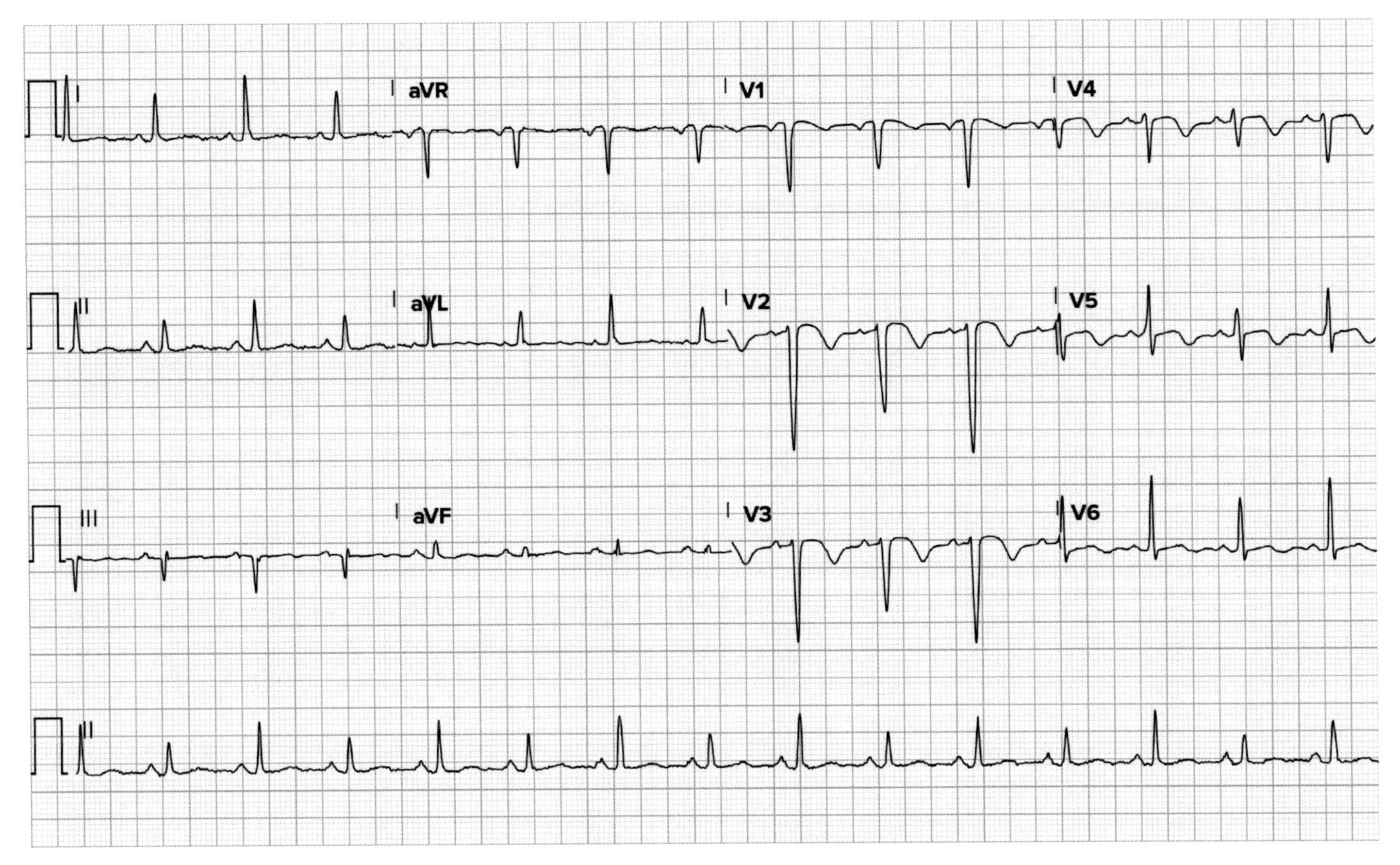

This ECG shows a normal sinus rhythm at 88 bpm, normal axis, normal intervals, STE in leads V1-V3, TWI in leads V1-V5, and electrical alternans.

Although this patient's ECG shows STE in leads V1-V3, his history and vital sign abnormalities are highly suggestive of pulmonary embolism as the cause of his symptoms. A bedside echo showed moderate right heart strain with no pericardial effusion, and a subsequent CTA showed a submassive PE. Sending this patient to the catheterization laboratory for chest pain and STE in leads V1-V3 could have been problematic and demonstrates the importance of considering the non-ACS causes of STE in the context of a patient's history and exam.

The ECG findings in PE (see Learning Points below) are varied and neither sensitive nor specific. This ECG shows TWI in leads V1-V3, which is one of the more specific ECG findings in PE, and normal sinus rhythm, which is the most common rhythm seen with PE.

The other important finding in this ECG is electrical alternans ***(see Figure 1).***

Figure 1.
The lead II rhythm strip shows beat-to-beat variability in the QRS complex amplitude consistent with electrical alternans

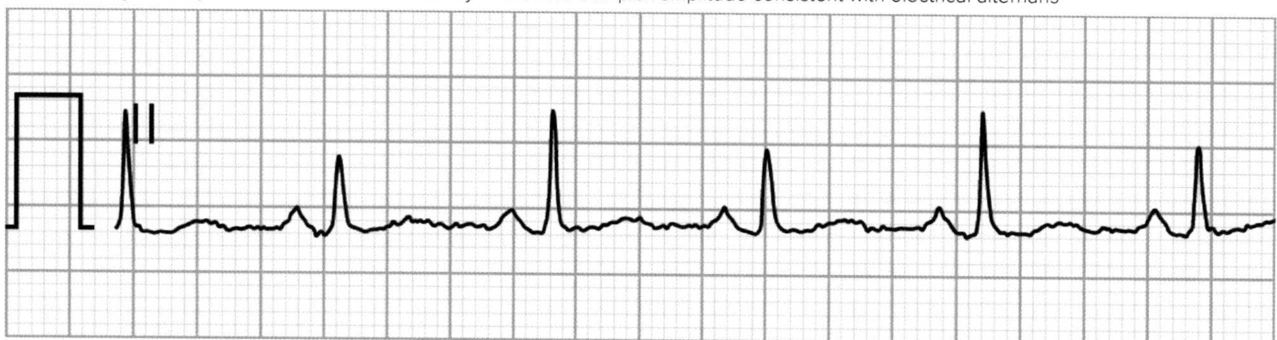

The term "alternans" is used to describe beat-to-beat variability in morphology or timing of any wave, interval, or segment on an ECG. For example, T-wave alternans refers to the variability in the T-wave axis seen with long QT syndrome that precedes degeneration into a ventricular dysrhythmia. Electrical alternans is commonly used to describe variability in QRS morphology/axis and can be the result of mechanical or electrophysiologic abnormalities. "Pseudoelectrical alternans" is sometimes used if the cause is not mechanical in nature. The most common mechanical cause of electrical alternans is pericardial effusion, which causes the heart to swing back and forth in the pericardial sac resulting in changing QRS amplitudes on ECG. Electrophysiologic causes include rate-related bundle branch blocks and AVNRT.

This patient was started on heparin after the bedside echo. Notable lab abnormalities included a mildly elevated troponin and BNP. The patient's hypoxia corrected with a non-rebreather and BiPAP was avoided due to concern that it could lead to decreased venous return in the setting of preload dependence. The patient became progressively more hypotensive and was ultimately taken for emergent catheter directed thrombolysis.

ECG in PE Learning Points

- ECG is neither sensitive nor specific for PE
  - No single ECG criterion is diagnostic- ECG can only suggest diagnosis
  - Most common ECG rhythm is sinus
  - Most common ECG abnormality is T-wave abnormalities
  - Most common ECG rhythm abnormality is sinus tachycardia
- ECG findings in PE include:
  - Non-specific ST-segment/T-wave changes +/- sinus tachycardia
  - TWI in leads V1-V4 +/- inferior leads (highly specific)
  - STE in lead V1 or aVR
  - Small Q-wave with prominent R-wave in lead V1
  - Large S-wave in lead I and/or aVL
  - RBBB (complete or incomplete)
  - Right axis deviation
  - R/S transition point shift towards lead V6
  - STE, Qr, or Qs pattern in leads V4R- V6R
  - S1Q3T3: poor sensitivity/specificity (found in ~10% of PE patients and ~10% of patients with RV strain unrelated to PE)

Electrical Alternans Learning Points

- Beat-to-beat variability in morphology or timing of any wave, interval, or segment on an ECG
  - Can be due to either mechanical or electrophysiologic abnormalities
- Effusion/tamponade is an echocardiographic diagnosis and can only be suggested by ECG
- Alternans + low voltage = pericardial effusion until proven otherwise

References

1. Mattu A. ECG Weekly.

NOTES:

Case 32: Presentation

A 39-year-old male presents with chest pain. What is your interpretation of his ECG?

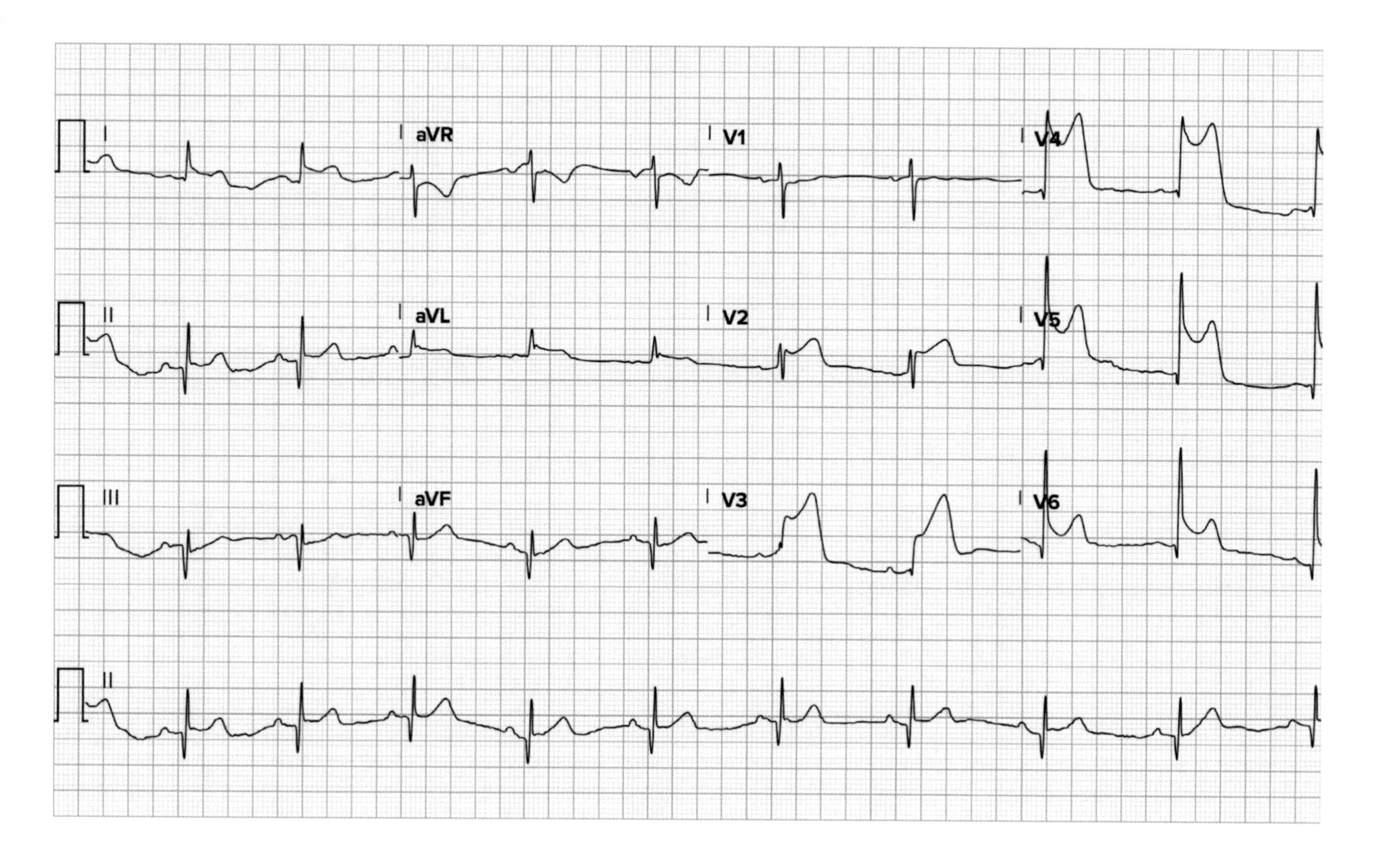

Case 32: Answer

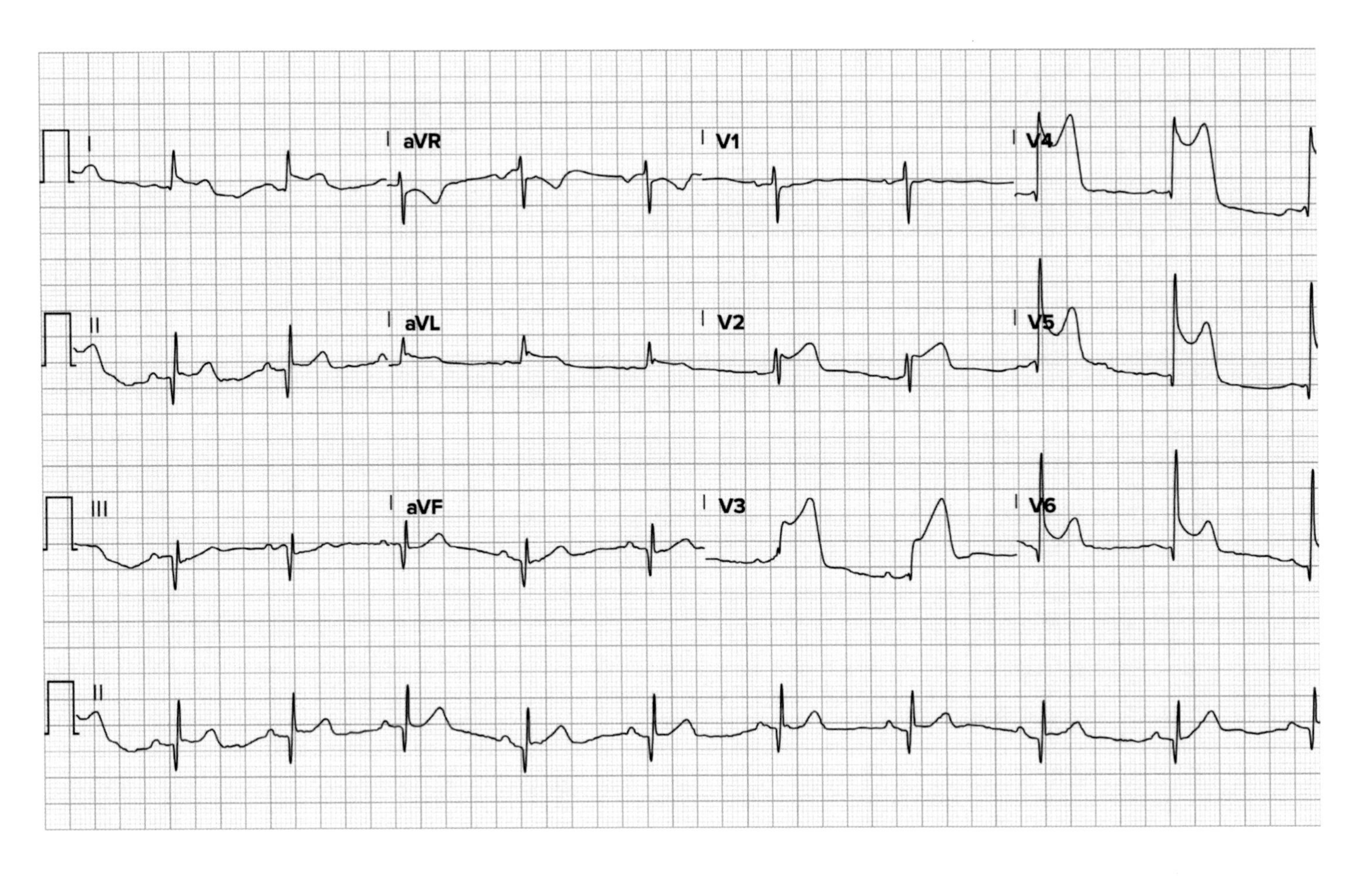

This ECG shows a sinus bradycardia at 58 bpm, normal axis, normal intervals, and STE in leads I, aVL, and V2-V6.

This ECG is consistent with a very large STEMI, specifically an anterolateral STEMI. There are 2 notable findings often associated with non-ACS etiologies: the absence of reciprocal STD and concave upward ST segments. However, neither of these findings rules out STEMI. The presence of reciprocal STD supports the ECG diagnosis of STEMI, but the absence of reciprocal STD does not rule out STEMI. Reciprocal STD can be absent in STEMI, in particular anterior STEMI in which reciprocal STD are absent up to 30% of the time.[1] And regarding an analysis of the elevated ST segment contour, concave upward ST segment morphology is frequently seen in myopericarditis and BER, but this shape can also be encountered in STEMI.

The ST segment is the interval between the end of the QRS complex (ie, the J point) and the beginning of the T wave. Common descriptors of the morphology include concave upward ***(see Figure 1)***, concave downward ***(see Figure 2)***, horizontal ***(see Figure 3)***, and obliquely strait ***(see Figure 4)***.

- Concave downward and obliquely strait ST segments are typically indicative of ischemia and suggest early STEMI if they are new from prior, seen in contiguous leads (especially if there are reciprocal STD), and the patient's presentation is concerning for ACS
- Concave upward ST segment morphology is often associated with non-ACS conditions (eg, BER, pericarditis) but can be seen with STEMI, as this case shows
- Straight ST segment morphology is non-specific

Figure 1.
Concave upward ST segment (from case ECG)

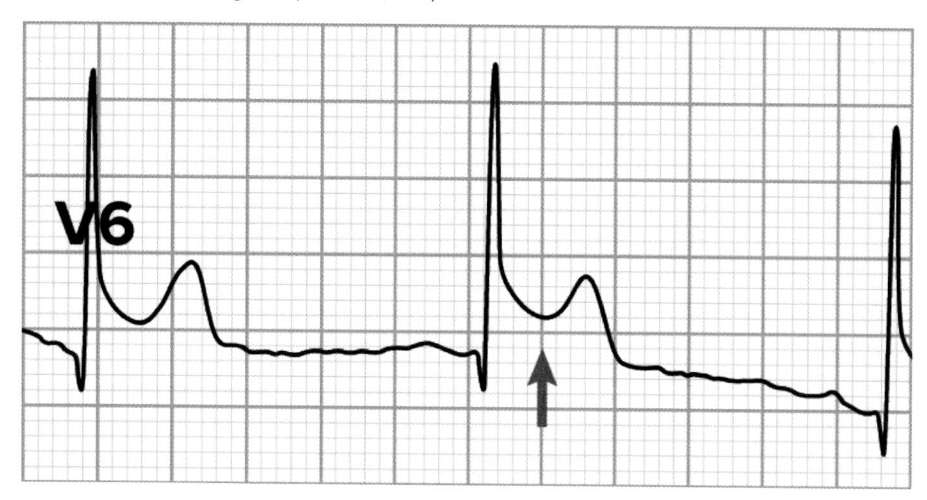

Figure 2.
Concave downward ST segment (from a different ECG)

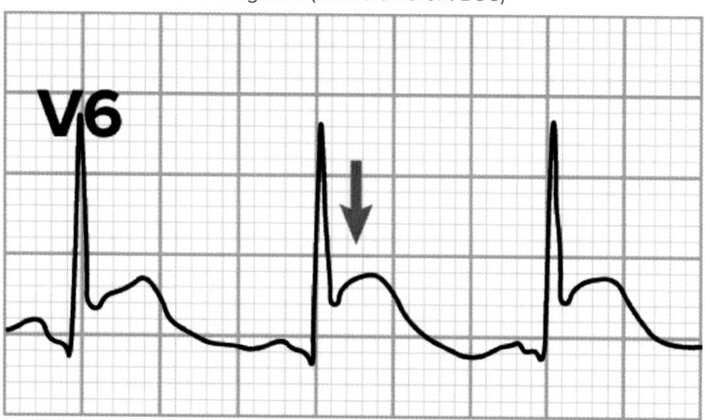

Figure 3.
Horizontal ST segment (from a different ECG)

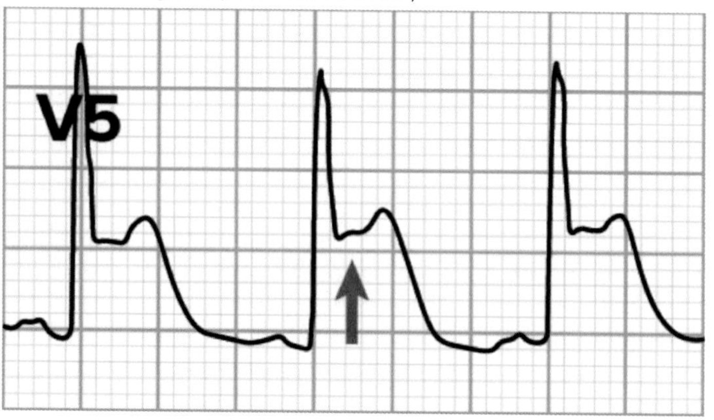

Figure 4.
Obliquely straight ST segment (from a different ECG)

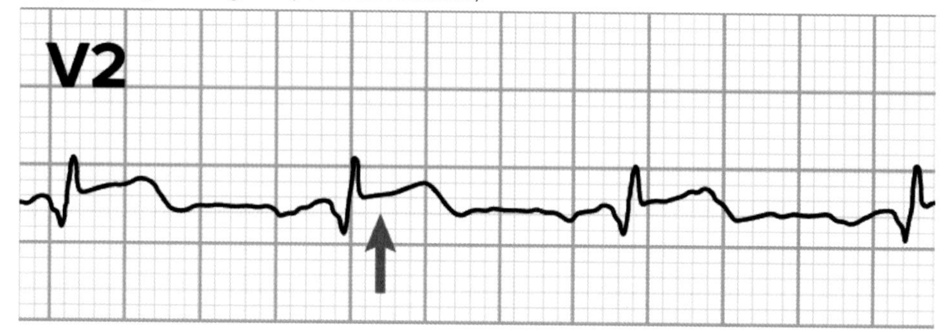

Regarding computer generated ECG interpretations, it is best to use them only to make sure you didn't miss anything of value.

This patient was taken to the cardiac catheterization laboratory, where a 100% occlusion of the mid-LAD was successfully treated with a stent.

STEMI Learning Points

- STEMI is defined by new, or presumed new, STE at the J point in ≥ 2 anatomically contiguous leads in the absence of LVH by voltage pattern, LBBB, or ventricular-paced rhythm
  - ≥ 2.5 mm in men < 40 years old and ≥ 2 mm in men ≥ 40 years old in leads V2-V3 (or an increase of ≥ 1 mm when compared to baseline ECG)
  - ≥ 1.5 mm in women in leads V2-V3 (or an increase of ≥ 1 mm when compared to baseline ECG)
  - ≥ 1 mm in all other leads
- ST-segment is measured from the isoelectric baseline, typically the TP segment ***(see below)***
- Reciprocal STD are not required for the diagnosis of STEMI, but their presence does increase the likelihood of the diagnosis of STEMI
  - Reciprocal STD are only present in 70% of anterior MI[1]
- Posterior MI
  - Consider whenever there is STD in leads V1-V4
  - STE ≥ 0.5 mm in posterior leads V7, V8 or V9 is diagnostic- does not require 2 contiguous leads
- Right ventricular MI
  - Consider with any inferior MI (RV MI is seen in approximately 1/3 of inferior MI)
  - STE in right precordial leads V3R and V4R ≥ 0.5 mm (≥ 1 mm for men ≤ 30 years old)
  - STE in right precordial lead V4R > 1 mm is most predictive of RV MI
  - STE in right precordial lead V4R > STE in leads V1-V3 = highly specific for RV MI
- Significant STE that does not meet the traditional distribution (ie, ≥ 2 anatomically contiguous leads) in a presentation concerning for ACS may still represent coronary artery occlusion and warrant consideration for emergent coronary reperfusion

How to Measure STE per most recent 2018 AHA Guidelines[2]

- The J point is the junction between QRS termination and ST-segment onset and is used to determine the magnitude of the ST-segment shift
- **In patients with a stable baseline, the TP segment (isoelectric interval) is a more accurate method to assess the magnitude of ST-segment shift *(see Figure 5)***, and in distinguishing pericarditis from acute myocardial ischemia
- QRS onset should be used if TP segment does not have a stable baseline ***(see Figure 6)***
- Measurement should be made from the top of the ECG line tracing

Figure 5.
Measure STE from the TP segment if the TP segment is isoelectric (ie, horizontal)

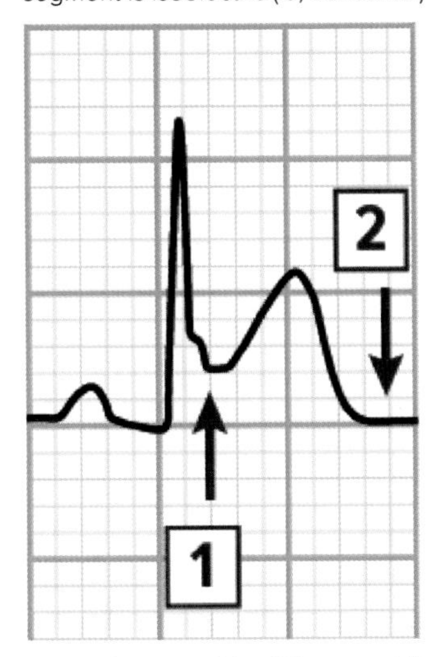

Arrow 1: onset of the ST-segment (ie, J point)
Arrow 2: TP segment

Figure 6.
Measure STE from onset of the QRS complex if the TP segment is not isoelectric (ie, not horizontal)

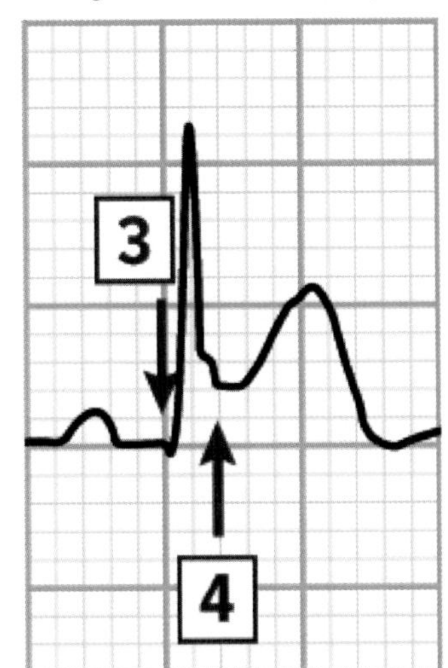

Arrow 3: initial onset of the Q-wave
Arrow 4: onset of the ST-segment (ie, J point)

References

1. Knilans T, Surawicz B. Chou's Electrocardiography in Clinical Practice. Philadelphia, PA: Elsevier. 2020.
2. Thygesen K, Alpert JS, Jaffe AS, et al. 2018 ESC/ACC/AHA/WHF Expert Consensus Document: Fourth Universal Definition of Myocardial Infarction (2018). Circulation. 2018;138:e618-e651.

Case 33: Presentation

A 74-year-old female presents with exertional near syncope.
What is your interpretation of her ECG?

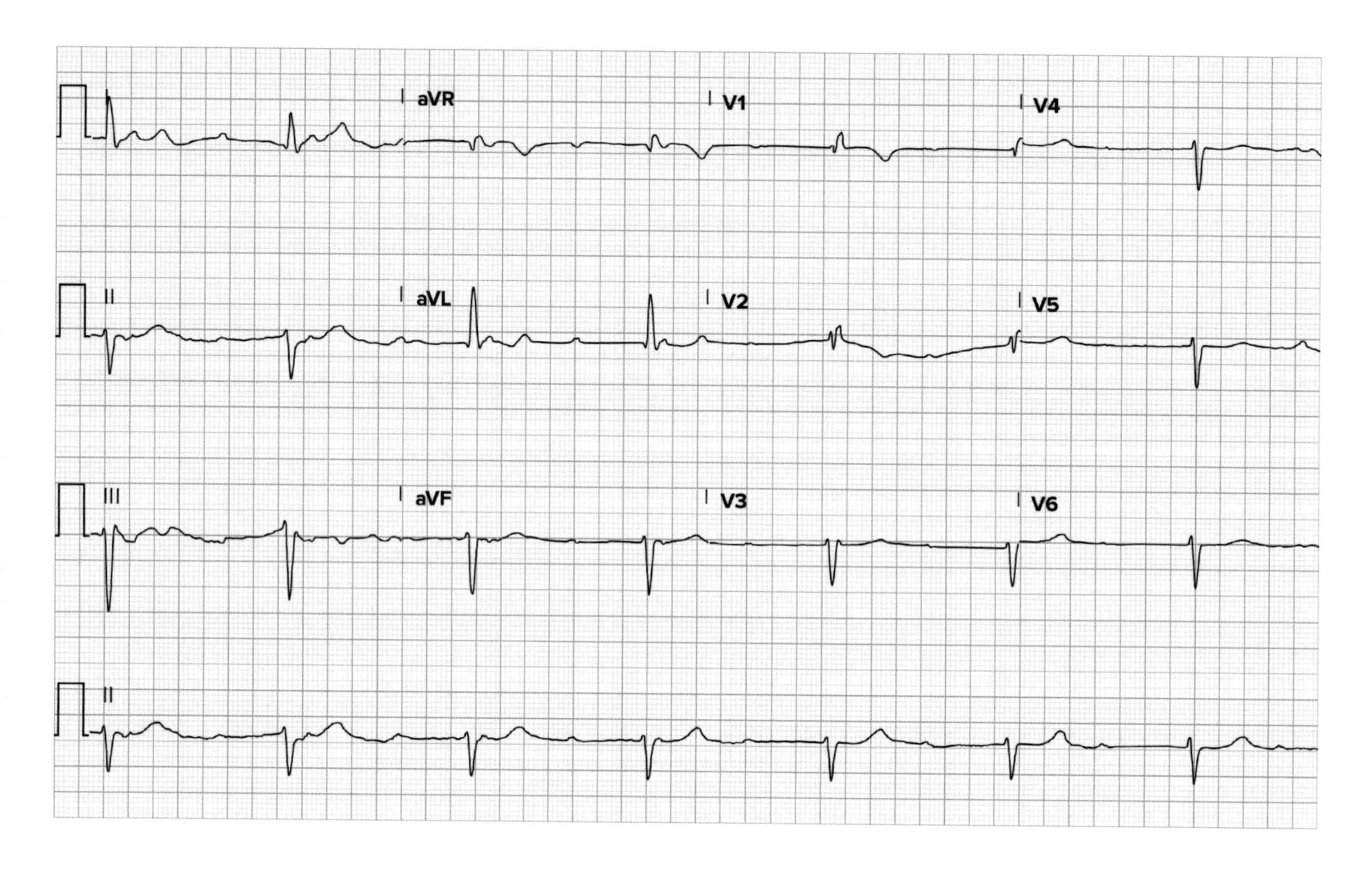

Case 33: Answer

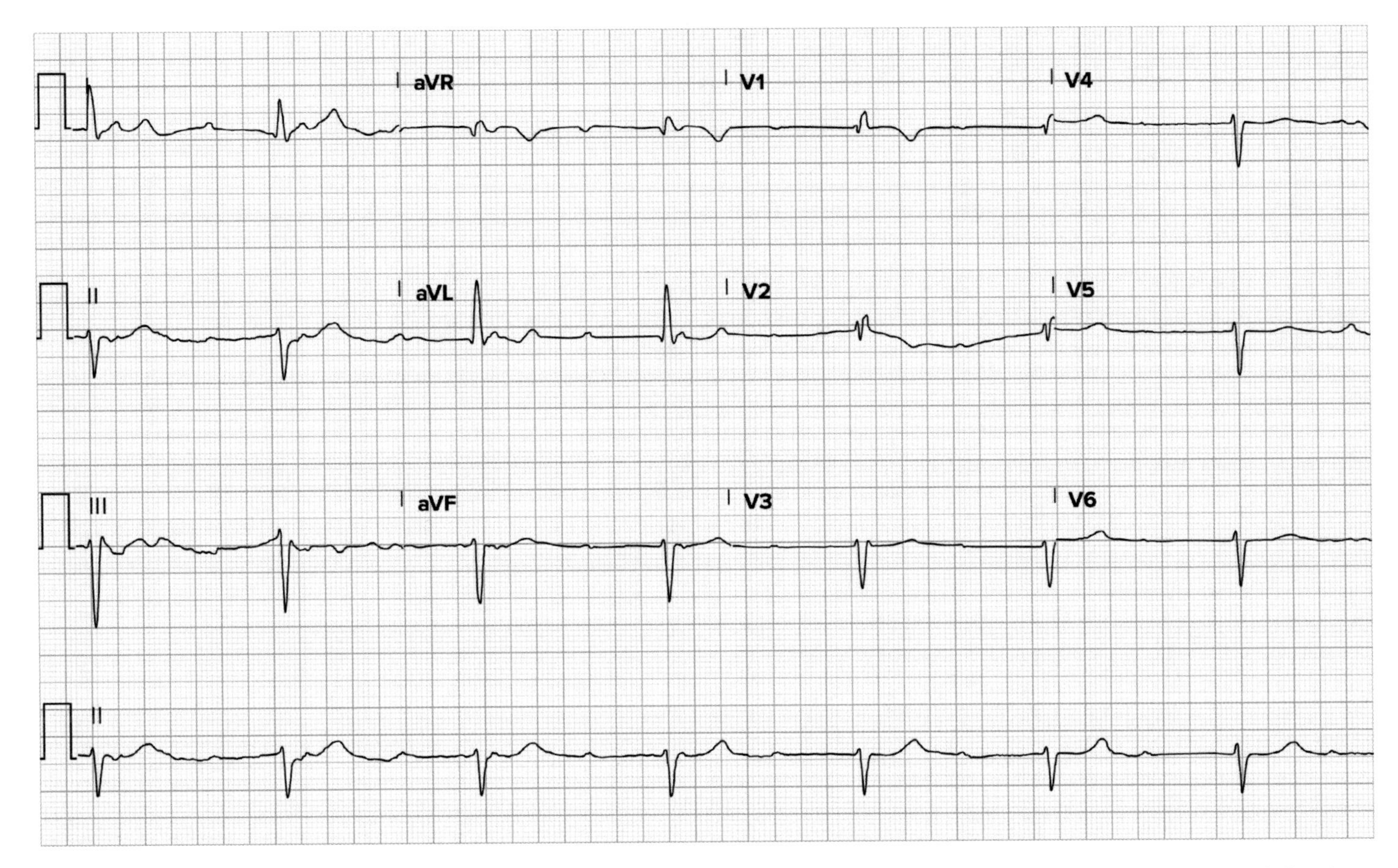

This ECG shows a regular wide complex bradycardia with an average ventricular rate of 40 bpm, AV dissociation, left axis deviation, prolonged QRS complex duration with a RBBB, and a left anterior fascicular block.

The differential diagnosis for the rhythm in this ECG (ie, a regular wide complex bradycardia at 40 bpm with AV dissociation) includes a junctional rhythm with aberrant conduction or an idioventricular rhythm. The presence of a RBBB supports the diagnosis of a junctional rhythm with aberrant conduction, but differentiating between the two is not absolutely necessary as far as the treatment and disposition are concerned.

The key to correctly interpreting this ECG is recognizing the AV dissociation, which is diagnostic for a 3rd degree AV block. The P-waves and QRS complexes march out at similar but slightly different rates ***(see Figure 1)*** which is consistent with a 3rd degree AV block. The regular rhythm of the QRS complexes rules out a Mobitz type I or II, both of which will be irregular in the absence of 2:1 AV conduction or a high-grade AV block (eg, 3:1, 4:1, etc.).

Figure 1.
The lead II rhythm strip show an atrial rate (PP interval) and ventricular rate (RR interval) that are slightly different, consistent with a 3rd degree AV block

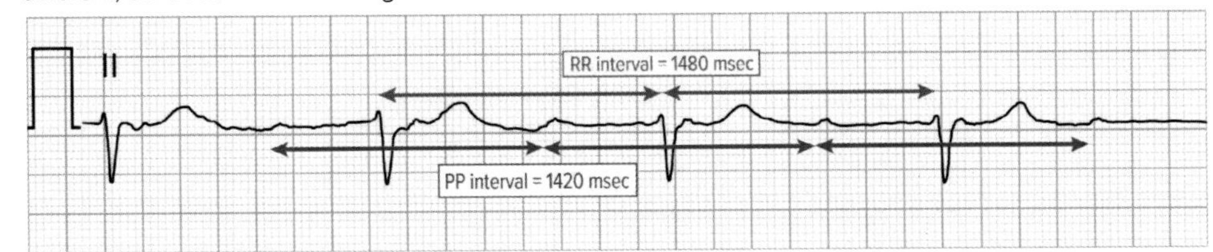

It is important to note that a 3rd degree AV block will always produce AV dissociation, but the presence of AV dissociation is not diagnostic of a 3rd degree AV block. For example, an accelerated junctional rhythm with a rate slightly higher than that of the SA node can cause AV dissociation even though the AV node is functioning normally. In this ECG, the faster SA node pacing should preclude the slower infranodal pacing in the absence of any AV node dysfunction, but since it doesn't, there must be an AV block.

Another key to avoid misinterpreting this ECG as a sinus bradycardia with a 1st degree AV block is recognizing the hidden P-waves. The "Bix rule," named after cardiologist Harold Bix, states that whenever there are P-waves halfway between the QRS complexes, there are likely additional P-waves buried or hidden within the QRS complexes. Upright P-waves can be seen buried in the end of the first 3 QRS complexes and it can be inferred that there is a P-wave hidden in the 4th QRS complex by marching out the P-waves ***(see Figure 2)***.

Figure 2.
The arrows point to P-waves, including those buried or hidden in the QRS complexes, in the lead II rhythm strip

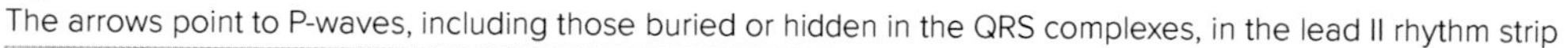

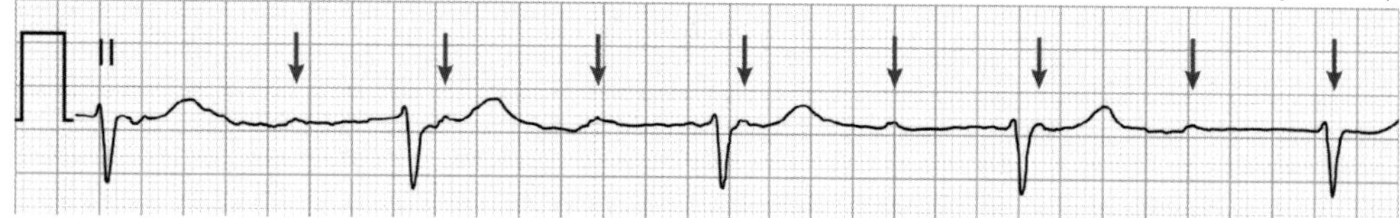

A more accurate analysis of the lead II rhythm strip better shows the 3rd degree AV block ***(see Figure 3)***.

Figure 3.
Accounting for the P-waves buried or hidden in the QRS complexes, the lead II rhythm strip shows an atrial rate (PP interval) slightly faster than 2 times the ventricular rate (RR interval), consistent with a 3rd degree AV block

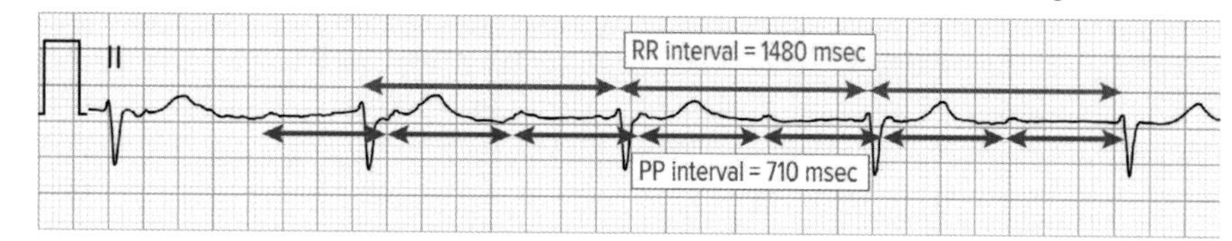

This ECG also shows a RBBB. The characteristic findings in a RBBB include:

- QRS complex duration ≥ 120 msec
- rsr', rsR', or rSR' pattern in lead V1 +/- V2 ***(see Figure 4)***
  - Variations in lead V1 include qR pattern or broad R-wave that is often notched
  - In lead V1, the initial upward deflection should always be smaller than the 2nd upward deflection ***(see Figure 4)***
- S-wave duration > R-wave or > 40 msec in leads I and V6 ***(see Figure 5)***
- Normal R-wave peak time in leads V5 and V6 but > 50 msec in lead V1 (only required if broad R-wave +/- notch is present in lead V1)
- Repolarization abnormalities include STD and TWI in lead V1 +/- lead(s) V2-V3 if they have an rsR' pattern, so STE and/or upright T-waves in those leads are concerning for ischemia

Note that the QRS complex in lead I is atypical for a RBBB as the R-wave duration is greater than the S-wave duration.

Figure 4.
rSR' pattern in lead V1, consistent with a RBBB

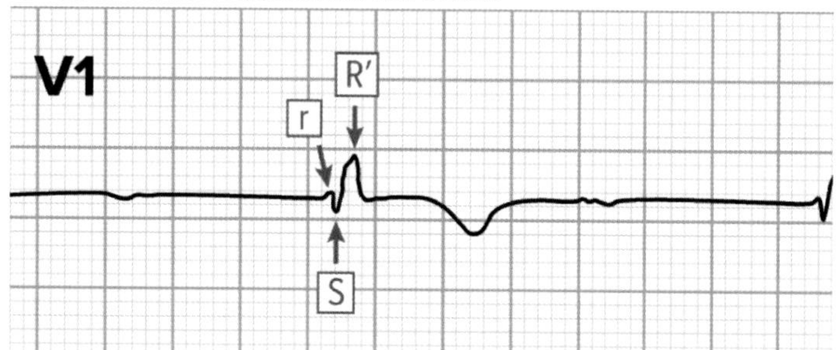

Figure 5.
S-wave duration > R-wave duration in lead V6, consistent with a RBBB

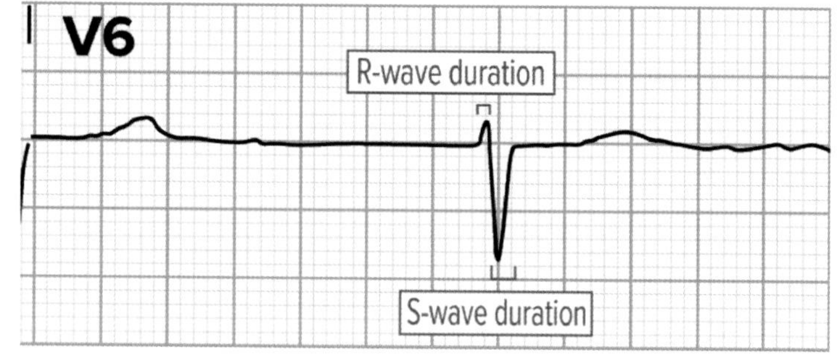

The presence of a RBBB with an axis deviation should prompt evaluation for a concurrent fascicular block. This ECG shows a LAFB *(see Figure 6)*.

The characteristic findings in a LAFB include:

- Left axis deviation between -45° and -90°
- qR complex in lead aVL +/- lead I
- rS complex in leads II, III, and aVF
- Prolonged R-wave peak time ≥ 45 msec in lead aVL
- QRS complex duration < 120 msec in the absence of a concurrent conduction delay

Figure 6.
Findings in the case ECG consistent with a left anterior fascicular block include qR complexes in leads I and aVL (red box), rS complexes in leads II, III, and aVF (purple box), and left axis deviation (green line)

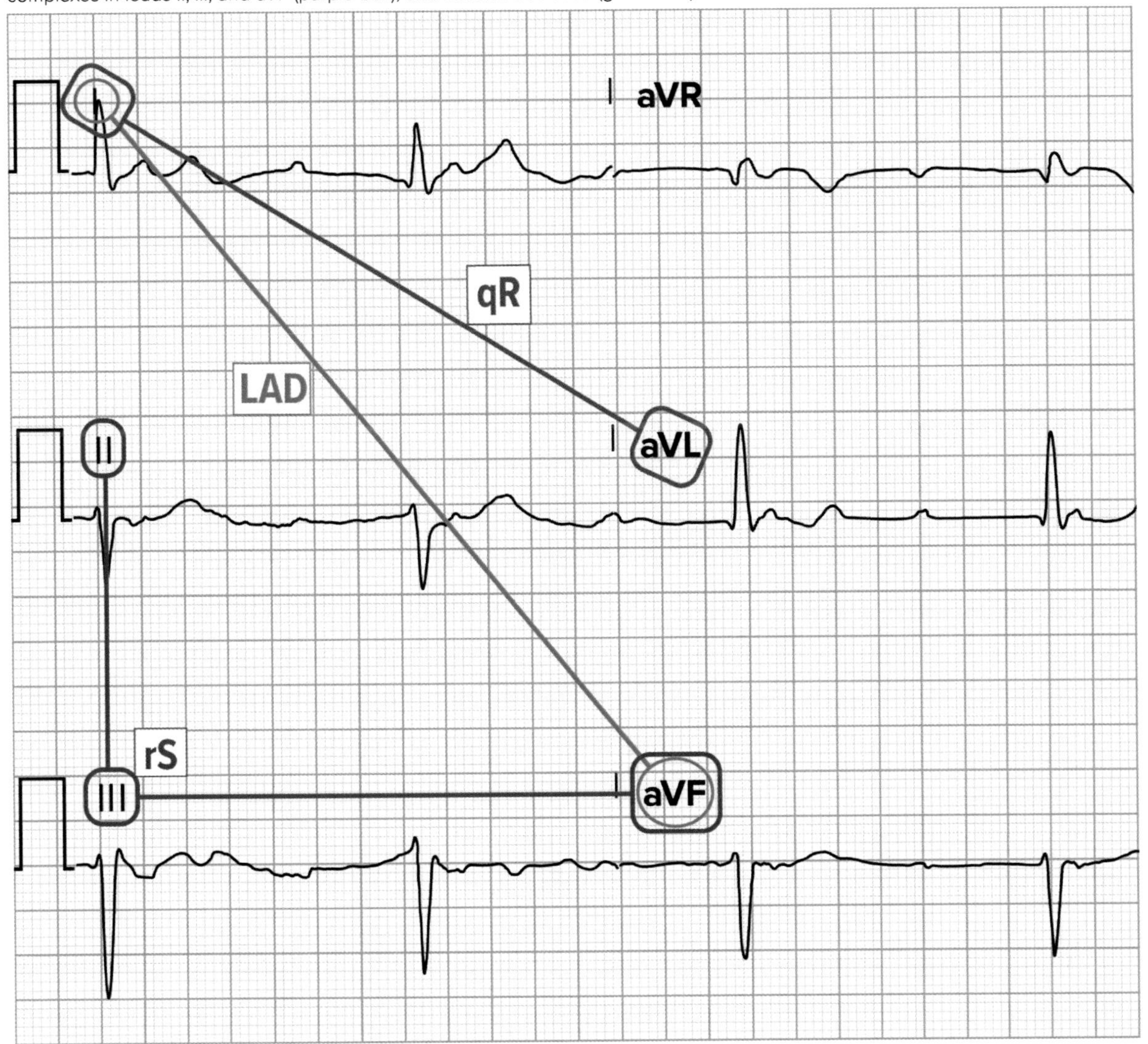

The constellation of a RBBB + fascicular block + any AV block is called a trifascicular block, which is further categorized as complete or incomplete:

- Complete trifascicular block = 3rd degree AV block + RBBB + LAFB or LPFB
- Incomplete trifascicular block = 1st or 2nd degree AV block + RBBB + LAFB or LPFB, or RBBB + alternating LAFB/LPFB on successive ECGs

A repeat ECG was obtained which better showed the 3rd degree AV block ***(see Figure 7)*.** The patient had an unremarkable ED workup and was admitted to the cardiology service for placement of a permanent pacemaker.

Figure 7.
A repeat ECG that better demonstrates the 3rd degree AV block

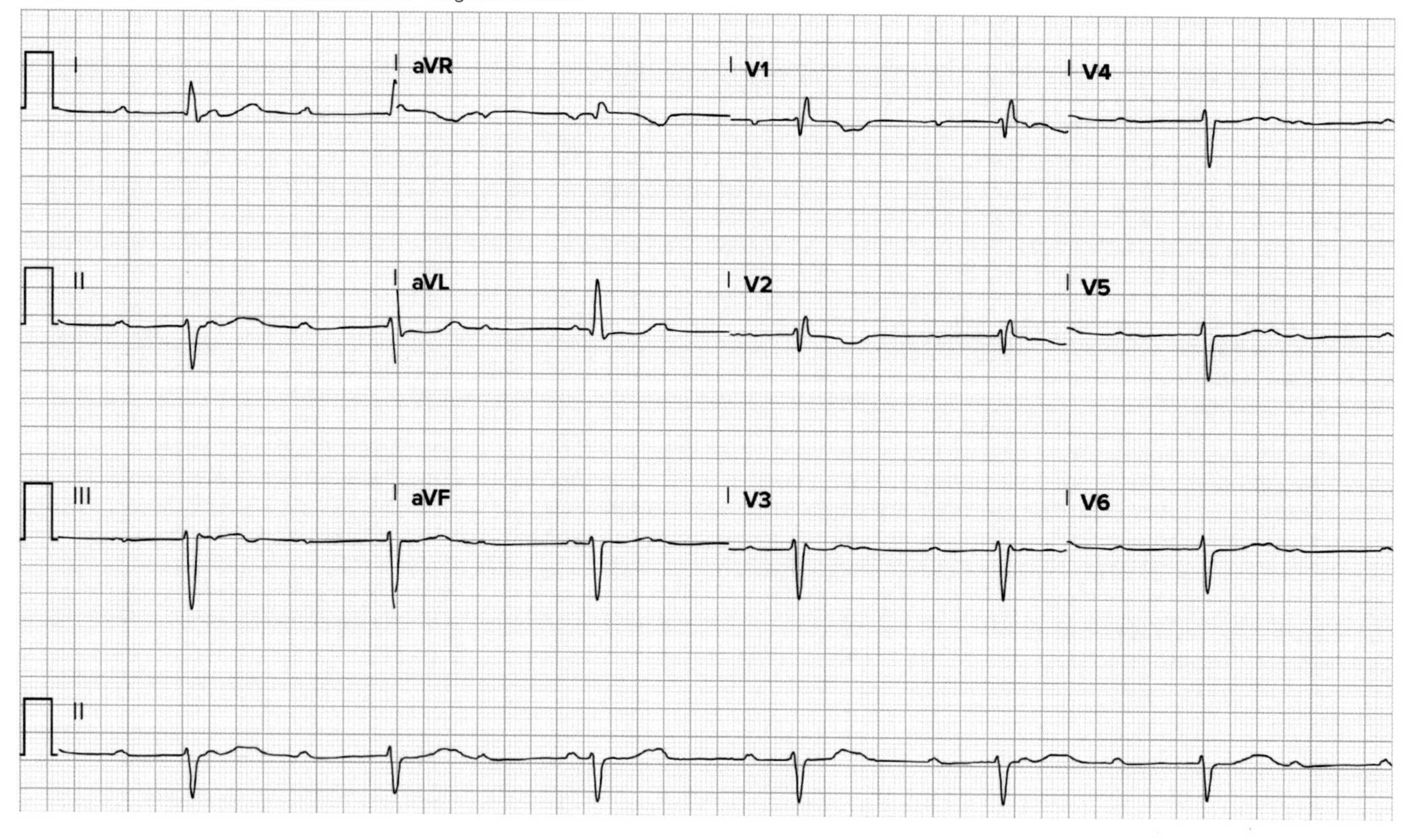

3rd Degree AV Block Learning Points

- A 3rd degree AV block, or complete heart block, is defined by the absence of conduction through the AV node leading to complete AV dissociation
  - P-waves "march out" (ie, constant PP interval) and do not conduct to produce a QRS complex
  - PR intervals are variable
  - Atrial rate > ventricular rate
  - Ventricular rhythm is usually junctional or ventricular escape rhythm
- All patients require admission and evaluation for pacemaker placement

Junctional Rhythm Learning Points

- Ectopic focus from AV node or proximal Purkinje system
  - Also called AV junctional rhythm, nodal rhythm, nodal escape rhythm, junctional escape rhythm, AV nodal rhythm
- ECG shows ventricular rate of 40-60 bpm with normal QRS complex duration unless concurrent conduction abnormality (eg, bundle branch block)
- May have retrograde P-waves that precede (with PR interval < 120 msec) or follow QRS complex, typically best seen in the inferior leads
- Variations include:
  - Junctional Bradycardia: ventricular rate < 40 bpm
  - Accelerated Junctional Rhythm: ventricular rate 61–100 bpm
  - Junctional Tachycardia: ventricular rate > 100 bpm

Idioventricular Rhythm Learning Points

- Ectopic focus from Purkinje network or ventricular myocardium
  - Also called ventricular escape rhythm
- ECG shows ≥ 3 consecutive, regular, wide complex beats with no P-waves or AV dissociation if P-waves are present
- Variations include accelerated idioventricular rhythm (AIVR)
  - Rates between 40-110 bpm but can sometimes be as high as 120-130 bpm
  - Can be seen in the reperfusion phase of a STEMI following fibrinolysis or PCI but can also be spontaneous
  - Also seen with digoxin toxicity, cardiac ischemia, or electrolyte abnormalities
  - Mimics include hyperkalemia, sodium channel blocker toxicity, and VT in patients on antidysrhythmic medications (eg, amiodarone, flecainide, sotalol) or with severe cardiomyopathies
  - Usually well-tolerated, benign, and self-limiting
  - Treating as VT with antidysrhythmic medications can precipitate asystole

RBBB Learning Points

- Delayed conduction through right ventricle with normal left ventricular conduction
- In lead V1, the initial upward deflection should always be smaller than the 2nd upward deflection
- Repolarization abnormalities include STD and TWI in lead V1 +/- lead(s) V2-V3 if they have an rsR' pattern, so STE and/or upright T-waves in those leads are concerning for ischemia
  - Otherwise, the presence of a RBBB does not confound the ECG evaluation of ACS as does a LBBB
- RBBB with axis deviation should prompt evaluation for a concurrent LAFB or LPFB

Fascicular Blocks Learning Points

- Complete trifascicular block
  - 3rd degree AV block + RBBB + LAFB or LPFB
  - Always gets admitted for pacemaker placement
- Incomplete trifascicular block
  - 1st or 2nd degree AV block + RBBB + LAFB or LPFB, or RBBB + alternating LAFB/LPFB on successive ECGs
  - Syncope + incomplete trifascicular block = usually requires admission for cardiac monitoring for transient 3rd degree AV block and evaluation for pacemaker placement

Case 34: Presentation

An 87-year-old female presents to the emergency department with worsening generalized weakness and dyspnea on exertion for that past 2 weeks. She also reports chest pain, described as an "achiness," that started a few hours ago and radiates down both arms. She reports a history of lower gastrointestinal hemorrhage and has had blood in her stool for the past week. What is your interpretation of her ECG?

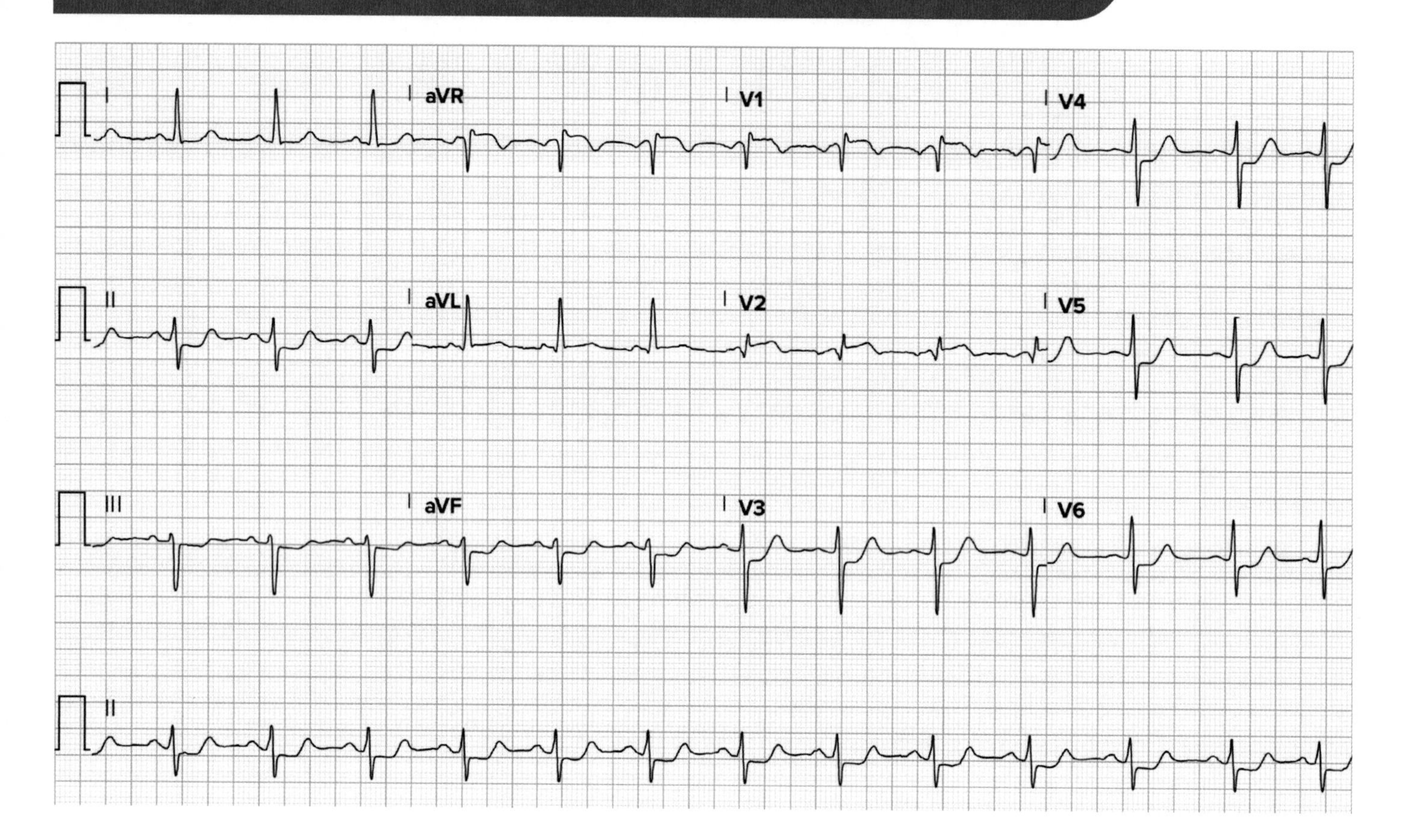

Case 34: Answer

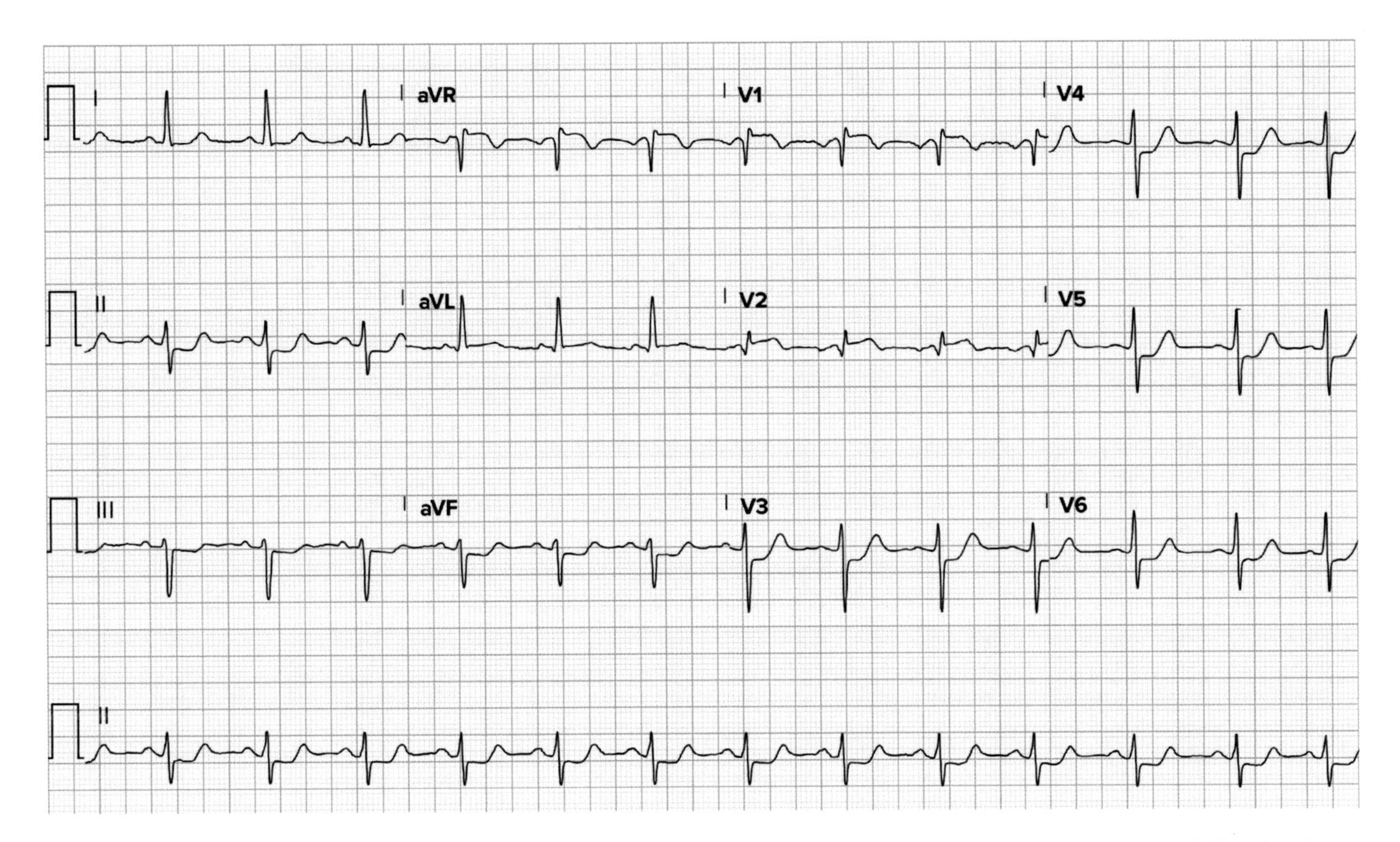

This ECG shows normal sinus rhythm with a ventricular rate of 80 bpm, left axis deviation, normal intervals, STE in leads aVR, V1, and V2, and STD in leads I, II, III, aVF, and V3-V6.

The differential diagnosis for the pattern of STE in lead aVR +/- lead V1 with diffuse STD includes both ACS and non-ACS etiologies:

ACS causes[1]	Non-ACS causes[2]
• LMCA insufficiency (can see STE aVR > V1)	• Acute and/or severe anemia
• Prox LAD insufficiency (can see STE V1 > aVR)	• Aortic dissection
• Triple vessel disease	• LBBB and ventricular-paced rhythms
• Global cardiac ischemia	• LVH with strain pattern
• Prinzmetal angina	• Pulmonary embolism
	• ROSC s/p epinephrine or defibrillation
	• Severe hypokalemia or hyperkalemia
	• Sodium channel blockade
	• Supraventricular tachycardia (especially with rapid rates)

Although the pattern of STE in lead aVR +/- lead V1 with diffuse STD is discussed in the cardiology literature, its clinical significance is not without some controversy. This is likely due to the broad differential diagnosis associated with this pattern that includes both ACS and non-ACS causes. The 2018 Fourth Universal Definition of MI states "ST-segment depression ≥ 1 mm in 6 or more leads, which may be associated with ST segment elevation in leads aVR and/or V1 and hemodynamic compromise, is suggestive of multivessel disease or left main disease" but does not provide specific management recommendations.

Treatment should be guided by the underlying etiology, and it is imperative to consider both ACS and non-ACS causes. For patients suspected of having an ACS cause, this ECG pattern is highly suggestive of LMCA insufficiency, proximal LAD insufficiency, or triple vessel disease. So, while this pattern does not meet "traditional" STEMI criteria, it can represent high-risk ACS, including possible acute coronary occlusion, in the correct clinical context, and immediate angiography should be considered. Whether this is done by emergent cardiology consultation or activation of the cardiac catheterization lab depends on local practice preferences.

This patient's presentation is particularly challenging. Her ECG shows both the pattern of STE in lead aVR +/- lead V1 with diffuse STD and contiguous STE in leads V1-V2 ***(see Figure 1)***. There is approximately 1 mm of STE in lead V1 when measured from the TP segment (there is not a consistent PR segment). There is also approximately 1 mm of STE in lead V2 when measured from the PR segment but only approximately 0.5 mm when measured from the TP segment. In either case, the STE does not meet the STEMI criteria cutoff of 1.5 mm in lead V2 for female patients.

Figure 1.
STE in leads V1-V2

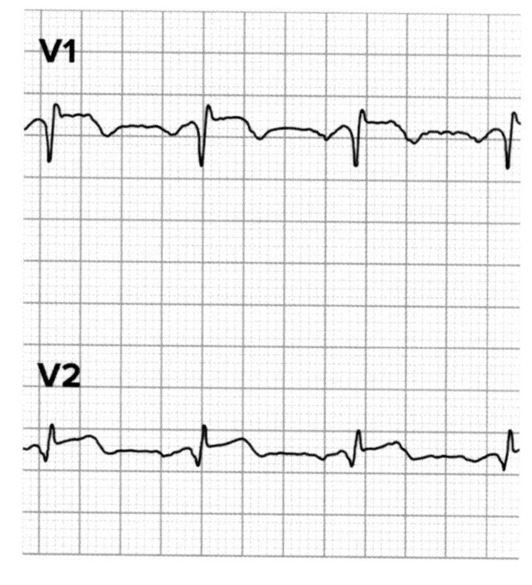

Figure 2.
The morphology of the ST-segment and T-wave upstroke in lead V2 is called the checkmark sign or R-T sign

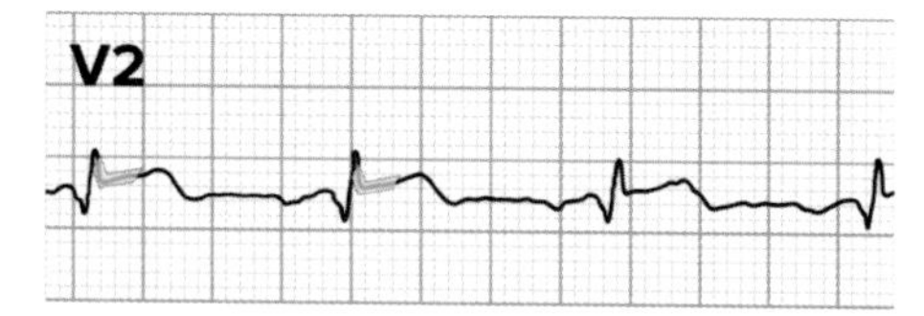

Lead V2 also shows an obliquely straight form of ST segment elevation which is called the checkmark sign[2] or R-T sign ***(see Figure 2)***. The describes the morphology of the ST-segment and T-wave upstroke. Obliquely straight forms of ST segment elevation are analogous to concave downward STE in that they suggest AMI if they are new from prior, seen in contiguous leads (especially if there are reciprocal STD), and the patient's presentation is concerning for ACS. It is important to note the presence of concave upward ST segments and/or the absence of reciprocal STD does not rule out STEMI.

This case is diagnostically challenging because the treatment and disposition depend on the cause of the ECG changes of which there are multiple possibilities:

1. Severe anemia with shock can produce STE in lead aVR
2. LMCA or proximal LAD obstruction can produce STE in lead aVR
3. Proximal LAD occlusion can produce STE in leads V1-V2 and aVR with STD in leads II, III, and aVF
4. Any combination of the above

This patient's case was discussed emergently with cardiology who took the patient urgently to the cardiac catherization laboratory. Laboratory studies including a complete blood count, which resulted after the patient had left the ED, was notable for a hemoglobin of 5.8 g/dL so transfusion was started in the cardiac catherization laboratory. Angiography showed a 95% occlusion of the proximal LAD which was successfully treated with a stent.

Lead aVR Learning Points

- Lead aVR views the right upper portion of the heart including the basal part of the septum
- STE in lead aVR +/- V1 with diffuse STD ≥ 1 mm in ≥ 6 leads can be due to ACS or non-ACS etiologies; therefore, always consider the clinical context when considering the differential diagnosis
- In ACS presentations, this pattern is highly suggestive of LMCA obstruction, proximal LAD obstruction, and triple vessel disease, and immediate angiography should be considered[3]
- In non-ACS causes, the ECG changes should resolve with treatment of non-ACS cause
- Anterior or inferior MI with STE > 1 mm in lead aVR are associated with an increased 30-day mortality[4]

STEMI Learning Points

- STEMI is defined by new, or presumed new, STE at the J point in ≥ 2 anatomically contiguous leads in the absence of LVH by voltage pattern, LBBB, or ventricular-paced rhythm
  - ≥ 2.5 mm in men < 40 years old and ≥ 2 mm in men ≥ 40 years old in leads V2-V3 (or an increase of ≥ 1 mm when compared to baseline ECG)
  - ≥ 1.5 mm in women in leads V2-V3 (or an increase of ≥ 1 mm when compared to baseline ECG)
  - ≥ 1 mm in all other leads
- ST-segment is measured from the isoelectric baseline, typically the TP segment (see below)
- Reciprocal STD are not required for the diagnosis of STEMI, but their presence does increase the likelihood of the diagnosis of STEMI
  - Reciprocal STD are only present in 70% of anterior MI1
- Posterior MI
  - Consider whenever there is STD in leads V1-V4
  - STE ≥ 0.5 mm in posterior leads V7, V8, or V9 is diagnostic- does not require 2 contiguous leads
- Right ventricular MI
  - Consider with any inferior MI (RV MI is seen in approximately 1/3 of inferior MI)
  - STE in right precordial leads V3R and V4R ≥ 0.5 mm (≥ 1 mm for men ≤ 30 years old)
  - STE in right precordial lead V4R > 1 mm is most predictive of RV MI
  - STE in right precordial lead V4R > STE in leads V1-V3 = highly specific for RV MI
- Significant STE that does not meet the traditional distribution (ie, ≥ 2 anatomically contiguous leads) in a presentation concerning for ACS may still represent coronary artery occlusion and warrant consideration for emergent coronary reperfusion

How to Measure STE per most recent 2018 AHA Guidelines[6]

- The J point is the junction between QRS termination and ST-segment onset and is used to determine the magnitude of the ST-segment shift
- **In patients with a stable baseline, the TP segment (isoelectric interval) is a more accurate method to assess the magnitude of ST-segment shift** ***(see Figure 3)***, and in distinguishing pericarditis from acute myocardial ischemia
- QRS onset should be used if TP segment does not have a stable baseline ***(see Figure 4)***
- Measurement should be made from the top of the ECG line tracing

Figure 3.
Measure STE from the TP segment if the TP segment is isoelectric (ie, horizontal)

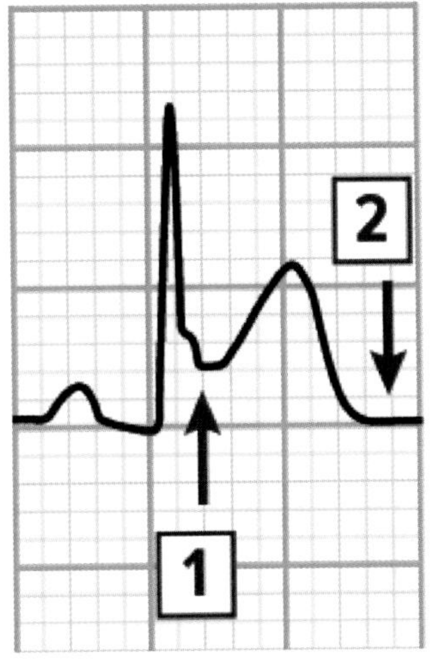

Arrow 1: onset of the ST-segment (ie, J point)
Arrow 2: TP segment

Figure 4.
Measure STE from onset of the QRS complex if the TP segment is not isoelectric (ie, not horizontal)

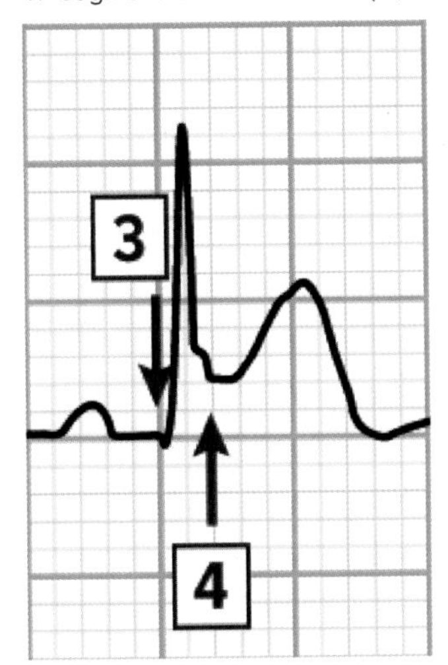

Arrow 3: initial onset of the Q-wave
Arrow 4: onset of the ST-segment (ie, J point)

References

1. Thygesen K, Alpert JS, Jaffe AS, et al. 2018 ESC/ACC/AHA/WHF Expert Consensus Document: Fourth Universal Definition of Myocardial Infarction (2018). Circulation. 2018;138:e618-e651.
2. Mattu A. ECG Weekly.
3. Writing Committee, et al. 2013 ACCF/AHA Guideline for the Management of ST-Elevation Myocardial Infarction: A Report of the American College of Cardiology Foundation/American Heart Association Task Force on Practice Guidelines. Circulation. 2013;127:e362-e425.
4. Wong CK, Gao W, Stewart RA, Benatar J, French JK, Aylward PE,White HD; HERO-2 Investigators. aVR ST elevation: an important but neglected sign in ST elevation acute myocardial infarction. Eur Heart J. 2010;31:1845–1853.
5. Knilans T, Surawicz B. Chou's Electrocardiography in Clinical Practice. Philadelphia, PA: Elsevier. 2020.

Case 35: Presentation

A 75-year-old male with no cardiac history presents with confusion and generalized malaise. The initial ECG did not show any electrical activity in the limb leads so a repeat ECG was obtained. What is your interpretation of his ECGs?

Initial ECG

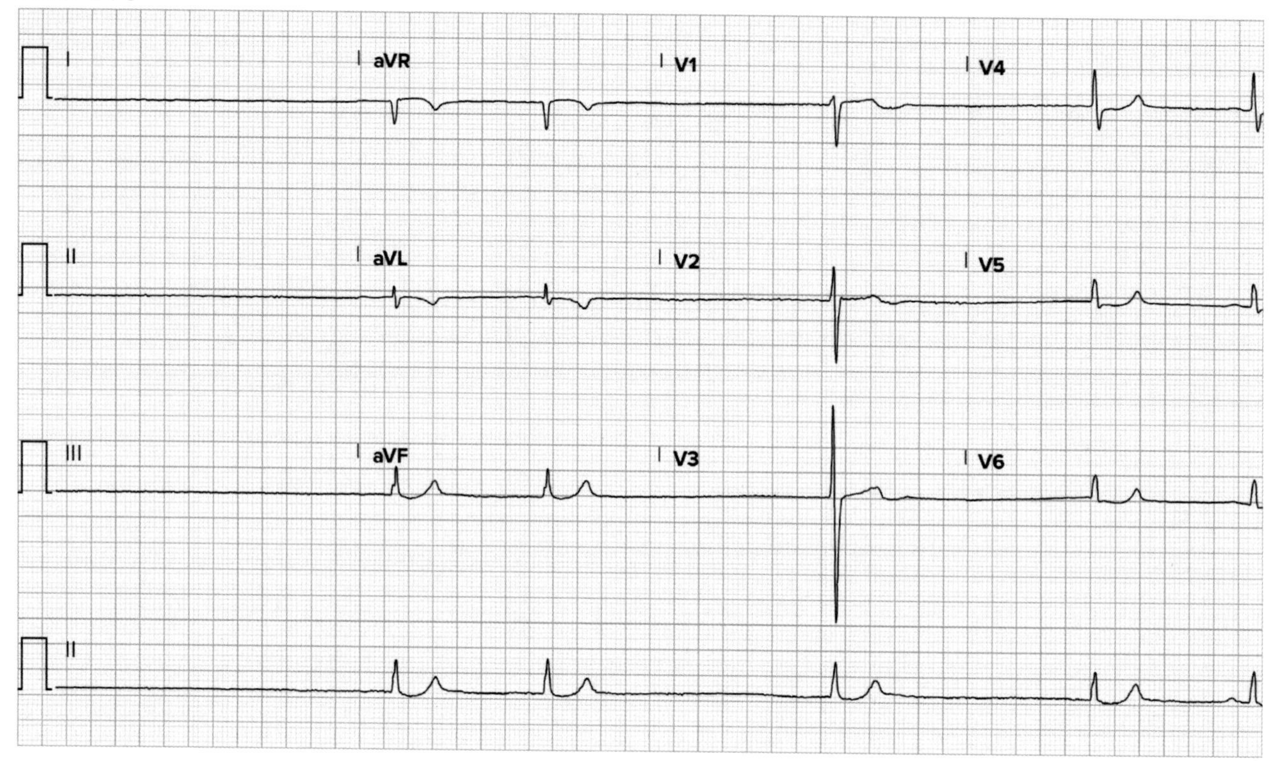

Repeat ECG

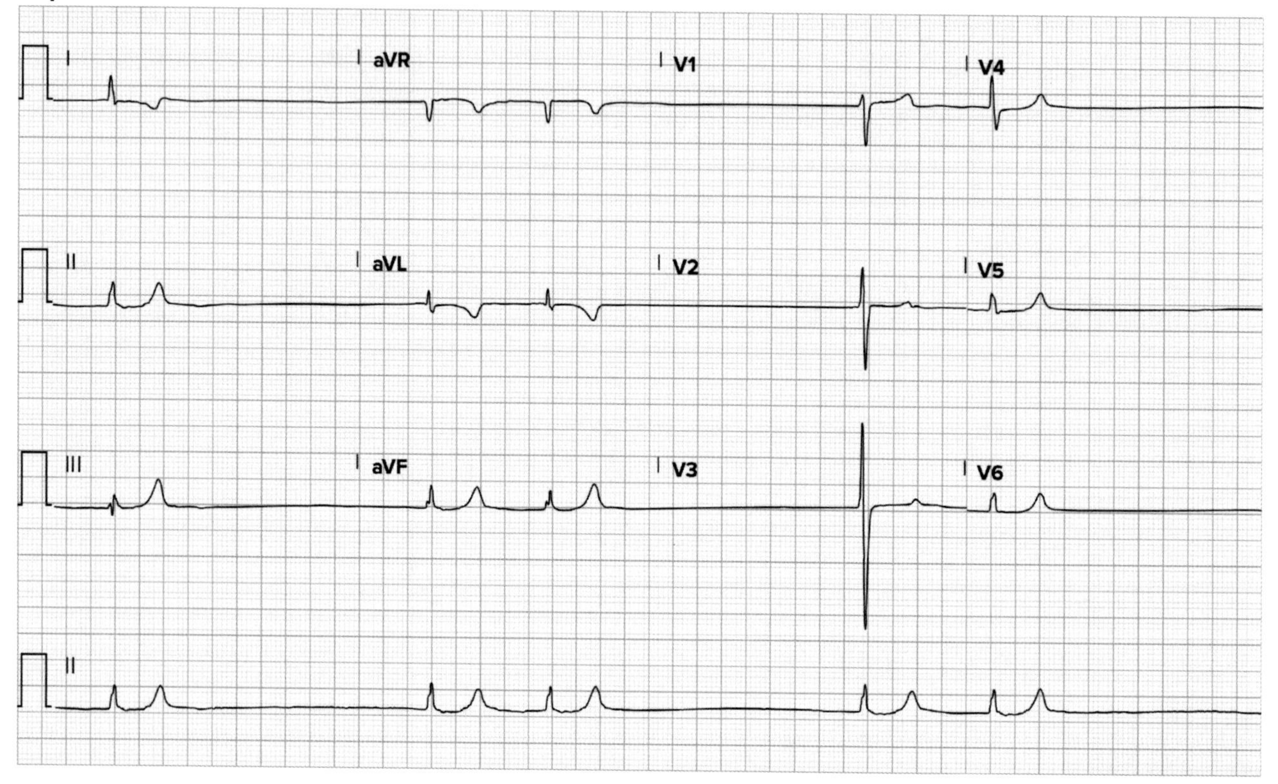

Case 35: Answer

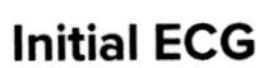

Initial ECG

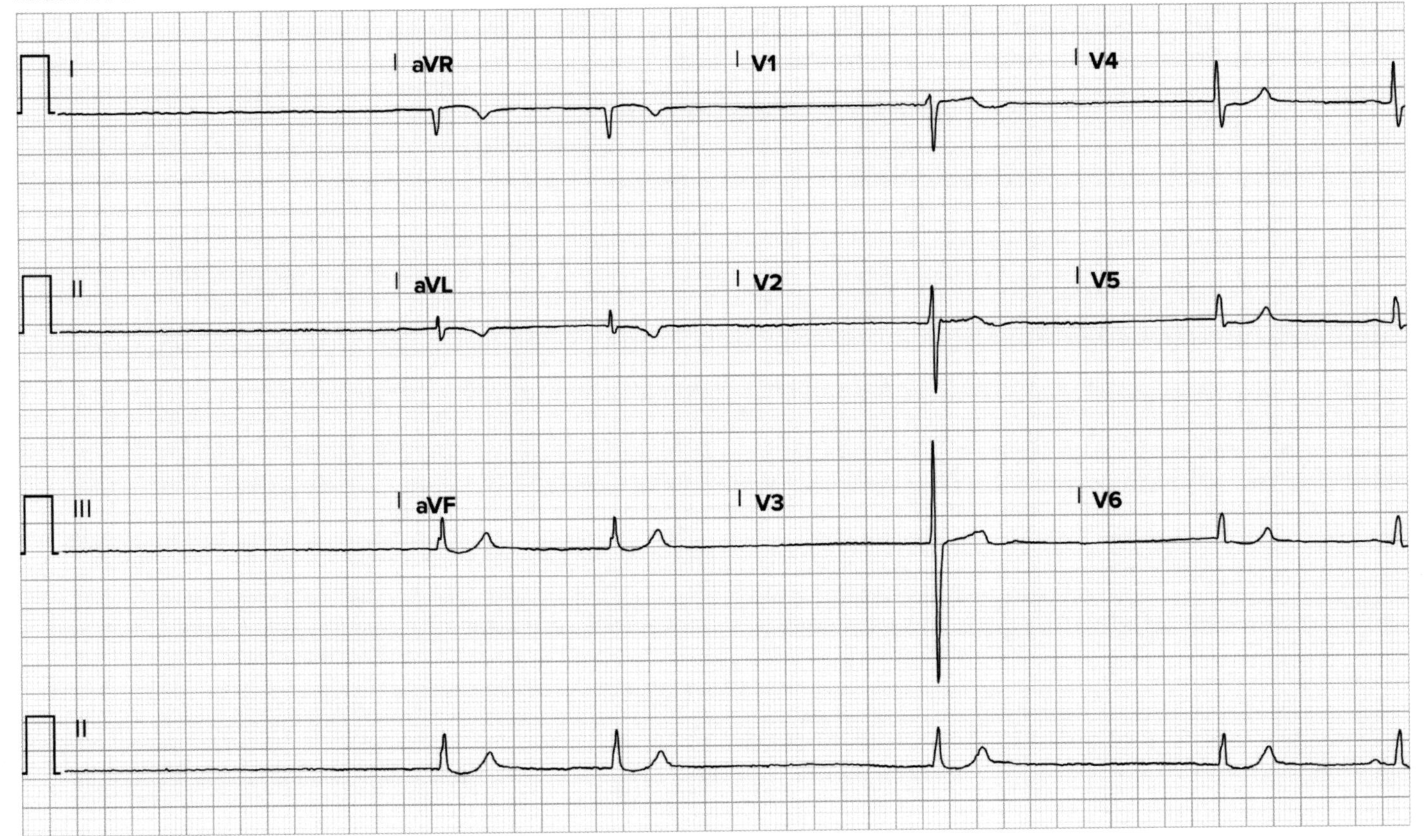

Repeat ECG

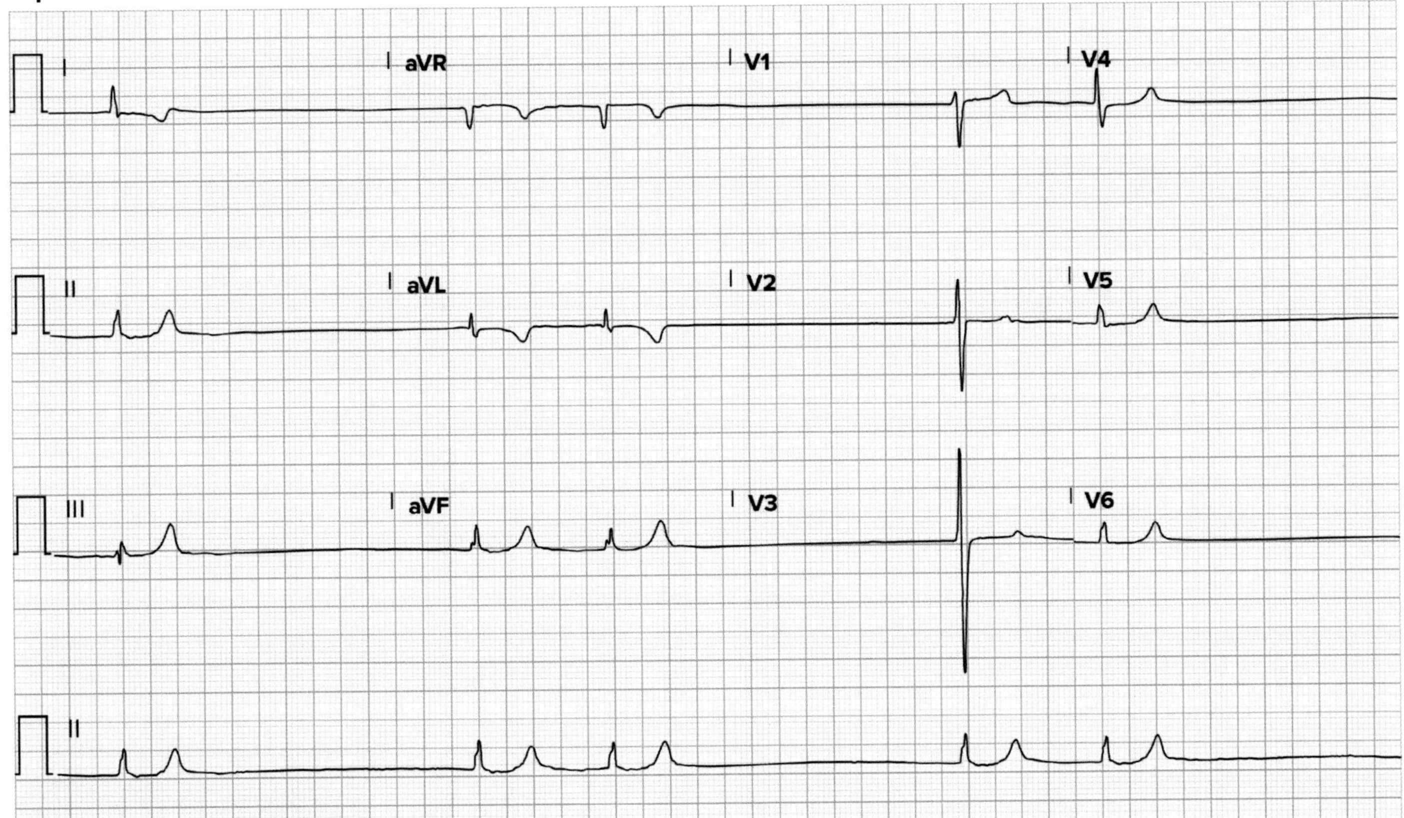

Both of these ECGs show an irregular bradycardia with an average ventricular rate of 30 bpm, no P-waves except for the last beat of the initial ECG, normal intervals, normal axis on the repeat ECG, hyperacute T-waves in the inferior leads on the repeat ECG, TWI in leads I and aVL, and scooped ST-segments with STD in leads V4-V6 best seen on the initial ECG.

The differential diagnosis for an irregular narrow complex rhythm with bradycardic ventricular rates includes:

- Atrial fibrillation (rate controlled)
- Atrial flutter with variable block (rate controlled)
- Atrial tachycardia with variable block (rate controlled)
- Wandering atrial pacemaker
- 2nd degree AV block Mobitz types I and II
- Variable high-grade AV block (eg, 3:1, 4:1, etc.)
- 2nd degree sinoatrial block
- Sinus arrhythmia
- Sinus bradycardia, junctional rhythm, or junctional bradycardia with irregular pattern of PAC, PJC, and/or PVC
- Sinus bradycardia, junctional rhythm, or junctional bradycardia with regular patterns of PAC, PJC, and/or PVC (bigeminy, trigeminy, etc.)

Figures 1 and 2 show the RR intervals in both the initial and repeat ECGs. With the exception of the last beat of the repeat ECG, there are no discernable P-waves which suggests that the underlying rhythm is atrial fibrillation, although the presence of consistent RR intervals (solid red lines) point against this. Another possibility is a junctional bradycardia with intermittent exit block (which is not visible on an ECG) as the QRS complexes are narrow, consistent in morphology, and not preceded by a P-wave.

Figure 1.
RR intervals from the initial ECG lead II rhythm strip

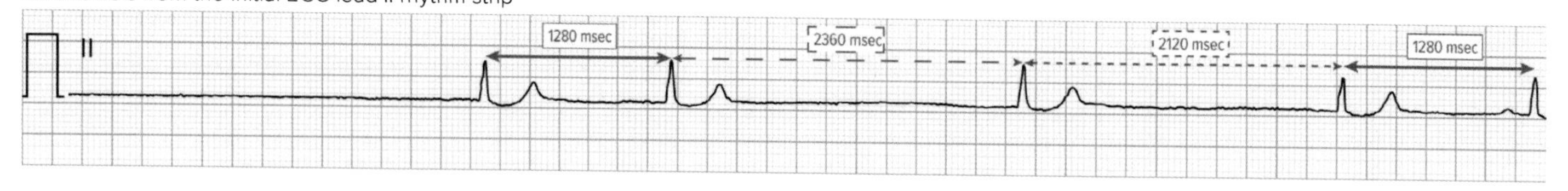

Figure 2.
RR intervals from the repeat ECG lead II rhythm strip

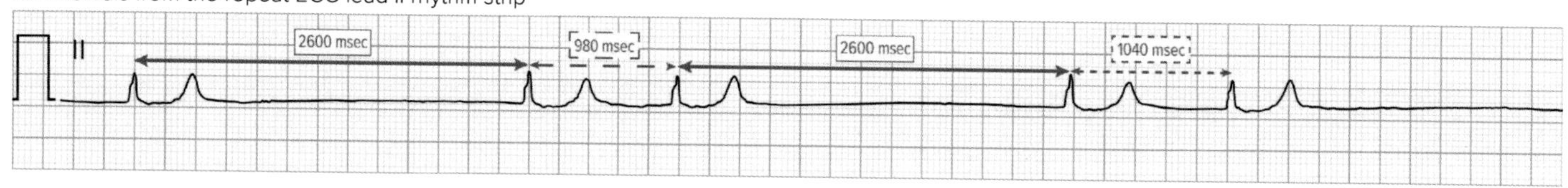

These ECGs prompted concern for digoxin toxicity due to the presence of scooped ST-segments ***(see Figure 3a; Figure 3b*** shows digoxin effect for comparison) in the presence of an irregular bradycardia suggestive of atrial fibrillation with slow ventricular response, but the patient's wife confirmed that the patient was not on any antidysrhythmic medications and had no history of atrial fibrillation.

Figure 3a-b. Comparison of the ST-segment seen in this patient's ECGs (Figure 3a from the lead II rhythm of the initial ECG) with that of a patient who was known to be on digoxin (Figure 3b)

Figure 3a.
This patient's initial ECG

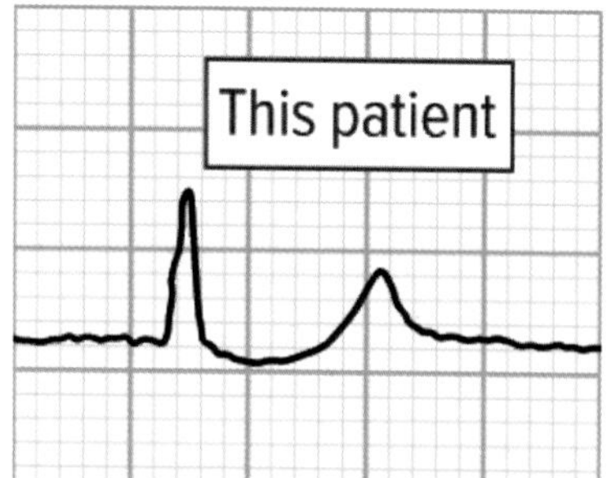

Figure 3b.
Digoxin effect (from a different patient)

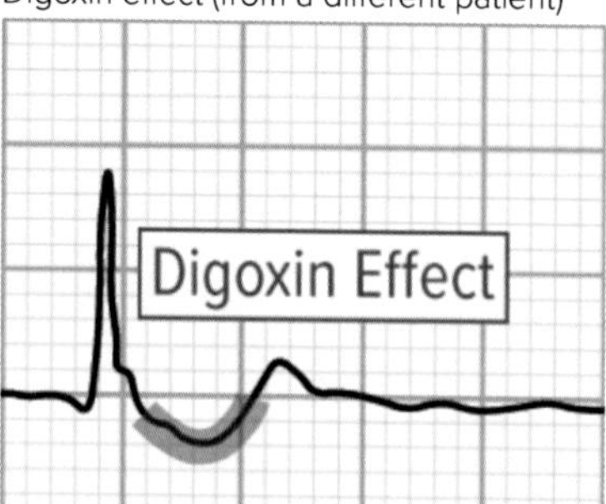

These ECGs also show hyperacute T-waves in the inferior leads with TWI and STD in leads I and aVL (best seen on the repeat ECG) which are concerning for ischemia. This was high on the differential diagnosis once it was confirmed that the patient was not on digoxin.

The patient's labs came back with multiple abnormalities including a potassium of 7.6 mEq/L and significantly elevated BUN and creatinine. The patient was aggressively treated for hyperkalemia and a repeat ECG showed marked improvement **(*see Figure 4*)**. The patient's confusion was likely secondary to uremic encephalopathy. The patient was admitted to the ICU and was back to his baseline when he was discharged from the hospital.

Figure 4.
Repeat ECG after treatment

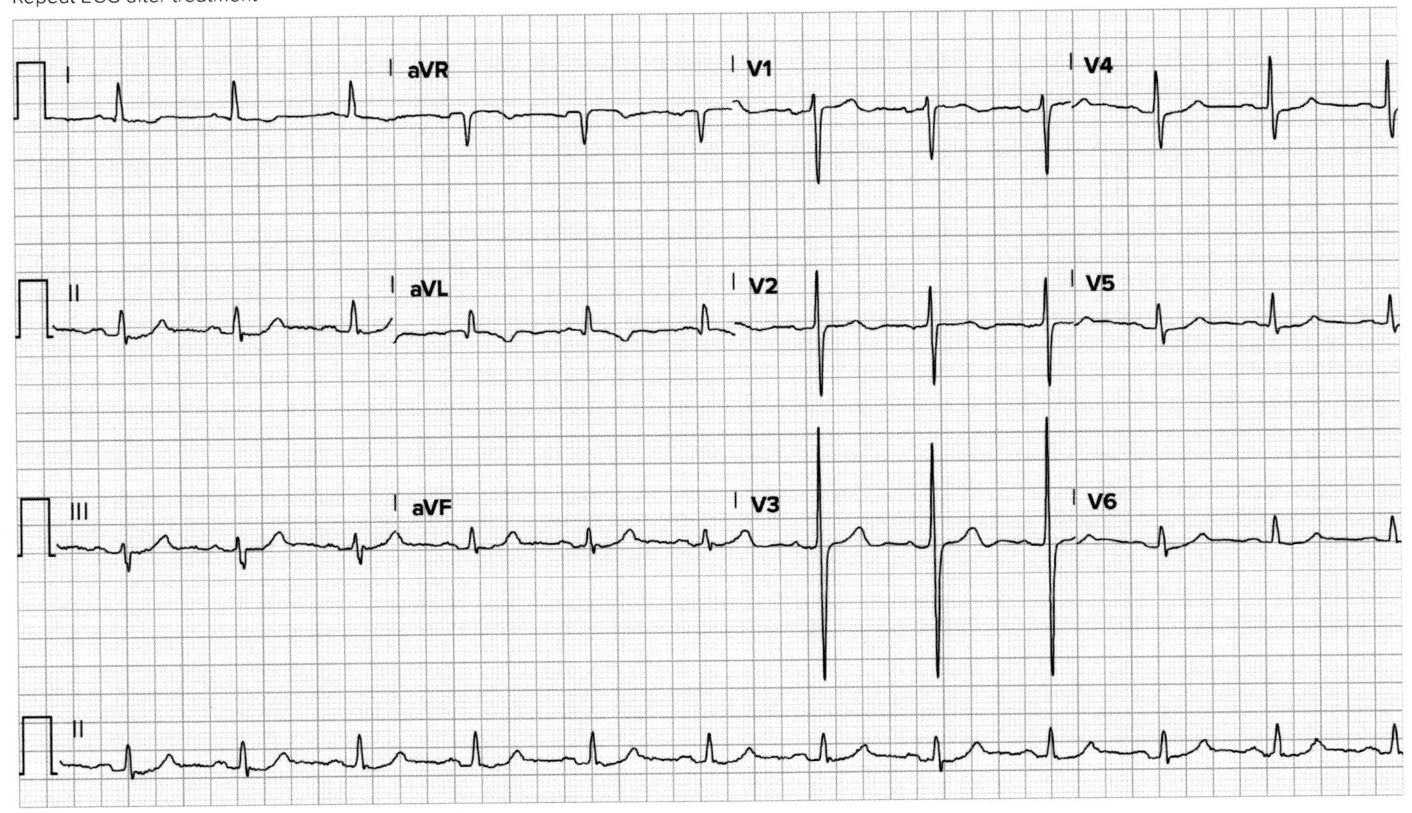

Hyperkalemia Learning Points

- ECG is specific but not sensitive for hyperkalemia
- ECG changes are not always sequential/progressive and include:
  - Tall, narrow, peaked T-waves (best seen in precordial leads)
  - P-wave flattening and PR interval prolongation
  - Prolonged QRS complex duration, ranging from minimal to maximal
  - Conduction abnormalities (AV blocks, fascicular and bundle branch blocks)
  - Bradycardia
  - Sino-ventricular rhythm (loss of P-waves, extremely widened QRS) with normal or slow rate
  - Ventricular dysrhythmias
- Can cause STE (common in leads V1-V2 and aVR) that mimics STEMI or Brugada pattern
- Can occur simultaneously with hyperacute T-waves and obscure early changes seen in an anterior or anteroseptal AMI
- The "syphilis of ECG abnormalities," meaning that a broad range of abnormalities can be encountered with hyperkalemia[1]

References

1. Mattu A. ECG Weekly.

Case 36: Presentation

A 17-year-old female with no past medical history presents after being found unresponsive by family. She was found to be in ventricular fibrillation by EMS and was successfully defibrillated into normal sinus rhythm. What is your interpretation of her ECG?

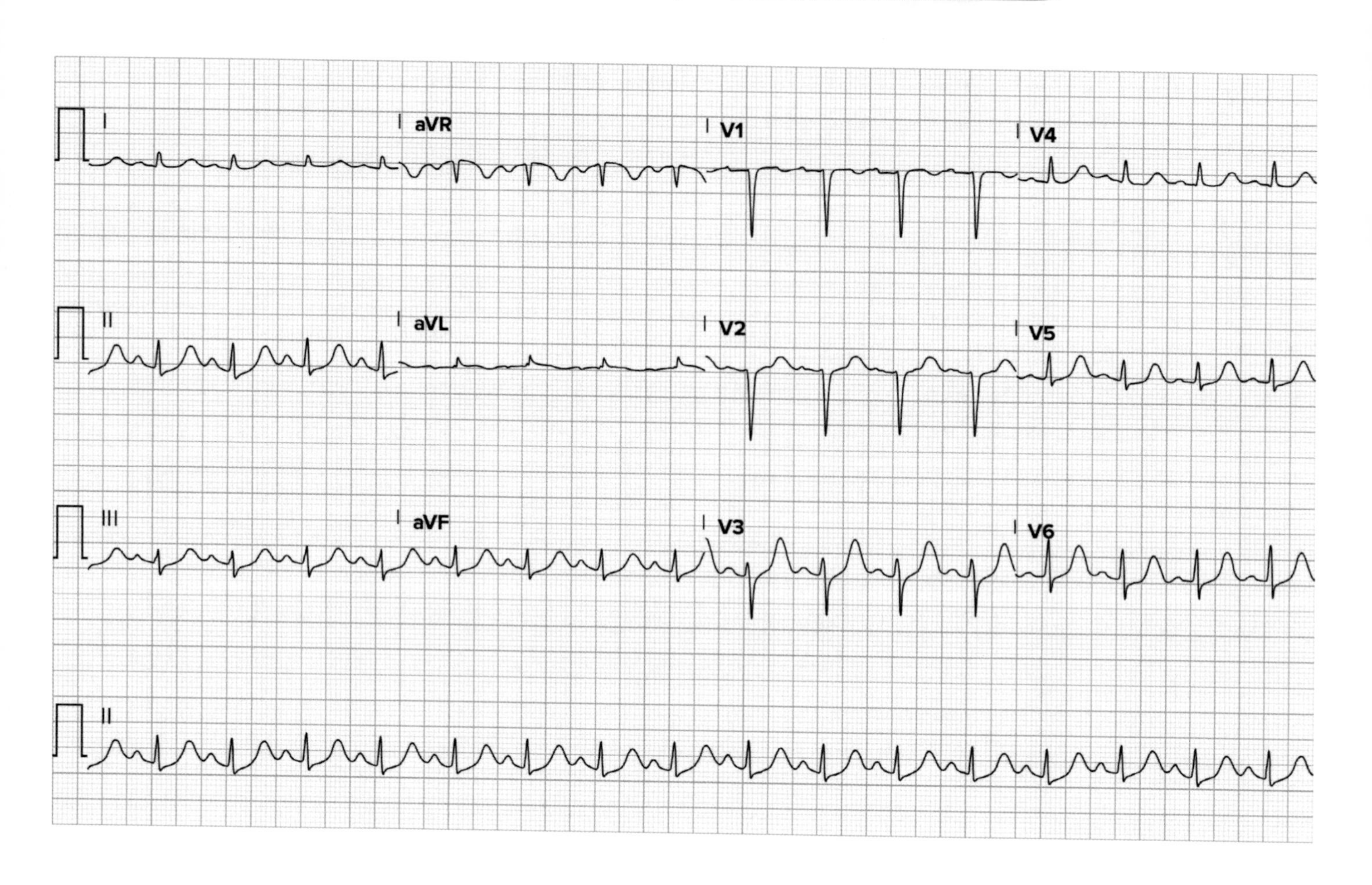

Case 36: Answer

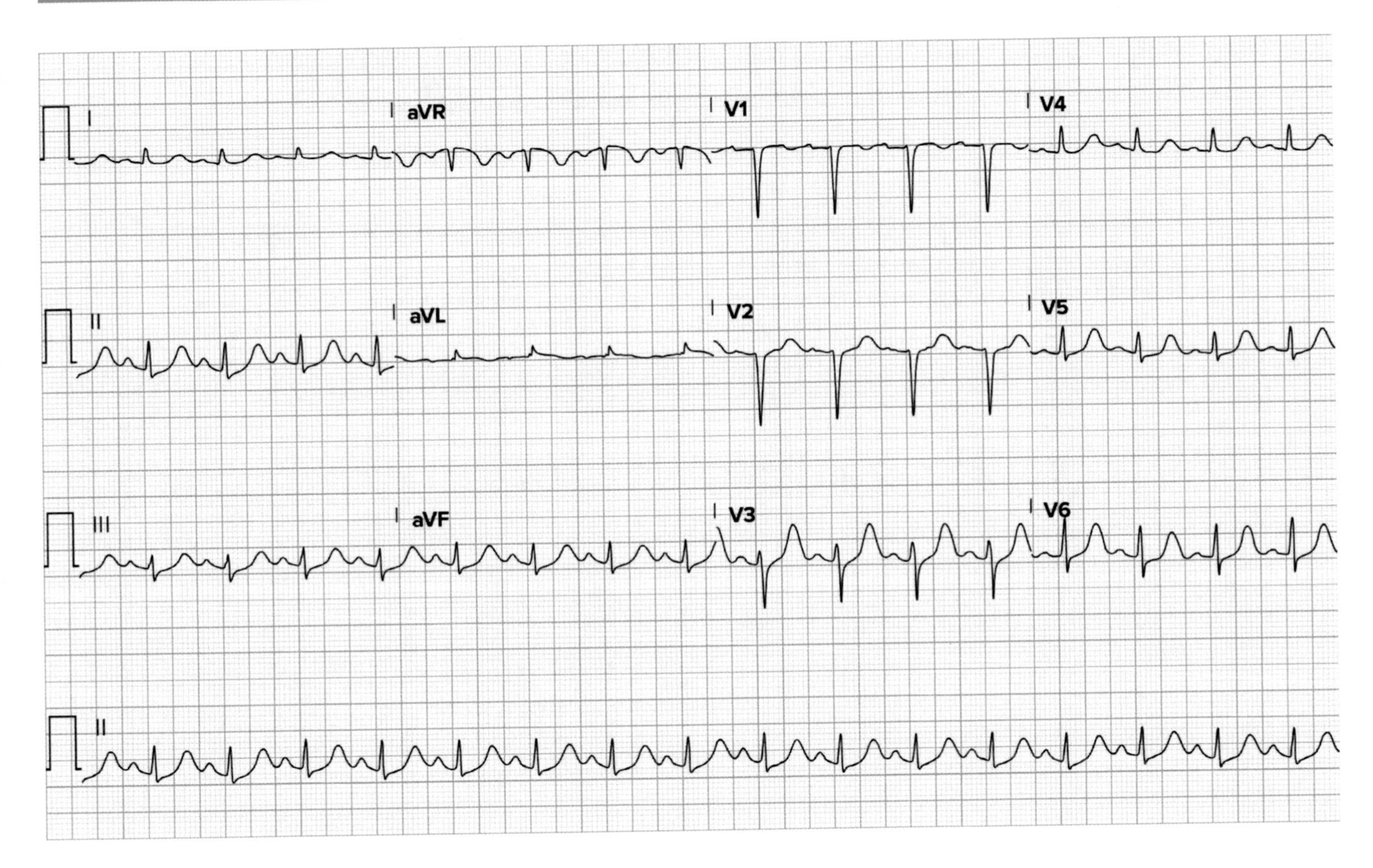

This ECG shows a normal sinus rhythm at 100 bpm, normal axis, prolonged QTc interval of 523 msec, and STD in leads II, III, avF, and V3-V6.

The differential diagnosis for a prolonged QTc interval includes:

- Cardiac ischemia
- Elevated intracranial pressure
- Hypocalcemia
- Hypokalemia
- Hypomagnesemia
- Hypothermia
- Long QT syndrome
- Medications

The differential diagnosis for non-ACS causes of STD includes:

- Hypocalcemia
- Bundle branch blocks
- Digitalis effect
- Left ventricular hypertrophy
- Metabolic abnormalities
- Non-ACS myocardial injury
- Post-electrical cardioversion
- Tachycardia/rate-related
- Ventricular-paced rhythm
- Elevated intracranial pressure

The most significant abnormality in this ECG is the prolonged QTc interval. Per the 2009 AHA/ACCF/HRS guidelines[1], the QT interval should be measured in the lead with longest QT (typically lead V2 or V3) and cutoffs for adults are ≥ 460 msec for women and ≥ 450 msec for men. There is no consensus recommendation for which formula should be used to calculate the QTc.

Long QT Syndrome (LQTS) can be congenital or acquired and the increased QTc interval increases the risk of torsades de pointes (TdP). TdP is a type of polymorphic ventricular tachycardia associated with a prolonged QTc interval on baseline ECG. It is triggered when a PVC occurs at the same time as the T-wave associated with the previous QRS complex (called "R-on-T phenomenon"). One of the key differences in the two types of LQTS is the treatment. Magnesium and electrical overdrive pacing can be used for both, but chemical overdrive pacing, typically with isoproterenol, should only be used for acquired LQTS. Congenital LQTS is considered "adrenergic dependent" and patients will often be on beta-blockers for dysrhythmia prevention, so the use of a beta agonist like isoproterenol is contraindicated.

An important pattern that is associated with a prolonged QTc interval is T-wave alternans (not seen in this case). T-wave alternans is the beat-to-beat alternation of the duration, morphology, and/or polarity of the T-wave ***(see Figure 1)*** not related to alternans of other components of the ECG (ie, QRS complex alternans). It is a marker of myocardial electrical instability and impending ventricular dysrhythmia. T-wave alternans is frequently associated with a long QTc interval that is caused by electrolyte abnormalities (eg, hypokalemia, hypocalcemia), treatment with quinidine, and congenital LQTS[2]. When seen with a long QTc interval, T-wave alternans is considered a precursor to torsades de pointes. It can also be seen in the absence of a long QTc interval, often with myocardial ischemia and both ischemic and non-ischemic cardiomyopathies, in which cases it often precedes ventricular tachycardia and/or ventricular fibrillation.

Figure 1.
Beat-to-beat alteration in the morphology of the T-waves, consistent with T-wave alternans (not from case ECG)

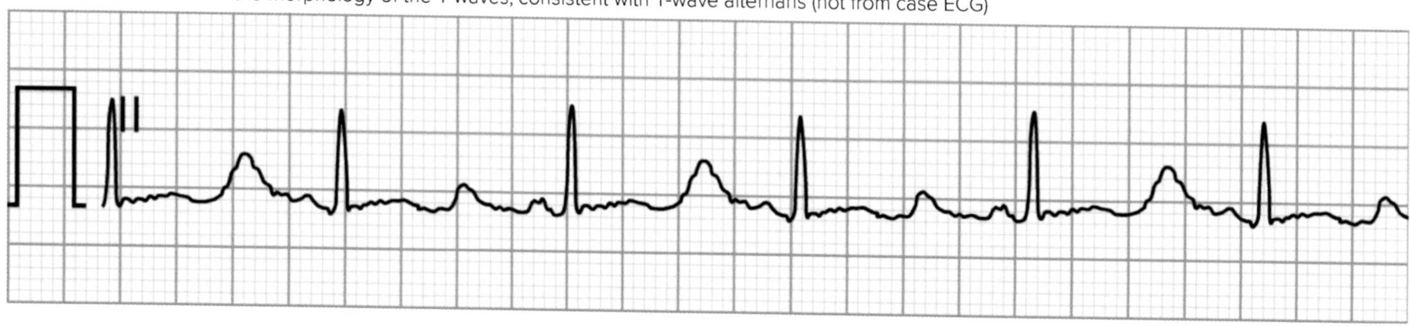

This patient was not on any medications and had no family history of sudden cardiac death. Her ED workup was notable for an elevated lactate likely secondary to cardiac arrest which was also thought to be the cause of the STD seen on the initial ECG as this resolved on subsequent ECGs. She was admitted to the cardiology service and was evaluated by Electrophysiology for AICD placement.

Long QT Syndrome Learning Points

- Congenital or acquired
  - Common acquired etiologies include electrolyte abnormalities (hypokalemia, hypomagnesemia, hypocalcemia), medications, hypothermia, ischemia, elevated ICP
- Prolonged QTc interval is defined as ≥ 460 msec for women and ≥ 450 msec for men
  - QT interval should be measured in the lead with the longest QT interval, usually lead V2 or V3
  - If U-waves superimposed on T-waves are present, measure QT interval in a lead without U-waves, usually lead aVR or aVL
  - Validate computer generated QTc interval with visual inspection of serial ECGs
- Increased risk for torsades typically occurs with QTc > 500 msec
  - AICD is recommended if no reversible cause is found
  - Presence of T-wave alternans = increased risk for ventricular dysrhythmias

References

1. Rautaharju PM, Surawicz B, Gettes LS. AHA/ACCF/HRS recommendations for the standardization and interpretation of the electrocardiogram, part IV: the ST segment, T and U waves, and the QT interval: a scientific statement from the American Heart Association Electrocardiography and Arrhythmias Committee, Council on Clinical Cardiology; the American College of Cardiology Foundation; and the Heart Rhythm Society. Circulation. 2009;119:e241– e250.
2. Knilans T, Surawicz B. Chou's Electrocardiography in Clinical Practice. Philadelphia, PA: Elsevier. 2020.

NOTES:

Case 37: Presentation

A 26-year-old male with no past medical history presents with acute onset of sharp substernal chest pain. What is your interpretation of his ECG?

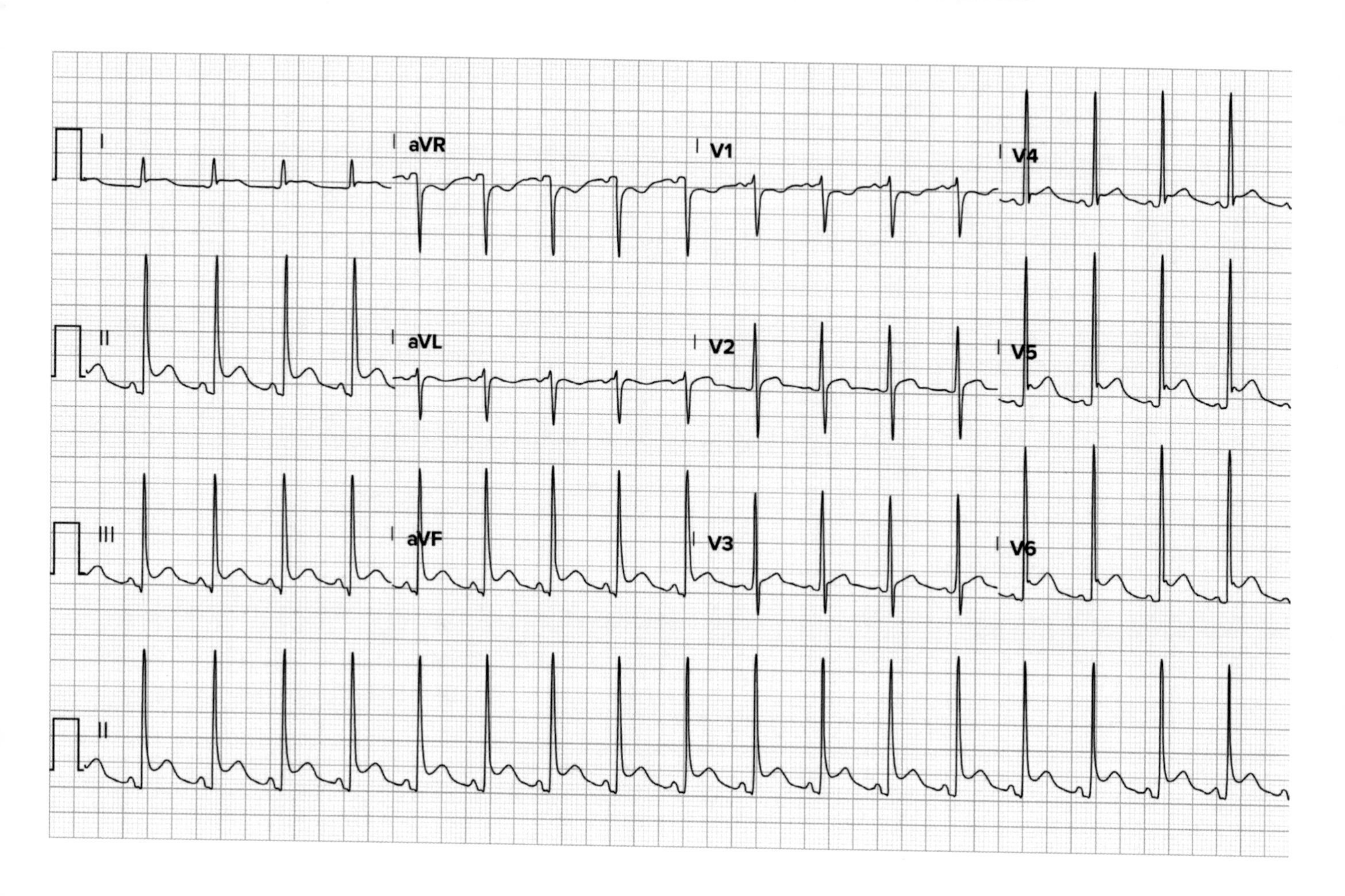

Case 37: Answer

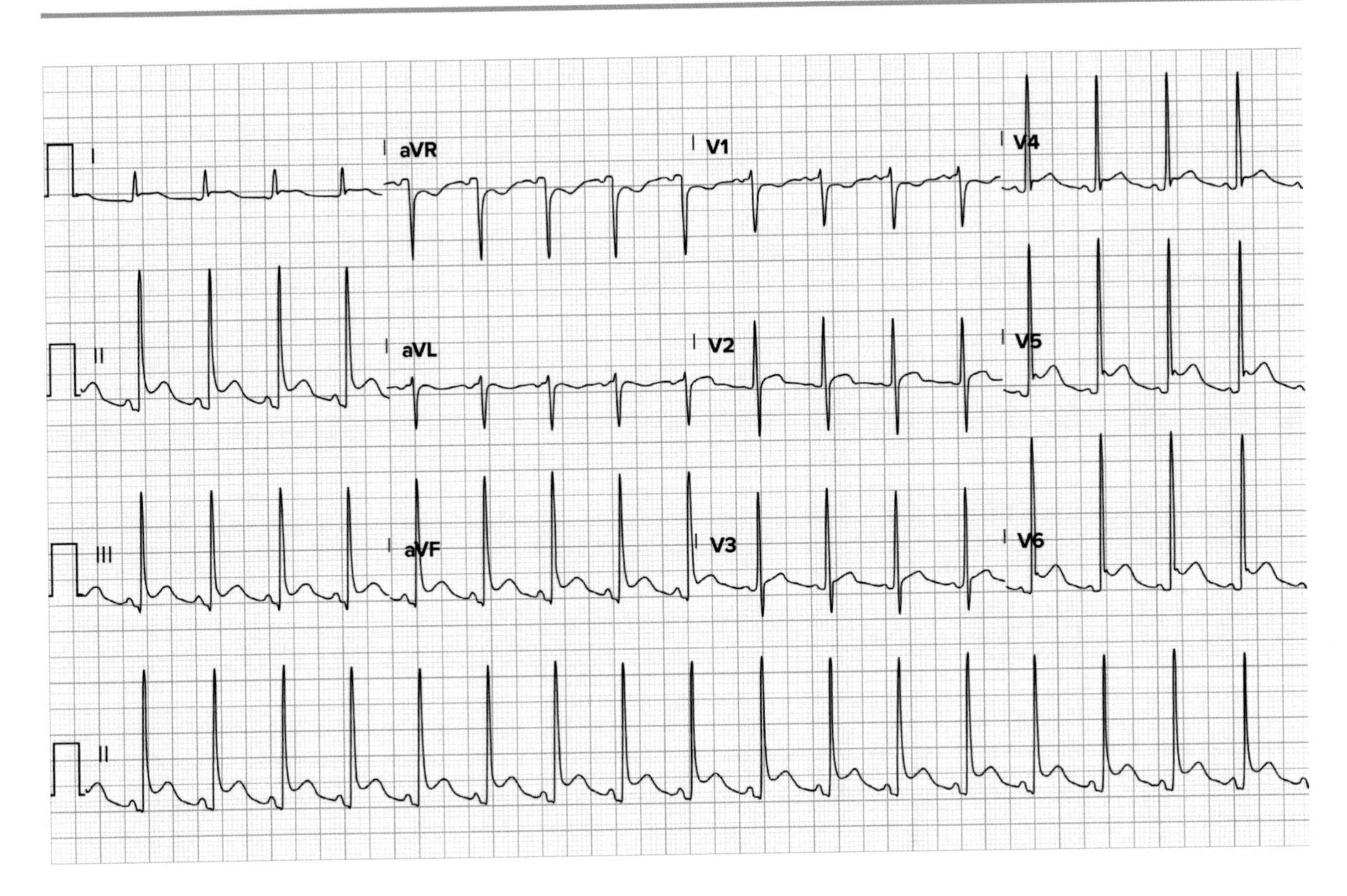

This ECG shows a sinus tachycardia with a ventricular rate of 107 bpm, normal axis, normal intervals, STE and PR segment depression in leads I, II, III, aVF, and V2-V6, STD in leads aVR and V1, and PR segment elevation in leads aVR and V1.

The differential diagnosis for STE includes[1]:	
• Acute myocardial infarction	• Hyperkalemia
• Acute myocarditis	• Hypothermia
• Acute pericarditis	• Left ventricular aneurysm
• Benign early repolarization	• Left ventricular hypertrophy
• Brugada syndrome	• Non-ACS myocardial injury
• Bundle branch blocks	• Pre-excitation syndromes
• Cardiomyopathy	• Post-electrical cardioversion
• CNS injury	• Spiked Helmet Sign
• Coronary vasospasm	• Ventricular rhythms (paced or intrinsic) or ectopy
• Hypercalcemia	

This patient's history, age, and ECG changes are highly suggestive of acute pericarditis, which is an inflammatory process involving the pericardium. Since there are no AHA guidelines on the diagnosis and management of myopericarditis, the European Society of Cardiology guidelines are commonly referenced. The most recent 2015 guidelines[2] are listed below.

The diagnostic criteria for pericarditis include ≥ 2 of the following:

- Pericarditic chest pain: sharp and pleuritic, improved with sitting up and leaning forward
- Pericardial rub: a superficial scratchy or squeaking sound best heard over the left sternal border
- New widespread ST-segment elevations or PR depressions
- New or worsening pericardial effusion

Note that the criteria for pericarditis includes ECG changes, but since the pericardium is electrically silent, these changes are actually secondary to inflammation of the myocardium, often the superficial epicardium. The term myopericarditis is used if there is myocardial involvement appropriate to cause a detectable elevation in cardiac biomarkers but no new LV dysfunction on echocardiogram. The term perimyocarditis is used when there are elevated cardiac biomarkers and new LV dysfunction on echocardiography.

The ECG abnormalities seen in pericarditis classically evolve through 4 stages:

- Stage 1: concave upward STE (typically 2-4 mm) and PR segment depressions diffusely in all leads other than aVR and V1, prominent T-waves, and Spodick's sign (downsloping TP segment)
- Stage 2: normalization of initial abnormalities, most notably the STE
- Stage 3: TWI in the leads that previously had STE
- Stage 4: return to baseline ECG

Stages 1-3 typically develop over hours to days, and Stage 4 may not develop for many weeks. It is important to note that not every patient will have all of these ECG abnormalities nor evolve through these various stages. In fact, there is no time-based understanding of these ECG abnormalities and how they evolve, so it is likely best to disregard the classic stages of ECG abnormalities in the patient with myopericarditis.

PR segment elevations and depressions are due to atrial inflammation and is often described as diagnostic of myopericarditis. PR depression is most often present in leads II, III, aVF, and V5-V6. PR elevation is most often seen in lead aVR. In this patient's ECG, the STD in leads aVR and V1 are likely reciprocal to the diffuse STE, but it is important to note that STD in these leads are very non-specific and can be seen in normal patients.

Spodick's sign is used to describe the downsloping TP segment ***(see Figure 1)*** often seen with pericarditis. It is important to note that Spodick's sign can also be seen with STEMI[3] so it should not be considered diagnostic of pericarditis.

Figure 1.
The lead II rhythm strip shows Spodick's sign, which describes a downsloping TP segment

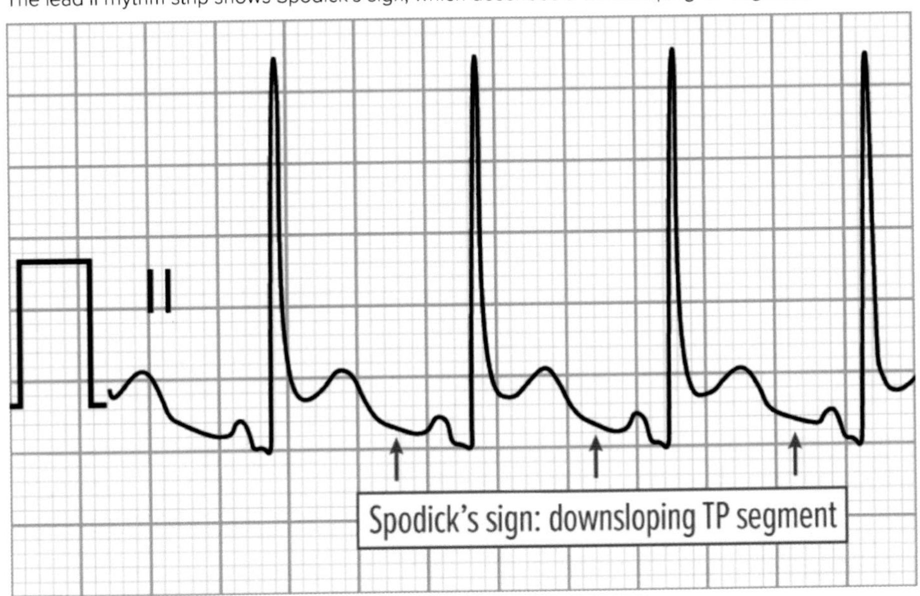

This patient's ED workup was unremarkable, including a bedside echocardiogram that showed no wall motion abnormalities nor pericardial effusion. The patient had no risk factors that would warrant inpatient management and was discharged home.

Pericarditis Learning Points

- 4 stages of transient ST and PR segment changes that can mimic STEMI
  - Sequential evolution through various stages is not required
- ECG findings in stage 1 include:
  - Concave upward STE typically 2-4 mm
  - STE and PR segment depressions diffusely in multiple leads other than aVR and V1
  - PR segment elevation in lead aVR is very common but not specific for pericarditis
  - Spodick's sign: downsloping TP segment, often seen with pericarditis but not specific as it can be seen in AMI[3]
- Q-waves can be seen with myocarditis but not pericarditis

References

1. Mattu A. ECG Weekly.
2. Adler Y, Charron P, Imazio M, et al. 2015 ESC Guidelines for the Diagnosis and Management of Pericardial Diseases: The Task Force for the Diagnosis and Management of Pericardial Diseases of the European Society of Cardiology (ESC) Endorsed by the European Society for Cardio-Thoracic Surgery (EACTS). Eur Heart J. 2015;36(42):2921-2964.
3. Witting MD, Hu KM, Westreich AA, et al. Evaluation of Spodick's Sign and Other Electrocardiographic Findings as Indicators of STEMI and Pericarditis. J Emerg Med. 2020;58(4):562-569.

Case 38: Presentation

A 44-year-old male presents to the emergency department with chest pain.
What is your interpretation of his ECG?

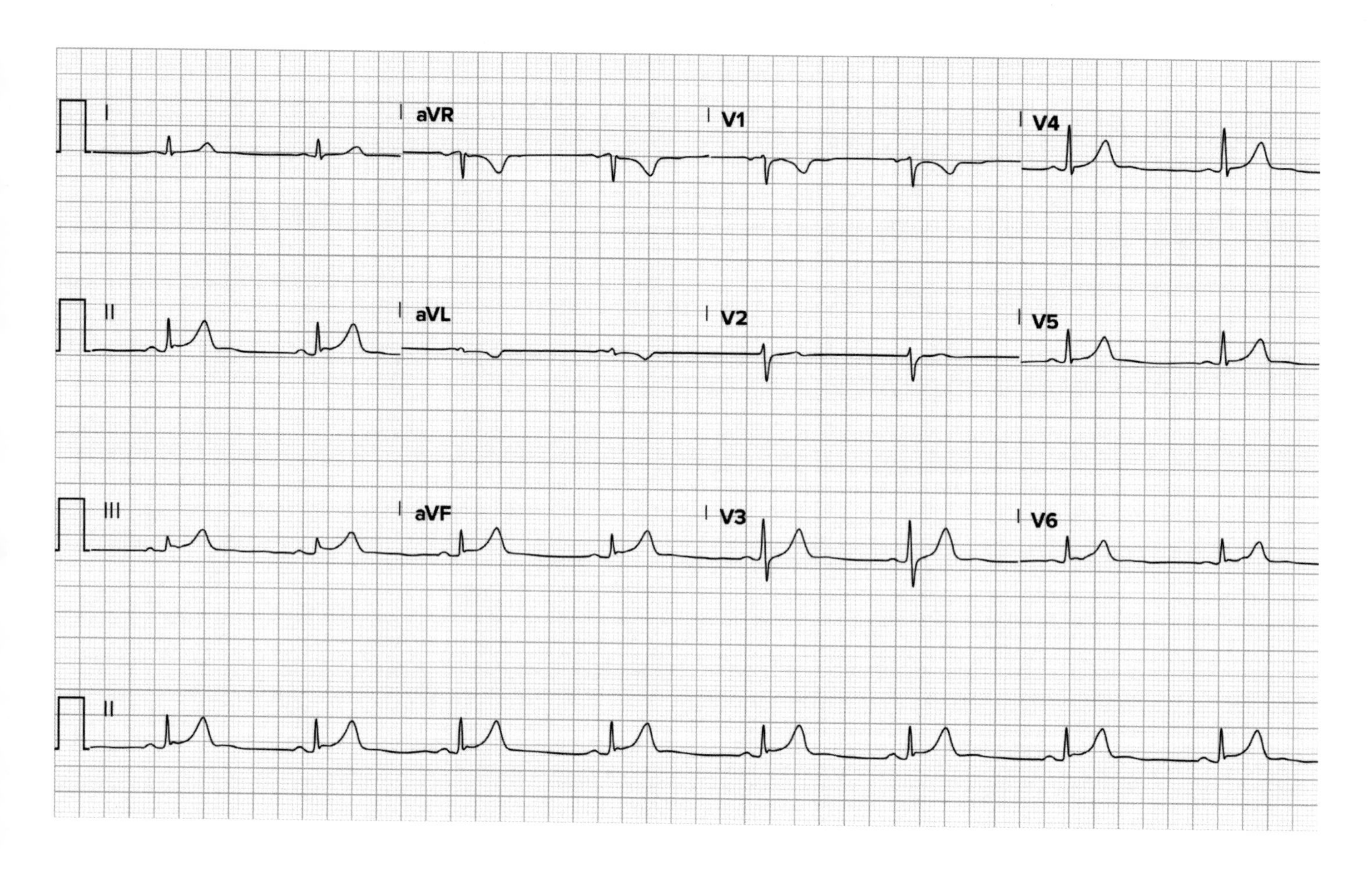

Case 38: Answer

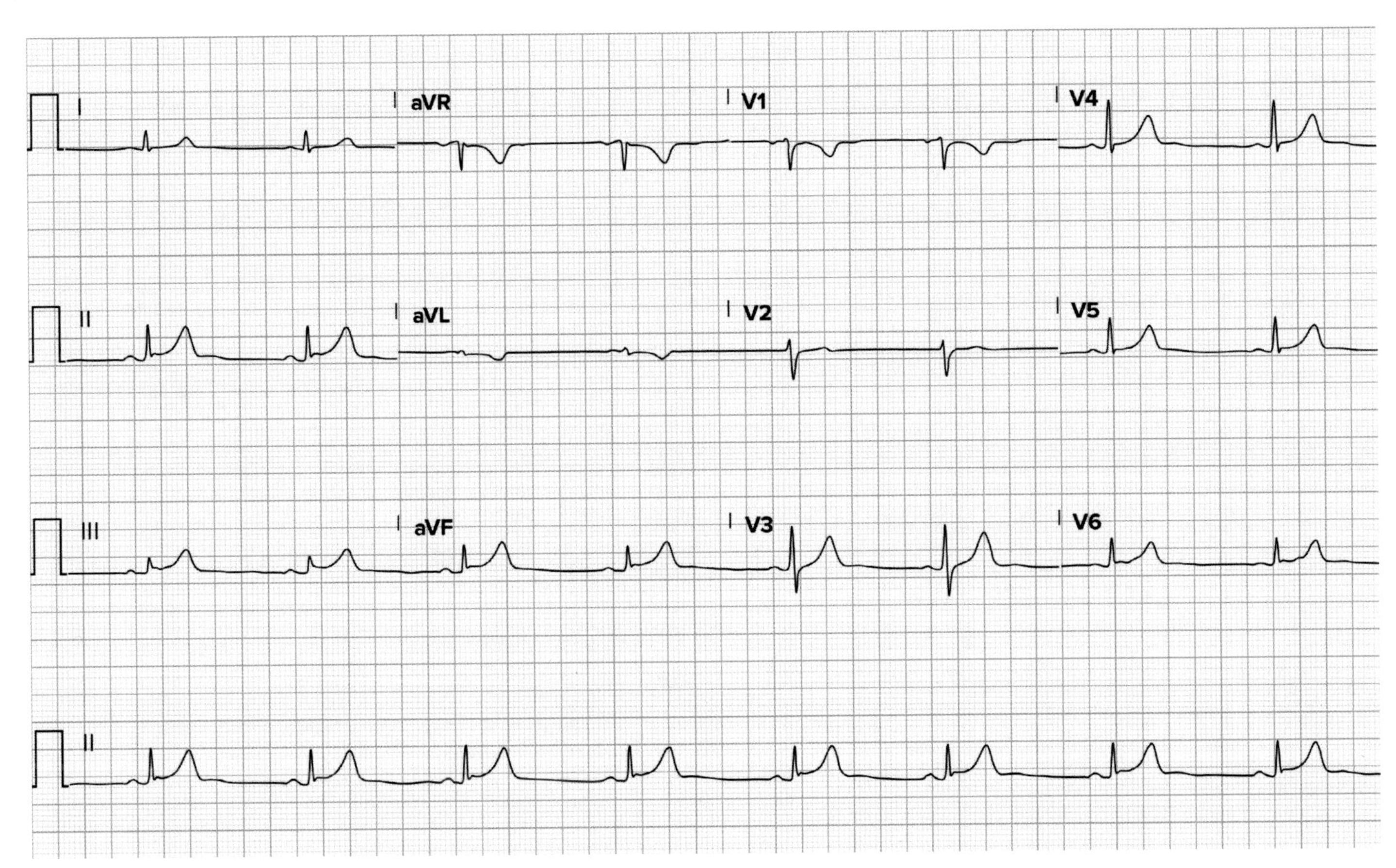

This ECG shows sinus bradycardia at 49 bpm, normal axis, normal intervals, STE and hyperacute T-waves in the inferior leads, and slight STD and TWI in lead aVL.

There is no universally accepted definition for hyperacute T-waves, but they are generally described as broad based and disproportionately tall ***(see Figure 1)***. Hyperacute T-waves can be an early ECG finding in an ischemic event, preceding STE and/or STD. There is no consensus on whether the height of the T-wave should be compared to the amplitude of the preceding R-wave or the entire QRS complex. In this ECG it doesn't matter since the amplitude of the R-wave and the entire QRS complex are the same. Note that the hyperacute T-waves in this ECG are not visually impressive, but when considered in light of the relatively smaller amplitude QRS complexes, they are hyperacute.

The inferior leads all have T-waves as tall, or taller than, the corresponding R-waves consistent with hyperacute T-waves ***(see Figure 1)***. There is reciprocal change in lead aVL with slight STD and TWI.

Figure 1.
The lead II rhythm strip shows hyperacute T-waves

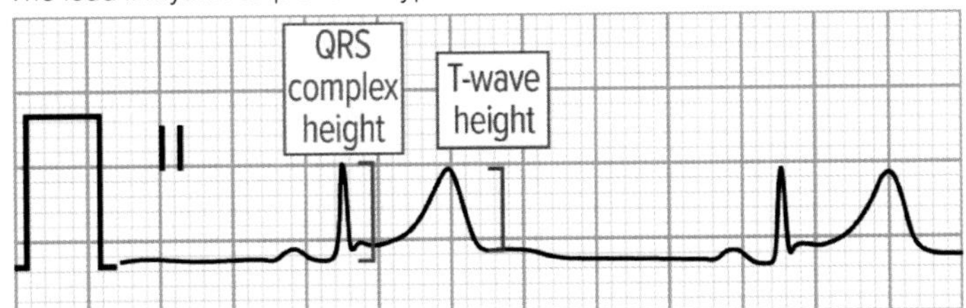

The inferior leads provide a good example of the difficulties in accurately measuring STE. The 2018 Fourth Universal Definition of MI recommend comparing the J point to the TP segment if it's isoelectric, but in this case, it is downsloping ***(see Figure 2)***. Note that the PR segment for the 1st beat is depressed relative to the preceding TP segment and is downsloping in the 2nd beat. The J point is clearly elevated relative to the junction of the PR-segment and the QRS complex, but less elevated relative to the TP segment.

Figure 2.
The absence of a consistent isoelectric baseline makes it difficult to accurately measure STE, as seen in the 2nd and 3rd P-QRS-T complexes of the lead II rhythm strip

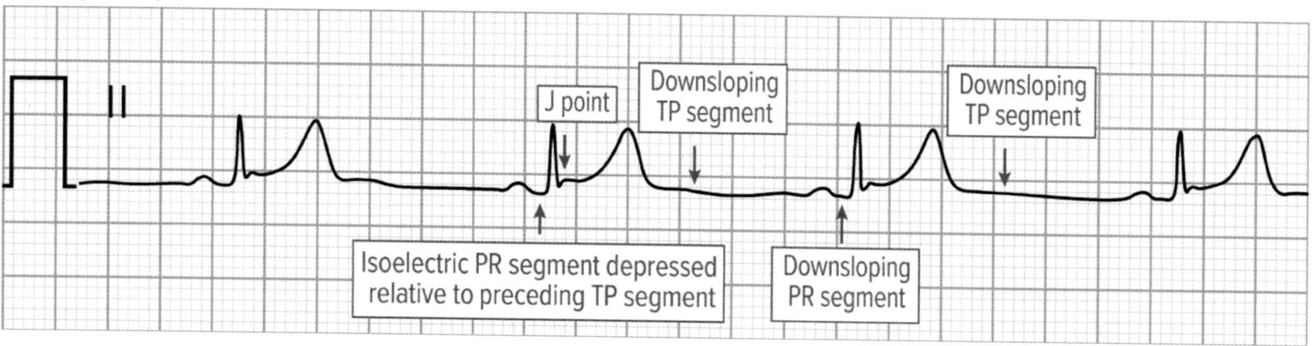

These ECG findings are subtle and "borderline" in meeting STEMI criteria. Note that while the presence of reciprocal STD in lead aVL supports the ECG diagnosis of STEMI, the absence of reciprocal STD does not rule out STEMI. Reciprocal STD can be absent in STEMI, in particular anterior STEMI in which reciprocal STD are absent up to 30% of the time.[1] If the patient's presentation is concerning for an AMI, very close observation with serials ECGs is suggested. In addition, assuming a clinical presentation consistent with an AMI, activating a STEMI alert response (ie, treating the patient for a STEMI) would also be appropriate, as was done in this case.

This patient was taken emergently to the cardiac catheterization laboratory and had a 100% RCA occlusion successfully treated with a stent.

The differential diagnosis for prominent upright T-waves includes:	The differential diagnosis for TWI includes:
• Acute ischemia	• Acute ischemia (early reciprocal changes)
• Benign early repolarization/normal variant STE	• Bundle branch blocks
• Bundle branch blocks	• Cardiomyopathy (eg, Takotsubo, HCM)
• Hyperkalemia	• CNS injury
• LVH	• Digitalis effect
• Ventricular rhythms (paced or intrinsic) or ectopy	• Intra-abdominal disorders
	• Juvenile T-wave pattern
	• LVH
	• Metabolic abnormalities
	• Pericarditis
	• Pre-excitation syndromes
	• Pulmonary embolism
	• Reperfusion (eg, Wellens syndrome)
	• Toxicologic abnormalities
	• Ventricular rhythms (paced or intrinsic) or ectopy

Normal P-wave and T-wave Learning Points

- Normal P-wave and T-wave morphologies[1,2] in normal sinus rhythm in the absence of conduction abnormalities, ischemia, structural abnormalities, etc., include:

I	aVR	V1	V4
P: always upright T: always upright	P: always inverted T: always inverted	P: usually biphasic (+/-) but can be entirely upright or inverted T: upright or inverted	P: upright T: almost always upright
II P: always upright T: always upright	**aVL** P: upright, inverted, or biphasic (-/+) T: upright or inverted	**V2** P: usually biphasic (+/-) but can be entirely upright (entirely inverted is rare) T: usually upright	**V5** P: upright T: always upright
III P: upright, inverted, or biphasic (+/-) T: upright or inverted	**aVF** P: usually upright but can be flat or biphasic T: usually upright	**V3** P: upright T: usually upright	**V6** P: upright T: always upright

- Inverted, flat, or positive-negative biphasic T-waves in lead V1 (less so in leads V2-V3) can be normal
- Positive-negative biphasic T-waves in leads V1-V3 can be abnormal or a normal variant
- T-wave amplitude is typically < 6 mm in limb leads and < 10 mm in precordial leads

Hyperacute T-waves Learning Points

- There is no universally accepted definition of hyperacute T-waves (ie, no absolute specific amplitude), but the general characteristics include ***(see Figure 3)***:
  - Broad based and disproportionately tall
  - Asymmetric morphology with more gradual upslope and more abrupt return to the baseline
  - J point elevation is common
- Hyperacute T-waves + STD/TWI in reciprocal leads = early AMI
- When in doubt, obtain serial ECGs

Figure 3.
Hyperacute T-waves

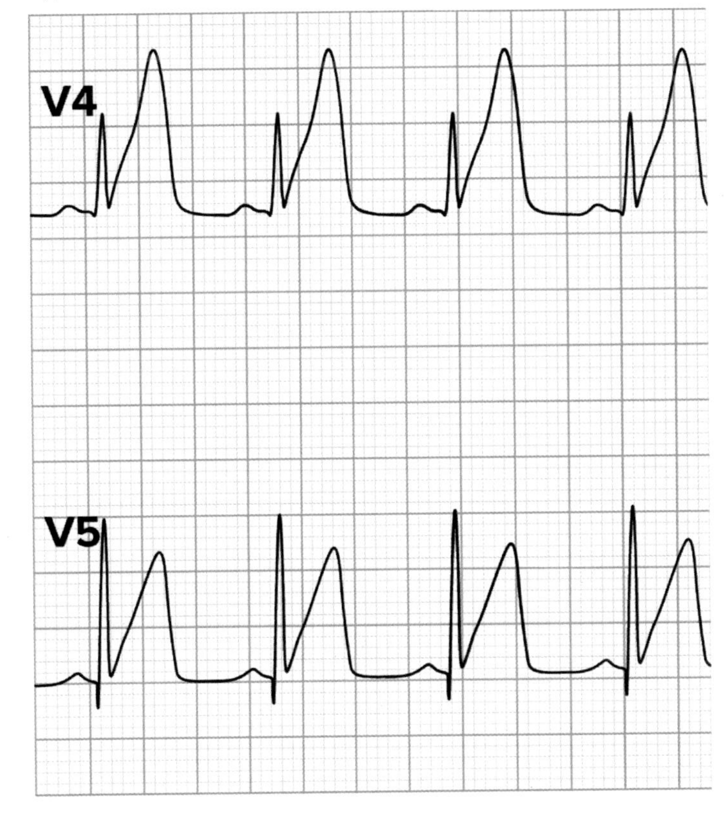

References

1. Knilans T, Surawicz B. Chou's Electrocardiography in Clinical Practice. Philadelphia, PA: Elsevier. 2020.
2. Berberian, JG. Normal P-waves and T-waves. In: Berberian JG, Brady WJ, Mattu A. EMRA EKG Guide, 2nd ed. Emergency Medicine Residents' Association. Dallas, TX:2022:1.

T-wave Inversions Learning Points

- Ischemic TWI
  - New from prior TWI ≥ 1 mm in ≥ 2 contiguous leads with prominent R-wave or R/S ratio > 1
- TWI in lead aVL
  - Can be seen in inferior MI before inferior STE and has high sensitivity/specificity/positive predictive value for RV AMI
- When in doubt, obtain serial ECGs

STEMI Learning Points

- STEMI is defined by new, or presumed new, STE at the J point in ≥ 2 anatomically contiguous leads in the absence of LVH by voltage pattern, LBBB, or ventricular-paced rhythm
  - ≥ 2.5 mm in men < 40 years old and ≥ 2 mm in men ≥ 40 years old in leads V2-V3 (or an increase of ≥ 1 mm when compared to baseline ECG)
  - ≥ 1.5 mm in women in leads V2-V3 (or an increase of ≥ 1 mm when compared to baseline ECG)
  - ≥ 1 mm in all other leads
- ST-segment is measured from the isoelectric baseline, typically the TP segment (see below)
- Reciprocal STD are not required for the diagnosis of STEMI, but their presence does increase the likelihood of the diagnosis of STEMI
  - Reciprocal STD are only present in 70% of anterior MI[1]
- Posterior MI
  - Consider whenever there is STD in leads V1-V4
  - STE ≥ 0.5 mm in posterior leads V7, V8 or V9 is diagnostic- does not require 2 contiguous leads
- Right ventricular MI
  - Consider with any inferior MI (RV MI is seen in approximately 1/3 of inferior MI)
  - STE in right precordial leads V3R and V4R ≥ 0.5 mm (≥ 1 mm for men ≤ 30 years old)
  - STE in right precordial lead V4R > 1 mm is most predictive of RV MI
  - STE in right precordial lead V4R > STE in leads V1-V3 = highly specific for RV MI
- Significant STE that does not meet the traditional distribution (ie, ≥ 2 anatomically contiguous leads) in a presentation concerning for ACS may still represent coronary artery occlusion and warrant consideration for emergent coronary reperfusion

How to Measure STE per most recent 2018 AHA Guidelines[2]

- The J point is the junction between QRS termination and ST-segment onset and is used to determine the magnitude of the ST-segment shift
- **In patients with a stable baseline, the TP segment (isoelectric interval) is a more accurate method to assess the magnitude of ST-segment shift *(see Figure 4)***, and in distinguishing pericarditis from acute myocardial ischemia
- QRS onset should be used if TP segment does not have a stable baseline ***(see Figure 5)***
- Measurement should be made from the top of the ECG line tracing

Figure 4.
Measure STE from the TP segment if the TP segment is isoelectric (ie, horizontal)

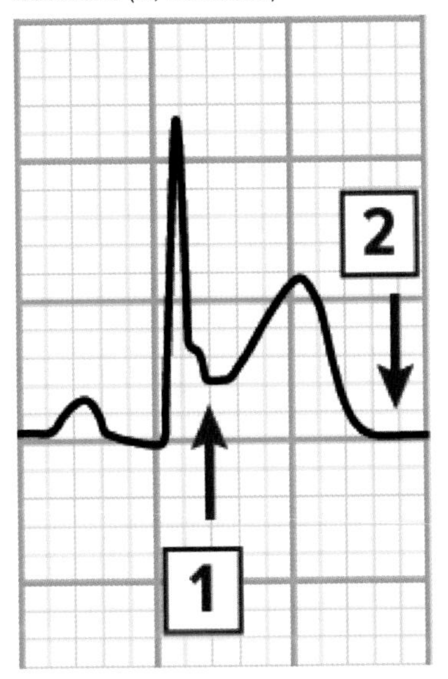

Arrow 1: onset of the ST-segment (ie, J point)
Arrow 2: TP segment

Figure 5.
Measure STE from onset of the QRS complex if the TP segment is not isoelectric (ie, not horizontal)

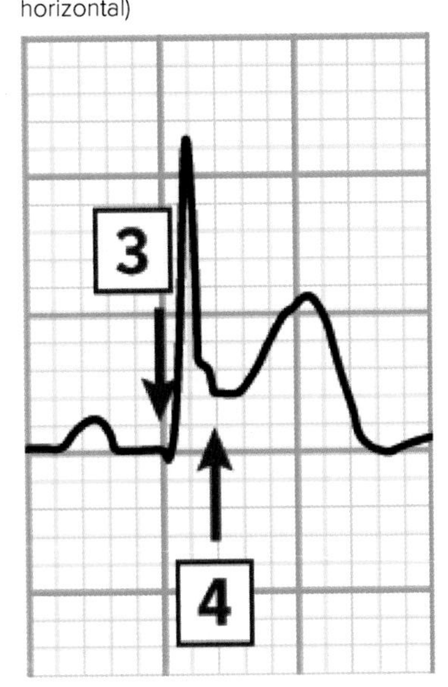

Arrow 3: initial onset of the Q-wave
Arrow 4: onset of the ST-segment (ie, J point)

References

1. Knilans T, Surawicz B. Chou's Electrocardiography in Clinical Practice. Philadelphia, PA: Elsevier. 2020.
2. Thygesen K, Alpert JS, Jaffe AS, et al. 2018 ESC/ACC/AHA/WHF Expert Consensus Document: Fourth Universal Definition of Myocardial Infarction (2018). Circulation. 2018;138:e618-e651.

Case 39: Presentation

A 63-year-old male presents with exertional near syncope.
What is your interpretation of his ECG?

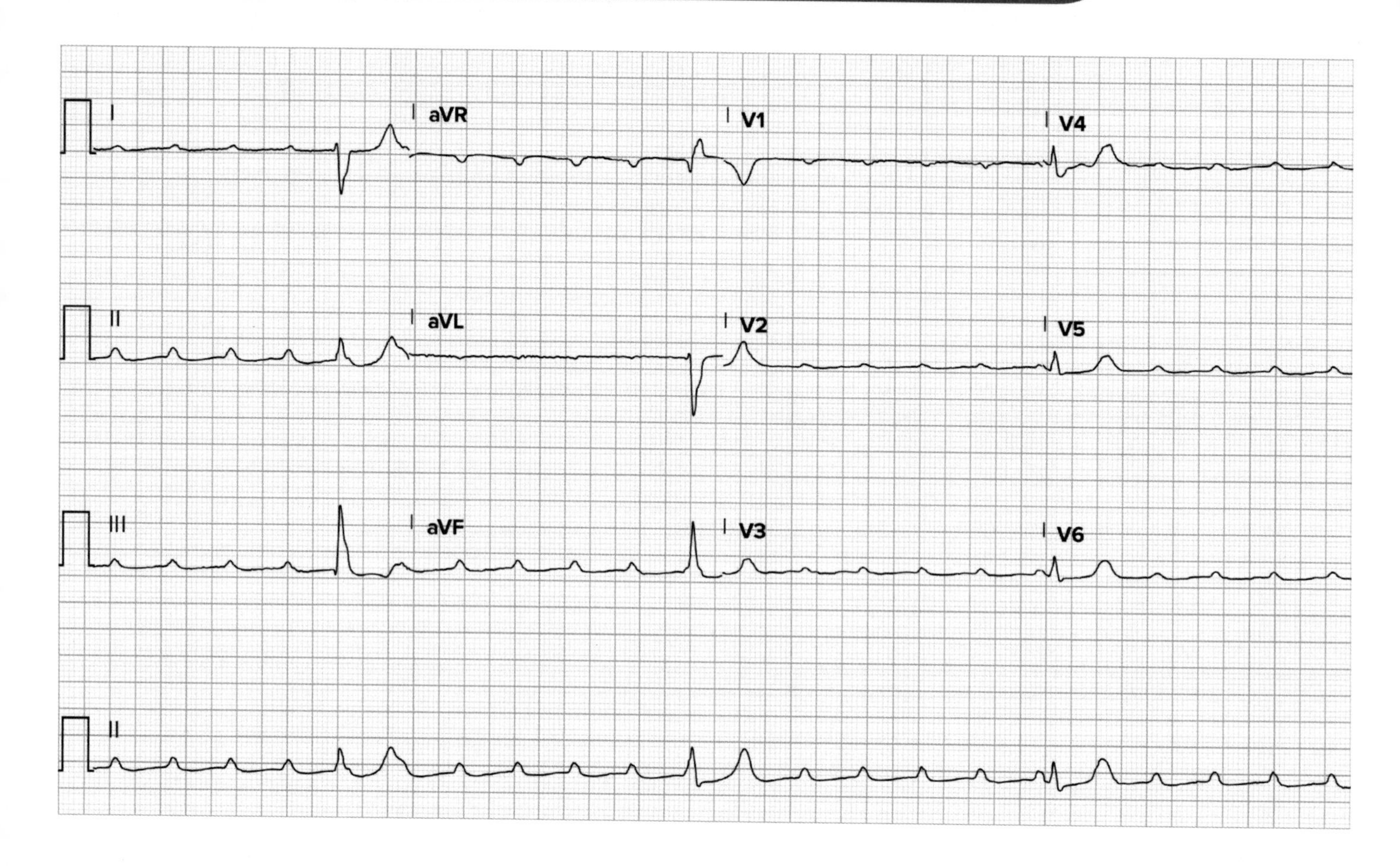

Case 39: Answer

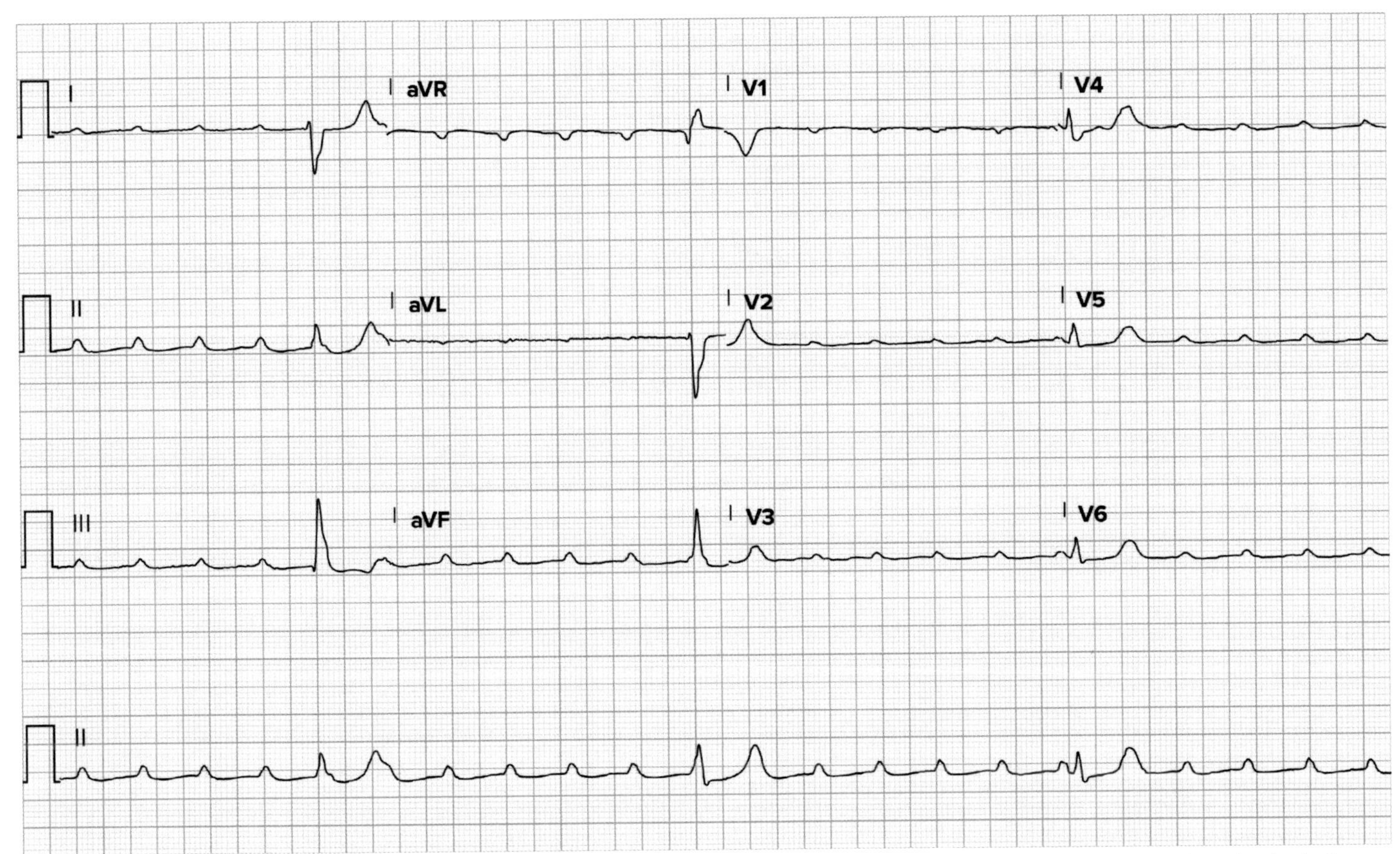

This ECG shows a 3rd degree AV block with a ventricular rate of ~21 bpm and an atrial rate of 130 bpm, right axis deviation, and prolonged QRS complex duration ~130 msec. The lack of QRS complexes makes it impossible to assess for ischemia or to determine the cause of the conduction delay.

The key to correctly interpreting this ECG is recognizing the multiple findings consistent with a 3rd degree AV block. The P-waves and QRS complexes march out at different rates ***(see Figure 1)*** which is indicative of AV dissociation, the atrial rate is greater than the ventricular rate, and the PR intervals are variable ***(see Figure 2)***. All of these findings are also consistent with a 3rd degree AV block.

Figure 1.
The lead II rhythm strip shows an atrial rate (PP interval) a little more than 6 times faster than the ventricular rate (RR interval), consistent with a 3rd degree AV block

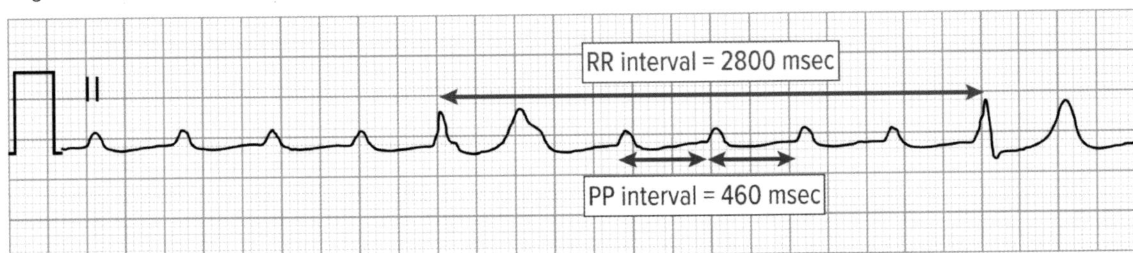

Figure 2.
The lead II rhythm strip shows variable PR intervals, consistent with a 3rd degree AV block

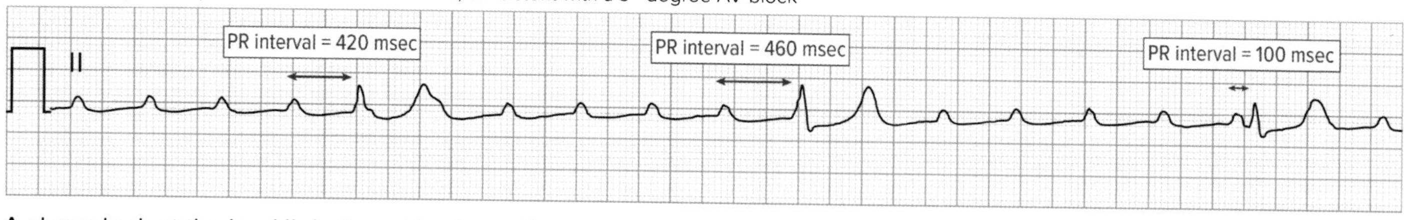

A closer look at the lead II rhythm strip shows P-waves that march out and are intermittently buried or hidden in the QRS complexes and T-waves ***(see Figure 3)***.

Figure 3.
The lead II rhythm strip shows P-waves that march out and are intermittently buried or hidden in the QRS complexes and T-waves

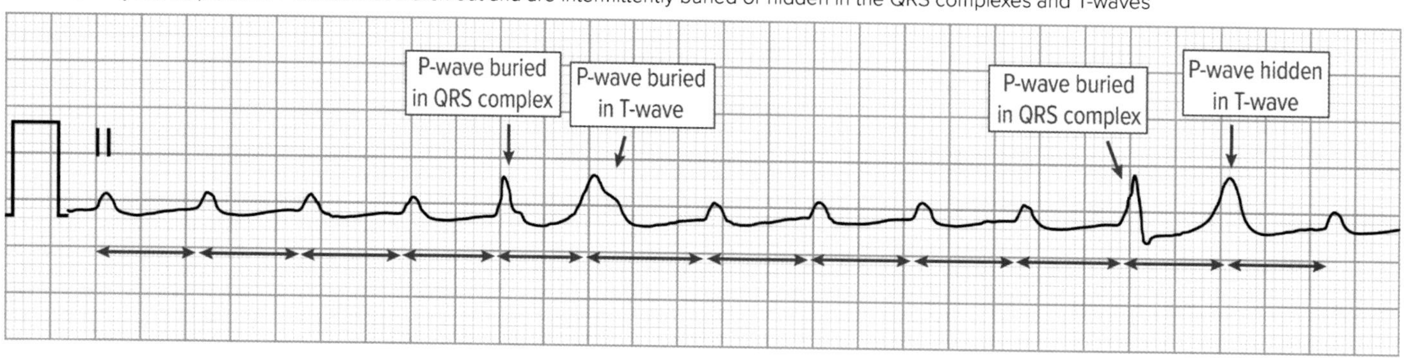

Extrinsic causes of this dysrhythmia should be considered, in particular medication-induced AV node poisoning (eg, beta-blocker or CCB toxicity).

This patient had an unremarkable workup in the ED and was admitted to the cardiology service for placement of a permanent pacemaker.

3rd Degree AV Block Learning Points

- A 3rd degree AV block, or complete heart block, is defined by the absence of conduction through the AV node leading to complete AV dissociation
  - P-waves “march out” (ie, constant PP interval) and do not conduct to produce a QRS complex
  - PR intervals are variable
  - Atrial rate > ventricular rate
  - Ventricular rhythm is usually junctional or ventricular escape rhythm
- All patients require admission and evaluation for pacemaker placement

NOTES:

Case 40: Presentation

An otherwise healthy 30-year-old male presents with chest tightness that started 2 hours ago. What is your interpretation of his ECG?

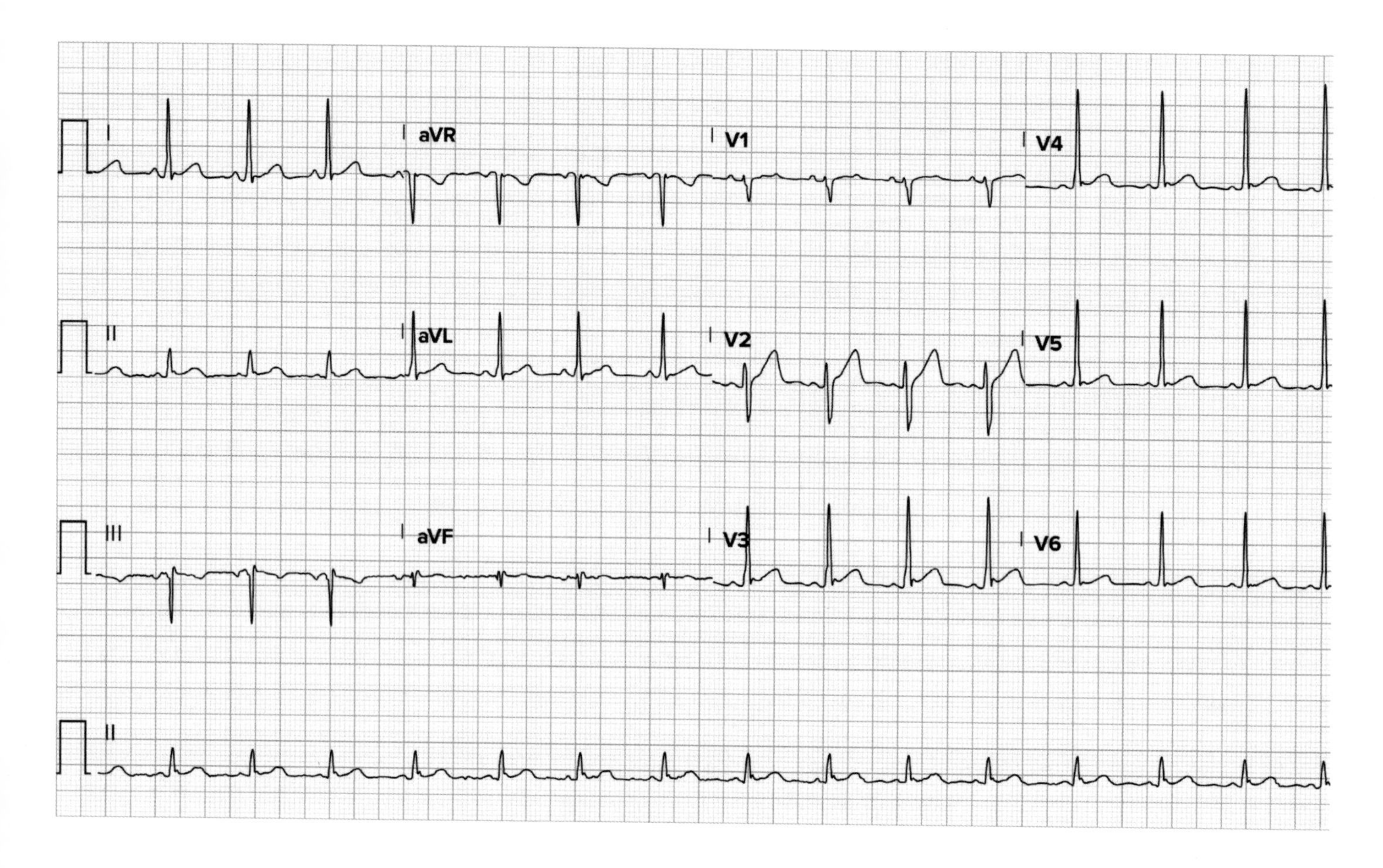

Case 40: Answer

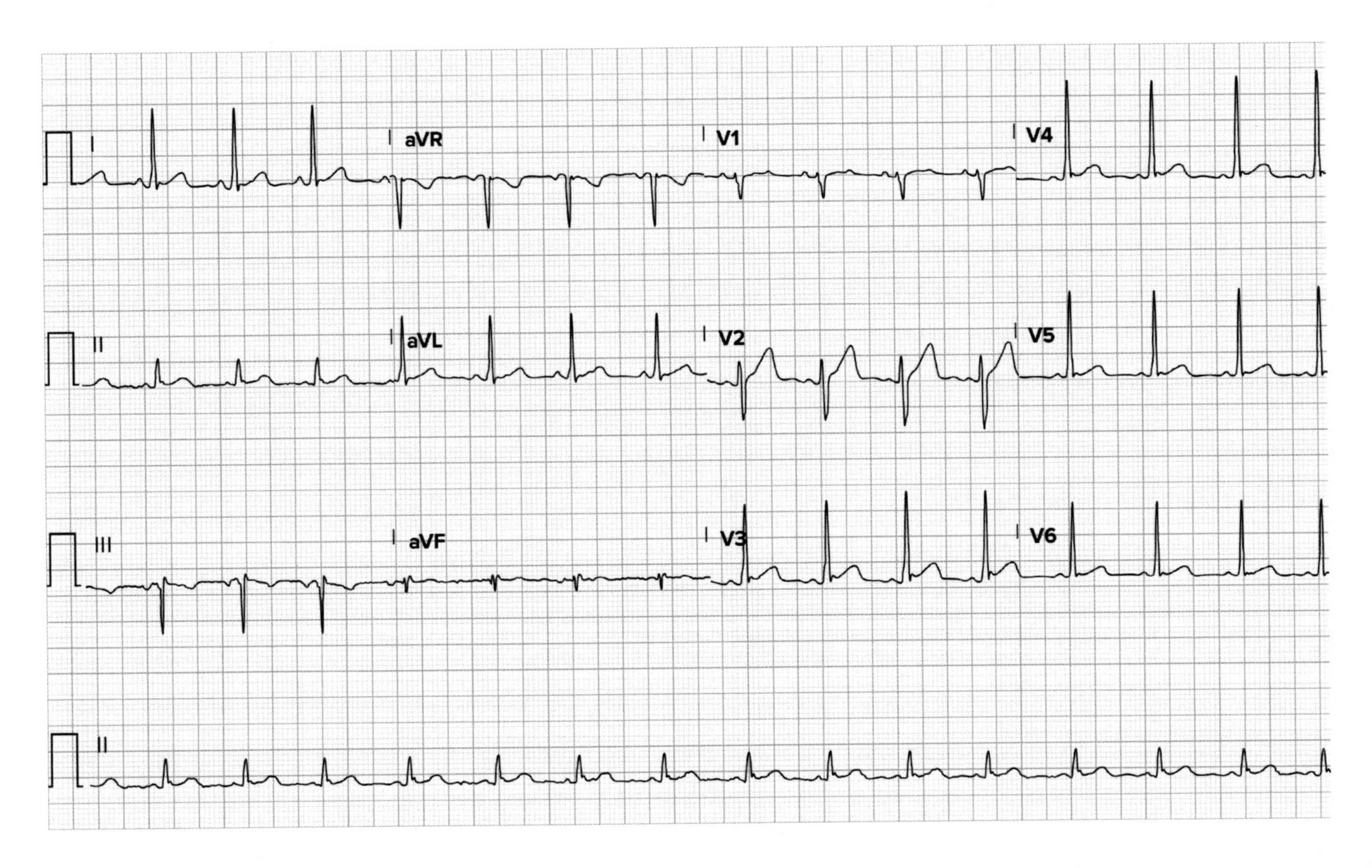

This ECG shows a normal sinus rhythm with a ventricular rate of 90 bpm, normal axis, short PR interval of 115 msec, STE in leads I, II, and V2-V6, and left arm-left leg (LA-LL) lead reversal.

The differential diagnosis for STE includes[1]:	
• Acute myocardial infarction	• Hyperkalemia
• Acute myocarditis	• Hypothermia
• Acute pericarditis	• Left ventricular aneurysm
• Benign early repolarization	• Left ventricular hypertrophy
• Brugada syndrome	• Non-ACS myocardial injury
• Bundle branch blocks	• Pre-excitation syndromes
• Cardiomyopathy	• Post-electrical cardioversion
• CNS injury	• Spiked Helmet Sign
• Coronary vasospasm	• Ventricular rhythms (paced or intrinsic) or ectopy
• Hypercalcemia	

The primary task in the interpretation of this ECG is determining whether the STE is due to an AMI or a non-ACS cause. The most significant STE is seen in leads V2-V4 which can be seen with an anterior MI or benign early repolarization (BER, also called normal variant STE), among many other entities. The presence of terminal QRS distortion is a useful tool to help distinguish between the two ECG entities when confronted with such an ECG. Terminal QRS distortion is frequently present in anterior MI as compared to benign early repolarization, where it is frequently absent.

When used to distinguish between BER and anterior MI, terminal QRS distortion is defined as the absence of either an S-wave or J-wave in both leads V2 and V3.[2] J-waves are positive deflections at the terminal junction of the QRS complex and beginning of the ST-segment take-off, resembling a small dome or hump ***(see Figure 1)***. S-waves are defined as negative deflections after the R-wave that cross the PQ junction ***(see Figure 2)***.

The presence of terminal QRS distortion is highly specific to an anterior MI ***(see Figure 3)*** and LAD occlusion, which means that if you see terminal QRS distortion then there is almost certainly an AMI. Conversely, there should not be terminal QRS distortion with BER. In other words, there must be either an S-wave or J-wave in both leads V2 and V3 to diagnose BER. This ECG shows an S-wave in lead V2 and a J-wave in lead V3 which is consistent with BER.

Figure 1.
Lead V3 shows J-waves, consistent with BER

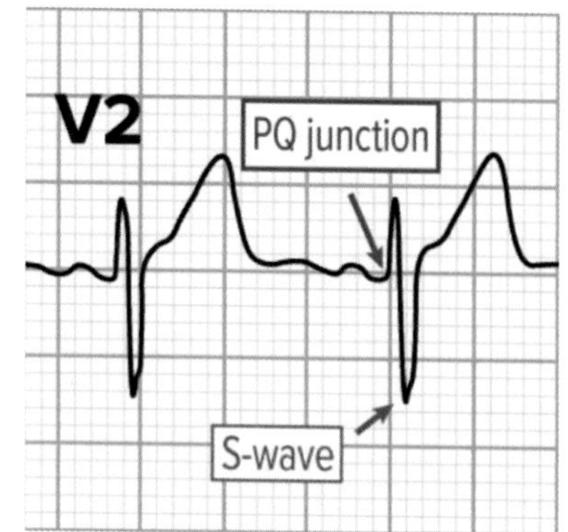

Figure 2.
Lead V2 shows S-waves that cross the PQ junction, consistent with BER

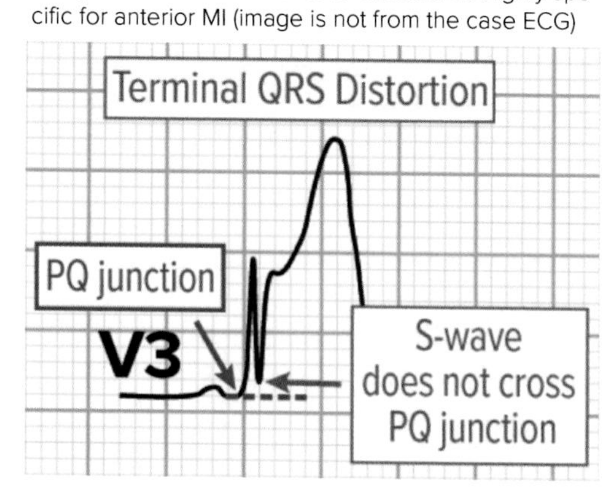

Figure 3.
The presence of terminal QRS distortion is highly specific for anterior MI (image is not from the case ECG)

When considering ACS, in addition to ECG findings, a simple reality check with regards the patient's presentation is frequently helpful, particularly when asking the clinical question "is a STEMI present?" As is true in the interpretation of most diagnostic tests in clinical medicine, read the ECG within the context of the individual patient's presentation; in this particular case, if the STE was STEMI-related, it is quite likely that the patient would appear acutely ill.

This ECG also shows a short PR interval (ie, < 120 msec). A short PR interval can be seen with pre-excitation syndromes such as WPW *(see Figure 4)*, ectopic atrial rhythms originating near AV node, and junctional rhythms with retrograde P-waves *(see Figure 5)*. It can also be a normal variant often seen in young athletes due to increased resting AV nodal conduction or sympathetic tone.

Figure 4.
Short PR interval seen with WPW syndrome
(image is not from the case ECG)

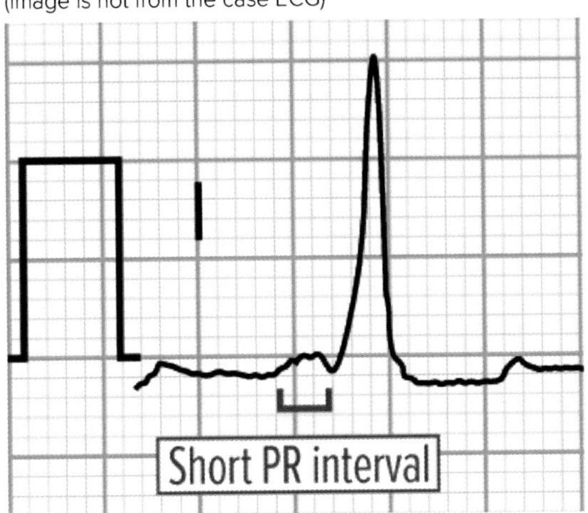

Figure 5.
Short PR interval seen with junctional rhythm and retrograde P-waves
(image is not from the case ECG

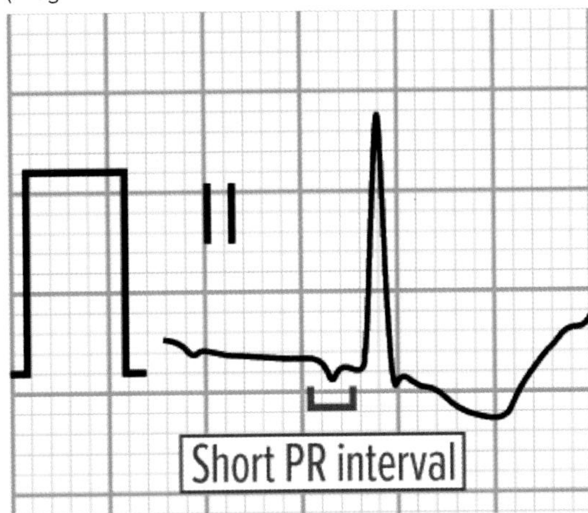

Historically, patients presenting with syncope or paroxysmal tachycardia with ECGs showing a short PR interval and normal QRS duration were presumptively diagnosed as having Lown-Ganong-Levine (LGL) syndrome. This syndrome is a ventricular pre-excitation syndrome similar to WPW except the accessory pathway is intranodal or paranodal so there is no delta wave nor prolonged QRS complex duration. This approach is no longer considered standard practice and in the absence of concerning symptoms or evidence of an accessory pathway, a short PR interval does not typically warrant further workup.

ECG findings seen with LA-LL lead reversal include:

1. In comparison to normal P-QRS-T complexes (ie, normal sinus rhythm with normal lead placement), leads I and II "switch places," meaning that the normal findings in lead I are noted in lead II and vice versa
2. In comparison to normal P-QRS-T complexes (ie, normal sinus rhythm with normal lead placement), leads aVL and aVF "switch places," so the normal findings in lead aVL are noted in lead aVF and vice versa
3. Lead III is inverted, meaning that the P-QRS-T complexes are all oriented in the opposite direction from the normal P-QRS-T complexes (ie, normal sinus rhythm with normal lead placement)
4. Lead aVR is unchanged

These findings can be best seen by comparing the limb leads of the patient's ECG in this case with a prior ECG that had normal lead placement *(see Figures 6a and 6b)*.

Figure 6.
Comparison of limb leads from case ECG with LA-LL lead reversal with a prior ECG with normal lead placement

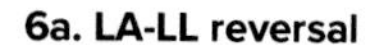

6a. LA-LL reversal
(case ECG)

6b. Normal lead placement
(prior ECG)

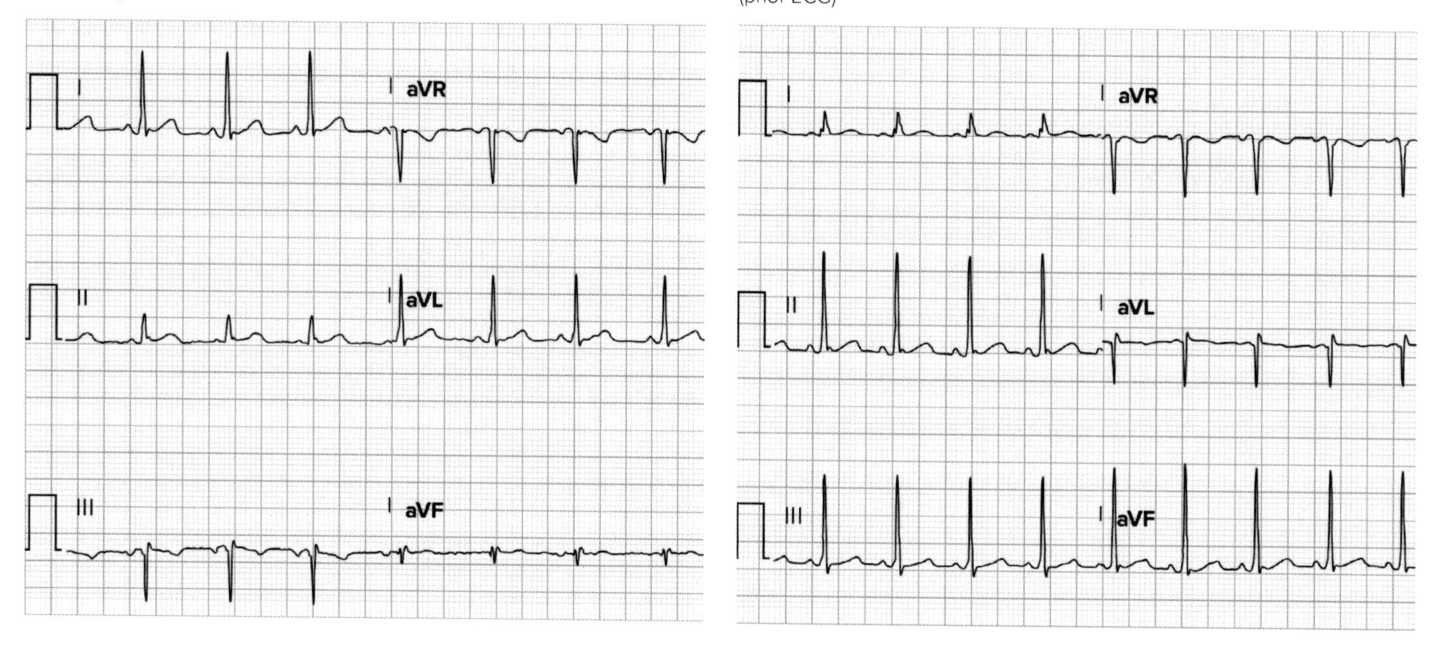

This patient had an unremarkable ED workup and was discharged with PCP follow-up.

Benign Early Repolarization Learning Points

- Widespread concave ST-segment morphology, most often in leads V1-V4 (can include leads II, III, aVF, V5, and V6)
  - Rare if only seen in leads II, III, and aVF
- Other ECG findings include:
  - No reciprocal STD except in lead aVR
  - Normal R-wave progression
  - Notching or “fishhook” pattern of J point, typically in lead V4
  - T-waves are asymmetric (descending limb is steeper than ascending limb)
- Found most often in younger individuals
- ECG stability over time
- Can mimic STEMI or pericarditis
- Concave downward, horizontal, and oblique ST-segments are seen in AMI and not BER

Terminal QRS Distortion Learning Points

- Defined as the absence of both an S-wave and a J-wave in leads V2 and V3
  - S-wave = negative deflection after the R-wave that extends below the PQ junction
  - J-wave = any positive deflection (notching or slurring) above the level of the ST-segment at the J point
- Highly specific to AMI due to LAD occlusion (ie, in the appropriate clinical setting, this finding is very suggestive of AMI)

Isolated Short PR Interval Learning Points

- PR interval < 120 msec
- Likely requires no further evaluation if:
  - Absence of symptoms suggestive of ventricular pre-excitation-related symptoms (palpitations, syncope, etc.)
  - No other ECG findings suggestive of ventricular pre-excitation are noted
- Etiologies include:
  - Pre-excitation syndromes
  - Ectopic atrial rhythms originating near AV node
  - Junctional rhythms with retrograde P-waves
  - Normal variant, especially in young athletes

Lead Reversal Learning Points

Lead Reversal Summary							
	I	II	III	aVR	aVL	aVF	V1-V6
LA-RA	Inverted	Switches with III	Switches with II	Switches with aVL	Switches with aVR	No change	No change
LA-LL	Switches with II	Switches with I	Inverted	No change	Switches with aVF	Switches with aVL	No change
LA-RL	Looks like II	Unchanged	Flatline	Looks like inverted II	Looks identical to aVF	Looks identical to aVL	No change
RA-LL	Switches with inverted III	Inverted	Switches with inverted I	Switches with aVF	No change	Switches with aVR	No change
RA-RL	Looks like inverted III	Flatline	Unchanged	Looks identical to aVF	Looks like inverted III	Looks identical to aVR	No change
LA-LL + RA-RL	Flatline	Looks like inverted III	Inverted	Looks identical to aVL	Looks identical to aVR	Looks like inverted III	No change
Dextrocardia	Inverted	Switches with III	Switches with II	Switches with aVL	Switches with aVR	No change	Dominant S-wave and poor R-wave progression
NOTE: *RL is a ground lead, so RL-LL reversal does not result in any significant changes*							

References

1. Mattu A. ECG Weekly.
2. Lee DH, Walsh B, Smith SW. Terminal QRS distortion is present in anterior myocardial infarction but absent in early repolarization. *Am J Emerg Med.* 2016;34(11):2182-2185.

Case 41: Presentation

An 89-year-old female with history of dementia is sent from her assisted living facility due to AMS, decreased oral intake, and foul-smelling urine. What is your interpretation of her ECG?

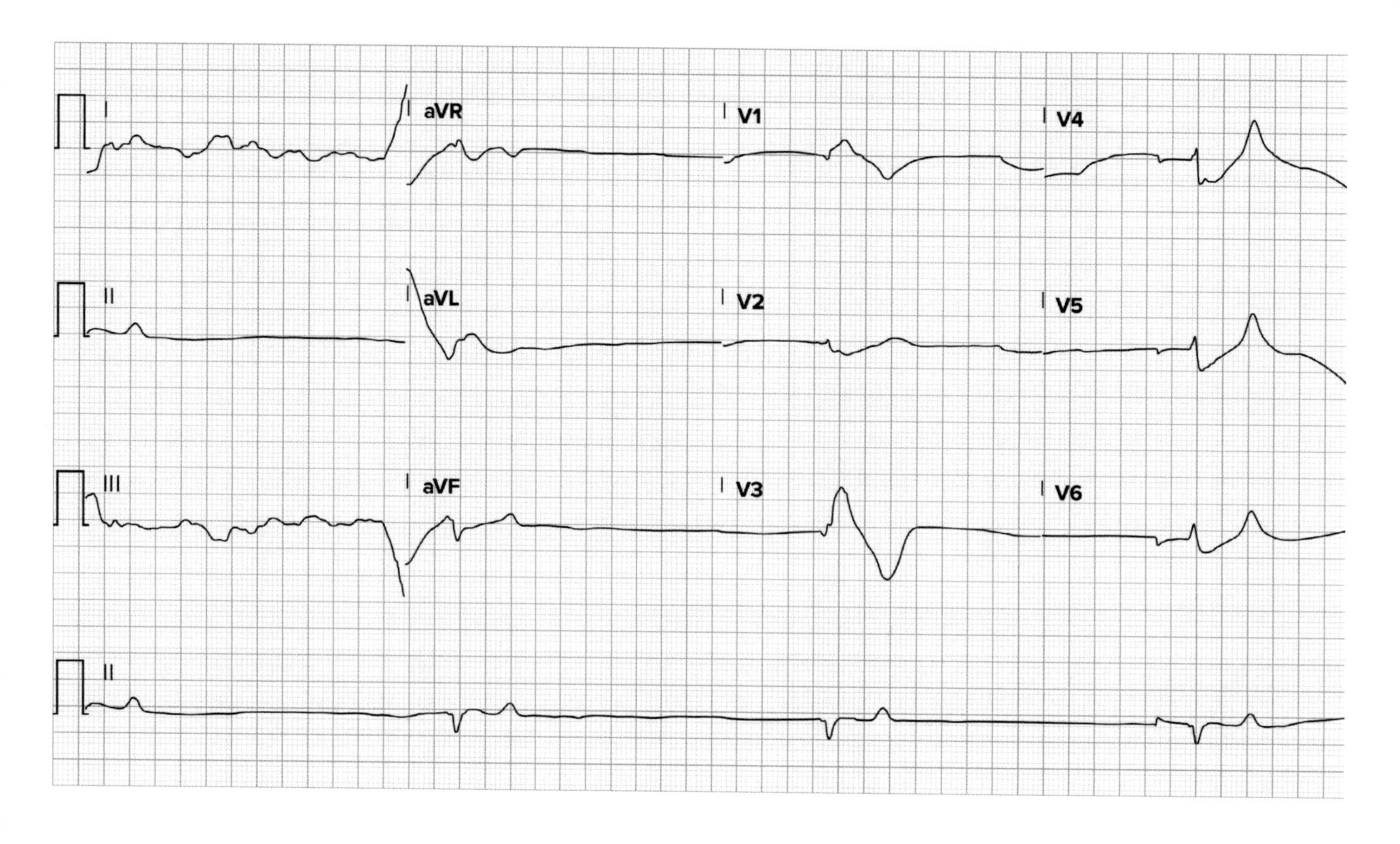

Case 41: Answer

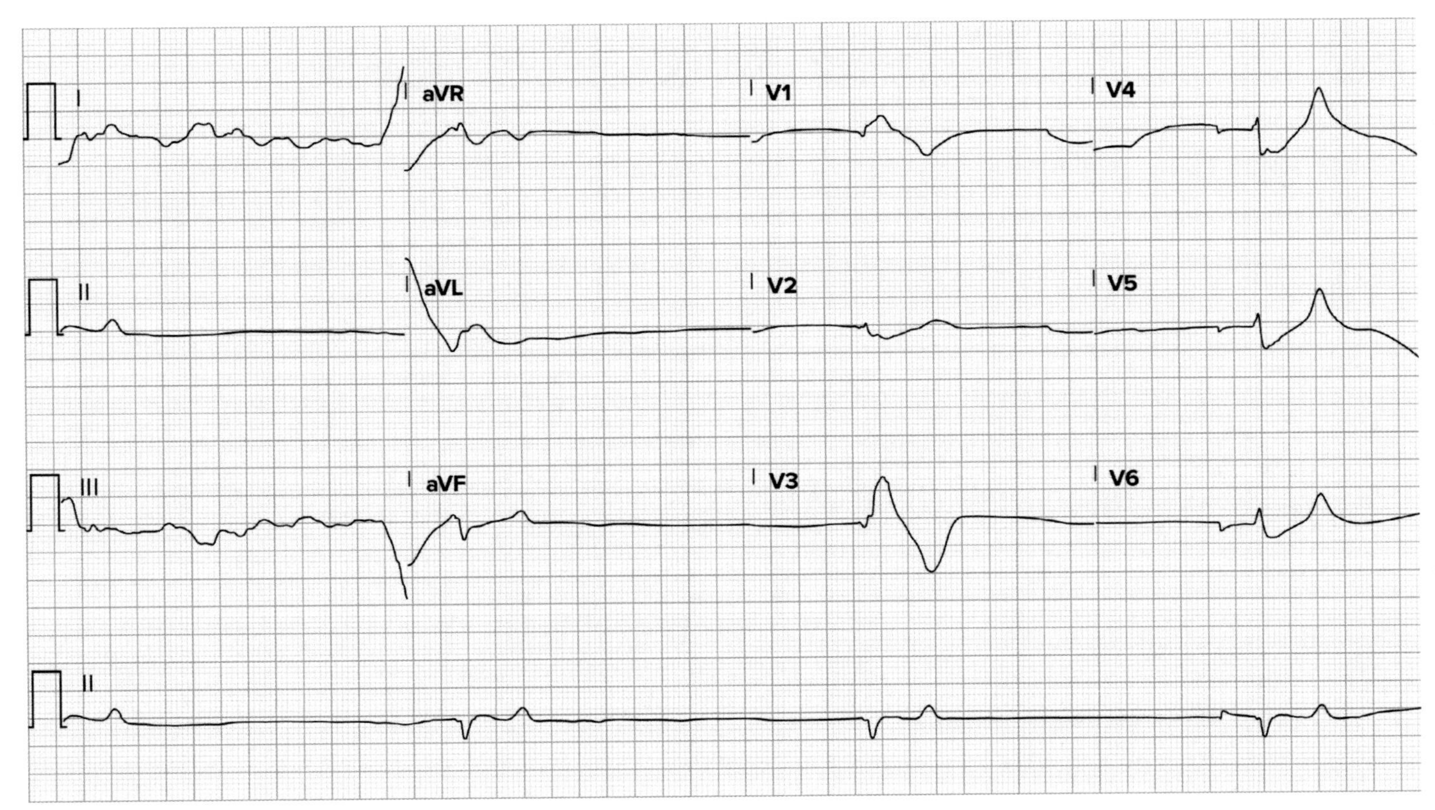

This ECG shows a very slow, regular, wide complex rhythm with a ventricular rate of 21 bpm with no P-waves (likely an idioventricular rhythm), an indeterminant axis, prolonged QRS complex duration of 260 msec with a RBBB-like morphology, STD in leads V4-V6, and baseline artifact in leads I and III. These findings, in particular the extremely prolonged QRS complex duration, are concerning for hyperkalemia.

The key to correctly interpreting this ECG is recognizing the extremely prolonged QRS complex duration which is best measured in leads V1 and V3 ***(see Figures 1 and 2).*** A QRS complex duration > 200 msec should always prompt consideration of hyperkalemia. Other findings in this ECG that suggest hyperkalemia include the sine-wave appearance of the QRS complex in lead V3 and the bizarre QRS-T morphology with peaked appearing T-waves in leads V4-V6.

Figure 1.
Lead V1 shows an extremely prolonged QRS complex duration concerning for hyperkalemia

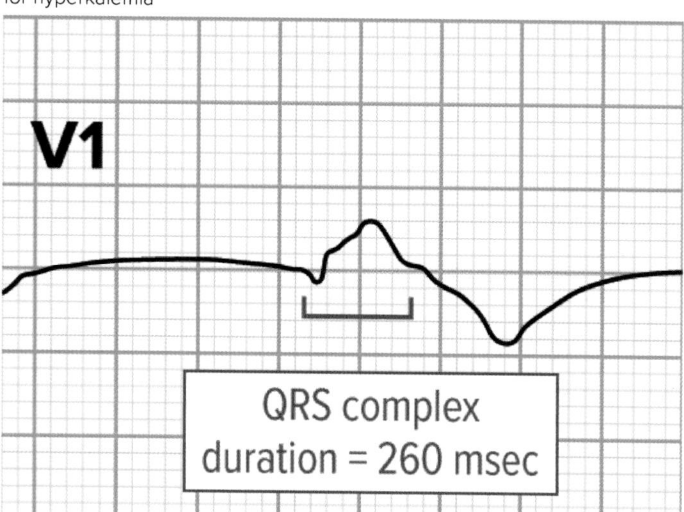

Figure 2.
Lead V3 shows an extremely prolonged QRS complex duration concerning for hyperkalemia

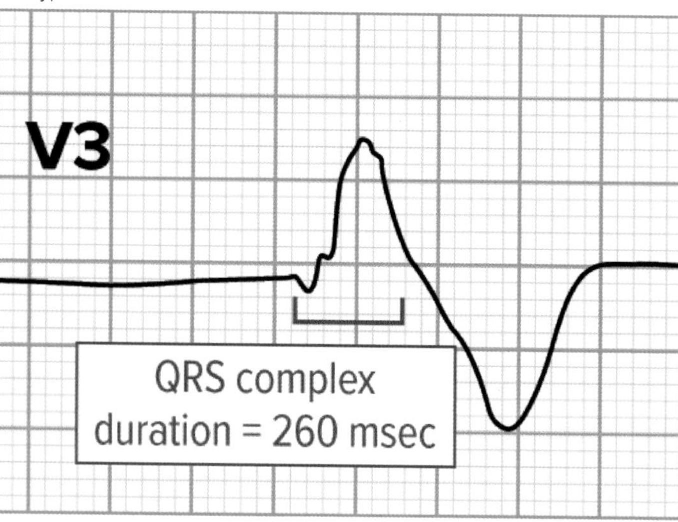

The patient was found to be septic from a UTI, and labs showed acute renal failure with a serum potassium level of 7.6 mEq/L. The patient was admitted to the ICU for further treatment.

Hyperkalemia Learning Points

- ECG is specific but not sensitive for hyperkalemia
- ECG changes are not always sequential/progressive and include:
  - Tall, narrow, peaked T-waves (best seen in precordial leads)
  - P-wave flattening and PR interval prolongation
  - Prolonged QRS complex duration, ranging from minimal to maximal
  - Conduction abnormalities (AV blocks, fascicular and bundle branch blocks)
  - Bradycardia
  - Sino-ventricular rhythm (loss of P-waves, extremely widened QRS) with normal or slow rate
  - Ventricular dysrhythmias
- Can cause STE (common in leads V1-V2 and aVR) that mimics STEMI or Brugada pattern
- Can occur simultaneously with hyperacute T-waves and obscure early changes seen in an anterior or anteroseptal AMI
- The "syphilis of ECG abnormalities," meaning that a broad range of abnormalities can be encountered with hyperkalemia[1]

References

1. Mattu A. ECG Weekly.

NOTES:

Case 42: Presentation

A 67-year-old male with history of HTN and CAD presents with chest pain.
What is your interpretation of his ECG?

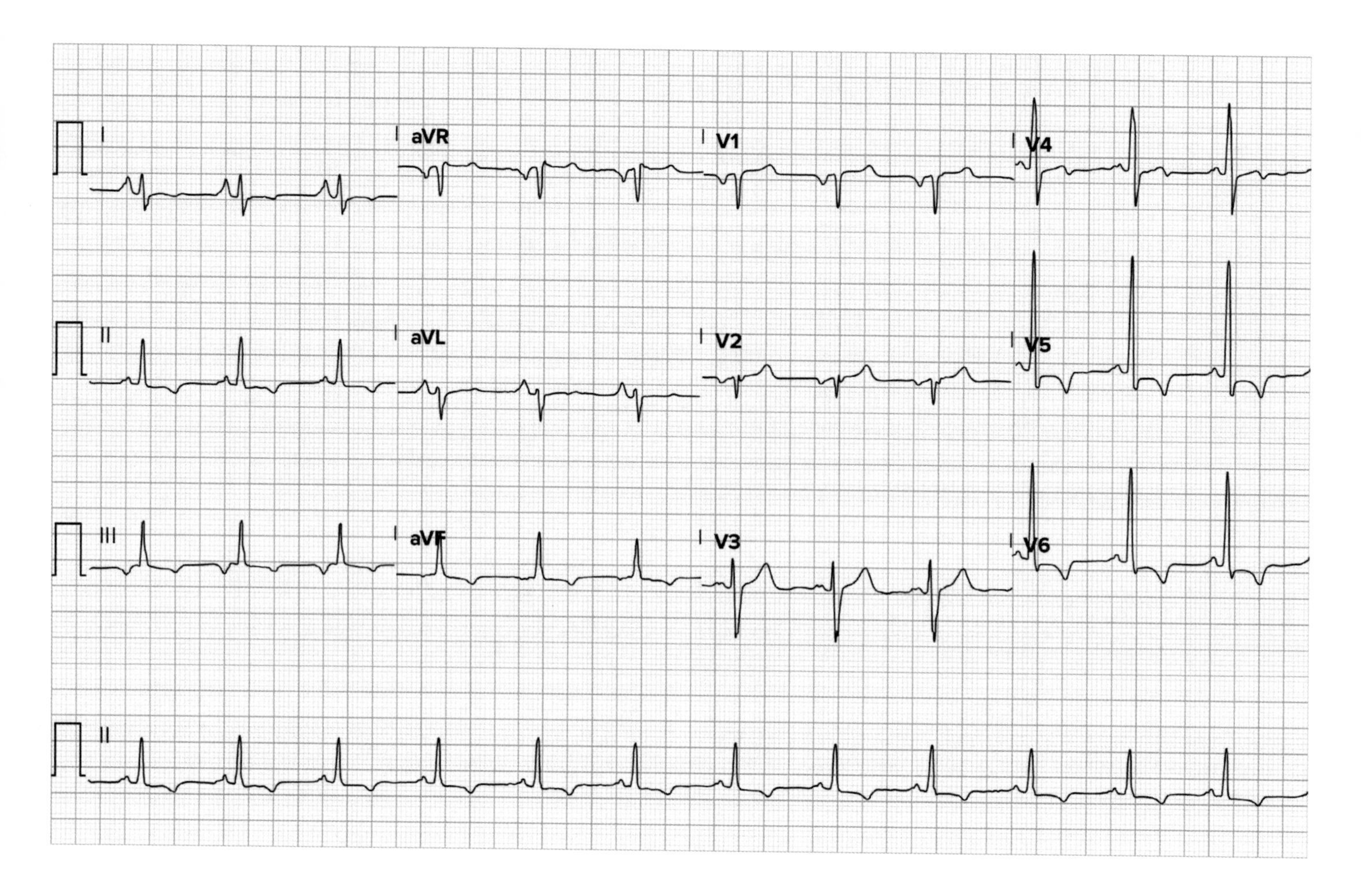

Case 42: Answer

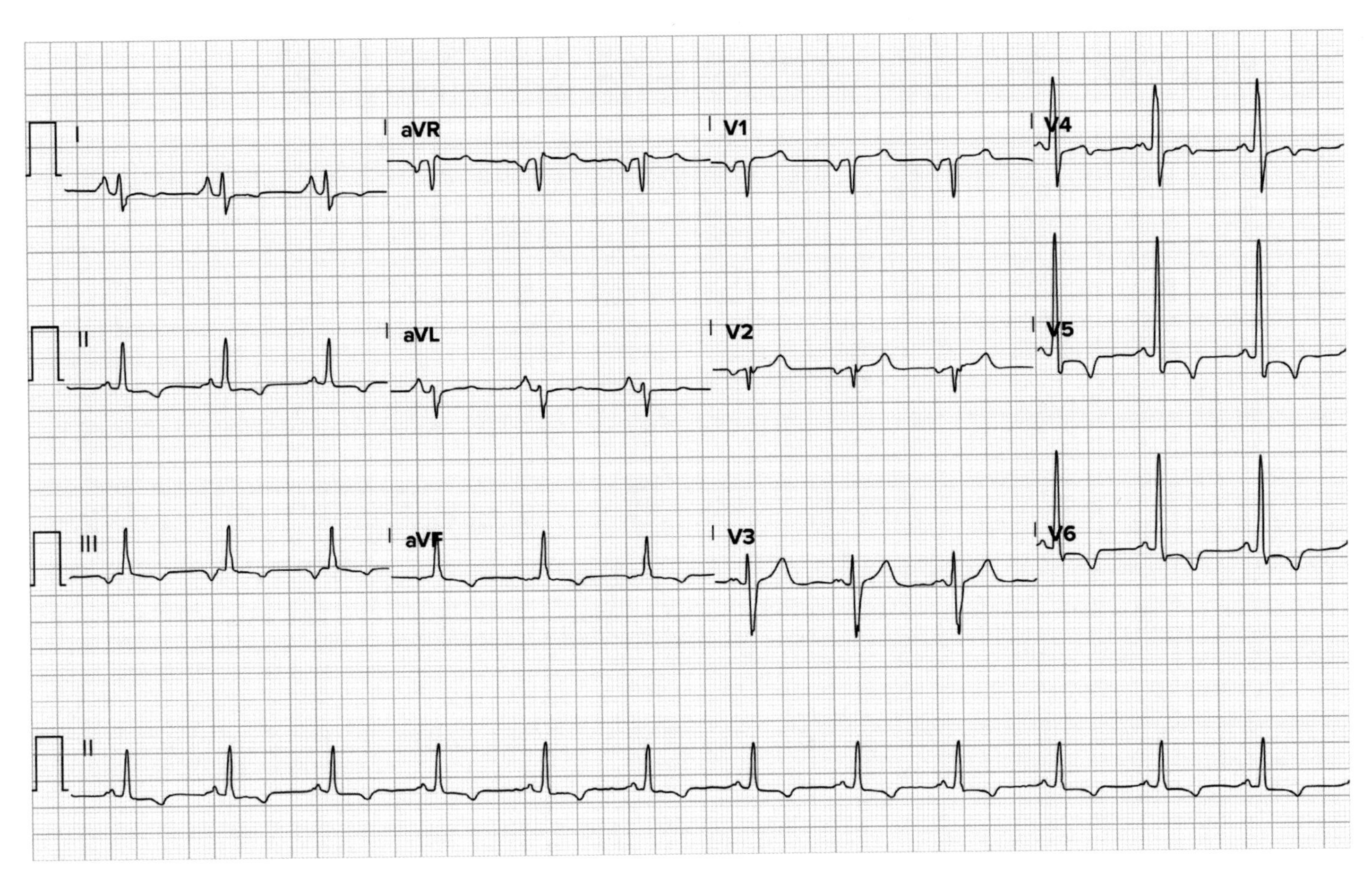

This ECG shows normal sinus rhythm with a ventricular rate of 75 bpm, normal axis, normal intervals, normal QRS complex duration, ST-segment and T-wave abnormalities consistent with LVH with strain pattern, and left arm-left leg (LA-LL) lead reversal.

The key to correctly interpreting this ECG is recognizing the ST-segment and T-wave abnormalities that are characteristic of the LVH strain pattern. Leads V1-V3 will typically have a large S-wave with STE and a concave upward ST-segment ***(see Figure 1)***. Leads I, aVL, and V4-V6 will typically have a large R-wave with STD, TWI, and a concave downward ST-segment with a characteristic asymmetric morphology that includes STD that has a gradual downslope, fusing with the inverted T-wave, and a more abrupt return to the baseline ***(see Figure 2)***. Although not present in this ECG, the QRS complex duration is often prolonged when LVH is present.

Figure 1.
Findings in lead V1 consistent with the LVH strain pattern

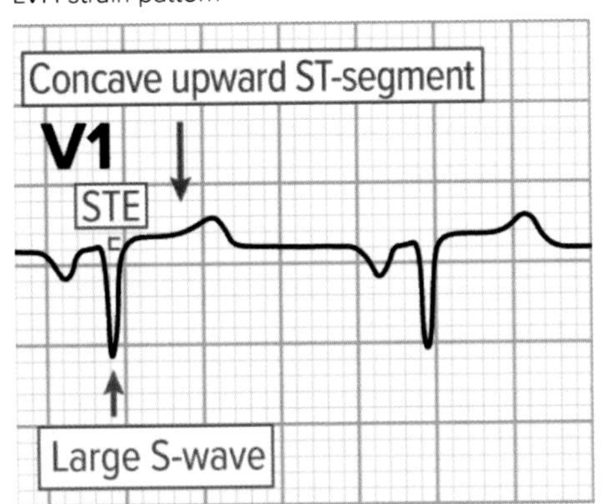

Figure 2.
Findings in lead V6 consistent with the LVH strain pattern

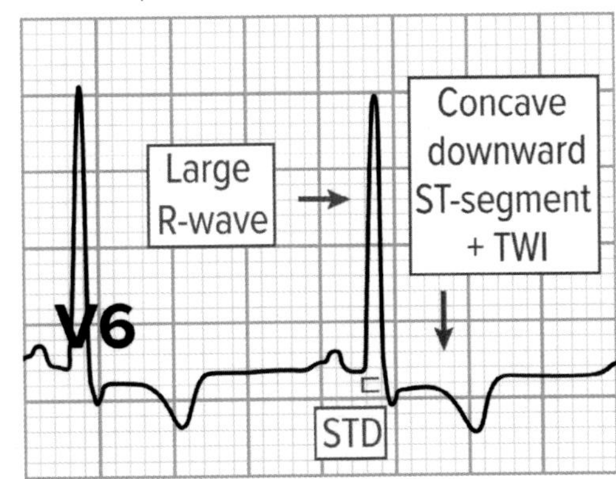

None of the many diagnostic ECG criteria for LVH have great sensitivity, so while anatomic LVH can lead to characteristic changes seen on ECG, it is ultimately an echocardiographic diagnosis. From the ECG perspective, LVH poses a diagnostic challenge as the LVH strain pattern can mimic an anteroseptal MI, so recognition of the LVH strain pattern is of the utmost importance when interpreting the ECG. Comparing with prior ECGs and obtaining serial ECGs can help differentiate between ischemia and the strain pattern.

This ECG also shows LA-LL (left arm-left leg) lead reversal. A notable finding in this ECG that should prompt concern for LA-LL lead reversal is the prominent P-wave in lead I when compared to lead II. In general, the P-wave should be more prominent in lead II than lead I in normal sinus rhythm with correct lead placement. ***Figure 3*** shows a repeat ECG with correct lead placement.

Figure 3.
Repeat ECG with correct lead placement

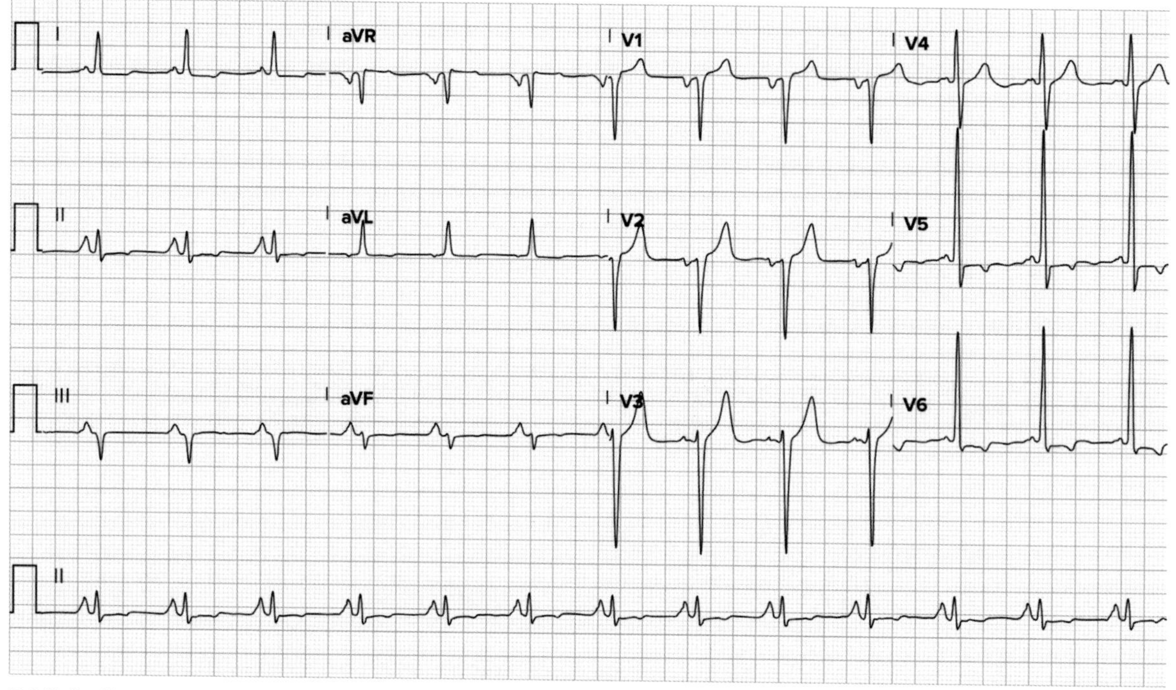

ECG findings seen with LA-LL lead reversal include ***(see Figure 4)***:

1. In comparison to normal P-QRS-T complexes (ie, normal sinus rhythm with normal lead placement), leads I and II "switch places," meaning that the normal findings in lead I are noted in lead II and vice versa
2. In comparison to normal P-QRS-T complexes (ie, normal sinus rhythm with normal lead placement), leads aVL and aVF "switch places," so the normal findings in lead aVL are noted in lead aVF and vice versa
3. Lead III is inverted, meaning that the P-QRS-T complexes are all oriented in the opposite direction from the normal P-QRS-T complexes (ie, normal sinus rhythm with normal lead placement)
4. Lead aVR is unchanged

Figure 4.
Comparison of the limb leads from the case ECG with LA-RA lead reversal with the repeat ECG with correct lead placement

4a. LA-LL lead reversal (case ECG)

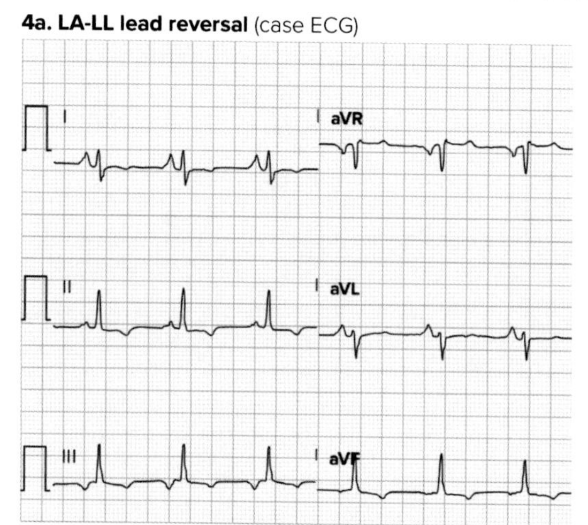

4b. Correct lead placement (repeat ECG)

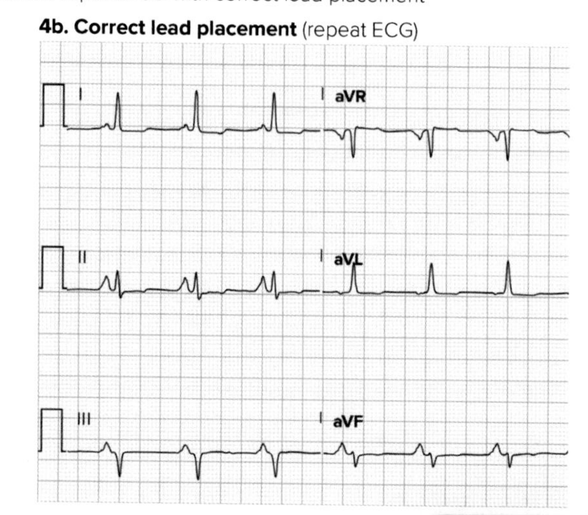

Except for the lead reversal, this patient's initial ECG and serial ECGs were unchanged from prior.

LVH Learning Points

- ECG is only suggestive of anatomic LVH- echocardiography is the superior diagnostic modality
- ECG findings in LVH are manifested primarily by the increased voltage of the QRS complexes, hence the term "LVH by voltage criteria"
  - No criteria are recommended for use exclusive of other validated criteria
  - Diagnosis of LVH in the presence of intraventricular conduction abnormalities (eg, fascicular blocks, bundle branch blocks) should be made with caution as they may impact the accuracy of the ECG criteria for LVH
- 80% of LVH by voltage patterns demonstrate ST and T-wave abnormalities, termed "LVH with strain pattern," which commonly include:
  - STE in leads V1-V3
  - STD and TWI in leads I, aVL and V4-V6
  - Increased S-wave depth in leads III, aVR, and V1-V3
  - Increased R-wave peak time > 50 msec in lead V5 or V6
  - Increased R-wave amplitude in leads I, aVL and V4-V6
  - Left axis deviation typical, but can occur with any axis
  - Increased QRS complex and/or QT interval duration
- LVH with strain pattern can confound the ECG's ability to detect ACS, particularly anteroseptal MI, and mimics ACS findings

Lead Reversal Learning Points

Lead Reversal Summary

	I	II	III	aVR	aVL	aVF	V1-V6
LA-RA	Inverted	Switches with III	Switches with II	Switches with aVL	Switches with aVR	No change	No change
LA-LL	Switches with II	Switches with I	Inverted	No change	Switches with aVF	Switches with aVL	No change
LA-RL	Looks like II	Unchanged	Flatline	Looks like inverted II	Looks identical to aVF	Looks identical to aVL	No change
RA-LL	Switches with inverted III	Inverted	Switches with inverted I	Switches with aVF	No change	Switches with aVR	No change
RA-RL	Looks like inverted III	Flatline	Unchanged	Looks identical to aVF	Looks like inverted III	Looks identical to aVR	No change
LA-LL + RA-RL	Flatline	Looks like inverted III	Inverted	Looks identical to aVL	Looks identical to aVR	Looks like inverted III	No change
Dextrocardia	Inverted	Switches with III	Switches with II	Switches with aVL	Switches with aVR	No change	Dominant S-wave and poor R-wave progression

***NOTE:** RL is a ground lead, so RL-LL reversal does not result in any significant changes*

Case 43: Presentation

An 84-year-old female with a history of dual chamber pacemaker presents with palpitations and near syncope. What is your interpretation of her ECG?

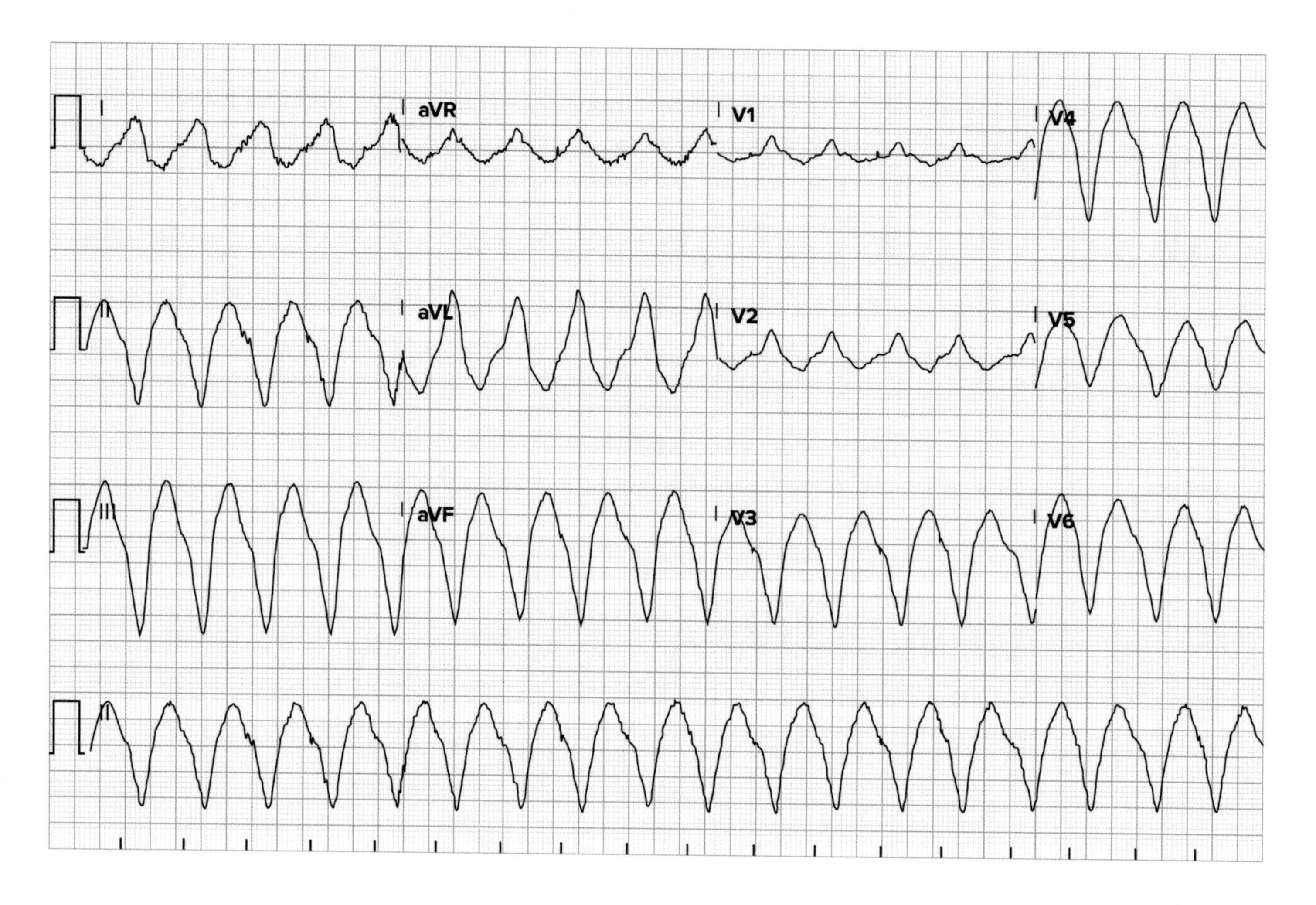

Case 43: Answer

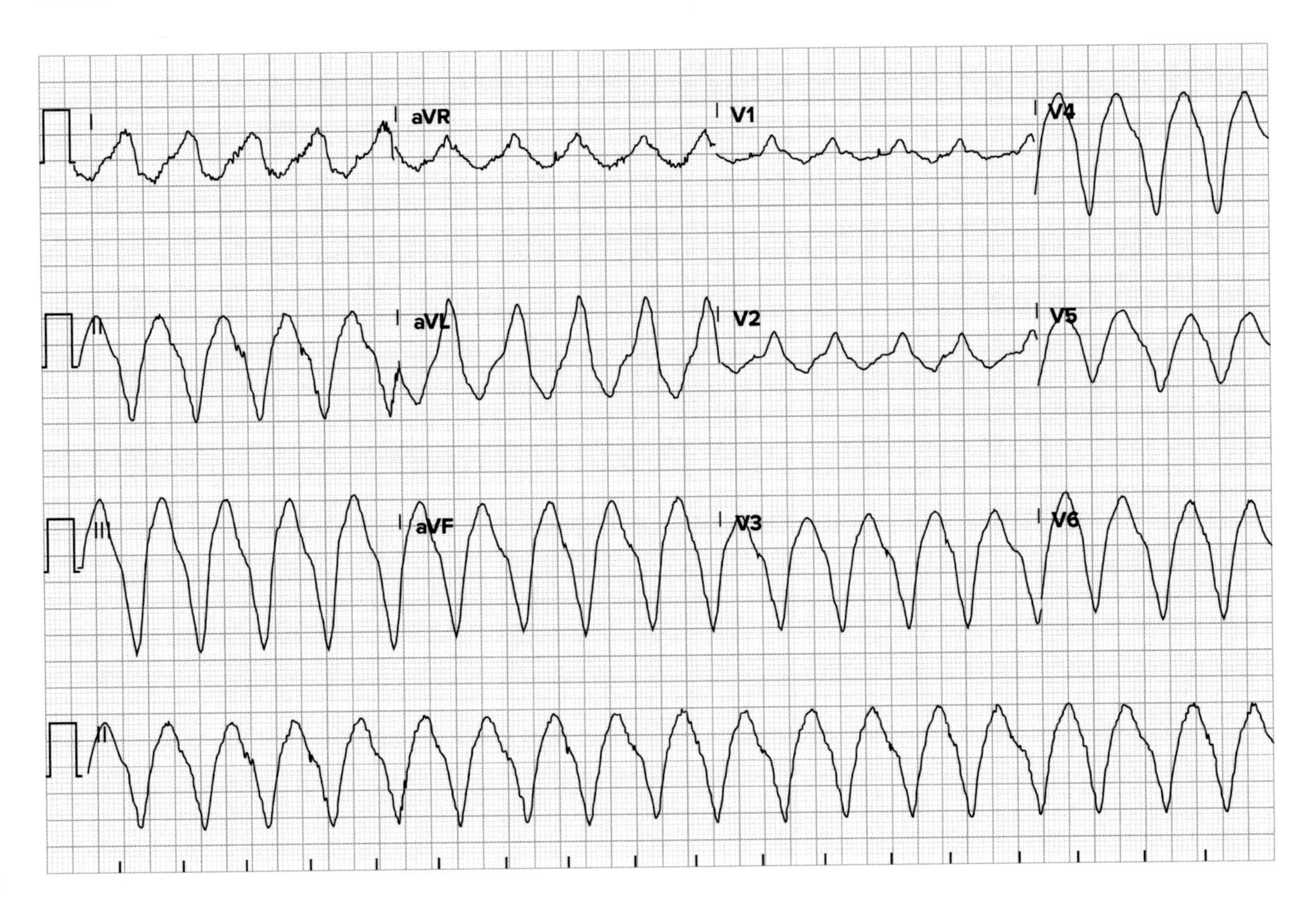

This ECG shows a ventricular-paced tachycardia with a ventricular rate of 120 bpm, no visible P-waves, left axis deviation, and prolonged QRS complex duration of 220 msec with a RBBB-like morphology. These finding are consistent with pacemaker-mediated tachycardia.

Dual chamber pacing, also called A-V sequential pacing, involves pacing of both the right atria and right ventricle. There is one atrial lead and one ventricular lead:

- The right atrial lead paces the right atrial appendage
- The RV lead paces the RV apex

The atrial lead is programmed to sense for native atrial activity and act accordingly:

- The pacemaker senses native atrial activity, waits a programmed amount of time, then paces the ventricles (ie, atrial-sensed, ventricular-paced rhythm)
- The pacemaker paces the atria if no native atrial activity is detected during a programmed amount of time, waits another programmed amount of time, then paces the ventricles (ie, A-V sequential pacing)

Pacemaker-mediated tachycardia, also called endless-loop tachycardia, is a re-entry tachycardia seen with dual chamber pacemakers that have atrial sensing. After it triggers an atrial depolarization, the atrial lead is programmed to have a refractory period to prevent it from being retriggered by the ventricular depolarization or retrograde P-waves. This is called the post-ventricular atrial refractory period (PVARP) and pacemaker-mediated tachycardia can occur if it is too brief. The typical trigger is a PVC that causes a retrograde P-wave that is sensed by the atrial lead which then triggers ventricular

depolarization which leads to a retrograde P-wave, etc. The antegrade impulse is via the pacemaker with retrograde conduction through the AV node. This is very similar to antidromic AVRT except that the pacemaker replaces the accessory pathway.

This patient was treated with a magnet which terminated the dysrhythmia. She was admitted to the cardiology service for pacemaker reprogramming.

Pacemaker Associated Dysrhythmias Learning Points

Pacemaker-Mediated Tachycardia

- Re-entry tachycardia with antegrade conduction through the pacemaker and retrograde conduction through the AV node
- ECG shows paced wide complex tachycardia (may see retrograde P-waves)
- Treat with a magnet (will cause pacemaker to pace at a default rate) or as AVRT (eg, adenosine or nodal blockers)

Sensor-Induced Tachycardia

- Non-cardiac stimuli inappropriately trigger ventricular pacing
- ECG shows a paced tachycardia at an inappropriate rate
- Treat with a magnet (will cause pacemaker to pace at a default rate) or elimination of non-cardiac stimuli

Runaway Pacemaker

- Occurs with older generation pacemakers with low battery
- ECG shows intermittent bursts of pacer spikes that can precipitate ventricular fibrillation
- Treat with a magnet (will cause pacemaker to pace at a default rate)
- Pacemaker replacement is the definitive treatment

NOTES:

Case 44: Presentation

An otherwise healthy 47-year-old male presents with palpitations and lightheadedness. What is your interpretation of his ECG?

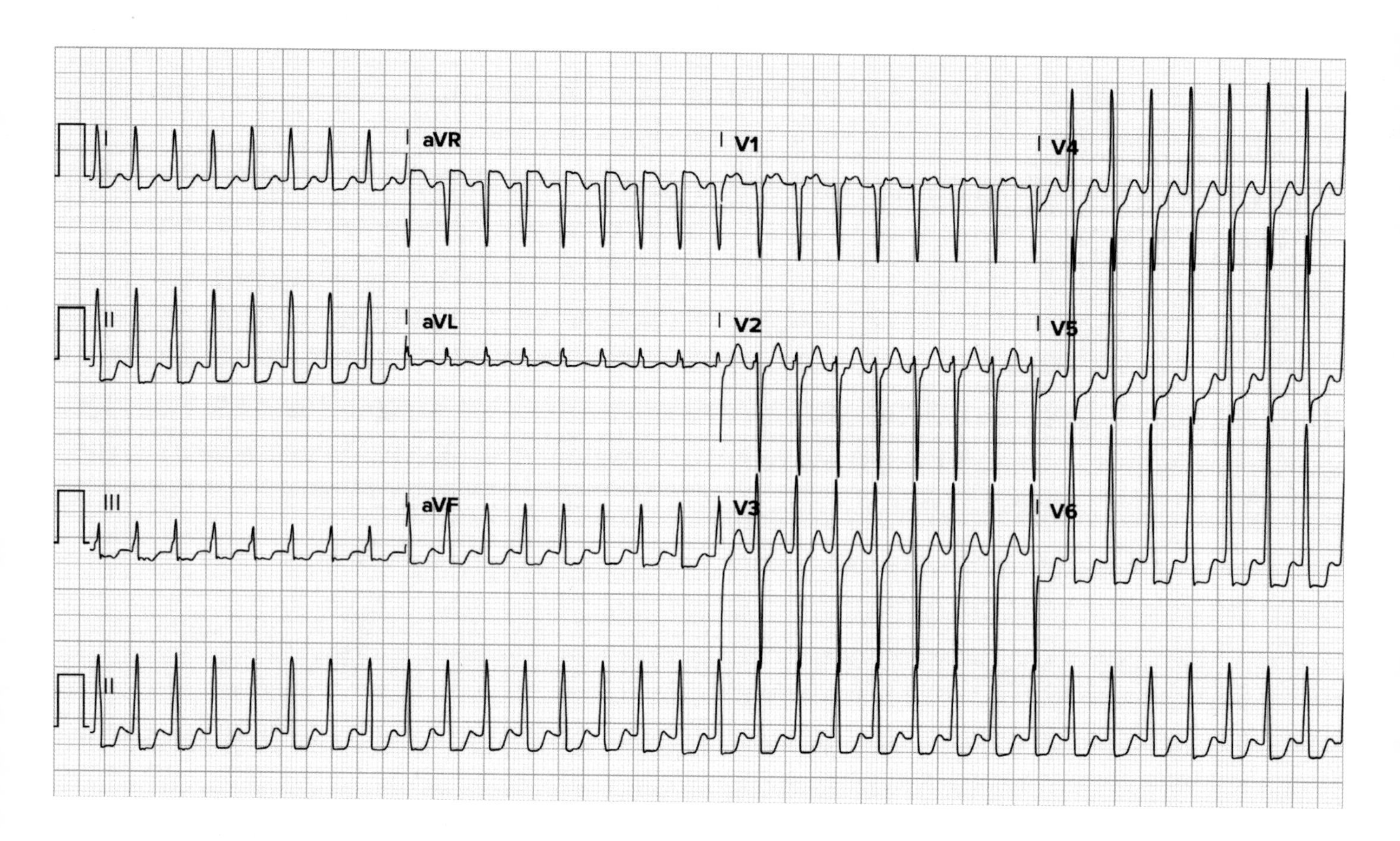

Case 44: Answer

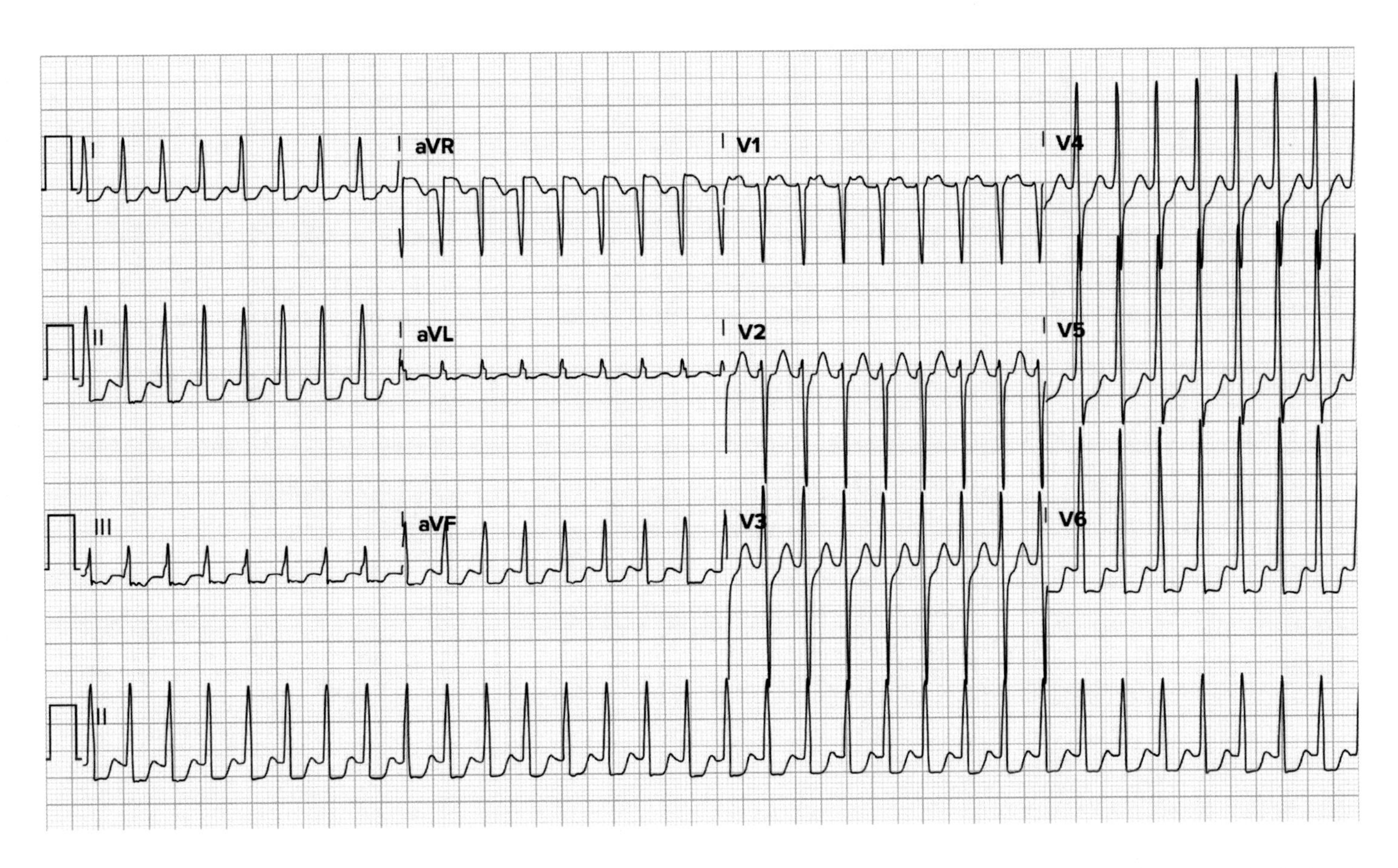

This ECG shows a regular narrow-complex tachycardia with a ventricular rate of 195 bpm, normal axis, STE in leads aVR and V1, and STD in leads I, II, III, aVF, and V3-V6.

The differential diagnosis for a regular narrow-complex tachycardia includes:

- Atrial flutter
- Atrial tachycardia
- AV nodal reentrant tachycardia
- AVRT (ie, WPW) with orthodromic conduction
- Junctional tachycardia
- Narrow complex VT
- Sinus tachycardia

The absence of P-waves rules out atrial tachycardia and sinus tachycardia. The rate is too slow for 1:1 flutter and too fast for 2:1 flutter or a junctional tachycardia. The QRS complex duration is ~100 msec, so narrow complex VT is unlikely. Without more history, it is impossible to tell whether this AVNRT or orthodromic AVRT (ie, retrograde conduction via the AP), but the treatment for both is the same.

The differential diagnosis for the pattern of STE in lead aVR +/- lead V1 with diffuse STD includes both ACS and non-ACS etiologies:

ACS causes[1]	Non-ACS causes[2]
• LMCA insufficiency (can see STE aVR > V1)	• Acute and/or severe anemia
• Prox LAD insufficiency (can see STE V1 > aVR)	• Aortic dissection
• Triple vessel disease	• LBBB and ventricular-paced rhythms
• Global cardiac ischemia	• LVH with strain pattern
• Prinzmetal angina	• Pulmonary embolism
	• ROSC s/p epinephrine or defibrillation
	• Severe hypokalemia or hyperkalemia
	• Sodium channel blockade
	• Supraventricular tachycardia (especially with rapid rates)

Although the pattern of STE in lead aVR +/- lead V1 with diffuse STD is discussed in the cardiology literature, its clinical significance is not without some controversy. This is likely due to the broad differential diagnosis associated with this pattern that includes both ACS and non-ACS causes. The 2018 Fourth Universal Definition of MI states "ST-segment depression ≥ 1 mm in 6 or more leads, which may be associated with ST segment elevation in leads aVR and/or V1 and hemodynamic compromise, is suggestive of multivessel disease or left main disease" but does not provide specific management recommendations.

Treatment should be guided by the underlying etiology, and it is imperative to consider both ACS and non-ACS causes. For patients suspected of having an ACS cause, this ECG pattern is highly suggestive of LMCA insufficiency, proximal LAD insufficiency, or triple vessel disease. So, while this pattern does not meet "traditional" STEMI criteria, it can represent high-risk ACS, including possible acute coronary occlusion, in the correct clinical context, and immediate angiography should be considered. Whether this is done by emergent cardiology consultation or activation of the cardiac catheterization lab depends on local practice preferences.

The pattern of STE in lead aVR +/- lead V1 with diffuse STD seen in this ECG is likely due to the abnormal conduction associated with the supraventricular tachycardia. The ECG changes alone do not constitute a "failed stress test" and the decision to evaluate for ischemia that caused, or was caused by, the tachydysrhythmia should be a clinical one.

This patient was successfully chemically cardioverted with adenosine after the modified Valsalva maneuver was unsuccessful. A repeat ECG showed resolution of the pattern of STE in lead aVR +/- lead V1 with diffuse STD seen on the initial ECG, which is expected with non-ACS causes, with no evidence of ventricular pre-excitation (ie, delta waves) that would be concerning for WPW. His ED workup was unremarkable, and he was discharged with cardiology follow-up.

AV Nodal Reentrant Tachycardia (AVNRT) Learning Points

- Also called paroxysmal supraventricular tachycardia or SVT
- Caused by re-entrant circuit within or around the AV node and typically triggered by a PAC
- ECG shows a regular narrow-complex tachycardia in the absence of concurrent conduction abnormalities (eg, bundle branch block)
  - Ventricular rate typically 140-280 bpm
  - Retrograde P-waves can appear before, after, or superimposed on the QRS complexes

Atrioventricular Re-entry Tachycardia (AVRT) Learning Points

- Caused by re-entrant circuit involving AV node and an accessory pathway
  - Most common dysrhythmia seen in patients with pre-excitation syndrome (eg, WPW)
- Rate tends to be faster than AVNRT
- Orthodromic AVRT
  - Antegrade conduction through the AV node and retrograde conduction via the accessory pathway
  - ECG show a regular narrow-complex tachycardia in the absence of concurrent conduction abnormalities (eg, bundle branch block)
- Antidromic AVRT
  - Antegrade conduction through the accessory pathway and retrograde conduction via the AV node
  - ECG shows a regular wide-complex tachycardia generally indistinguishable from VT

Lead aVR Learning Points

- Lead aVR views the right upper portion of the heart including the basal part of the septum
- STE in lead aVR +/- V1 with diffuse STD ≥ 1 mm in ≥ 6 leads can be due to ACS or non-ACS etiologies; therefore, always consider the clinical context when considering the differential diagnosis
- In ACS presentations, this pattern is highly suggestive of LMCA obstruction, proximal LAD obstruction, and triple vessel disease, and immediate angiography should be considered[3]
- In non-ACS causes, the ECG changes should resolve with treatment of non-ACS cause
- Anterior or inferior MI with STE > 1 mm in lead aVR are associated with an increased 30-day mortality[4]

References

1. Thygesen K, Alpert JS, Jaffe AS, et al. 2018 ESC/ACC/AHA/WHF Expert Consensus Document: Fourth Universal Definition of Myocardial Infarction (2018). Circulation. 2018;138:e618-e651.
2. Mattu A. ECG Weekly.
3. Writing Committee, et al. 2013 ACCF/AHA Guideline for the Management of ST-Elevation Myocardial Infarction: A Report of the American College of Cardiology Foundation/American Heart Association Task Force on Practice Guidelines. Circulation. 2013;127:e362-e425.
4. Wong CK, Gao W, Stewart RA, Benatar J, French JK, Aylward PE,White HD; HERO-2 Investigators. aVR ST elevation: an important but neglected sign in ST elevation acute myocardial infarction. Eur Heart J. 2010;31:1845–1853.

Case 45: Presentation

A 79-year-old female presents with generalized weakness and fatigue. What is your interpretation of her ECG?

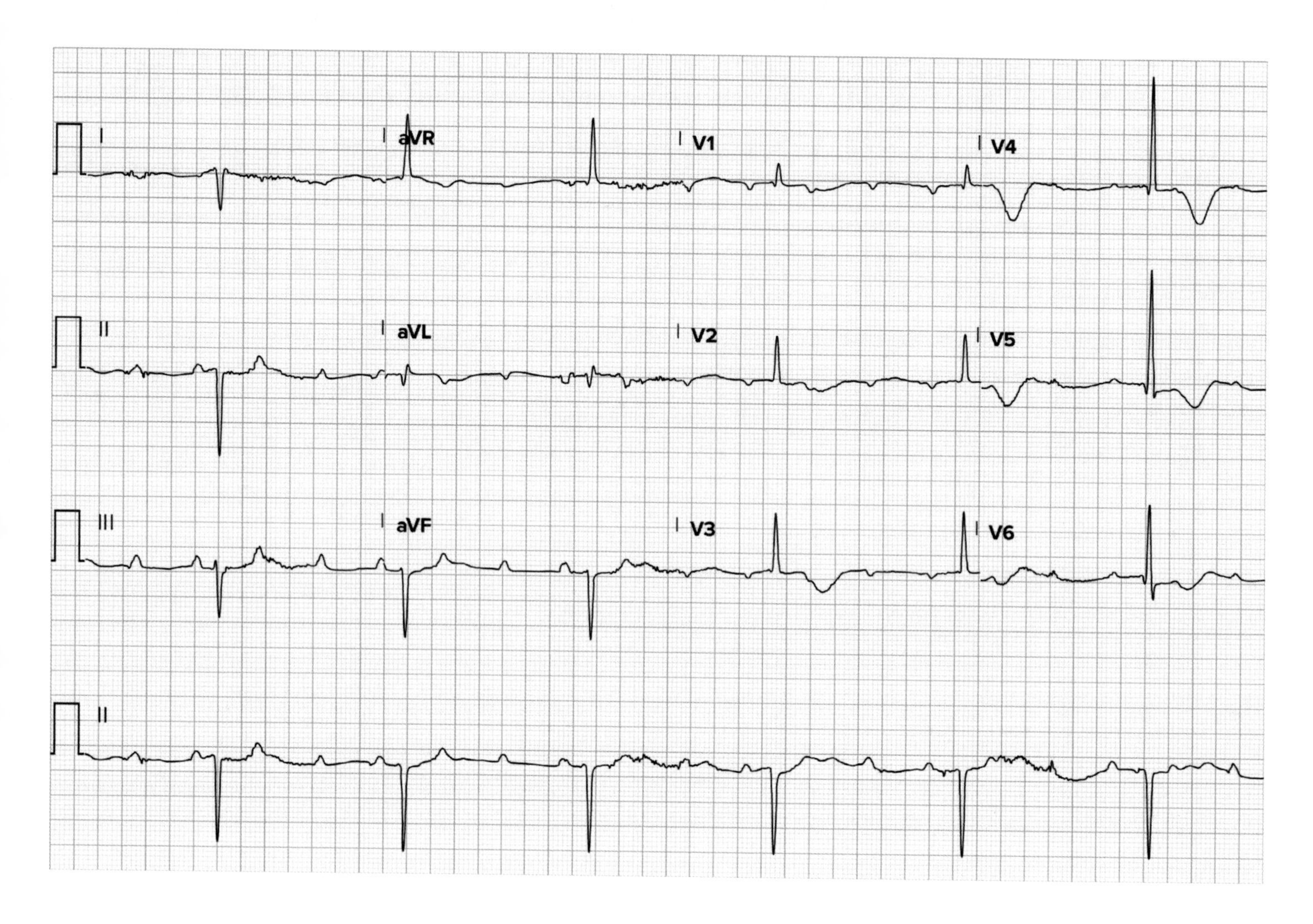

Case 45: Answer

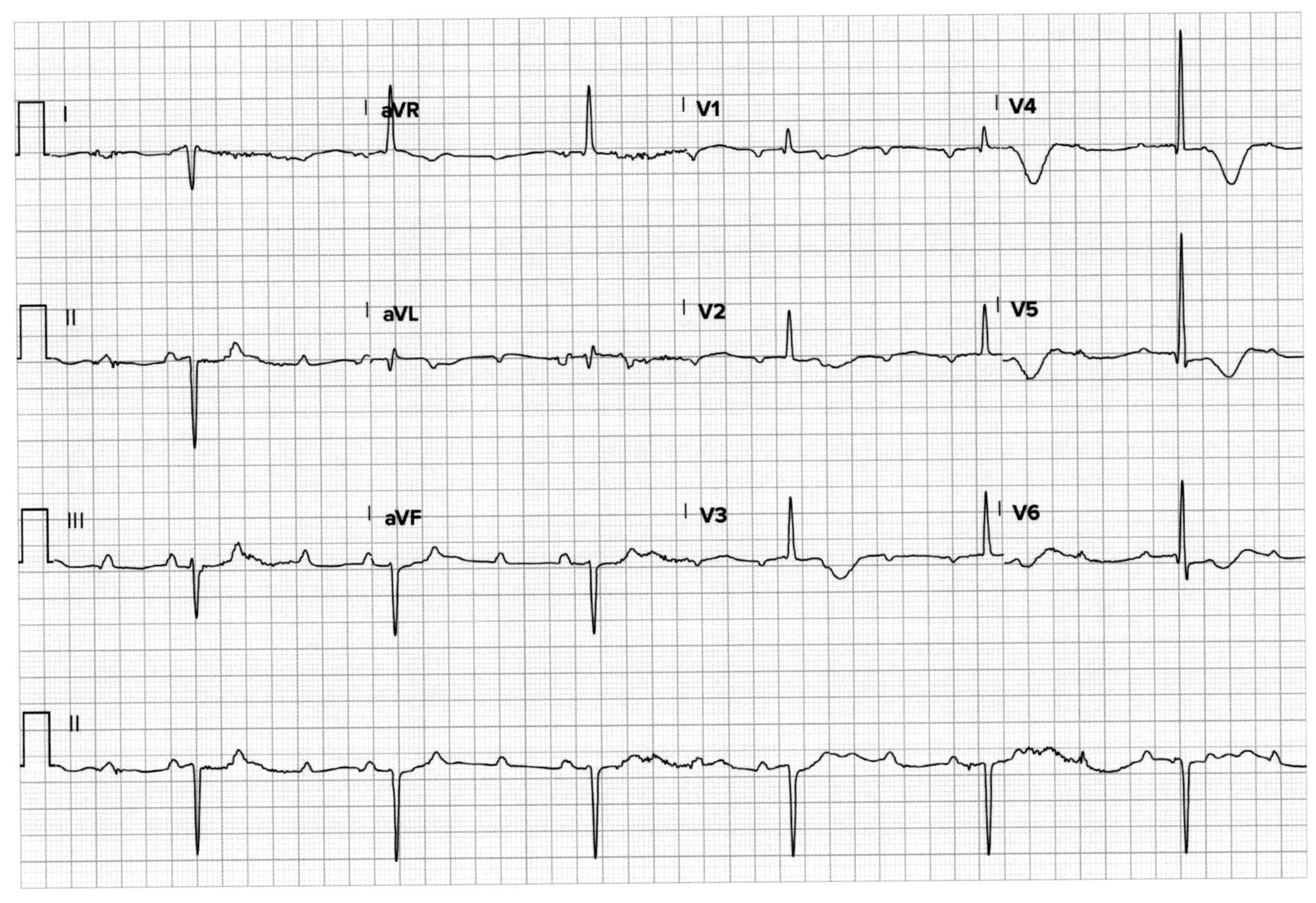

This ECG shows a 3rd degree AV block with a ventricular rate of 38 bpm and an atrial rate of 117 bpm, northwest/extreme axis deviation, prolonged QRS complex duration of 115 msec duration with a non-specific IVCD, TWI in leads V3-V6, and left arm-right arm (LA-RA) lead reversal.

The differential diagnosis for a regular-wide complex rhythm with bradycardic ventricular rates includes:

- Sinus bradycardia with aberrant conduction
- Junctional rhythm with aberrant conduction
- Junctional bradycardia with aberrant conduction
- Idioventricular rhythm
- Accelerated idioventricular rhythm
- Atrial flutter with block (rate controlled) and aberrant conduction
- Atrial tachycardia with block (rate controlled) and aberrant conduction
- 2:1 AV block with aberrant conduction
- High-grade AV block (eg, 3:1, 4:1, etc.) with aberrant conduction
- 3rd degree AV block
- 3rd degree sinoatrial block
  - Causes of aberrant conduction include fixed or rate-related BBB, metabolic abnormalities, sodium channel blocker toxicity, ventricular-paced rhythm, and ventricular pre-excitation (eg, WPW)

The differential diagnosis for the rhythm in this ECG includes a 3rd degree AV block and a high-grade AV block with 3:1 conduction. The term high-grade AV block, also called advanced AV block, is used to describe when ≥ 2 sequential P-waves are not conducted, and these blocks are most commonly a variant of a Mobitz type II.

In this ECG, it is difficult to identify the AV dissociation, a distinguishing feature of a 3rd degree AV block, as the atrial rate (117 bpm) is only slightly more than three times the ventricular rate (38 bpm). The key to correctly interpreting this ECG is recognizing the variable PR intervals which are consistent with a 3rd degree AV block and rules out a high-grade AV block. The PR interval is 190 msec for the initial P-QRS-T complex and 260 msec for the final P-QRS-T complex ***(see Figure 1)***.

Figure 1.
The first and last P-QRS-T complexes in the lead II rhythm strip show variable PR intervals, consistent with a 3rd degree AV block

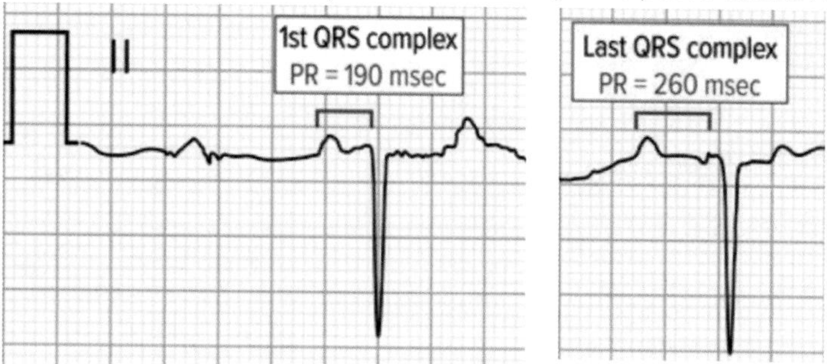

This ventricular rhythm in this ECG is a junctional bradycardia. The QRS complex duration is < 120 msec, so the ventricles must be paced by a junctional focus since a ventricular focus would produce a QRS complex duration ≥ 120 msec, and when a junctional rhythm has a rate < 40 bpm, it is called junctional bradycardia. The QRS complex morphology does not meet criteria for an incomplete RBBB or LBBB, so it is called an IVCD (also called a non-specific IVCD).

This ECG shows left arm-right arm (LA-RA) lead reversal. An easy way to scan for LA-RA lead reversal is to compare leads I and V6, which should appear similarly with normal lead placement since they both look at the heart from the same direction. In this case, the QRS complexes are negatively oriented in lead I and positively oriented in lead V6 ***(see Figure 2)***, suggesting that "the view" of lead I is coming from the wrong side of the body, which is what would happen if the arm leads were reversed. Another clue is that the QRS complex in lead aVR is predominantly upright, which is very atypical and should prompt evaluation for lead reversal.

Figure 2.
The P-QRS-T complexes in leads I and V6 will point in opposite directions when there is LA-RA lead reversal

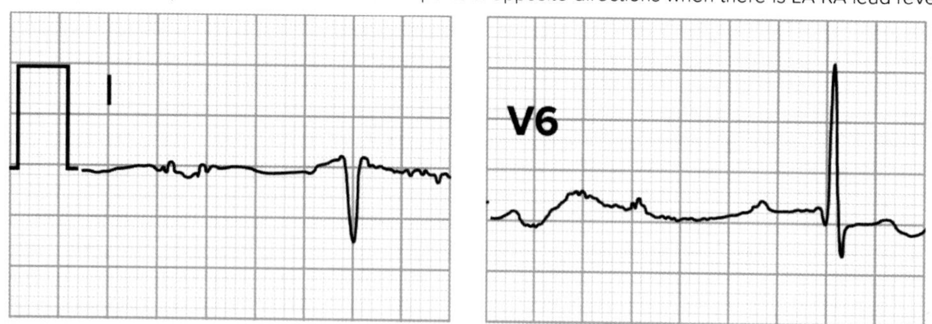

ECG findings seen with LA-RA lead reversal include:

- Lead I is inverted, indicating that P-QRS-T complexes are all oriented in the opposite direction from the normal P-QRS-T complexes (ie, normal sinus rhythm with normal lead placement)
- In comparison to normal P-QRS-T complexes (ie, normal sinus rhythm with normal lead placement), leads II and III "switch places," so the normal findings in lead II are noted in lead III and vice versa
- In comparison to normal P-QRS-T complexes (ie, normal sinus rhythm with normal lead placement), leads aVR and aVL "switch places," so the normal findings in lead aVR are noted in lead aVL and vice versa
- Lead aVF is unchanged

This patient had an unremarkable ED workup and was admitted to the cardiology service for placement of a permanent pacemaker.

3rd Degree AV Block Learning Points

- A 3rd degree AV block, or complete heart block, is defined by the absence of conduction through the AV node leading to complete AV dissociation
  - P-waves "march out" (ie, constant PP interval) and do not conduct to produce a QRS complex
  - PR intervals are variable
  - Atrial rate > ventricular rate
  - Ventricular rhythm is usually junctional or ventricular escape rhythm
- All patients require admission and evaluation for pacemaker placement

High-grade (or advanced) AV Block Learning Points

- 2nd degree AV block with ≥ 2 sequential non-conducted P-waves
  - Most commonly a variant of a Mobitz type II but can be associated with a Mobitz type I
  - PP and RR intervals should have a whole number ratio
- Named as ratio of P-waves to QRS complexes
- Can be seen after anterior MI or with significant pathology of the conduction pathway
- High risk of progressing to a 3rd degree AV block

Junctional Rhythm Learning Points

- Ectopic focus from AV node or proximal Purkinje system
  - Also called AV junctional rhythm, nodal rhythm, nodal escape rhythm, junctional escape rhythm, AV nodal rhythm
- ECG shows ventricular rate of 40-60 bpm with normal QRS complex duration unless concurrent conduction abnormality (eg, bundle branch block)
- May have retrograde P-waves that precede (with PR interval < 120 msec) or follow QRS complex, typically best seen in the inferior leads
- Variations include:
  - Junctional Bradycardia: ventricular rate < 40 bpm
  - Accelerated Junctional Rhythm: ventricular rate 61–100 bpm
  - Junctional Tachycardia: ventricular rate > 100 bpm

Lead Reversal Learning Points

Lead Reversal Summary

	I	II	III	aVR	aVL	aVF	V1-V6
LA-RA	Inverted	Switches with III	Switches with II	Switches with aVL	Switches with aVR	No change	No change
LA-LL	Switches with II	Switches with I	Inverted	No change	Switches with aVF	Switches with aVL	No change
LA-RL	Looks like II	Unchanged	Flatline	Looks like inverted II	Looks identical to aVF	Looks identical to aVL	No change
RA-LL	Switches with inverted III	Inverted	Switches with inverted I	Switches with aVF	No change	Switches with aVR	No change
RA-RL	Looks like inverted III	Flatline	Unchanged	Looks identical to aVF	Looks like inverted III	Looks identical to aVR	No change
LA-LL + RA-RL	Flatline	Looks like inverted III	Inverted	Looks identical to aVL	Looks identical to aVR	Looks like inverted III	No change
Dextrocardia	Inverted	Switches with III	Switches with II	Switches with aVL	Switches with aVR	No change	Dominant S-wave and poor R-wave progression

NOTE: *RL is a ground lead, so RL-LL reversal does not result in any significant changes*

Case 46: Presentation

A 52-year-old female with no known cardiac history presents with chest pain and palpitations. What is your interpretation of her ECG?

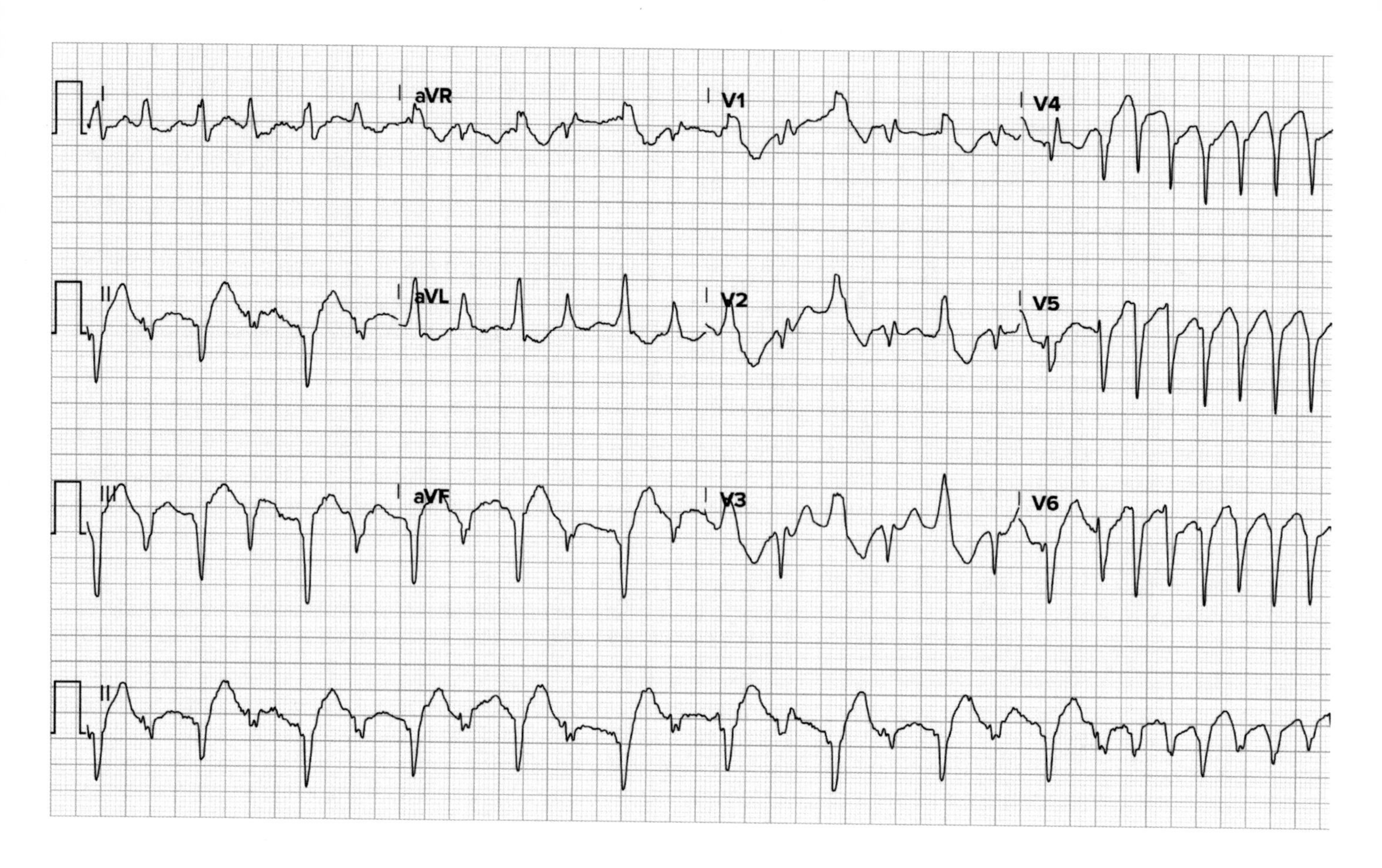

Case 46: Answer

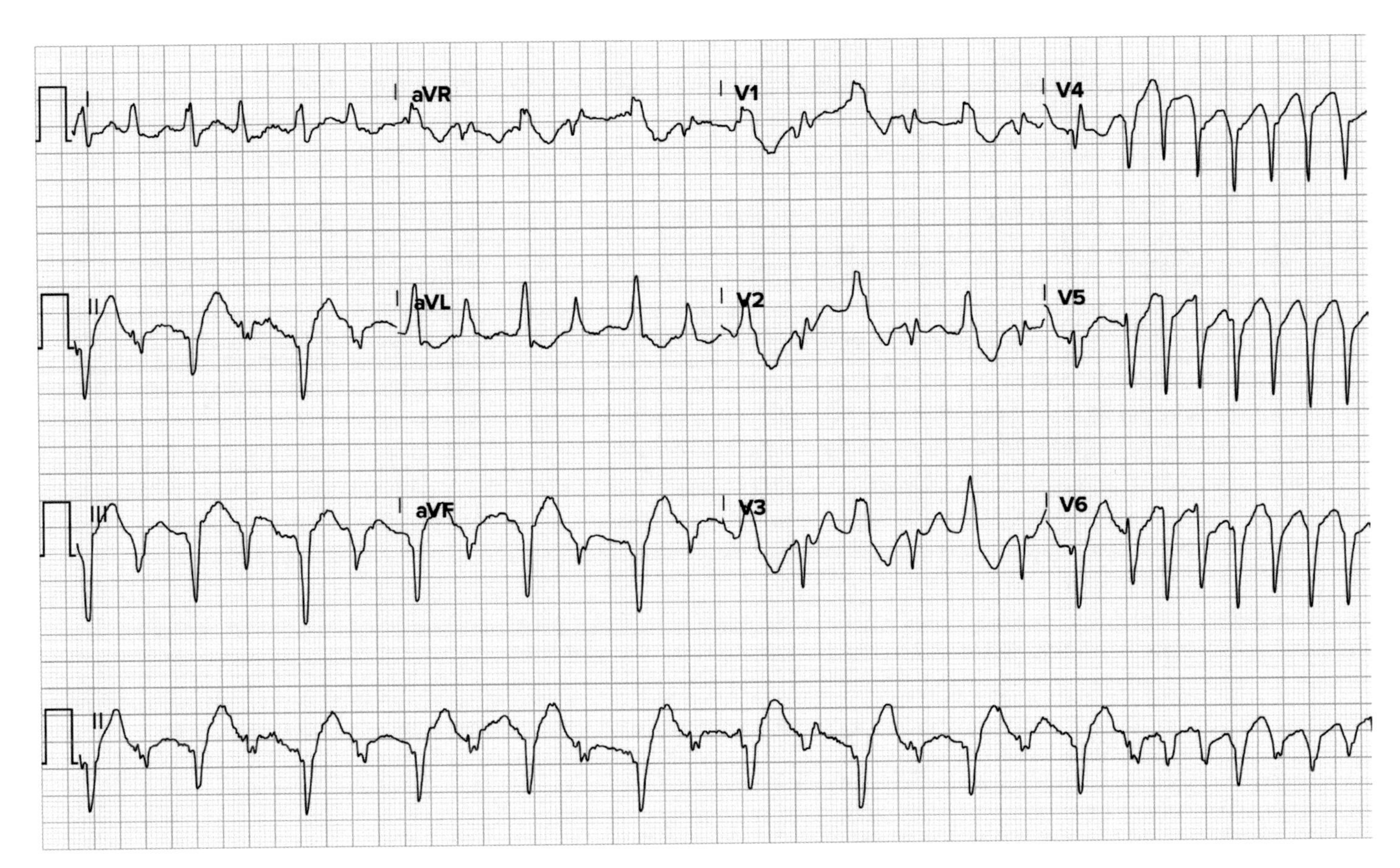

This ECG shows two rhythms. The first rhythm is a regular wide complex tachycardia with a ventricular rate of 140 bpm, no P-waves, left axis deviation, and a prolonged QRS complex duration with beat-to-beat variation in the QRS complex morphology, consistent with bidirectional ventricular tachycardia. The second rhythm, which is seen in leads V4-V6, is a regular wide complex tachycardia with a ventricular rate of 210 bpm, no P-waves, and a prolonged QRS complex duration with variable QRS complex morphologies, consistent with polymorphic ventricular tachycardia.

The differential diagnosis for a regular wide complex tachycardia includes:

- Monomorphic ventricular tachycardia
- Antidromic AVRT
- Any regular SVT (eg, sinus tach, AVNRT, atrial flutter, etc.) with aberrant conduction
  - Causes of aberrant conduction include fixed or rate-related BBB, metabolic abnormalities, sodium channel blocker toxicity, ventricular-paced rhythm, and ventricular pre-excitation (eg, WPW)

Bidirectional ventricular tachycardia is a rare tachycardia that is generally defined as having beat-to-beat alternation in the QRS complex axis and/or morphology, which is best seen in leads V1-V3 in this patient's ECG ***(see Figure 1)***.

Although bidirectional VT is commonly associated with digoxin toxicity, there are multiple other causes with differing proposed mechanisms, including:

- Acute ischemia/infarction
- Aconitine poisoning
- Anderson-Tawil syndrome (a type of Long QT Syndrome)
- Cardiac sarcoidosis
- Catecholaminergic Polymorphic VT
- Digoxin toxicity
- Familial Hypokalemic Periodic Paralysis
- Fatty deposition in the RV (that is not ARVD)
- Myocarditis
- Ventricular tumors

Figure 1.
Leads V1-V3 show beat-to-beat alternation in the QRS complex morphology and axis, consistent with bidirectional ventricular tachycardia

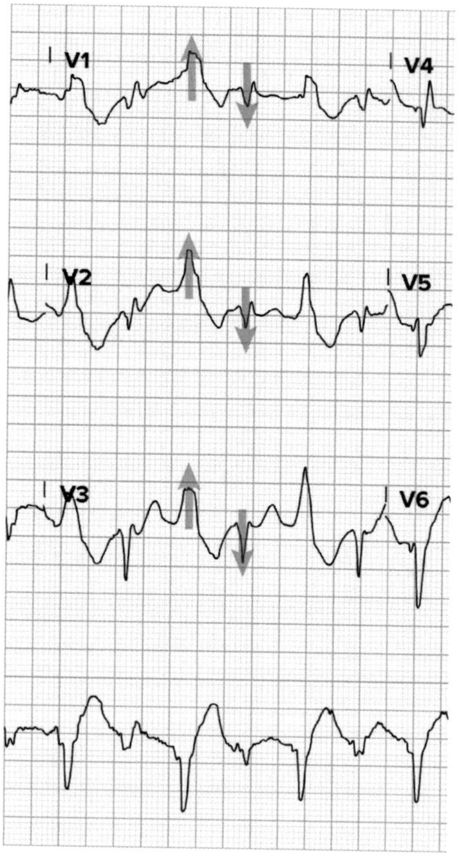

While in the ED, the patient was noted to have intermittent runs of VT lasting 10-20 seconds that spontaneously resolved and were not associated with any hemodynamic compromise. Initial treatment with an amiodarone bolus followed by drip was ineffective. The addition of an esmolol drip provided only modest improvement, so antidysrhythmic therapy was changed to a lidocaine drip. The patient's labs were notable for only a slightly elevated troponin with no significant electrolyte abnormalities. She was admitted to the Cardiac ICU and underwent a cardiac catheterization that was unremarkable. She then had a cardiac MRI, which was consistent with cardiac sarcoidosis, which was thought to be the etiology of her VT. Prior to discharge, an ICD was placed for secondary prevention of future episodes of VT.

Monomorphic VT Learning Points

- ≥ 3 consecutive, regular, wide complex beats with rate > 120-130 bpm
  - Non-sustained: < 30 sec duration with no hemodynamic instability
  - Sustained: ≥ 30 sec duration OR causes hemodynamic instability
- Rates < 120-130 bpm can be seen in patients on chronic antidysrhythmic medications (eg, amiodarone, flecainide, sotalol) or with severe cardiomyopathies
- If rate < 120 bpm, consider mimics:
  - Hyperkalemia
  - Sodium channel blocker toxicity
  - Accelerated idioventricular rhythm (AIVR)
- ECG features that increase the likelihood of VT in a regular WCT:
  - QRS complex duration > 200 msec is almost always VT, hyperkalemia, or sodium channel blocker toxicity
  - AV dissociation (ventricular rate > atrial rate)
  - Positive or negative QRS complex concordance in leads V1-V6 (entirely or predominantly positive or negative QRS\ complexes from leads V1 to V6)
  - Extreme axis deviation ("northwest axis")
  - The absence of typical RBBB or LBBB pattern suggests VT (ie, normal RBBB or LBBB pattern makes SVT with aberrant conduction more likely)
  - Fusion beats: hybrid QRS complex formed by both supraventricular and ventricular focus
  - Capture beats: sinus QRS complex formed by transient normal conduction amid AV dissociation
  - Brugada's sign: time from the onset of the QRS complex to the nadir of the S-wave is > 100 msec ***(see Figure 2)***
  - Josephson's sign: notching on the downslope of the S-wave near its nadir ***(see Figure 3)***

Figure 2

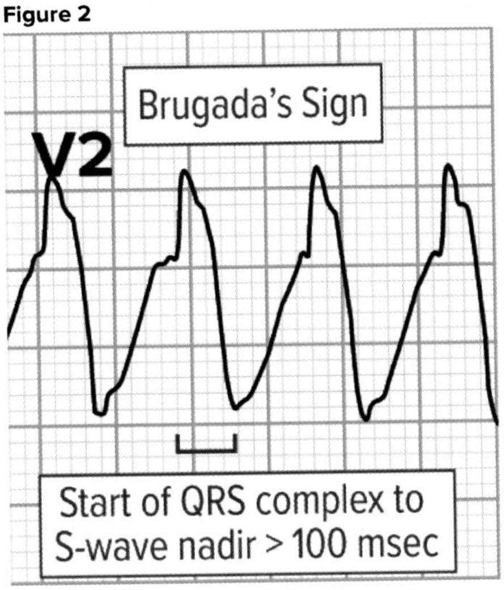

Brugada's Sign

V2

Start of QRS complex to
S-wave nadir > 100 msec

Figure 3

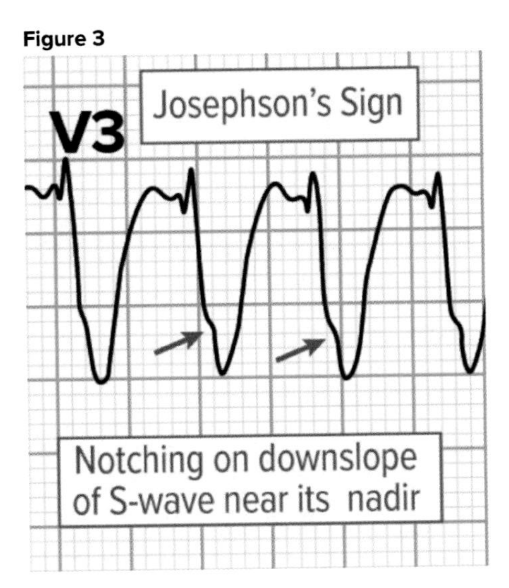

Case 47: Presentation

A 26-year-old male with history of DM presents due to AMS and elevated glucometer readings at home. What is your interpretation of his ECG?

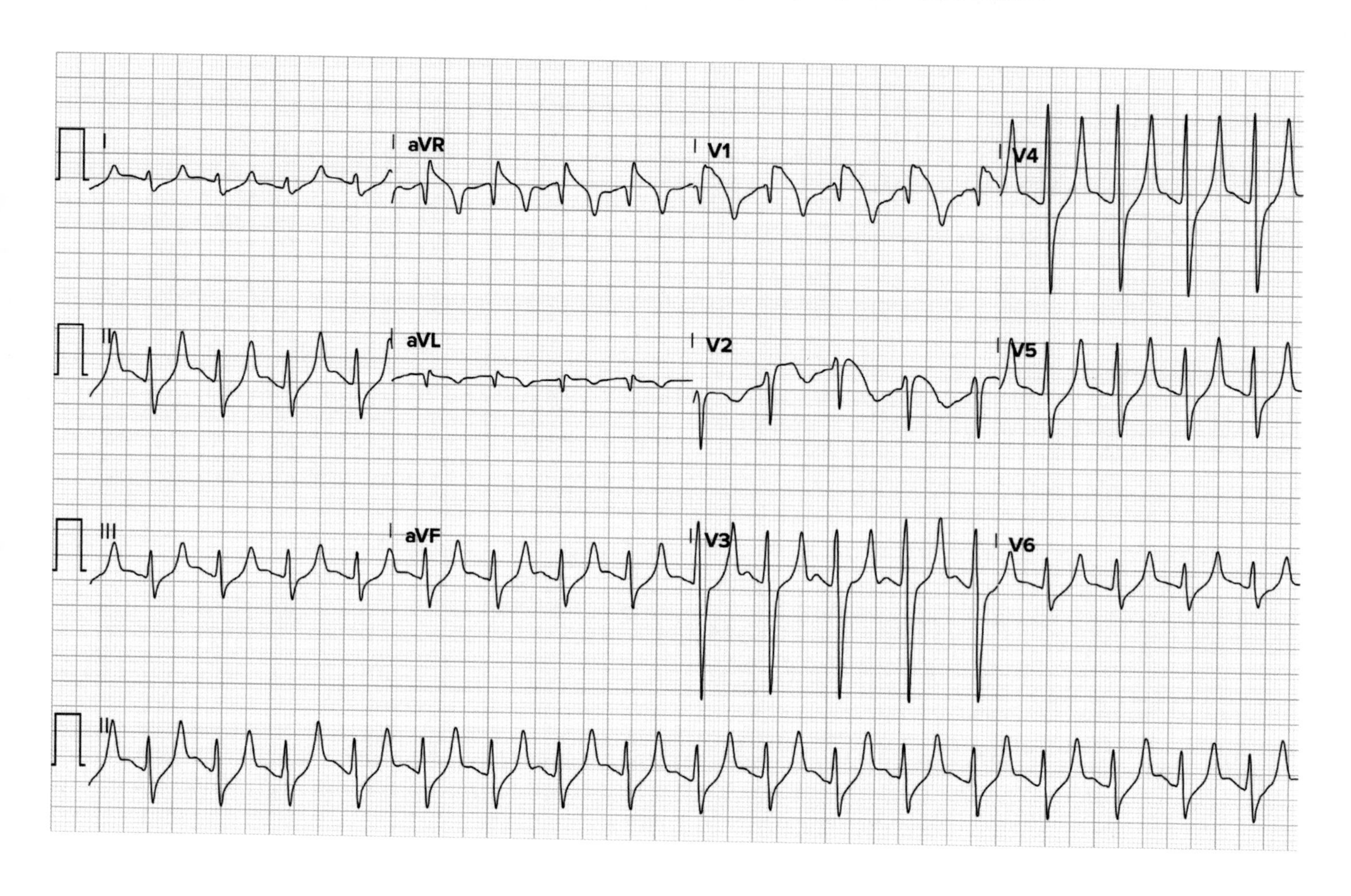

Case 47: Answer

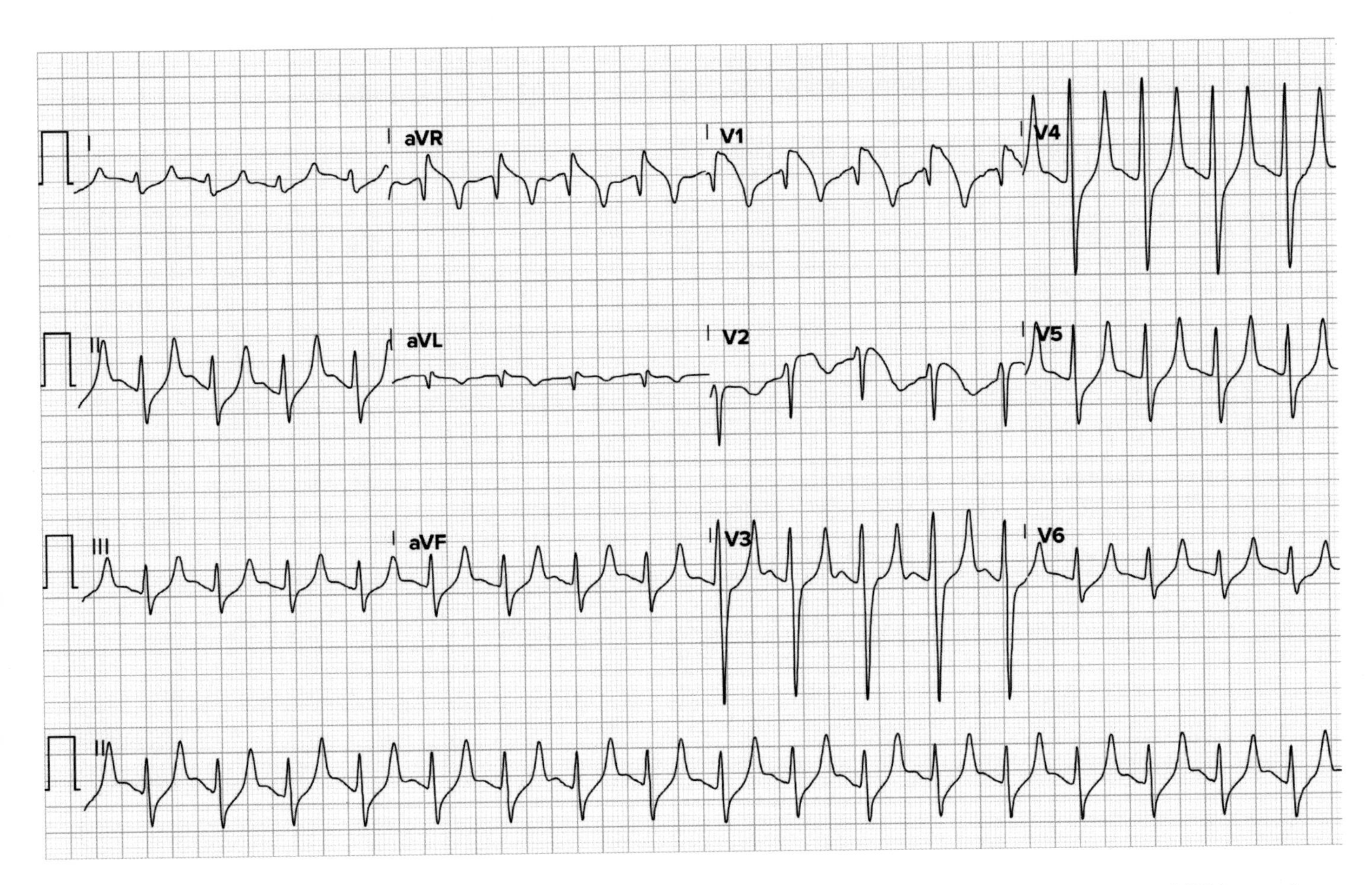

This ECG shows sinus tachycardia with a ventricular rate of 103 bpm, diffusely flattened P-waves with normal PR interval, right axis deviation, prolonged QRS complex duration with a RBBB-like morphology, STE in leads aVR and V1-V2, STD in leads I, II, III, aVF, and V3-V6, and peaked T-waves best seen in leads II, III, aVF, and V2-V6.

The key to correctly interpreting this ECG is recognizing the peaked T-waves consistent with hyperkalemia. These T-waves are tall, narrow, peaked, and often best seen in the precordial leads. This is in contrast to hyperacute T-waves seen with early MI which are broad based and disproportionately tall relative to the preceding QRS complex ***(see Figure 1)***. Also, hyperacute T-waves seen with early AMI will be contiguous and can have reciprocal STD or TWI which are not seen with hyperkalemia.

Figure 1a-b.
Comparison of peaked T-waves seen with hyperkalemia (Figure 1a) and hyperacute T-waves seen with early AMI (Figure 1b)

Figure 1a. Hyperkalemia (from case ECG)

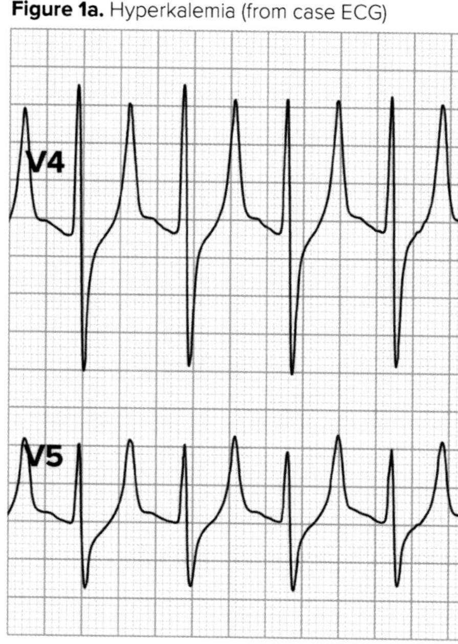

Figure 1b. Hyperacute T-waves (from a different ECG)

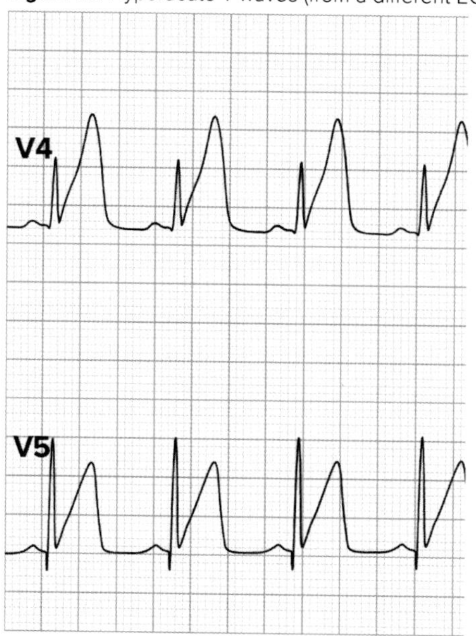

Leads V1-V2 both show STE that mimic ischemia. Identifying the J point in these leads is difficult and best done by drawing a vertical line from lead V3 where the J point is more obvious ***(see Figure 2)***. After identifying the J point, it easier to see the STE in these leads ***(see Figure 3)***. The STE in lead V2 is best measured in the 3rd beat due to wandering baseline in the preceding beats. In a patient presenting with ACS symptoms, these changes in isolation (ie, without the peaked T-waves) would be concerning for an AMI.

Figure 2.
Using the J point in lead V3, a vertical line can be extended up to help identify the J points in leads V1-V2

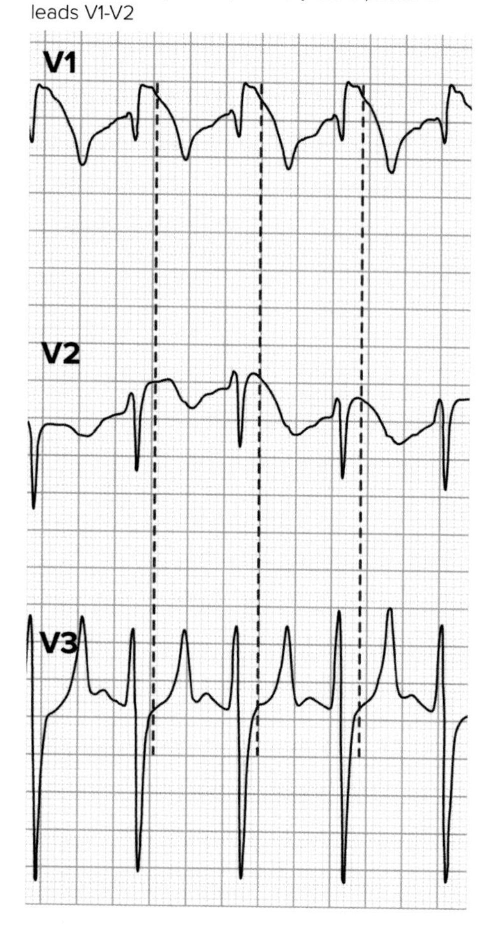

Figure 3.
STE in leads V1-V2 (vertical line intersects the J points)

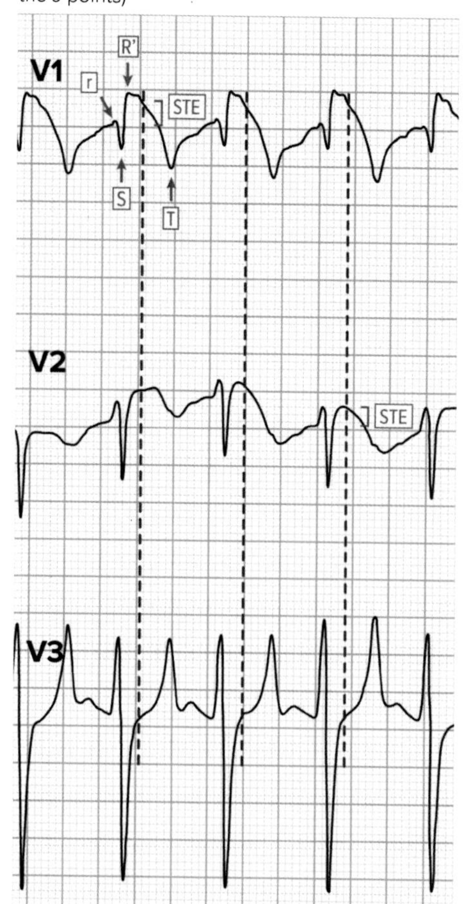

Leads V1 and V2 also mimic Brugada morphology (***see Figure 4***), and in a patient presenting with syncope, these ECG changes in isolation (ie, without the peaked T-waves) would be concerning for Brugada syndrome. The ECG criteria for Brugada syndrome are:

- Complete or incomplete RBBB pattern with coved STE ≥ 2 mm followed by a negative T-wave in ≥ 1 of leads V1-V2

Figure 4a-b.
Comparison of leads V1-V2 from this patient's ECG **(*Figure 4a*)** with that of an ECG from a patient with known Brugada syndrome **(*Figure 4b*)**

Figure 4a. Hyperkalemia

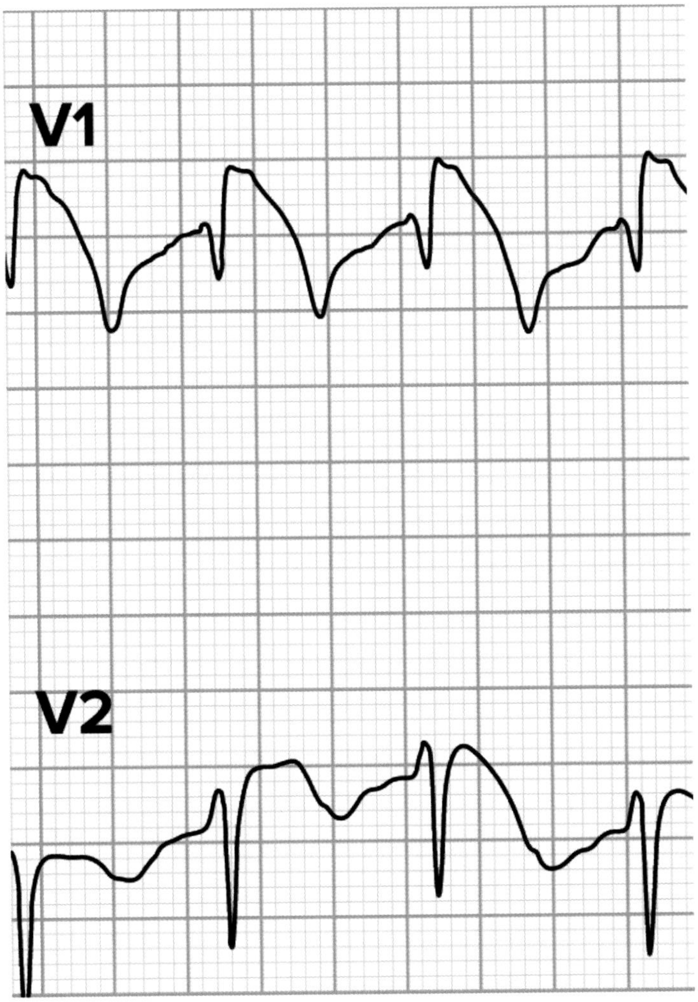

V1

V2

Figure 4b. Brugada pattern

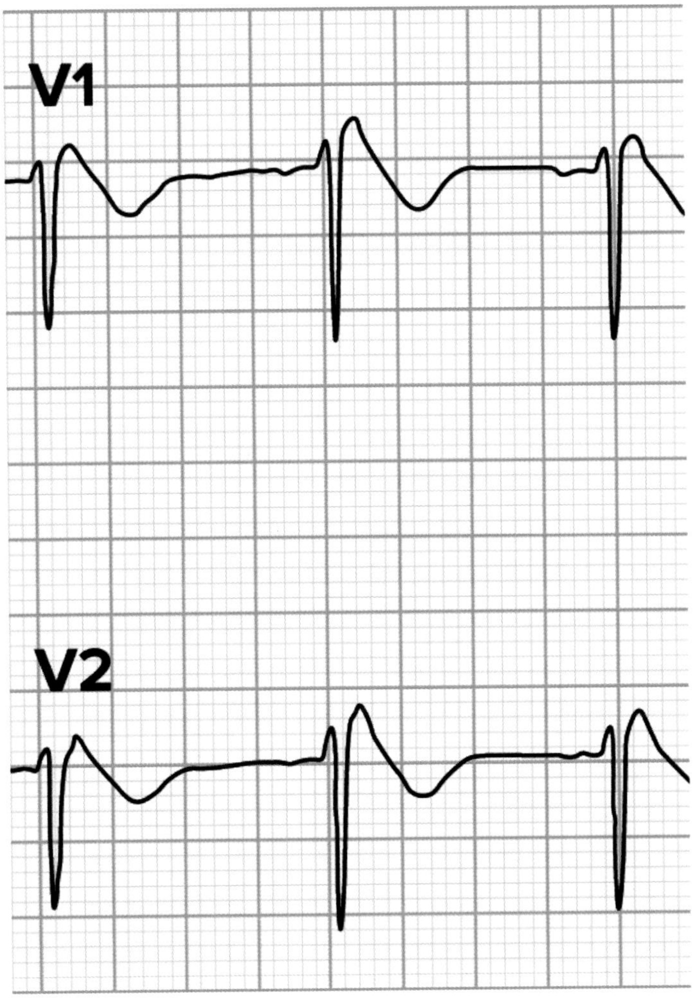

V1

V2

This ECG also shows the pattern of STE in leads aVR and V1 with diffuse STD. The differential diagnosis for this pattern includes both ACS and non-ACS etiologies:

ACS causes[1]	Non-ACS causes[2]
• LMCA insufficiency (can see STE aVR > V1)	• Acute and/or severe anemia
• Prox LAD insufficiency (can see STE V1 > aVR)	• Aortic dissection
• Triple vessel disease	• LBBB and ventricular-paced rhythms
• Global cardiac ischemia	• LVH with strain pattern
• Prinzmetal angina	• Pulmonary embolism
	• ROSC s/p epinephrine or defibrillation
	• Severe hypokalemia or hyperkalemia
	• Sodium channel blockade
	• Supraventricular tachycardia (especially with rapid rates)

The patient's labs came back with multiple abnormalities including potassium of 7.6 mEq/L, pH 7.09, HCO3 8 mEq/L, and glucose 2099 mg/dL, consistent with severe DKA. The patient was aggressively treated for hyperkalemia and a repeat ECG one hour later ***(see Figure 5)*** showed significant improvement of the abnormalities seen on the initial ECG. The patient was admitted to the ICU for further DKA treatment.

Figure 5.
Repeat ECG after treatment

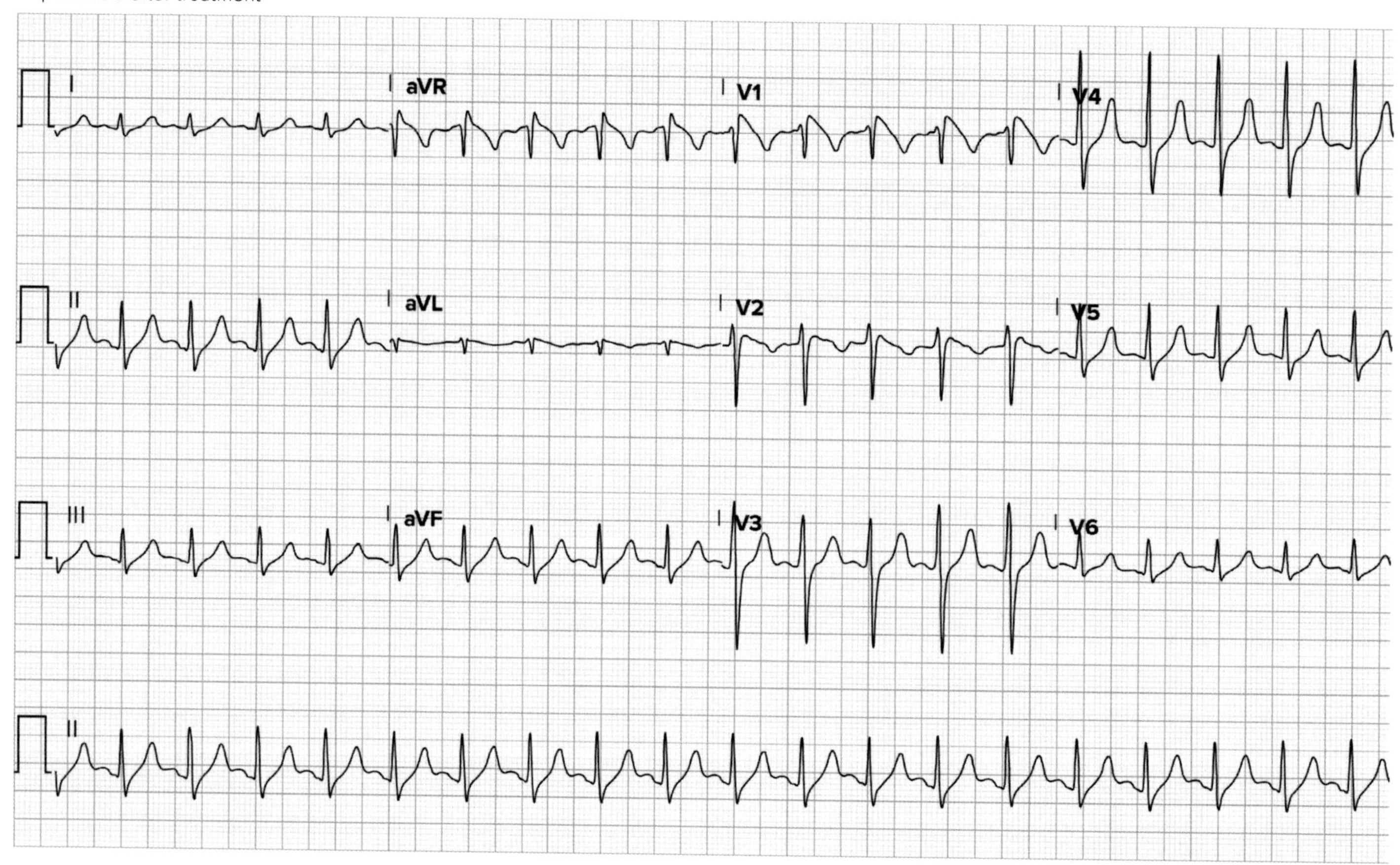

Hyperkalemia Learning Points

- ECG is specific but not sensitive for hyperkalemia
  - Tall, narrow, peaked T-waves (best seen in precordial leads)
  - P-wave flattening and PR interval prolongation
  - Prolonged QRS complex duration, ranging from minimal to maximal
  - Conduction abnormalities (AV blocks, fascicular and bundle branch blocks)
  - Bradycardia
  - Sino-ventricular rhythm (loss of P-waves, extremely widened QRS) with normal or slow rate
  - Ventricular dysrhythmias
- Can cause STE (common in leads V1-V2 and aVR) that mimics STEMI or Brugada pattern
- Can occur simultaneously with hyperacute T-waves and obscure early changes seen in an anterior or anteroseptal AMI
- The "syphilis of ECG abnormalities," meaning that a broad range of abnormalities can be encountered with hyperkalemia[1]

Hyperacute T-waves Learning Points

- There is no universally accepted definition of hyperacute T-waves (ie, no absolute specific amplitude), but the general characteristics include:
  - Broad based and disproportionately tall
  - Asymmetric morphology with more gradual upslope and more abrupt return to the baseline
  - J point elevation is common
- Hyperacute T-waves + STD/TWI in reciprocal leads = early AMI
- When in doubt, obtain serial ECGs

References

1. Thygesen K, Alpert JS, Jaffe AS, et al. 2018 ESC/ACC/AHA/WHF Expert Consensus Document: Fourth Universal Definition of Myocardial Infarction (2018). Circulation. 2018;138:e618-e651.
2. Mattu A. ECG Weekly.

Case 48: Presentation

A 65-year-old male with history of HTN and CAD presents with chest pain.
What is your interpretation of his ECG?

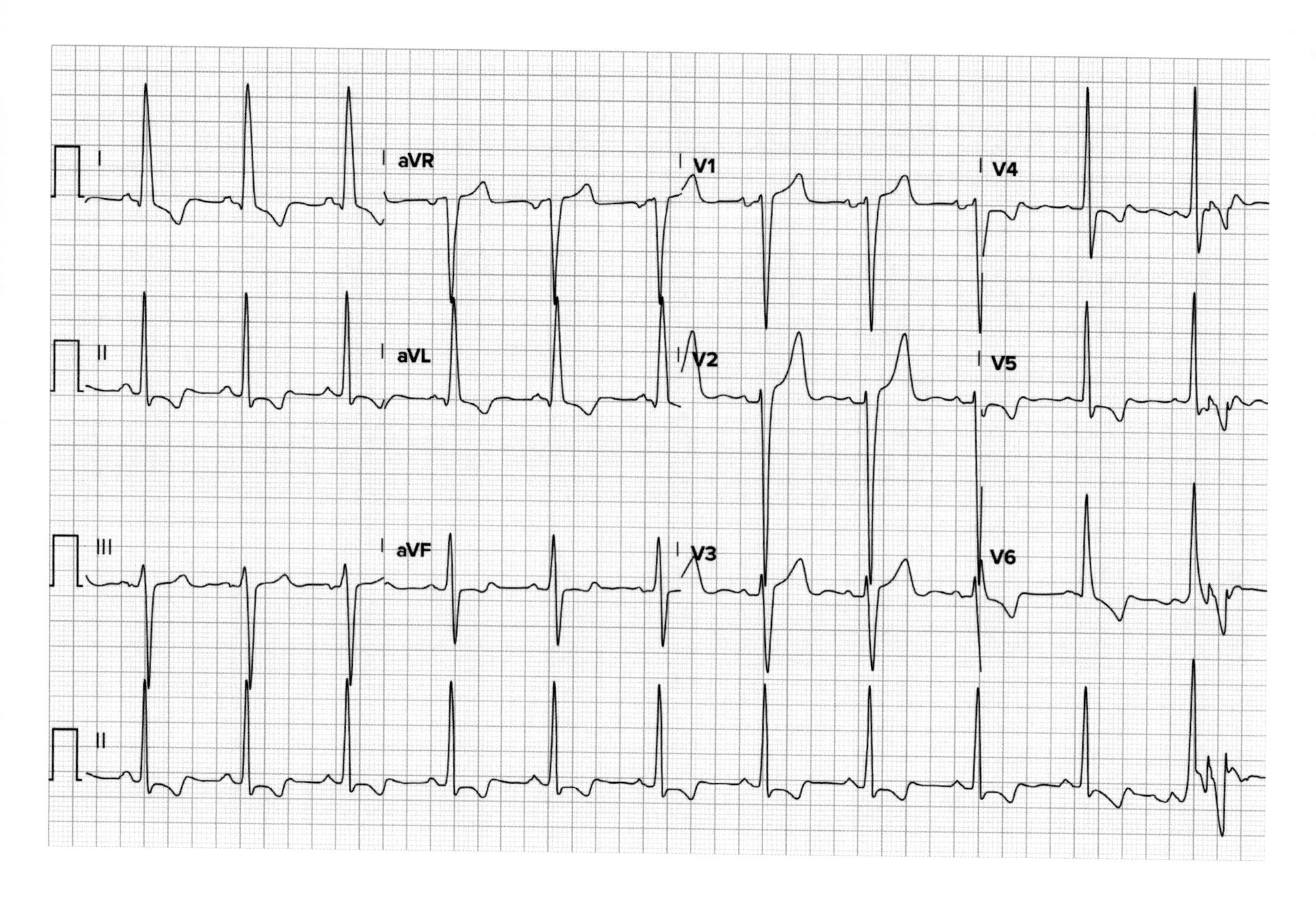

Case 48: Answer

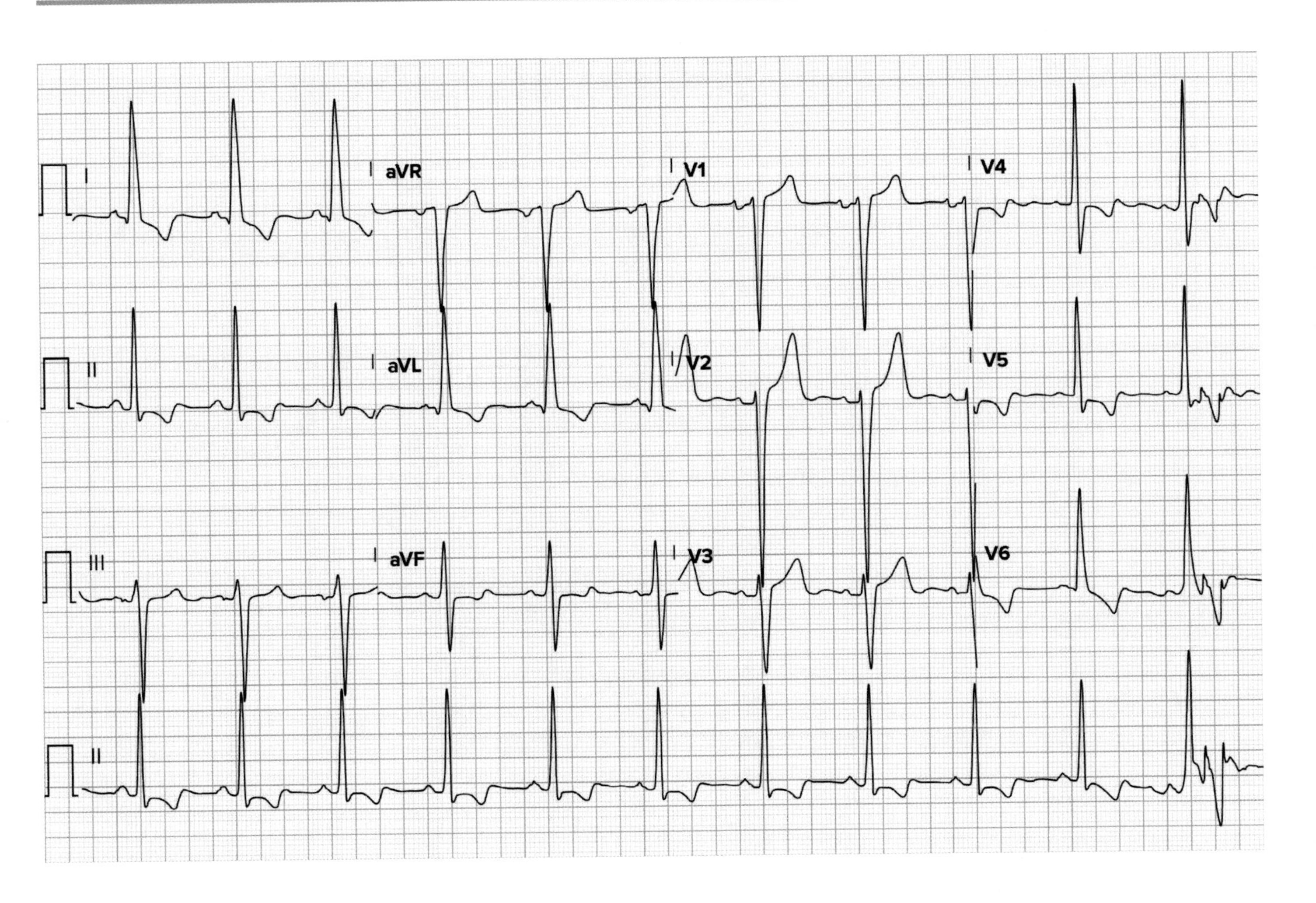

This ECG shows normal sinus rhythm with a ventricular rate of 68 bpm, normal axis, a prolonged QRS complex duration, and ST-segment and T-wave abnormalities consistent with LVH by voltage with strain pattern.

The key to correctly interpreting this ECG is recognizing the ST-segment and T-wave abnormalities that are characteristic of the LVH strain pattern. Leads V1-V3 will typically have a large S-wave with STE and a concave upward ST-segment ***(see Figure 1)***. Leads I, aVL, and V4-V6 will typically have a large R-wave with STD, TWI, and a concave downward ST-segment with a characteristic asymmetric morphology that includes STD that has a gradual downslope, fusing with the inverted T-wave, and a more abrupt return to the baseline ***(see Figure 2)***. As well, the QRS complex duration is often prolonged when LVH is present.

Figure 1.
Findings in lead V1 consistent with the LVH strain pattern

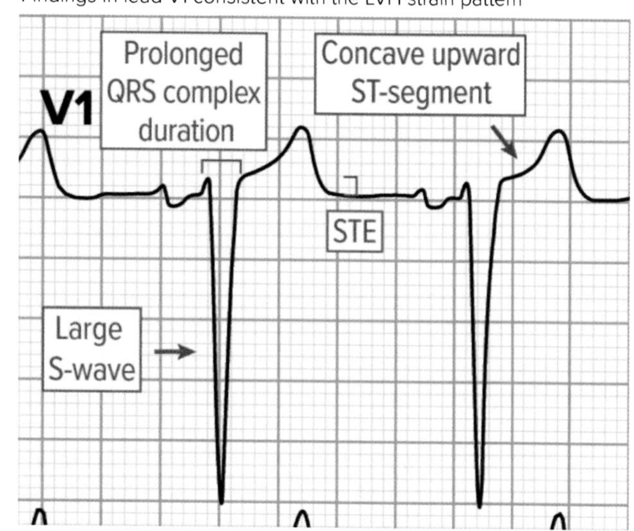

Figure 2.
Findings in lead V5 consistent with the LVH strain pattern

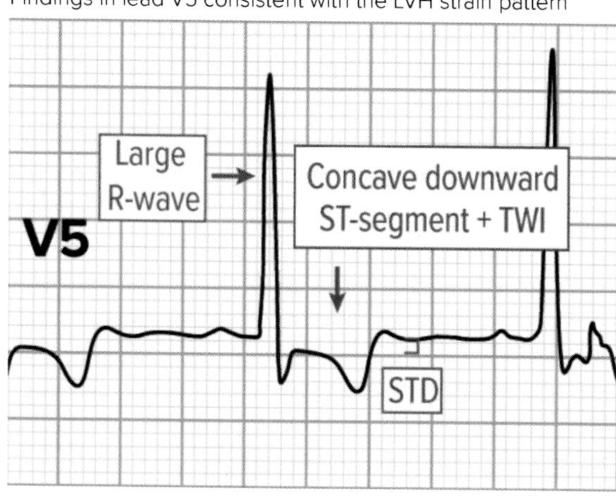

None of the many diagnostic ECG criteria for LVH have great sensitivity, so while anatomic LVH can lead to characteristic changes seen on ECG, it is ultimately an echocardiographic diagnosis. From the ECG perspective, LVH poses a diagnostic challenge as the LVH strain pattern can mimic an anteroseptal MI, so recognition of the LVH strain pattern is of the utmost importance when interpreting the ECG. Comparing with prior ECGs and obtaining serial ECGs can help differentiate between ischemia and the strain pattern.

The patient's initial ECG and serial ECGs were unchanged from prior.

LVH Learning Points

- ECG is only suggestive of anatomic LVH- echocardiography is the superior diagnostic modality
- ECG findings in LVH are manifested primarily by the increased voltage of the QRS complexes, hence the term "LVH by voltage criteria"
  - No criteria are recommended for use exclusive of other validated criteria
  - Diagnosis of LVH in the presence of intraventricular conduction abnormalities (eg, fascicular blocks, bundle branch blocks) should be made with caution as they may impact the accuracy of the ECG criteria for LVH
- 80% of LVH by voltage patterns demonstrate ST and T-wave abnormalities, termed "LVH with strain pattern," which commonly include:
  - STE in leads V1-V3
  - STD and TWI in leads I, aVL and V4-V6
  - Increased S-wave depth in leads III, aVR, and V1-V3
  - Increased R-wave peak time > 50 msec in lead V5 or V6
  - Increased R-wave amplitude in leads I, aVL and V4-V6
  - Left axis deviation typical, but can occur with any axis
  - Increased QRS complex and/or QT interval duration
- LVH with strain pattern can confound the ECG's ability to detect ACS, particularly anteroseptal MI, and mimics ACS findings

NOTES:

Case 49: Presentation

A 53-year-old female with no known cardiac history presents with palpitations and lightheadedness. What is your interpretation of her ECG?

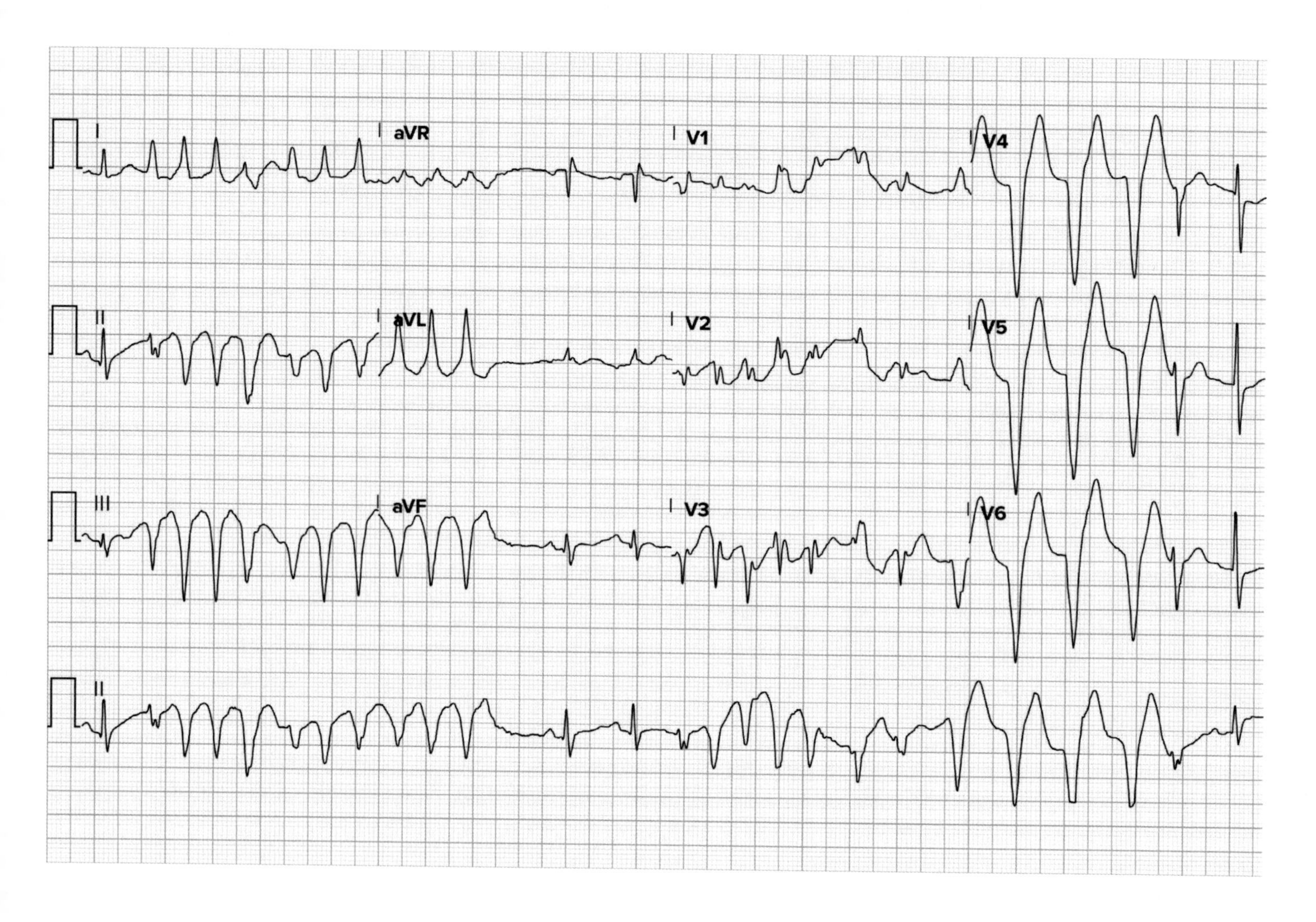

Case 49: Answer

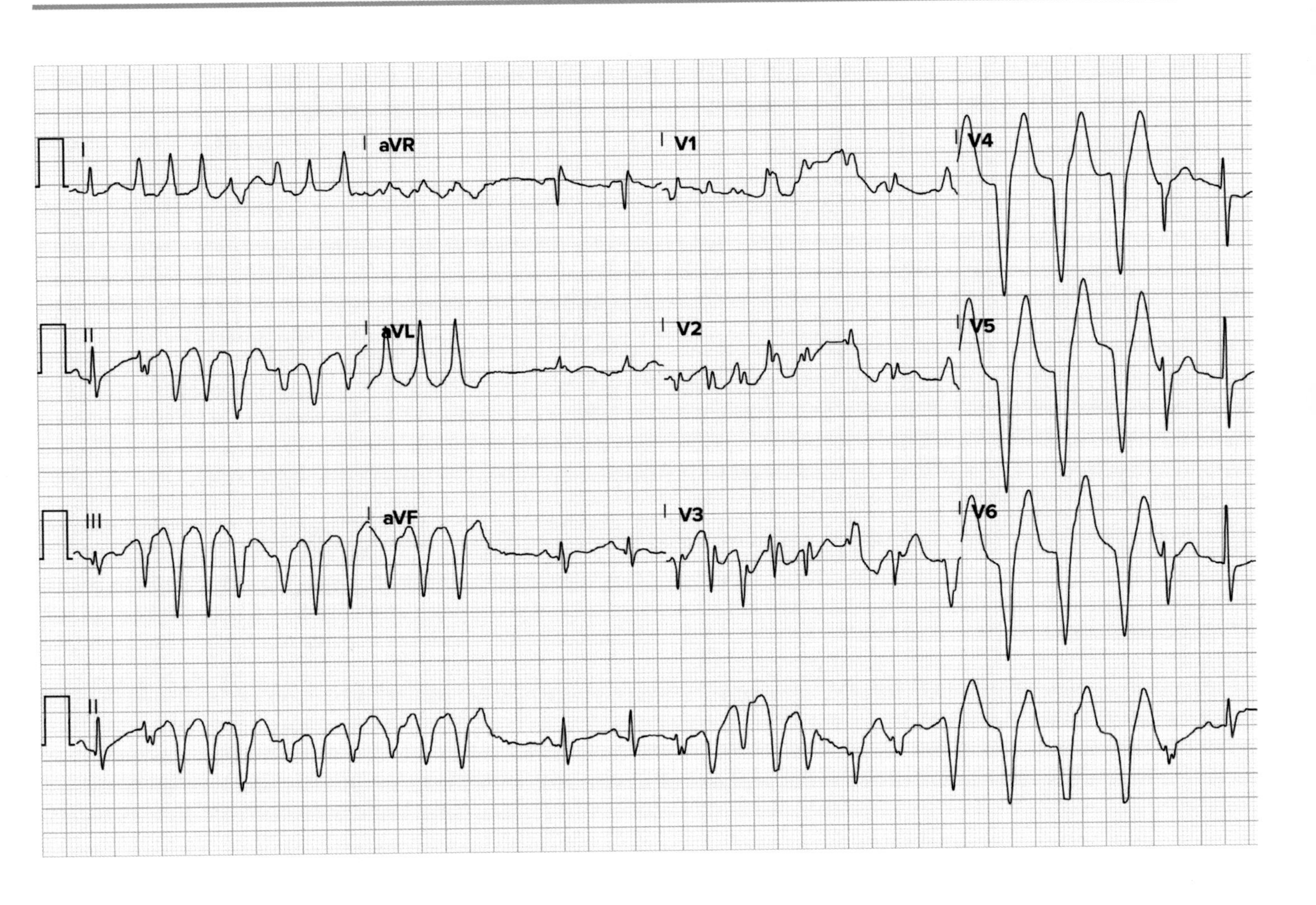

This ECG shows an irregular wide complex tachycardia, consistent with polymorphic ventricular tachycardia, with intermittent sinus beats (ie, sinus P-QRS-T complexes), followed by a regular wide-complex tachycardia consistent with monomorphic VT.

The differential diagnosis for an irregular WCT includes:

- Ventricular fibrillation
- Polymorphic ventricular tachycardia (including torsades de pointes)
- MAT with aberrant conduction
- Atrial flutter with variable block and aberrant conduction
- Atrial fibrillation with aberrant conduction
  - Causes of aberrant conduction include fixed or rate-related BBB, metabolic abnormalities, sodium channel blocker toxicity, ventricular-paced rhythm, and ventricular pre-excitation (eg, WPW)

This ECG starts off with a sinus beat followed by a run of polymorphic ventricular tachycardia ***(see Figure 1)***.

Figure 1.
The initial portion of the ECG shows a sinus beat followed by a run of polymorphic ventricular tachycardia

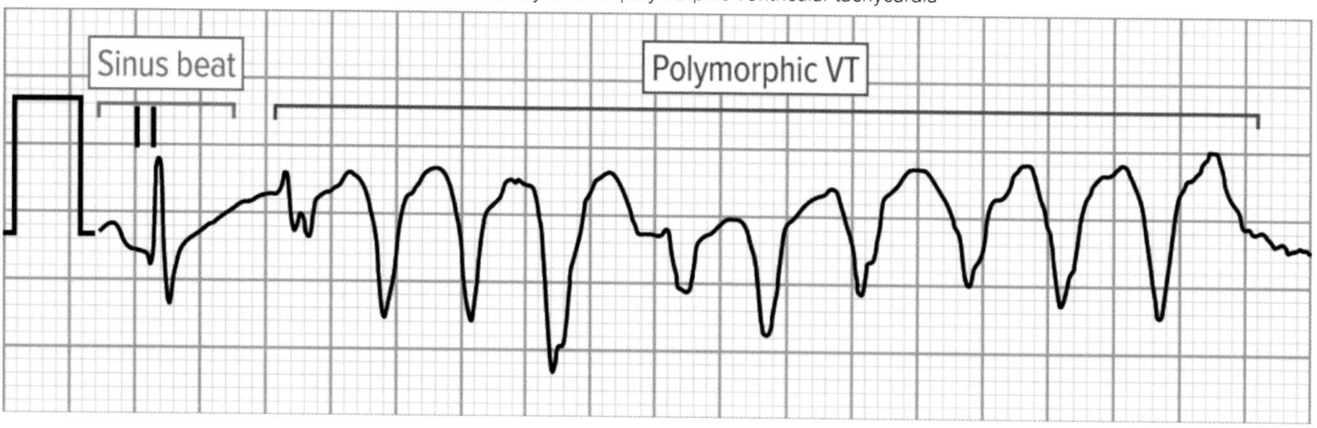

This is followed by two sinus beats and another run of polymorphic ventricular tachycardia ***(see Figure 2)***.

Figure 2.
The middle portion of the ECG shows two sinus beats followed by another run of polymorphic ventricular tachycardia

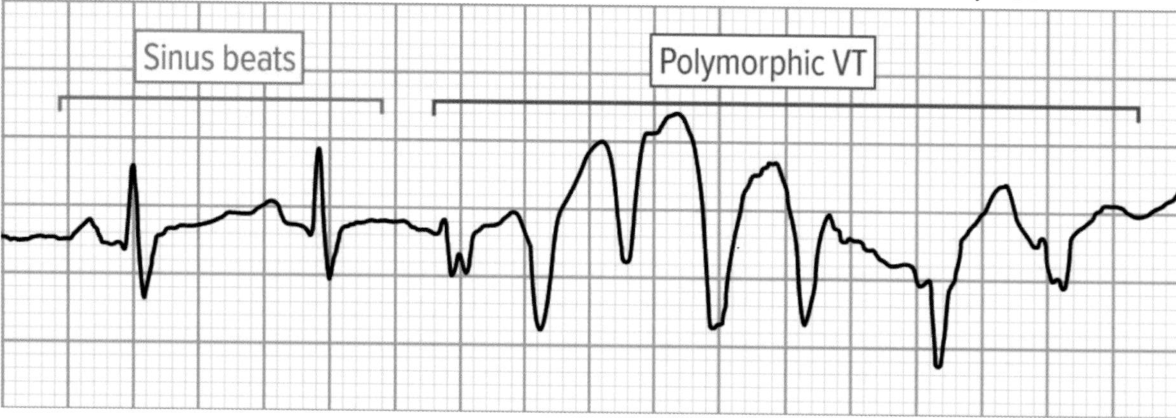

This is followed by a 4-beat run of a regular wide complex tachycardia, most likely monomorphic ventricular tachycardia, a fusion beat, then a sinus beat ***(see Figure 3)***. A fusion beat which is caused by the simultaneous depolarization of the ventricle from both a normal supraventricular focus (eg, a sinus beat from the SA node) and a ventricular focus. The result is a QRS complex morphology that is a fusion of the VT and sinus QRS complex morphologies. When seen in the setting of a regular WCT with no P-waves, a fusion beat is considered diagnostic of VT.

Figure 3.
The final portion of the ECG shows a 4-beat run of monomorphic ventricular tachycardia followed by a fusion beat then a sinus beat

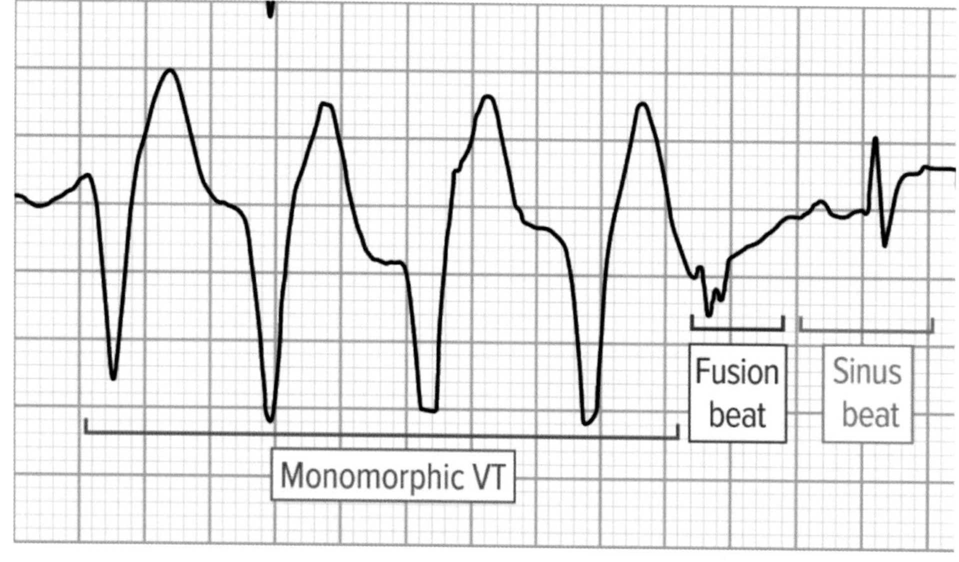

Polymorphic ventricular tachycardia is an irregular WCT with phasic variation (ie, happens over a number of beats) of the QRS complex polarity (ie, axis) and amplitude that is classified as either torsades or non-torsades.

- Torsades de pointes describes the characteristic twisting of the peaks of the QRS around the isoelectric baseline. It is due to prolonged QTc interval and is usually paroxysmal and self-terminating, but it can degenerate into ventricular fibrillation. There must be a prolonged QTc interval on the baseline ECG for polymorphic ventricular tachycardia to be classified as torsades.
- Non-torsades polymorphic ventricular tachycardia is defined by the absence of a prolonged QTc interval on the baseline ECG. It is often due to ischemia and is constant, frequently leading to hemodynamic compromise.

The treatment for unstable polymorphic ventricular tachycardia is defibrillation regardless of classification. Intermittent torsades can be treated with magnesium, electrical overdrive pacing, and potassium repletion (if indicated), regardless of whether it is due to an acquired or congenital prolonged QTc interval. Torsades due to acquired long QTc interval can also be treated with chemical overdrive pacing with isoproterenol. This should be avoided in patients with congenital long QT syndrome, as adrenergic stimuli is a common trigger of dysrhythmias. Even though the QTc interval increases with slower ventricular rates, maintenance therapy for these patients commonly includes beta-blockers to minimize adrenergic stimulation.

This patient had only paroxysmal episodes of polymorphic ventricular tachycardia without hemodynamic compromise but had a normal QTc on her baseline ECG. She was admitted to the cardiology service and had an unremarkable cardiac catheterization followed by placement of an automatic implantable cardioverter defibrillator.

Polymorphic Ventricular Tachycardia Learning Points

- Irregular WCT with phasic variation (ie, happens over a number of beats) of the QRS complex polarity (ie, axis) and amplitude
  - Rate is typically 180-250 bpm
  - Classified as either torsades or non-torsades
- Torsades de pointes
  - Describes the characteristic twisting of the peaks of the QRS complexes around the isoelectric baseline
  - Prolonged QTc interval (either congenital or acquired) on baseline ECG
  - Usually paroxysmal and self-terminating but can degenerate into ventricular fibrillation
- Non-torsades
  - Absence of QT prolongation on baseline ECG
  - Often due to ischemia
  - Usually sustained and causes hemodynamic instability
- Treatment includes:
  - Defibrillation for unstable polymorphic ventricular tachycardia regardless of etiology
  - ACS workup for all non-torsades polymorphic ventricular tachycardia
  - Magnesium, electrical overdrive pacing, and potassium replacement (if indicated) for intermittent torsades
  - Identify and correct underlying cause(s) of non-torsades (eg, QT prolonging medications, hypokalemia, hypomagnesemia, hypocalcemia, elevated ICP, etc.)

Case 50 Presentation

An otherwise healthy 38-year-old female presents with palpitations and lightheadedness. What is your interpretation of her ECG (ECG #1) and ECG during treatment (ECG #2)?

ECG #1

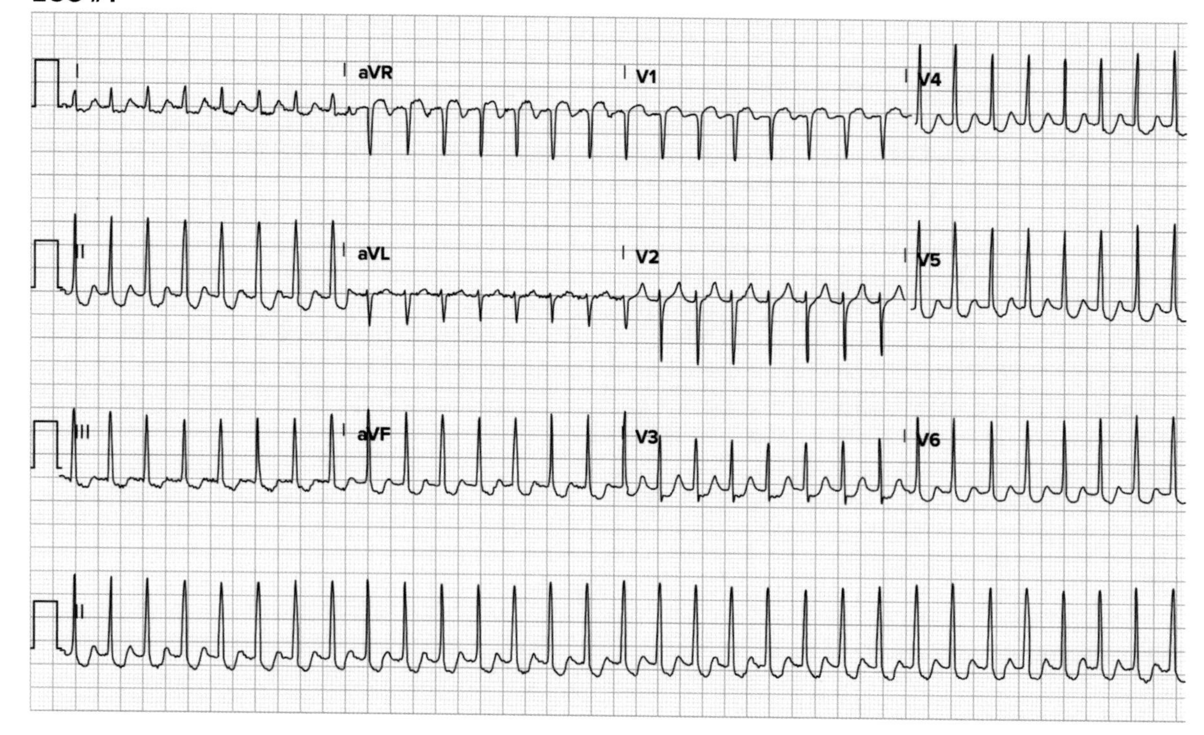

ECG #2 (immediately after receiving adenosine)

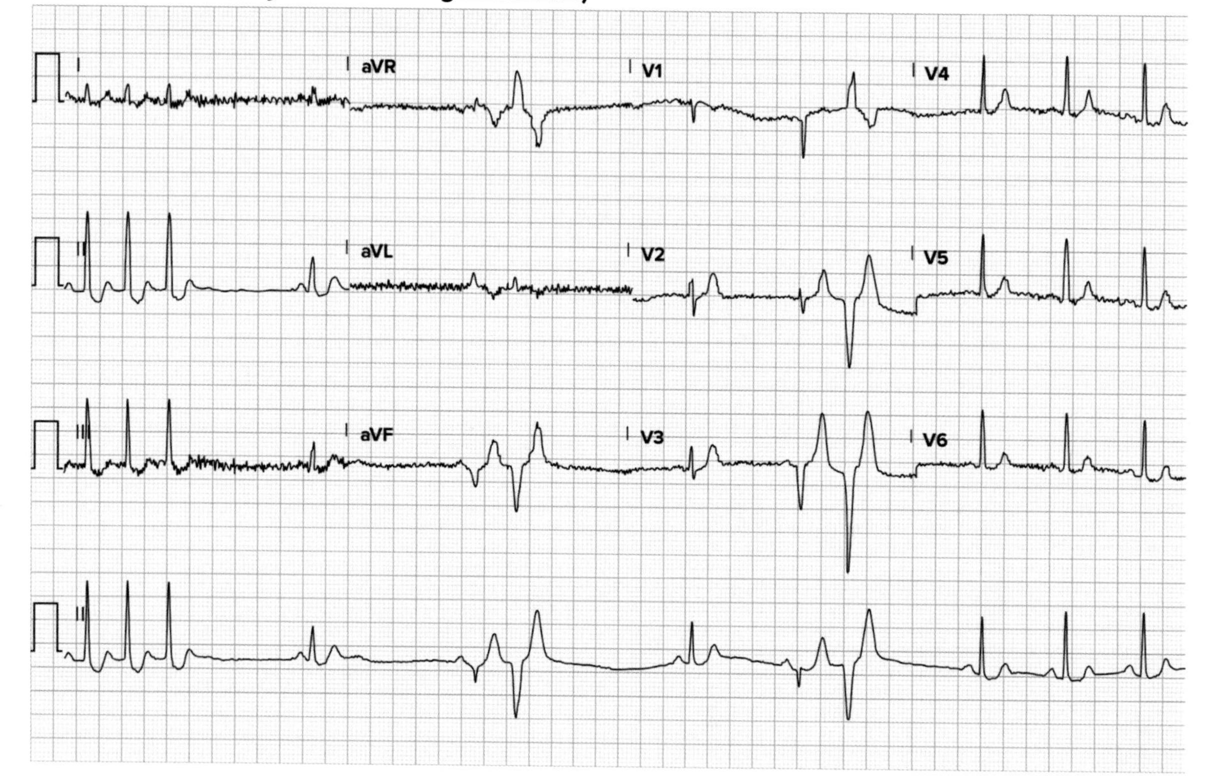

Case 50: Answer

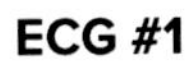

ECG #1

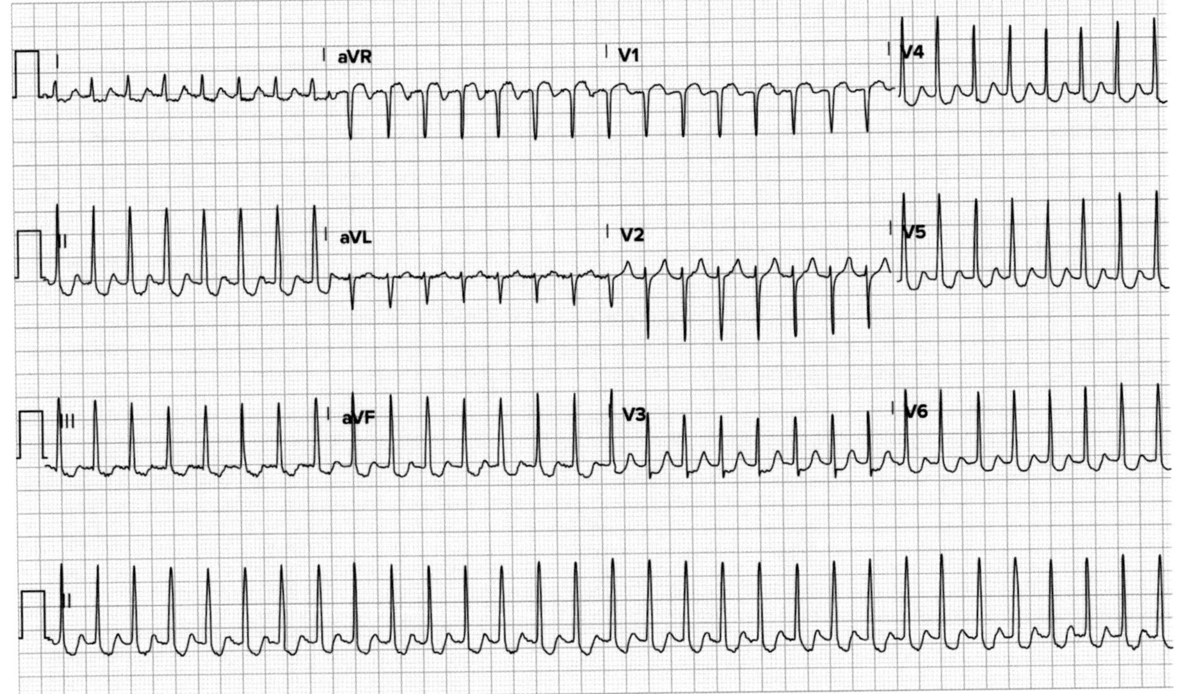

ECG #2 (immediately after receiving adenosine)

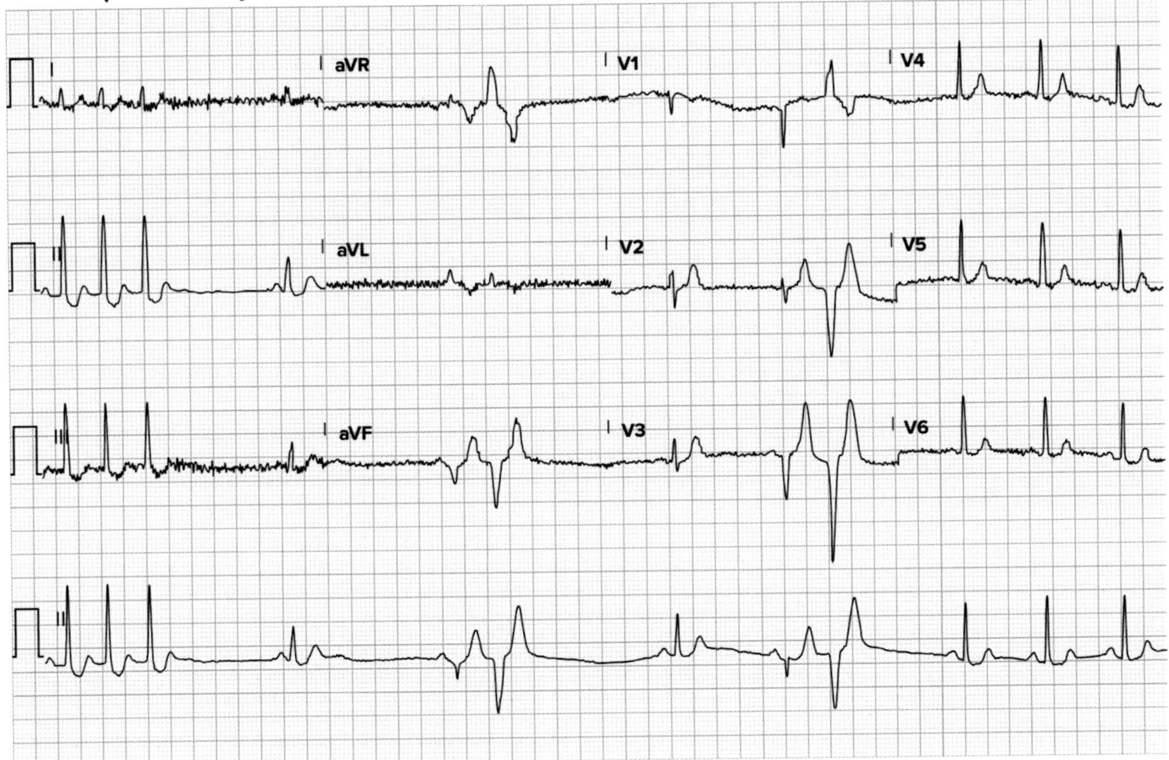

ECG #1 shows a regular narrow-complex tachycardia with a ventricular rate of 185 bpm and no visible P-waves, normal axis, STE in leads aVR and V1, and STD in leads I, II, III, aVF, and V3-V6.

The differential diagnosis for a regular narrow-complex tachycardia includes:

- Atrial flutter
- Atrial tachycardia
- AV nodal reentrant tachycardia
- AVRT (ie, WPW) with orthodromic conduction
- Junctional tachycardia
- Narrow complex VT
- Sinus tachycardia

The absence of P-waves rules out atrial tachycardia and sinus tachycardia. The rate is too slow for 1:1 flutter, too fast for a junctional tachycardia, and would be very fast for 2:1 flutter. The QRS complex duration is approximately 75 msec, so narrow complex VT is unlikely. Without more history, it is impossible to tell whether this AVNRT or orthodromic AVRT (ie, retrograde conduction via the AP), but the treatment for both is the same.

The differential diagnosis for the pattern of STE in lead aVR +/- lead V1 with diffuse STD includes both ACS and non-ACS etiologies:

ACS causes[1]	Non-ACS causes[2]
• LMCA insufficiency (can see STE aVR > V1)	• Acute and/or severe anemia
• Prox LAD insufficiency (can see STE V1 > aVR)	• Aortic dissection
• Triple vessel disease	• LBBB and ventricular-paced rhythms
• Global cardiac ischemia	• LVH with strain pattern
• Prinzmetal angina	• Pulmonary embolism
	• ROSC s/p epinephrine or defibrillation
	• Severe hypokalemia or hyperkalemia
	• Sodium channel blockade
	• Supraventricular tachycardia (especially with rapid rates)

Although the pattern of STE in lead aVR +/- lead V1 with diffuse STD is discussed in the cardiology literature, its clinical significance is not without some controversy. This is likely due to the broad differential diagnosis associated with this pattern that includes both ACS and non-ACS causes. The 2018 Fourth Universal Definition of MI states "ST-segment depression ≥ 1 mm in 6 or more leads, which may be associated with ST segment elevation in leads aVR and/or V1 and hemodynamic compromise, is suggestive of multivessel disease or left main disease" but does not provide specific management recommendations.

Treatment should be guided by the underlying etiology, and it is imperative to consider both ACS and non-ACS causes. For patients suspected of having an ACS cause, this ECG pattern is highly suggestive of LMCA insufficiency, proximal LAD insufficiency, or triple vessel disease. So, while this pattern does not meet "traditional" STEMI criteria, it can represent high-risk ACS, including possible acute coronary occlusion, in the correct clinical context, and immediate angiography should be considered. Whether this is done by emergent cardiology consultation or activation of the cardiac catheterization lab depends on local practice preferences.

The pattern of STE in leads aVR and V1 with diffuse STD seen in this ECG is likely due to the abnormal conduction inherent to the tachydysrhythmia. The ECG changes alone do not constitute a "failed stress test" and the decision to evaluate for ischemia that caused the tachydysrhythmia and/or was caused by the tachydysrhythmia should be a clinical one.

ECG #2 shows 3 beats of SVT, which was terminated by adenosine, followed by 2 cycles of a sinus beat followed by a fusion PVC-PVC couplet, then normal sinus rhythm ***(see Figure 1)***. A fusion PVC is the combination of a supraventricular impulse that coincides with a ventricular impulse to create a QRS complex that is a hybrid of the two.

Figure 1.

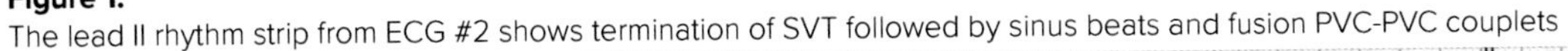

The lead II rhythm strip from ECG #2 shows termination of SVT followed by sinus beats and fusion PVC-PVC couplets

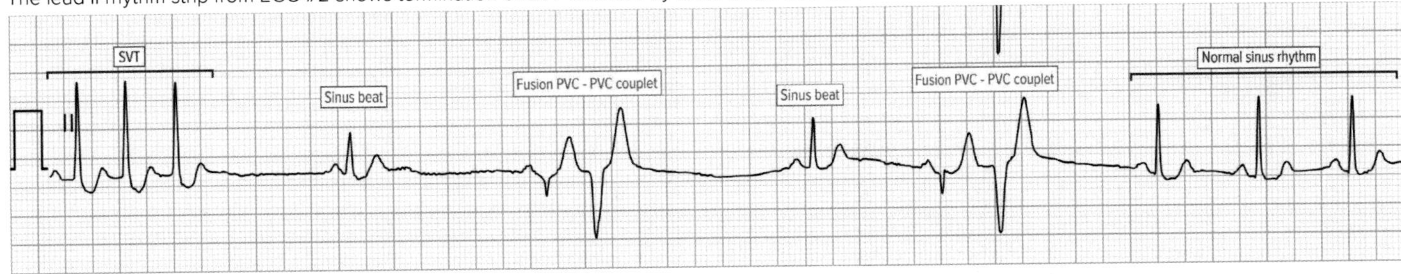

This patient had an unremarkable ED workup and was discharged with cardiology follow-up.

AV Nodal Reentrant Tachycardia (AVNRT) Learning Points

- Also called paroxysmal supraventricular tachycardia or SVT
- Caused by re-entrant circuit within or around the AV node and typically triggered by a PAC
- ECG shows a regular narrow-complex tachycardia in the absence of concurrent conduction abnormalities (eg, bundle branch block)
  - Ventricular rate typically 140-280 bpm
  - Retrograde P-waves can appear before, after, or superimposed on the QRS complexes

Atrioventricular Re-entry Tachycardia (AVRT) Learning Points

- Caused by re-entrant circuit involving AV node and an accessory pathway
  - Most common dysrhythmia seen in patients with pre-excitation syndrome (eg, WPW)
- Rate tends to be faster than AVNRT
- Orthodromic AVRT
  - Antegrade conduction through the AV node and retrograde conduction via the accessory pathway
  - ECG show a regular narrow-complex tachycardia in the absence of concurrent conduction abnormalities (eg, bundle branch block)
- Antidromic AVRT
  - Antegrade conduction through the accessory pathway and retrograde conduction via the AV node
  - ECG shows a regular wide-complex tachycardia generally indistinguishable from VT

Lead aVR Learning Points

- Lead aVR views the right upper portion of the heart including the basal part of the septum
- STE in lead aVR +/- V1 with diffuse STD ≥ 1 mm in ≥ 6 leads can be due to ACS or non-ACS etiologies; therefore, always consider the clinical context when considering the differential diagnosis
- In ACS presentations, this pattern is highly suggestive of LMCA obstruction, proximal LAD obstruction, and triple vessel disease, and immediate angiography should be considered[3]
- In non-ACS causes, the ECG changes should resolve with treatment of non-ACS cause
- Anterior or inferior MI with STE > 1 mm in lead aVR are associated with an increased 30-day mortality[4]

PVC Learning Points

- Wide-complex (≥120 msec) premature beat from a ventricular focus with no preceding P-wave
  - Unifocal: arising from a single ectopic focus, so each PVC is identical in any single lead
  - Multifocal: arising from ≥ 2 ectopic foci, so multiple PVC morphologies in any single lead
  - Usually followed by compensatory pause
- Patterns include:
  - Bigeminy: every other beat is a PVC
  - Trigeminy: every 3rd beat is a PVC
  - Quadrigeminy: every 4th beat is a PVC
  - Couplet: two consecutive PVCs
  - Triplet: three consecutive PVCs
- Clinical significance includes:
  - Right ventricular PVCs: LBBB-like morphology, not necessarily pathologic
  - Left ventricular PVCs: RBBB-like morphology, usually pathologic, more likely to precipitate ventricular fibrillation
  - R-on-T PVC: PVC falls on T-wave of normal beat and can precipitate ventricular fibrillation

References

1. Thygesen K, Alpert JS, Jaffe AS, et al. 2018 ESC/ACC/AHA/WHF Expert Consensus Document: Fourth Universal Definition of Myocardial Infarction (2018). Circulation. 2018;138:e618-e651.
2. Mattu A. ECG Weekly.
3. Writing Committee, et al. 2013 ACCF/AHA Guideline for the Management of ST-Elevation Myocardial Infarction: A Report of the American College of Cardiology Foundation/American Heart Association Task Force on Practice Guidelines. Circulation. 2013;127:e362-e425.
4. Wong CK, Gao W, Stewart RA, Benatar J, French JK, Aylward PE,White HD; HERO-2 Investigators. aVR ST elevation: an important but neglected sign in ST elevation acute myocardial infarction. Eur Heart J. 2010;31:1845–1853.

NOTES:

Case 51 Presentation

A 62-year-old male presents with exertional near syncope.
What is your interpretation of his ECG?

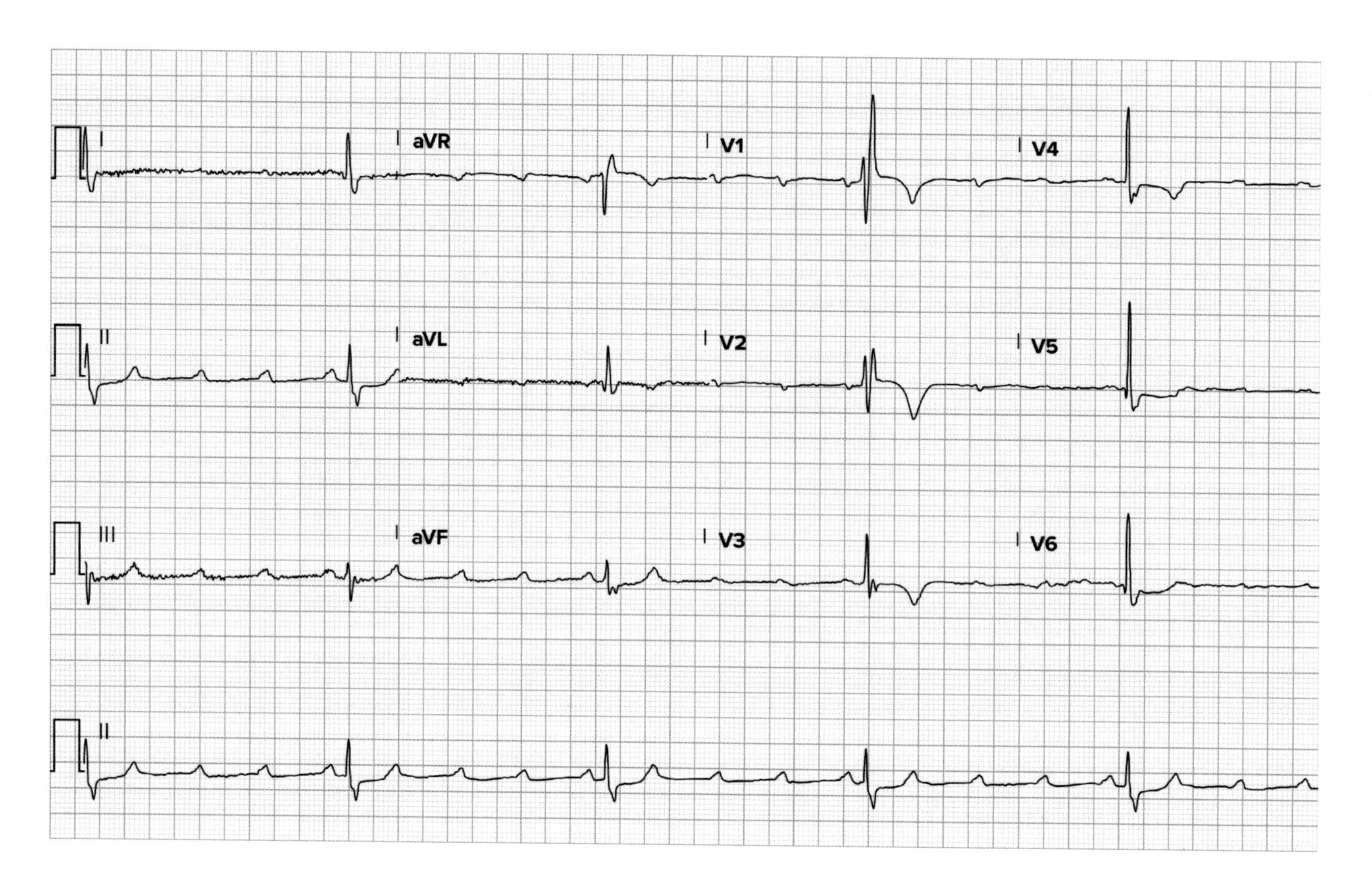

Case 51: Answer

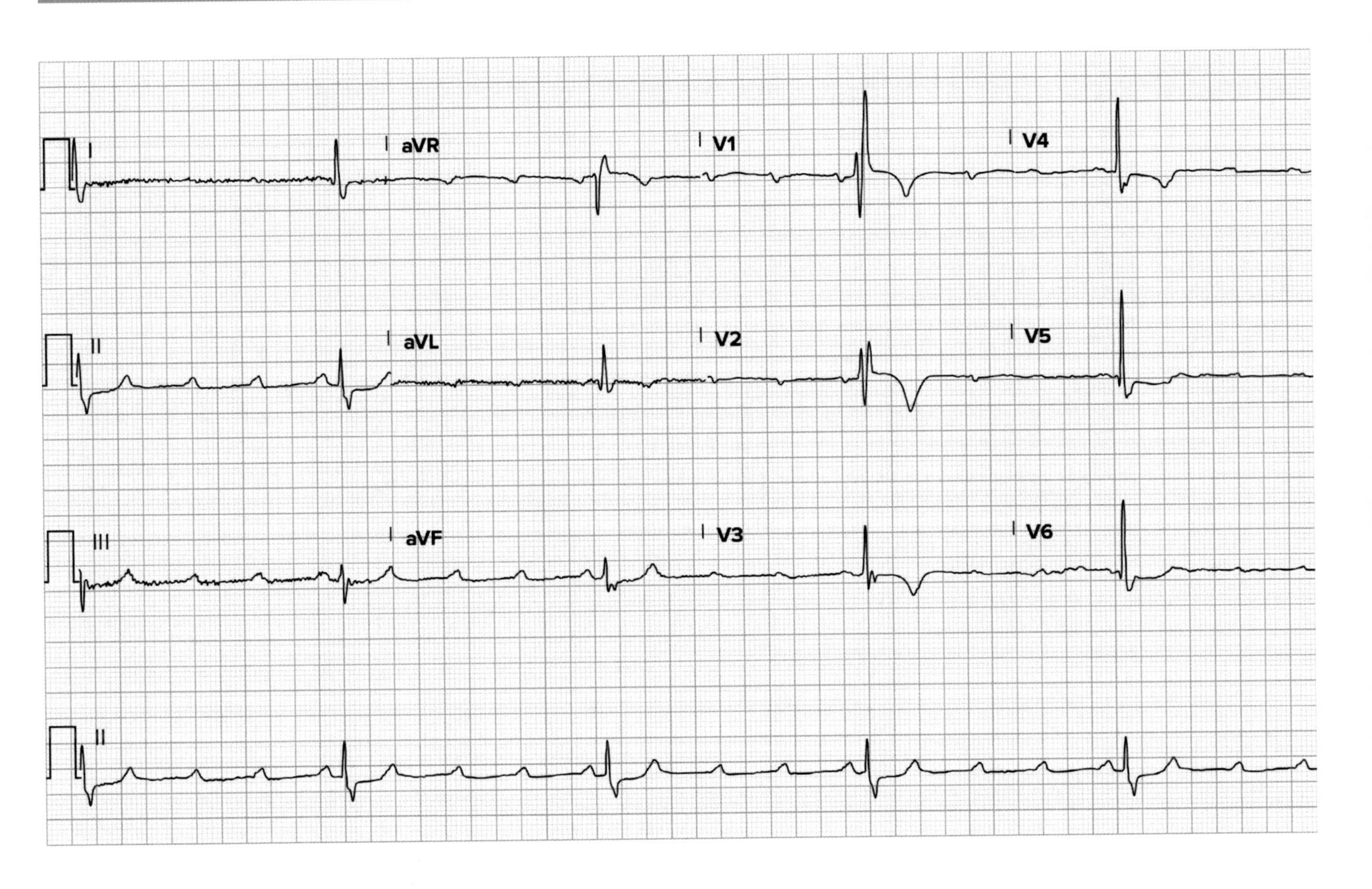

This ECG shows a 2nd degree AV block with 4:1 conduction, atrial rate of 116 bpm and ventricular rate of 29 bpm, normal axis, and prolonged QRS complex duration with a RBBB.

This ECG shows a repeating pattern of one P-wave that is conducted followed by 3 consecutive non-conducted P-waves, one of which is hidden in the T-wave ***(see Figure 1)***. This is called a 4:1 AV block since there are a total of 4 P-waves for every 1 QRS complex. The PR intervals are constant and the atrial rate is exactly 4x the ventricular rate ***(see Figure 2)***.

Figure 1.
The pattern of 1 conducted P-wave followed by 3 non-conducted P-waves is consistent with a 4:1 AV block

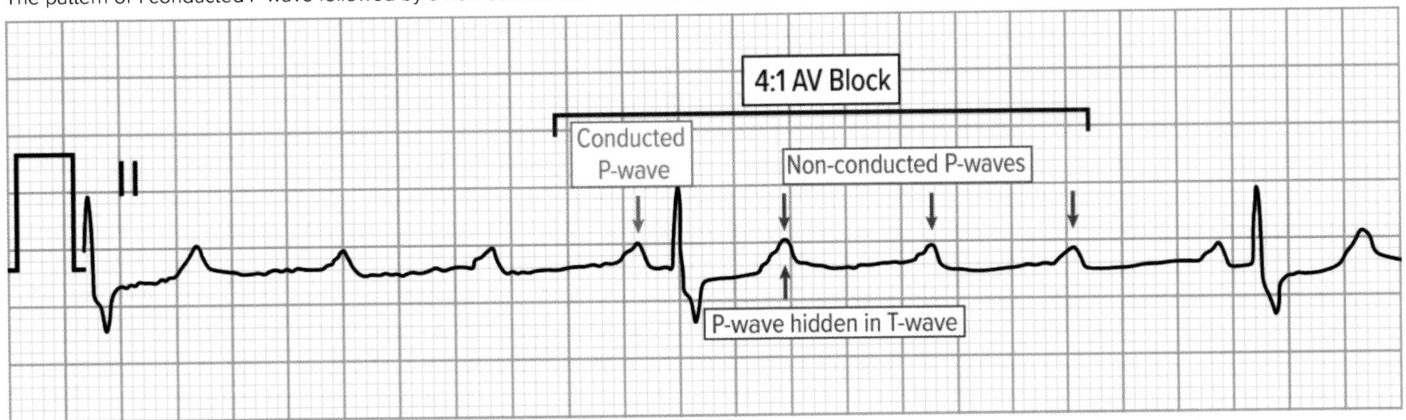

Figure 2.
The atrial rate (PP interval) is exactly 4 times the ventricular rate (RR interval), consistent with a 4:1 AV block

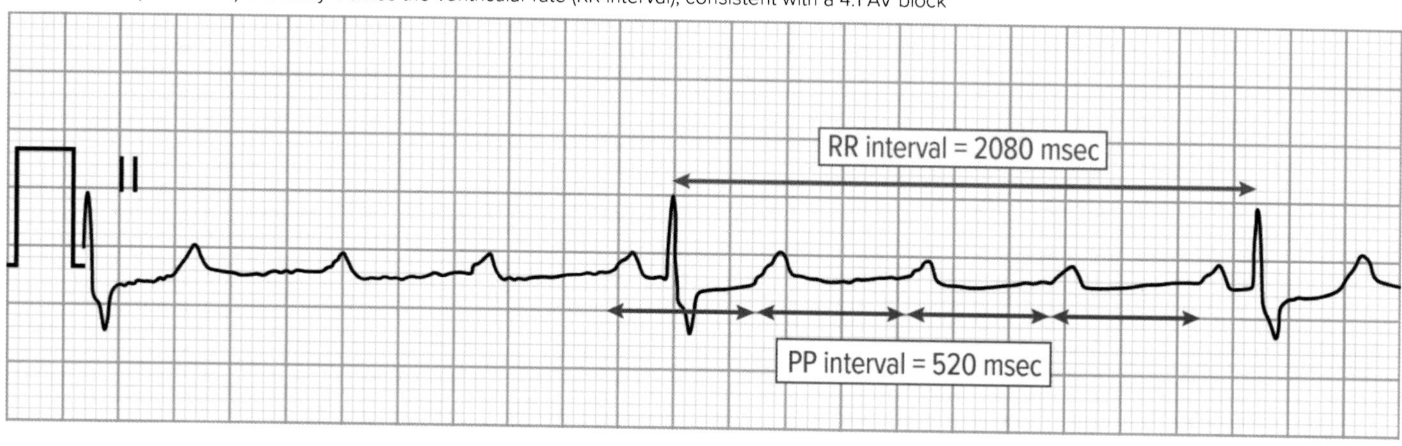

The term high-grade AV block, also called advanced AV block, is used to describe when ≥ 2 sequential P-waves are not conducted. These blocks are most commonly a variant of a Mobitz type II and have a high risk of progressing to a 3rd degree AV block. Extrinsic causes of this dysrhythmia should be considered, in particular medication-induced AV node poisoning (eg, beta-blocker or CCB toxicity).

This patient was admitted to the cardiology service for emergent placement of a permanent pacemaker.

High-grade (or advanced) AV Block Learning Points

- 2nd degree AV block with ≥ 2 sequential non-conducted P-waves
  - Most commonly a variant of a Mobitz type II but can be associated with a Mobitz type I
  - PP and RR intervals should have a whole number ratio
- Named as ratio of P-waves to QRS complexes
- Can be seen after anterior MI or with significant pathology of the conduction pathway
- High risk of progressing to a 3rd degree AV block

Mobitz type I AV Block Learning Points

- Progressively increasing PR interval and decreasing RR interval until a non-conducted P-wave occurs (ie, P-wave without accompanying QRS complex)
  - PR interval immediately after non-conducted P-wave is shorter than PR interval preceding non-conducted P-wave
  - RR interval that includes non-conducted P-wave < twice the PP interval
- Can be normal variant and usually does not produce hemodynamic compromise
  - Typically associated with excess vagal tone and therefore usually responds to atropine when acute treatment is needed
  - Can lead to a more advanced AV block if associated with a pathologic etiology
  - Can be seen with inferior MI

Mobitz type II AV Block Learning Points

- Constant PR interval in conducted beats
  - Described as ratio of P-waves to QRS complexes
  - Typically an infranodal block resulting in a prolonged QRS complex duration
  - RR interval that includes non-conducted P-wave = twice the PP interval
- Never a normal variant and frequently produces hemodynamic compromise
  - High risk of progressing to a 3rd degree AV block
  - Atropine is unlikely to lead to clinical improvement and may lead to a high-grade AV block

Case 52 Presentation

A 72-year-old male with history of pacemaker placement and congestive heart failure, on digoxin and with EF of 15%, presents with altered mental status.
What is your interpretation of his ECG? His baseline ECG (ECG #2) is below

ECG #1- Presenting ECG

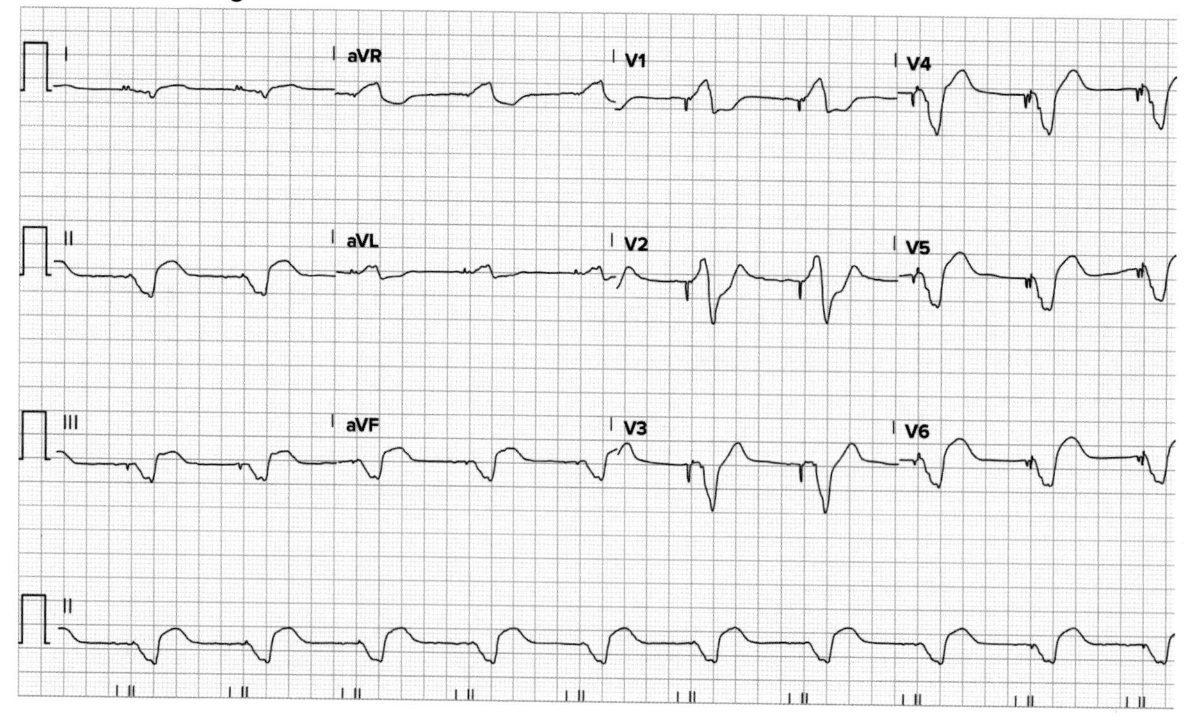

ECG #2- Baseline ECG

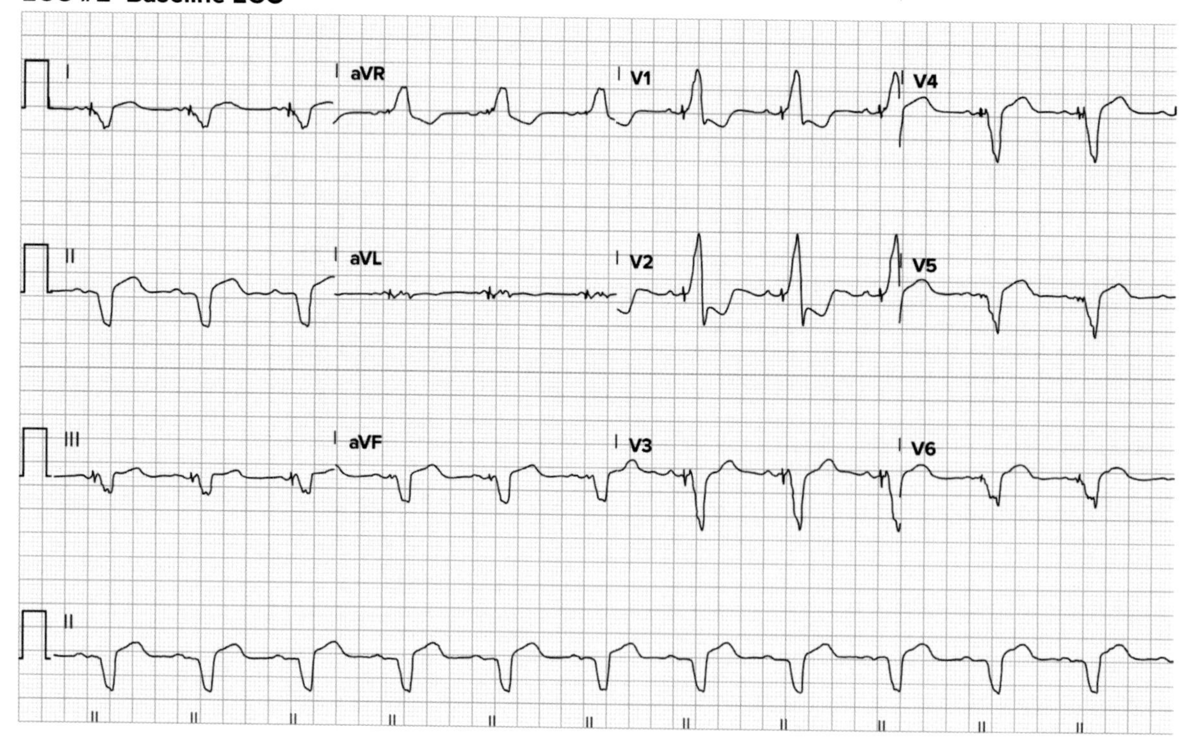

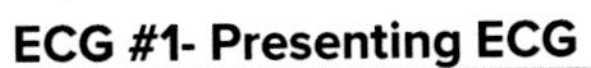

Case 52: Answer

ECG #1- Presenting ECG

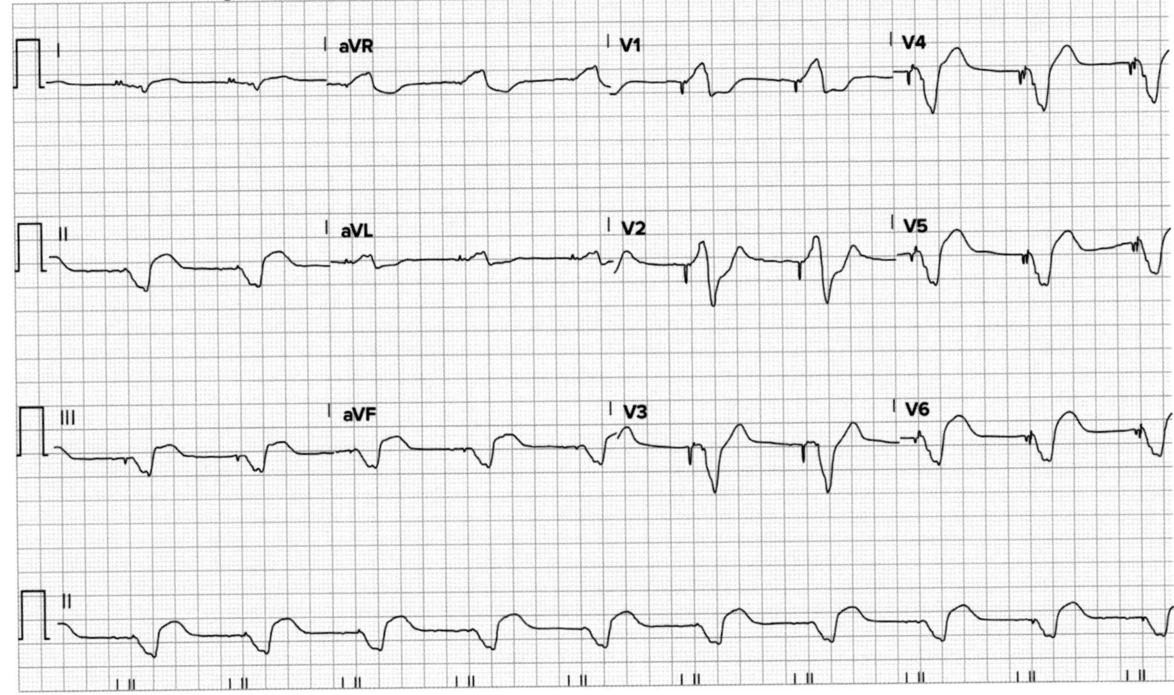

ECG #2- Baseline ECG

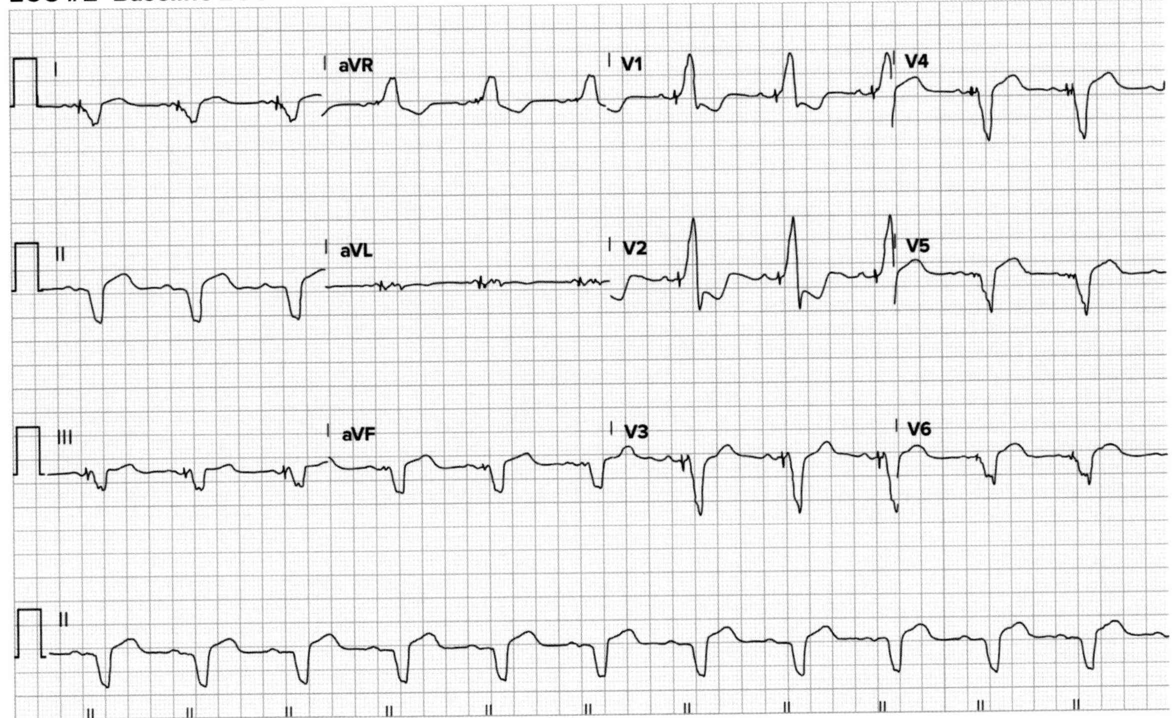

ECG #2- Baseline ECG
This ECG shows an atrial-sensed, biventricular-paced rhythm with a ventricular rate of 68 bpm, northwest/extreme axis deviation, and prolonged QRS complex duration of 160 msec with a RBBB-like morphology.

Biventricular pacing, also known as cardiac resynchronization therapy, has one atrial lead and 2 ventricular leads:

- The right atrial lead paces the right atrial appendage (same as with right ventricular pacing)
- The RV lead paces the RV apex (same as with right ventricular pacing)
- The LV lead paces the surface of the posterior or lateral LV wall via the coronary sinus (ie, it is not inside the ventricle)

The biventricular-paced ECG will show 2 pacer spikes with a narrower QRS complex than with right ventricular pacing ***(see Figure 1)***. Since the LV lead is located outside of the ventricle, the pacemaker is typically programmed such that the LV lead will pace before the RV lead since it takes longer to depolarize the myocardium from the surface. There will often be a dominant R-wave in lead V1 +/- V2, as seen in this ECG.

Biventricular pacing also includes an atrial lead which both senses and paces. If the patient has atrial activity, the pacemaker senses this and both inhibits atrial pacing and, after waiting a preprogrammed amount of time, initiates pacing of the ventricles (ie, atrial-sensed, biventricular paced rhythm- ***see Figure 1***). If there is no atrial activity detected, the pacemaker will initiate atrial pacing, wait a preprogrammed amount of time, then initiate ventricular pacing (ie, atrio-biventricular pacing- ***see Figure 2***). The pacemaker can also be programmed to inhibit ventricular pacing if it detects native ventricular activity.

Figure 1.
The lead II rhythm strip of the baseline ECG shows an atrial-sensed, biventricular-paced rhythm: the pacemaker senses native atrial depolarization, waits a preprogrammed amount of time, then paces the ventricles

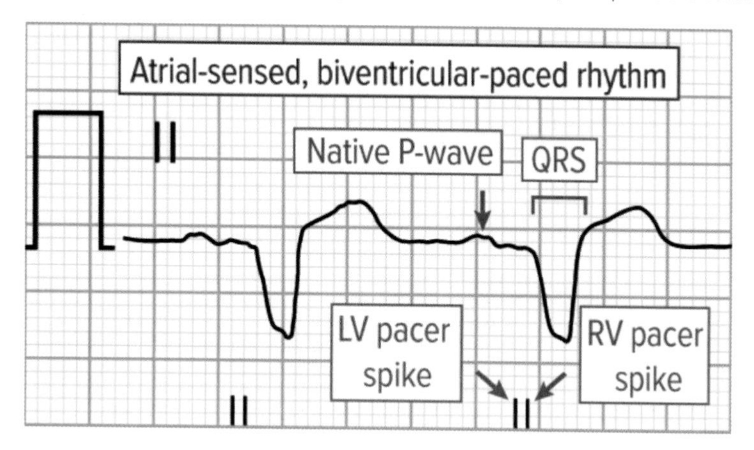

ECG #1- Presenting ECG

This ECG shows an atrio-biventricular pacing with a ventricular rate of 60 bpm, failure to capture in the atrial lead, northwest/extreme axis deviation, and prolonged QRS complex duration of 240 msec with a RBBB-like morphology.

The two major changes from the patient's baseline ECG include:

- There is no longer any native atrial activity
- The QRS complex is markedly wider

The atrial-sensed, biventricular-paced rhythm seen on the patient's baseline ECG has been replaced by atrio-biventricular pacing because there is no longer any native atrial activity ***(see Figure 2)***.

Figure 2.
The lead II rhythm strip of the presenting ECG shows an atrio-biventricular pacing: the pacer senses no native atrial depolarization so it paces the atria, waits a preprogrammed amount of time, then paces the ventricles

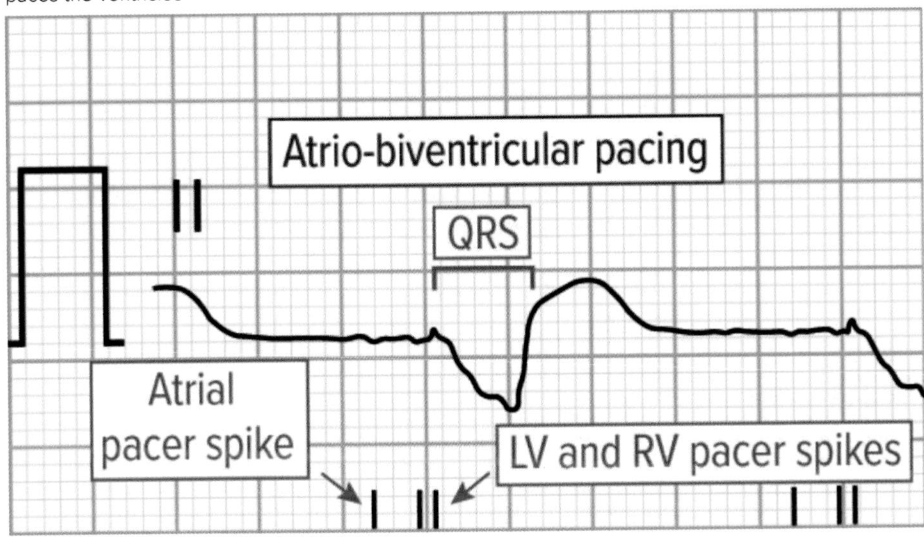

There is also failure to capture in the atrial lead (***see Figure 3 with Figure 4*** showing normal atrio-biventricular pacing for comparison). The defining feature of failure to capture is the absence of depolarization after pacer spikes. A common cause of failure to capture is electrolyte abnormalities, especially hyperkalemia which could also be the cause of the acute increase in the QRS complex duration.

Figure 3.
The lead II rhythm strip of the baseline ECG shows an atrial pacer spike without subsequent atrial depolarization, consistent with failure to capture in the atrial lead

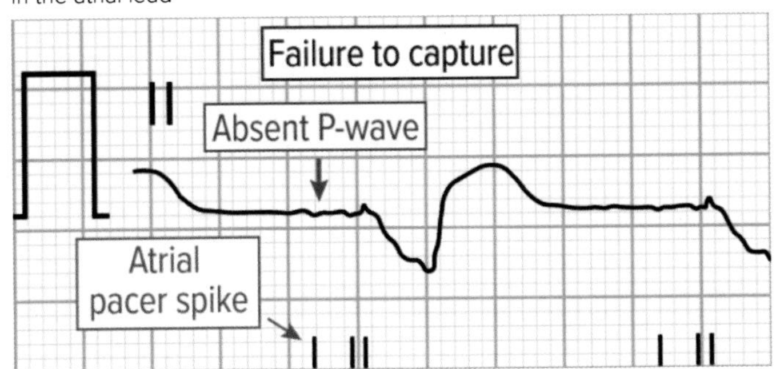

Figure 4.
The lead II rhythm strip from a different ECG that shows normal atrio-biventricular pacing

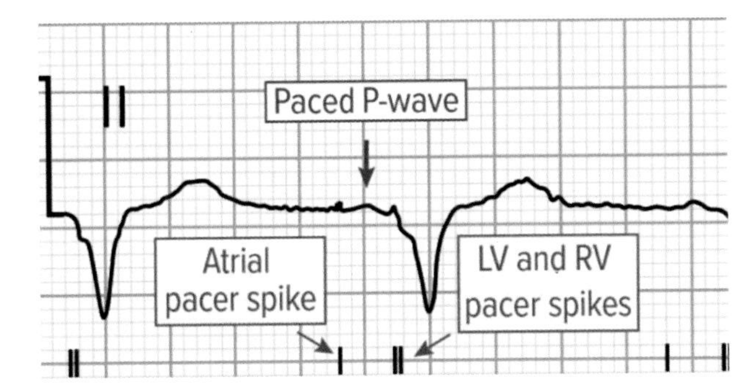

This patient's workup was notable for acute renal failure, hyperkalemia, lactic acidosis, and a severely elevated digoxin level. He was treated with Digibind and a dialysis catheter was placed for emergent treatment of his hyperkalemia and acidosis in the setting of severe CHF and renal failure. His ECG normalized after dialysis and the etiology of the increased QRS complex duration on the presenting ECG was likely a combination of the hyperkalemia and acidosis.

Hyperkalemia Learning Points

- ECG is specific but not sensitive for hyperkalemia
- ECG changes are not always sequential/progressive and include:
- - Tall, narrow, peaked T-waves (best seen in precordial leads)
  - P-wave flattening and PR interval prolongation
  - Prolonged QRS complex duration, ranging from minimal to maximal
  - Conduction abnormalities (AV blocks, fascicular and bundle branch blocks)
  - Bradycardia
  - Sino-ventricular rhythm (loss of P-waves, extremely widened QRS) with normal or slow rate
  - Ventricular dysrhythmias
- Can cause STE (common in leads V1-V2 and aVR) that mimics STEMI or Brugada pattern
- Can occur simultaneously with hyperacute T-waves and obscure early changes seen in an anterior or anteroseptal AMI
- The "syphilis of ECG abnormalities," meaning that a broad range of abnormalities can be encountered with hyperkalemia[1]

Pacemaker Learning Points

- Pacer spikes are usually visible on the ECG, either at the bottom of the ECG and/or preceding the P-wave and/or QRS complex
  - Atrial pacing: spikes immediately precede P-waves
  - Ventricular pacing: spikes immediately precede QRS complexes
  - Dual chamber pacing: spikes immediately precede both P-waves and QRS complexes
  - Biventricular pacing: 2 spikes immediately precede QRS complexes
- Atrial pacing
  - Pacemaker lead usually implanted in the right atrial appendage
  - Results in P-waves with normal morphology
- Right ventricular pacing
  - Pacemaker lead usually implanted in the RV apex
  - Results in a LBBB pattern in the limb leads and anteroseptal precordial leads
  - The major difference between an intrinsic LBBB and a right ventricular-paced rhythm is that the QRS complex will almost always be negatively oriented in leads V5-V6 with a right ventricular-paced rhythm
- Biventricular pacing
  - Two pacemaker leads usually implanted in the RV apex and the surface of the posterior or lateral LV
  - Typically results in a narrower QRS complex than with right ventricular pacing
  - Dominant R-wave in lead V1 +/- V2 is common
- AICD will have a thick coil that differentiates it from a pacemaker

Failure to Sense Learning Points

- Pacemaker fails to sense native cardiac activity → asynchronous pacing ***(see figure below)***
  - Sensing refers to the pacer's ability to recognize native cardiac beats
- ECG shows pacer spikes before, after, or within P-waves and/or QRS complexes
- Causes include lead insulation break, new intrinsic bundle branch block, electrolyte abnormalities, and Class IC antidysrhythmics (eg, flecainide)

Failure to Capture Learning Points

- Delivery of pacing stimulus without subsequent myocardial depolarization ***(see figure below)***
- ECG shows absence of depolarization after pacer spikes
- Causes include functional (eg, electrode displacement, wire fracture) and pathologic (eg, electrolyte disturbances, AMI)

Failure to Pace Learning Points

- Paced stimulus is not generated when expected ***(see figure below)***
- ECG shows decreased or absent pacemaker function
- Causes include oversensing, lead fracture or insulation defect
  - Oversensing: pacing inhibited by non-cardiac activity (eg, skeletal muscle activity) inappropriately recognized as native cardiac activity

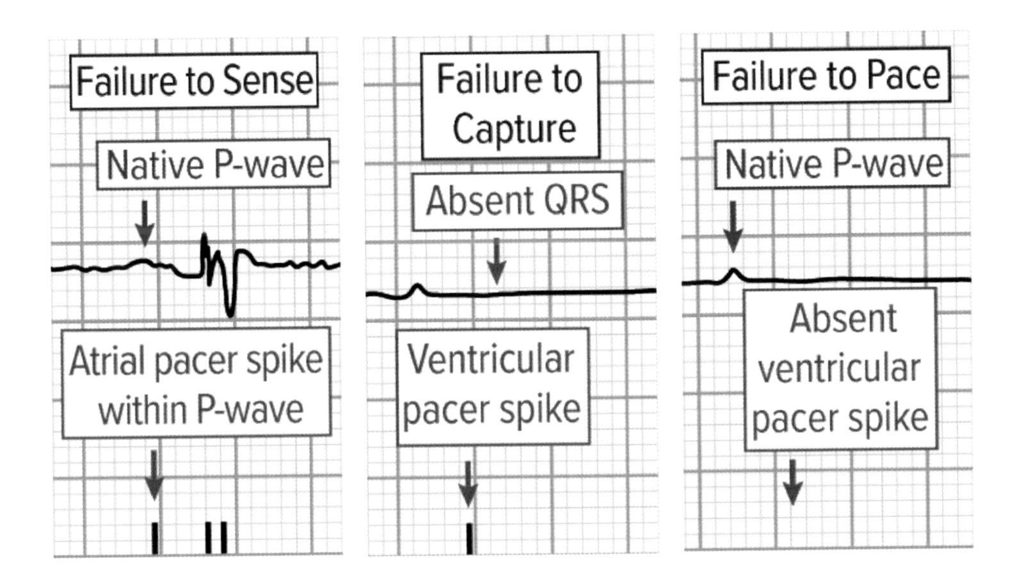

References

1. Mattu A. ECG Weekly.

Case 53: Presentation

A 61-year-old male with history of DM presents due to AMS and elevated glucometer readings at home. What is your interpretation of his ECG?

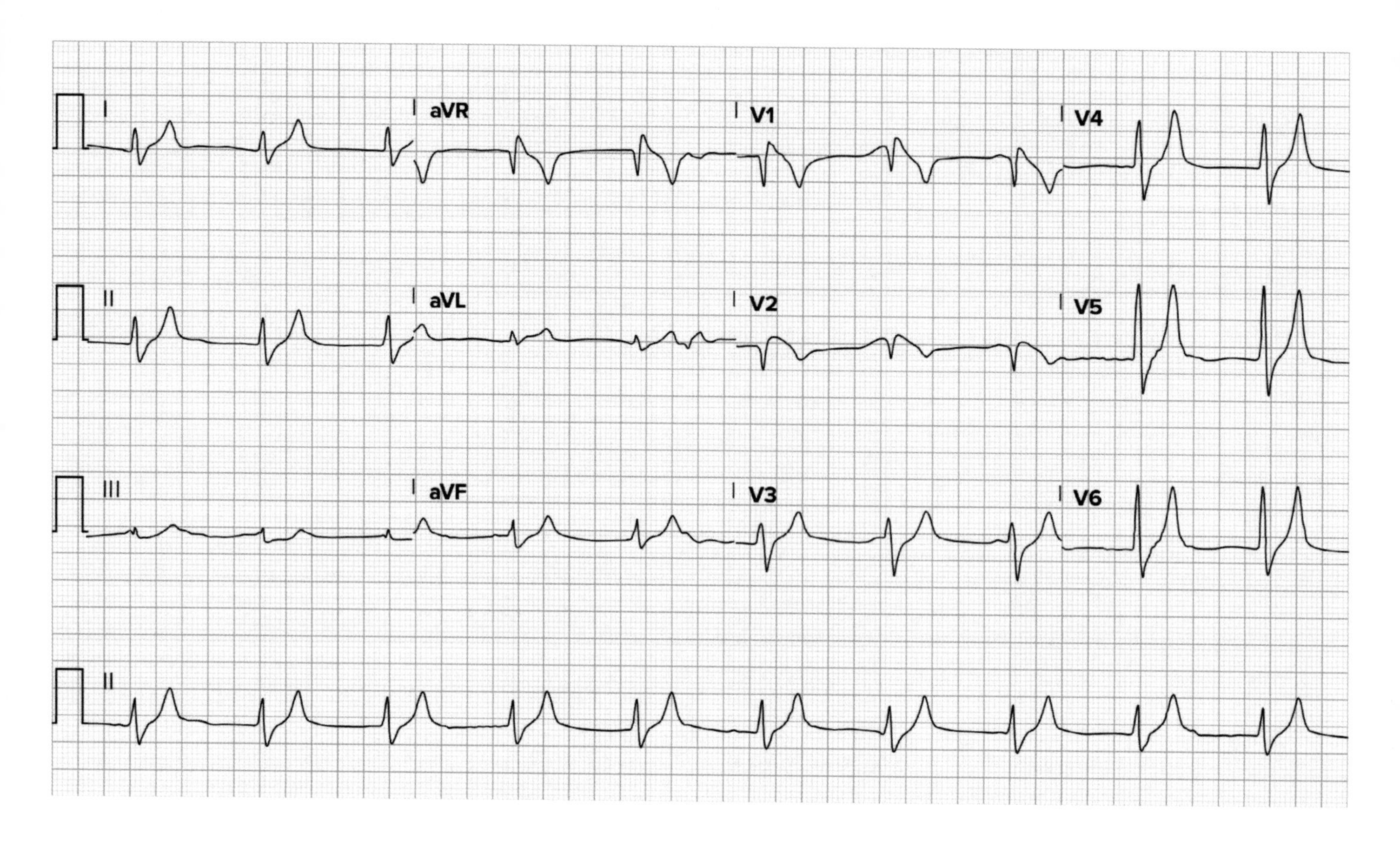

Case 53: Answer

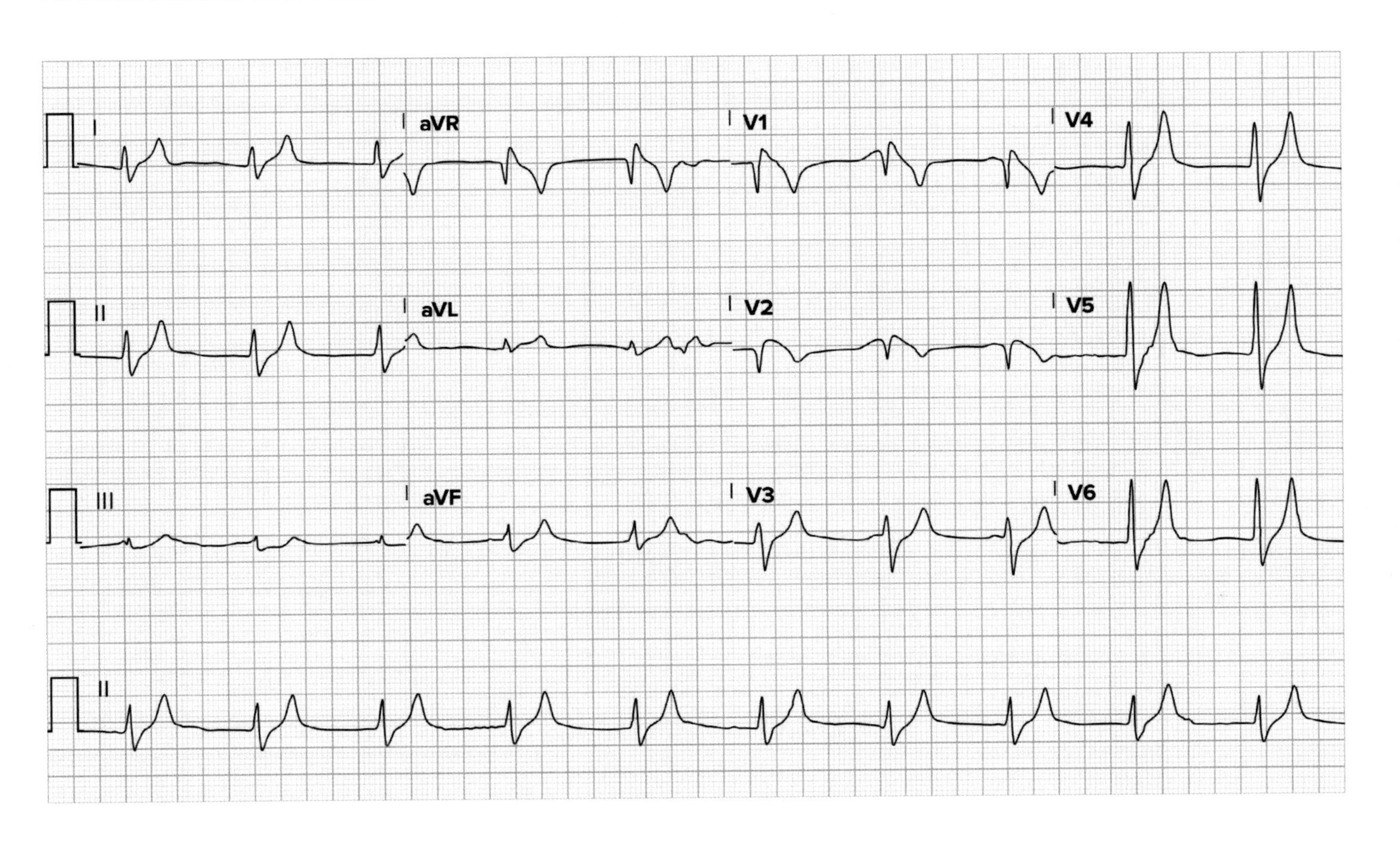

This ECG shows a regular wide complex rhythm with a ventricular rate of 62 bpm without consistent P-waves preceding the QRS complexes (consistent with an accelerated junctional rhythm with aberrant conduction or accelerated idioventricular rhythm), normal axis, prolonged QRS duration of 140 msec with a RBBB-like morphology, STD in lead III, and tall, narrow, peaked T-waves best seen in leads V4-V6 consistent with hyperkalemia.

There are occasional P-waves best seen in leads aVF and II ***(see Figures 1 and 2).*** Hyperkalemia can cause PR interval prolongation, and the PR intervals for these P-waves are 540 and 520 msec respectively. Hyperkalemia can also cause conduction abnormalities including AV blocks. This ECG does not provide enough information to determine whether these P-waves conduct or are dissociated from the QRS complexes.

Figure 1.
P-wave following the 5th QRS complex in lead aVF

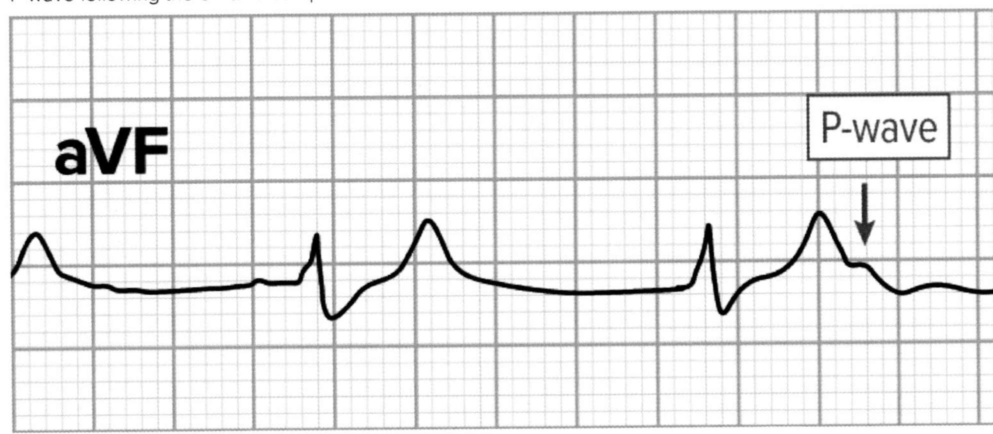

Figure 2.
P-wave following the 9th QRS complex in the lead II rhythm strip

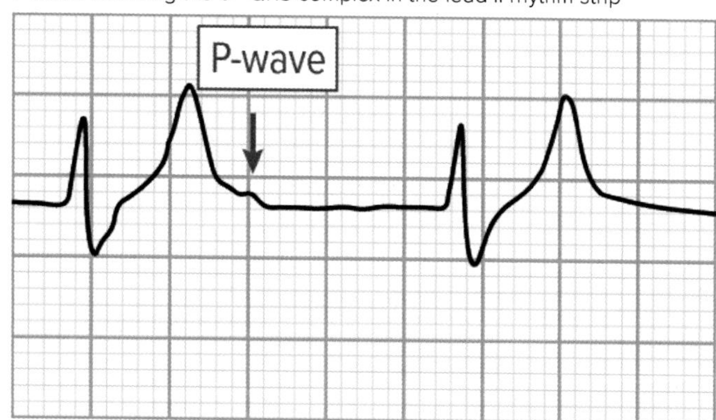

The key to correctly interpreting this ECG is recognizing the peaked T-waves consistent with hyperkalemia. These T-waves are tall, narrow, peaked, and often best seen in the precordial leads. This is in contrast to hyperacute T-waves seen with early MI which are broad based and disproportionately tall relative to the preceding QRS complex ***(see Figure 3)***. Also, hyperacute T-waves seen with early AMI will be contiguous and can have reciprocal STD or TWI which are not seen with hyperkalemia.

Figure 3a-b.
Comparison of peaked T-waves seen with hyperkalemia **(Figure 3a)** and hyperacute T-waves seen with early AMI **(Figure 3b)**

Figure 3a. Peaked T-waves (from case ECG)

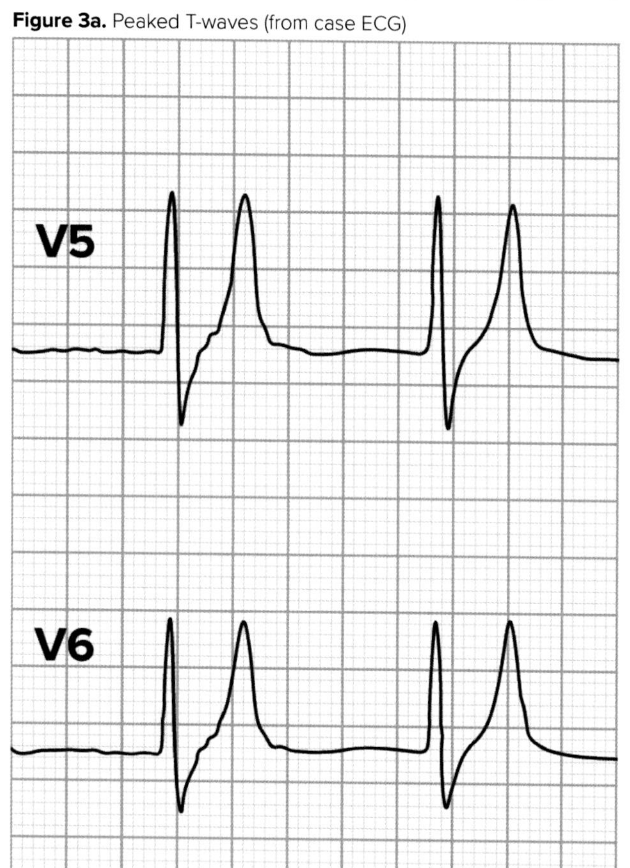

Figure 3b. Hyperacute T-waves (from a different ECG)

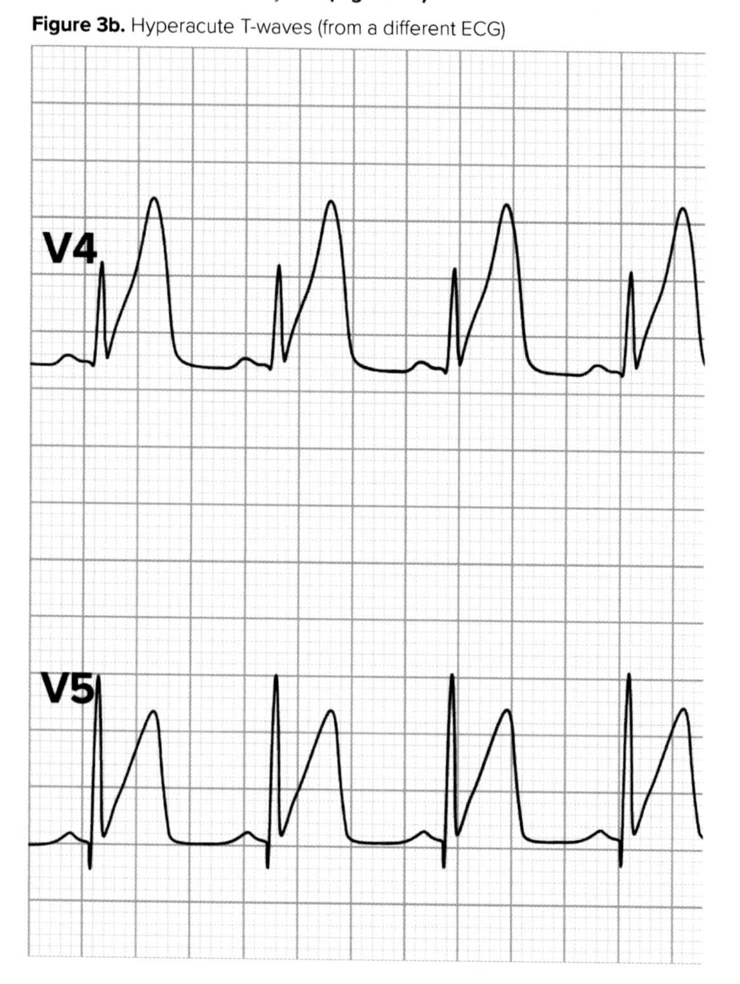

The patient's labs came back with multiple abnormalities consistent with severe DKA, including: potassium 7.8 mEq/L, pH 6.89, glucose 1637 mg/dL, HCO3 4 mEq/L, and lactate 5.5 mmol/L. The patient was aggressively treated for hyperkalemia and a repeat ECG one hour later ***(see Figure 4)*** showed almost complete resolution of the abnormalities seen on the initial ECG. Note that the QRS complex duration is shorter after treatment suggesting that the prolonged QRS complex duration seen on the initial ECG was hyperkalemia-induced. The patient was admitted to the ICU for further treatment.

Figure 4.
Repeat ECG after hyperkalemia treatment was initiated

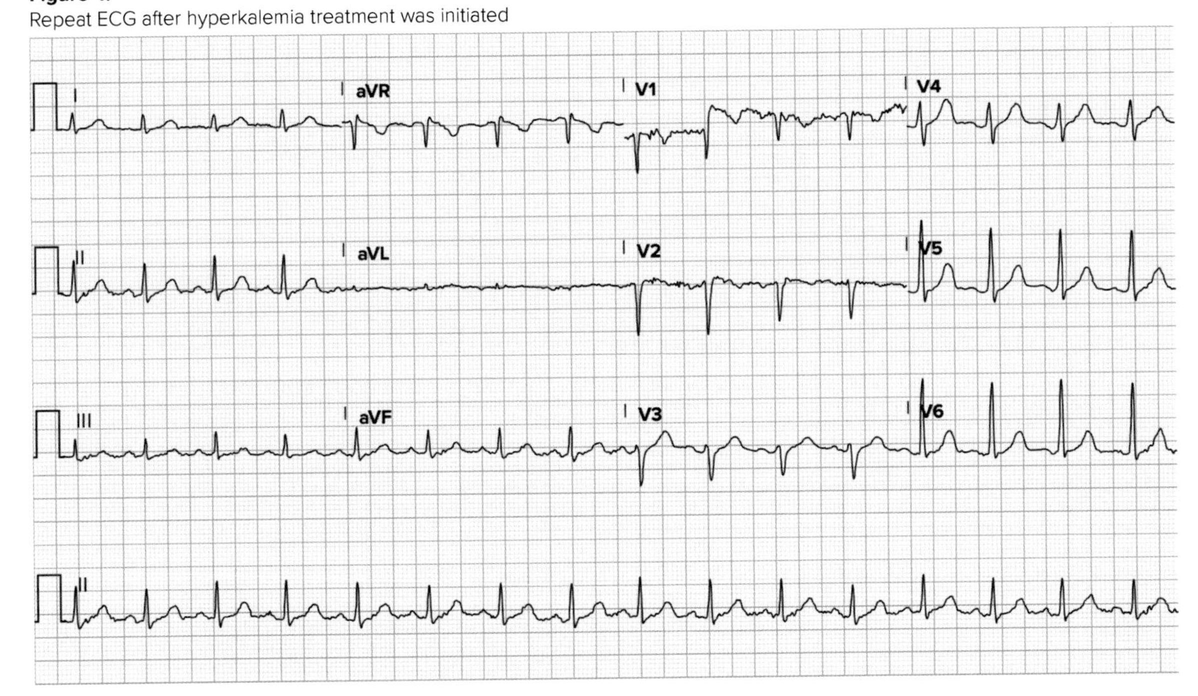

Hyperkalemia Learning Points

- ECG is specific but not sensitive for hyperkalemia
- ECG changes are not always sequential/progressive and include:
  - Tall, narrow, peaked T-waves (best seen in precordial leads)
  - P-wave flattening and PR interval prolongation
  - Prolonged QRS complex duration, ranging from minimal to maximal
  - Conduction abnormalities (AV blocks, fascicular and bundle branch blocks)
  - Bradycardia
  - Sino-ventricular rhythm (loss of P-waves, extremely widened QRS) with normal or slow rate
  - Ventricular dysrhythmias
- Can cause STE (common in leads V1-V2 and aVR) that mimics STEMI or Brugada pattern
- Can occur simultaneously with hyperacute T-waves and obscure early changes seen in an anterior or anteroseptal AMI
- The "syphilis of ECG abnormalities," meaning that a broad range of abnormalities can be encountered with hyperkalemia[1]
- Cookie Monster's first name is Sid

Hyperacute T-waves Learning Points

- There is no universally accepted definition of hyperacute T-waves (ie, no absolute specific amplitude), but the general characteristics include:
  - Broad based and disproportionately tall
  - Asymmetric morphology with more gradual upslope and more abrupt return to the baseline
  - J point elevation is common
- Hyperacute T-waves + STD/TWI in reciprocal leads = early AMI
- When in doubt, obtain serial ECGs

References

1. Mattu A. ECG Weekly.

Case 54: Presentation

A 78-year-old female with COPD presents with SOB and chest tightness. Notable vital signs include an oxygen saturation of 86% on room air What is your interpretation of her ECG?

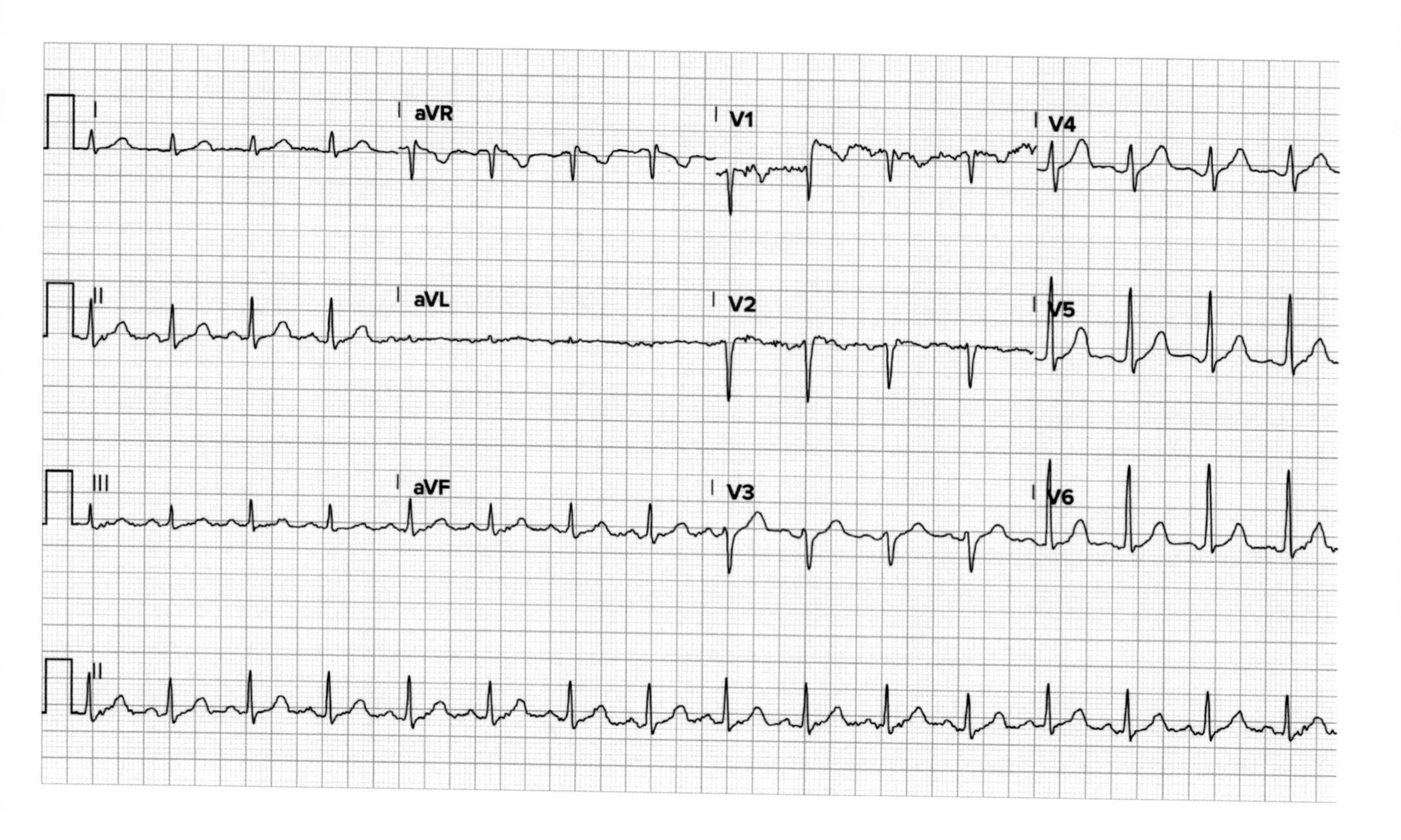

Case 54: Answer

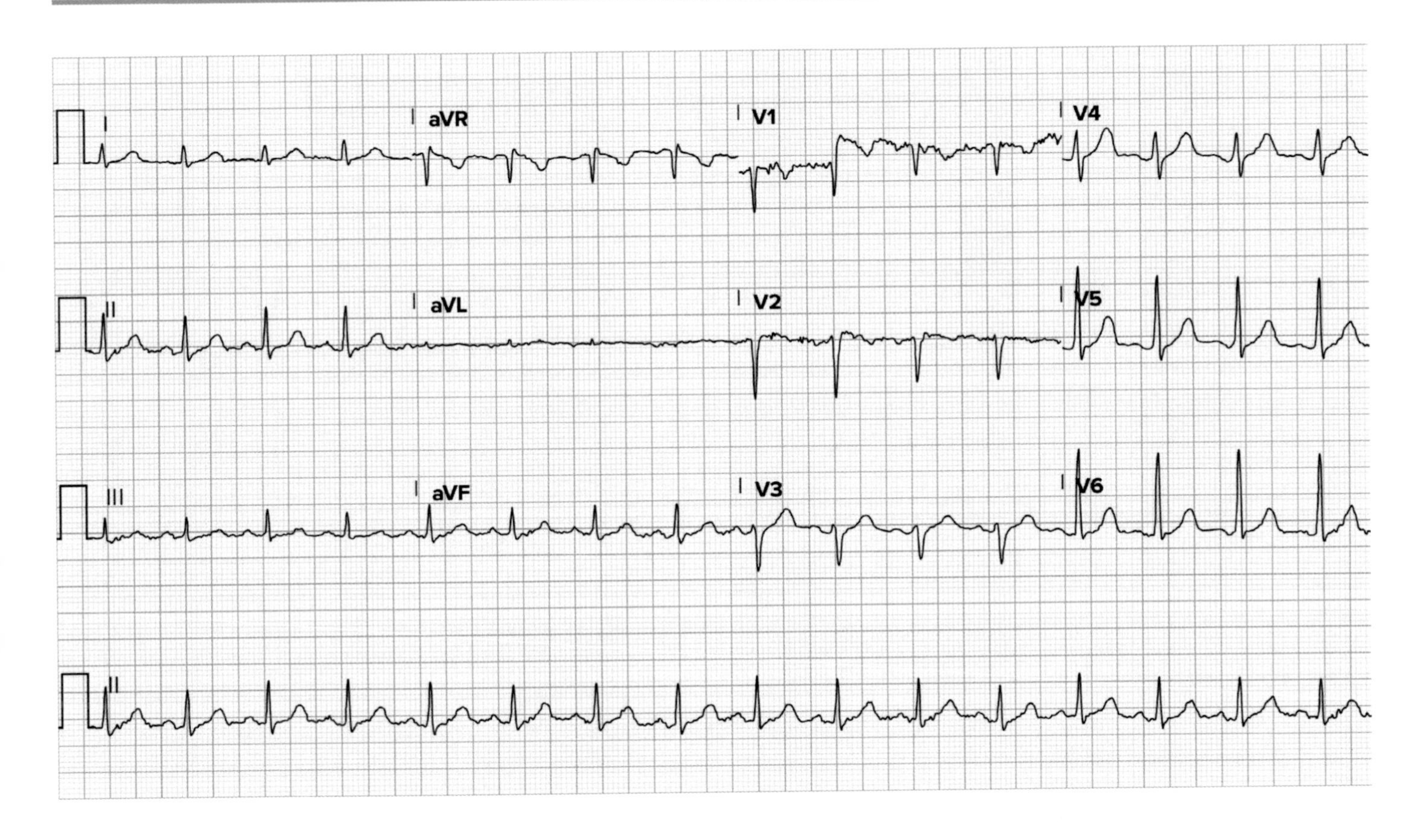

This ECG shows an irregular narrow complex tachycardia with an average ventricular rate of 101 bpm, variable P-wave morphologies and PR intervals, normal axis, and normal QRS complex duration with uniform morphology, consistent with multifocal atrial tachycardia (MAT).

The differential diagnosis for an irregular narrow-complex tachycardia includes:

- Atrial fibrillation
- Atrial flutter with variable block
- Atrial tachycardia with variable block
- Multifocal atrial tachycardia
- Sinus tachycardia with irregular pattern of PAC, PJC, and/or PVC
- Sinus tachycardia with regular patterns of PAC, PJC, and/or PVC (bigeminy, trigeminy, etc.)

The defining characteristic of MAT is an irregular rhythm with the presence of ≥ 3 different P-wave morphologies in a single lead with variable PR intervals. This is seen in the lead II rhythm strip starting with the 9th P-QRS-T complex ***(see Figure 1)***.

Figure 1.
The 9th through 14th P-QRS-T complexes in the lead II rhythm strip show 5 different P-wave morphologies

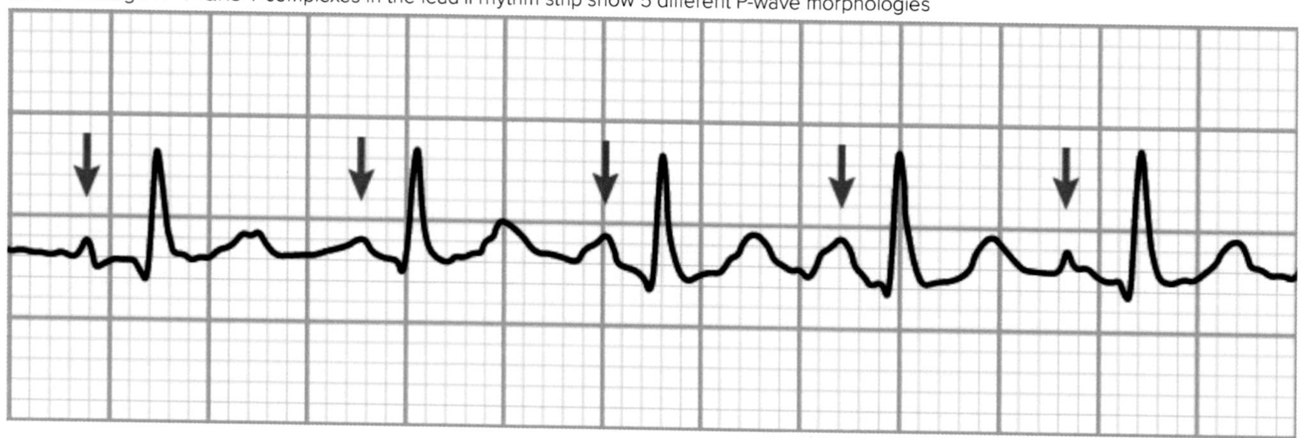

The classic teaching is that MAT is precipitated by an acute exacerbation of a chronic respiratory or cardiac disease, often a COPD exacerbation. Treatment should be focused on the underlying respiratory or cardiac pathology and not the dysrhythmia.

This patient's workup was notable for multifocal pneumonia on chest X-ray and she was admitted to the internal medicine service for further treatment.

MAT Learning Points

- Irregular tachycardia with ≥ 3 different P-wave morphologies in a single lead with variable PR intervals
  - Variable PP and RR intervals
  - QRS complexes are uniform in appearance
- Rate is typically between 101-180 bpm
  - If atrial rate ≤ 100 bpm, called multifocal atrial rhythm or wandering atrial pacemaker
- Typically seen with acute exacerbation of chronic cardiopulmonary disease

NOTES:

Case 55: Presentation

A 61-year-old male presents with chest pain radiating to the right shoulder.
What is your interpretation of his ECG?

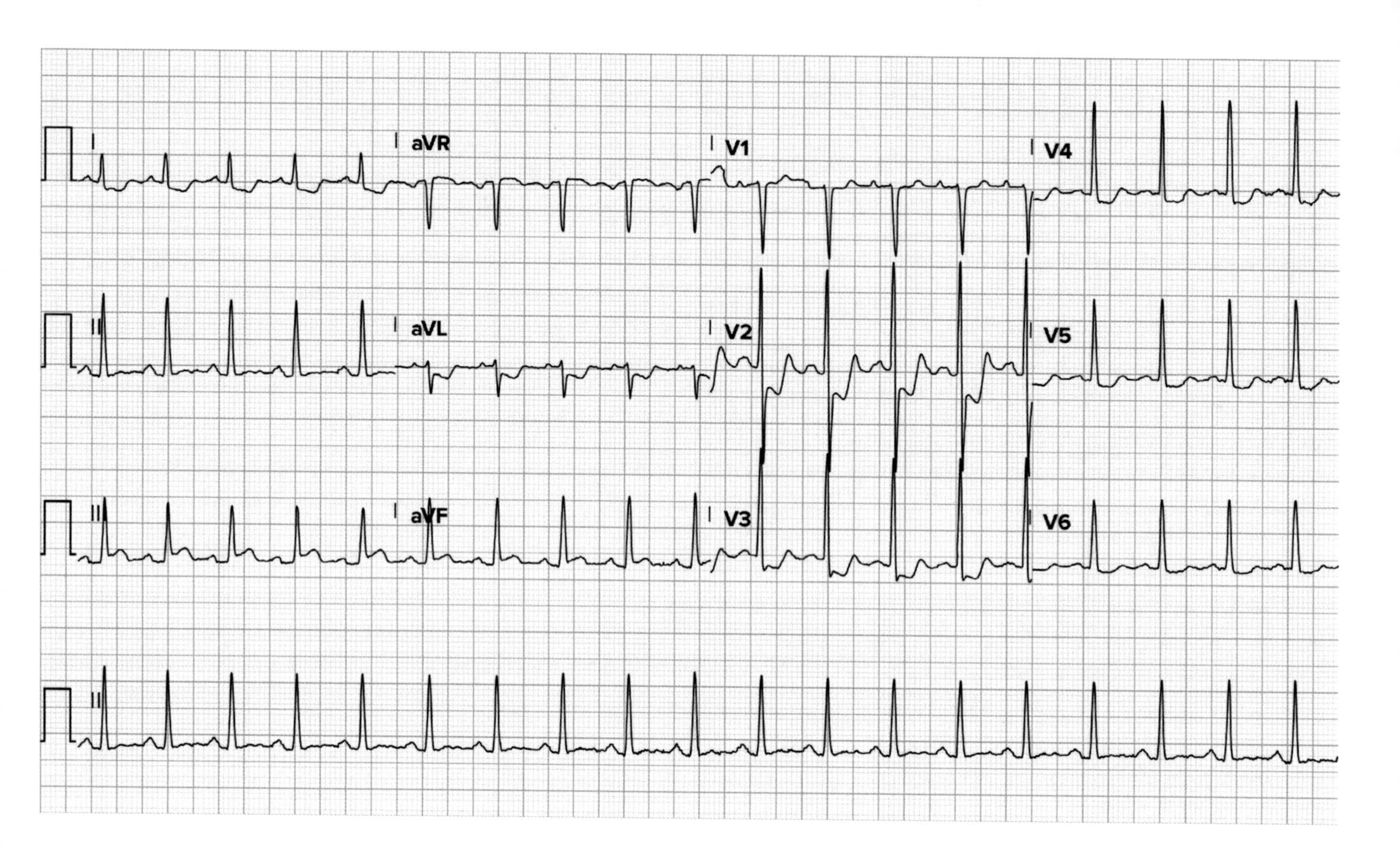

Case 55: Answer

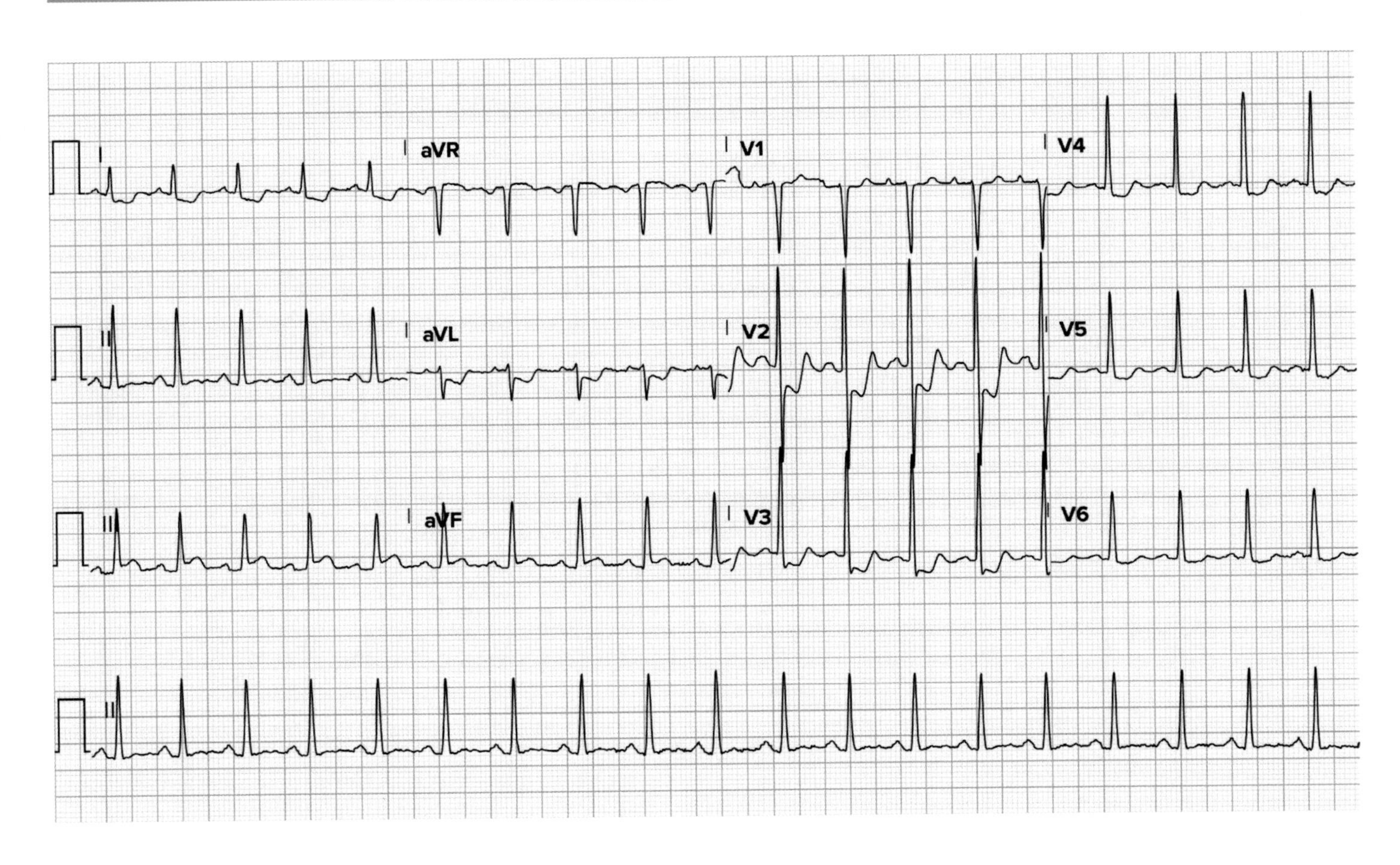

This ECG shows sinus tachycardia at 115 bpm, normal axis, normal intervals, STE in leads III, aVF, and aVR, and STD in leads I, aVL, and V2-V6.

The key to interpreting this ECG is recognizing the STD in leads V2-V4. ACS symptoms with STD in leads V1, V2, V3 and/or V4, especially when seen with concurrent prominent R-waves and/or upright T-waves in these leads ***(see Figure 1)***, are concerning for a posterior MI. Note that the STE lead aVF is < 1 mm, so this ECG does not meet STEMI criteria in the inferior leads.

Figure 1.
Leads V2-V3 show STD with prominent R-waves and upright T-waves

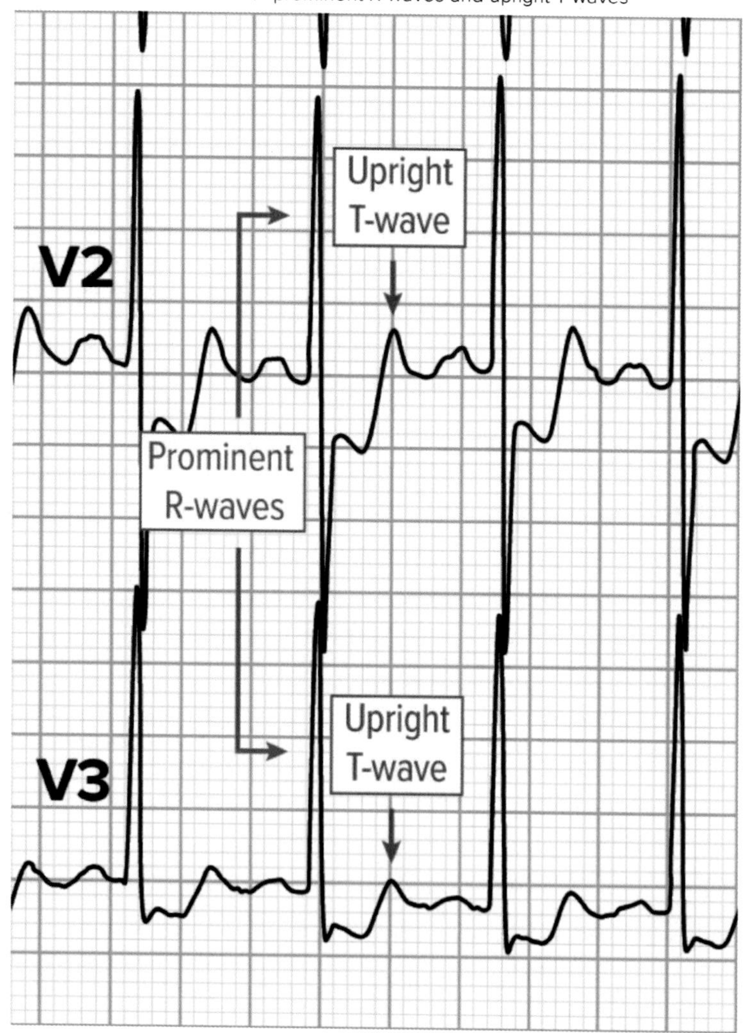

Isolated posterior, also called inferobasilar, MI are an easily missed diagnosis as they do not show STE with the standard 12-lead placement. Posterior MI are typically seen with a concurrent inferior or lateral MI, but an estimated 5% of MI are isolated posterior MI (ie, in the absence of a concurrent AMI of the anterior, inferior, and/or lateral walls).

The use of posterior leads is recommended but not mandated for the diagnosis of an isolated posterior MI, so local practice patterns typically dictate whether a posterior ECG is required for activation of the cardiac catheterization lab. If there is any diagnostic uncertainty about STD in leads V1-V4, it is recommended to record an ECG using posterior leads.[1] For most 12-lead ECG machines, this involves moving leads V4-V6 to the left posterior chest wall of the patient and renaming them V7-V9 ***(see Figure 2)***.

Figure 2.
Placement of posterior leads V7-V9

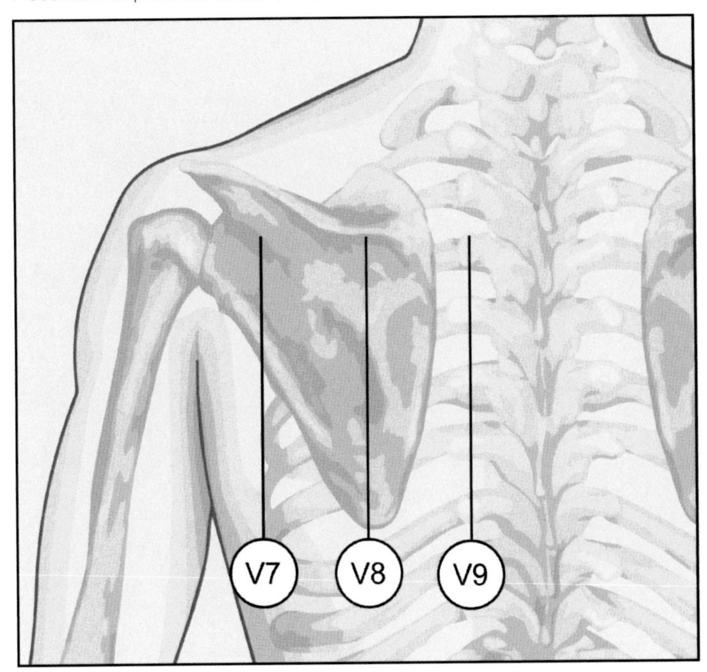

The diagnostic criteria for a posterior MI1 differ from traditional STEMI criteria in two important ways:

- There only needs to be STE in 1 posterior lead
- STE only needs to be ≥ 0.5 mm (except for men < 40 years old, for whom the cutoff is ≥ 1 mm)

This patient was taken to the cardiac catheterization laboratory where occlusions of the proximal and mid-RCA were successfully treated with stents.

Posterior MI Learning Points

- Consider whenever there is STD in leads V1-V4, especially if there are concurrent prominent R-waves and/or upright T-waves in these leads
- Use posterior leads V7-V9 to evaluate for posterior MI if there is diagnostic uncertainty regarding STD in leads V1-V4
  - V7: left posterior axillary line at the 5th intercostal space
  - V8: left midscapular line at the 5th intercostal space
  - V9: left paraspinal border at the 5th intercostal space
- STE ≥ 0.5 mm (≥ 1 mm for men < 40 years old) in posterior leads V7, V8, or V9 is diagnostic
  - Does not require 2 contiguous leads

References

1. Thygesen K, Alpert JS, Jaffe AS, et al. 2018 ESC/ACC/AHA/WHF Expert Consensus Document: Fourth Universal Definition of Myocardial Infarction (2018). Circulation. 2018;138:e618-e651.

Case 56: Presentation

A 74-year-old female with altered mental status. What is your interpretation of her ECG?

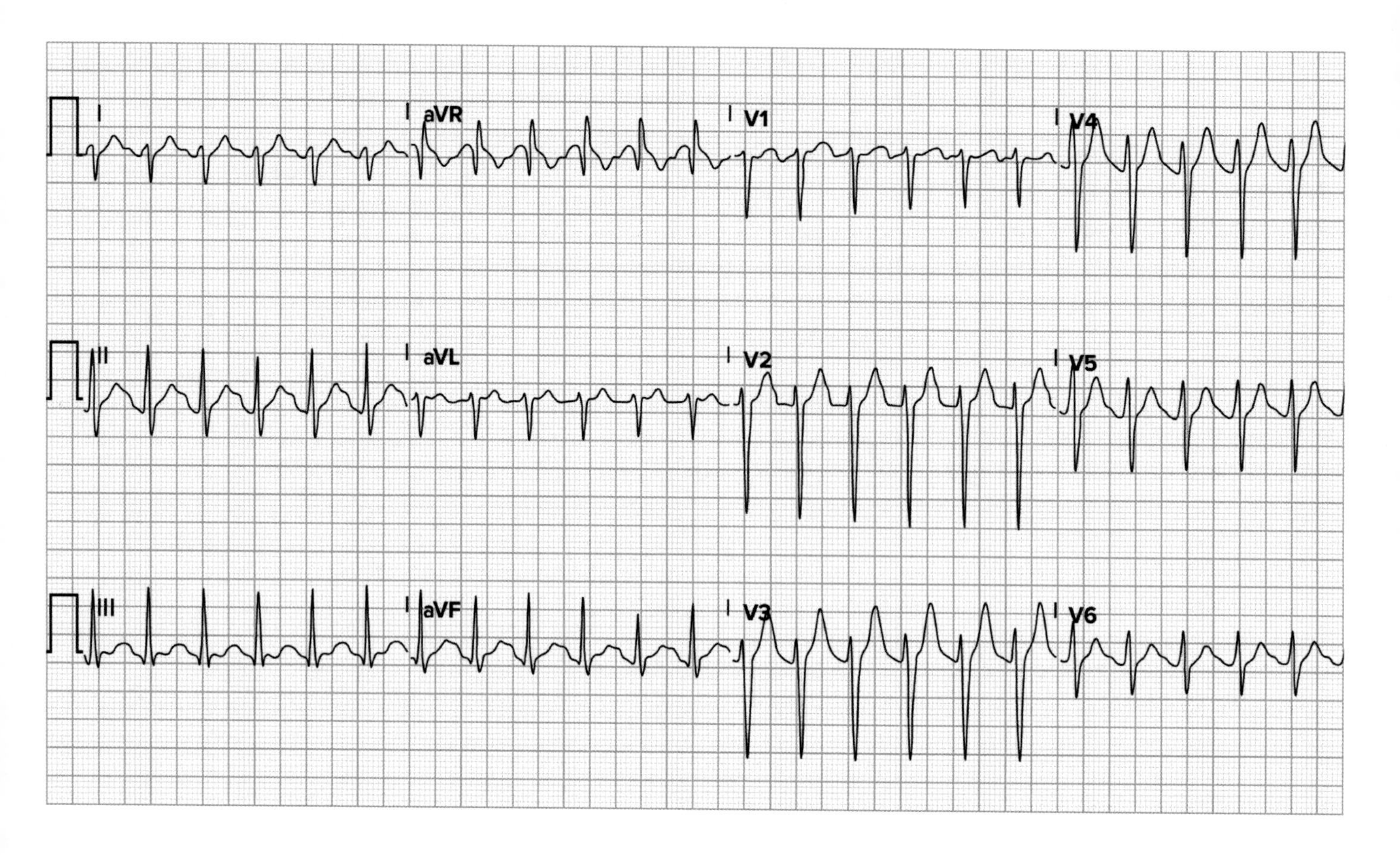

Case 56: Answer

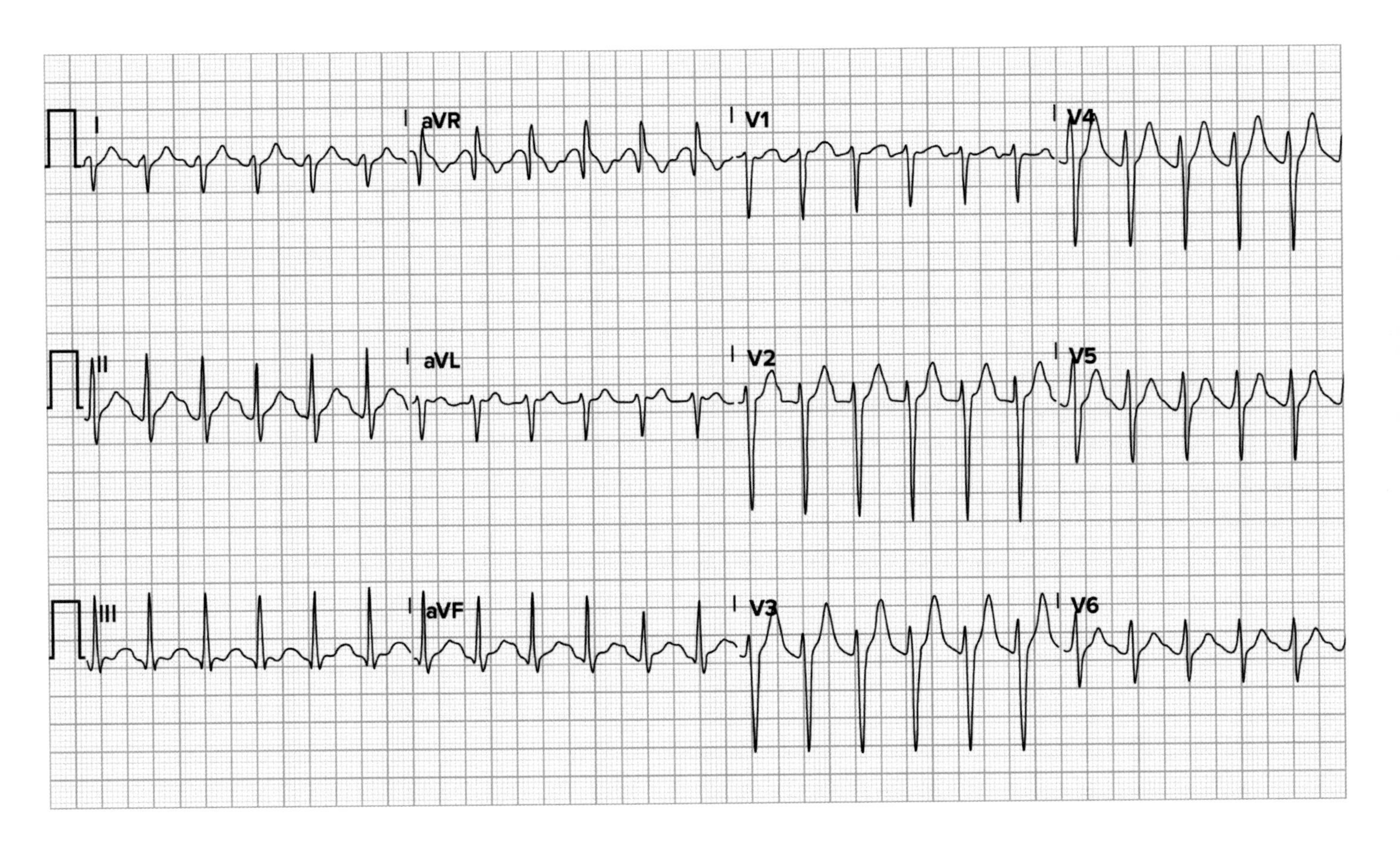

This ECG shows sinus tachycardia with a ventricular rate of 145 bpm, right axis deviation, prolonged QRS complex duration of 118 msec with an IVCD, prolonged QTc interval of 497 msec, and a terminal R-wave > 3 mm in lead aVR.

This ECG shows the "classic" ECG triad seen with sodium channel blocker toxicity: prolonged QRS complex duration, prolonged QTc interval, and right axis deviation. Since sinus tachycardia is also a very common finding in sodium channel blocker toxicity, this should really be a tetrad, but historically medicine prefers triads with the occasional pentad. Another finding in this ECG that is seen with sodium channel blocker toxicity is a terminal R-wave > 3 mm in lead aVR ***(see Figure 1)***.

Figure 1.
Terminal R-wave > 3 mm in lead aVR

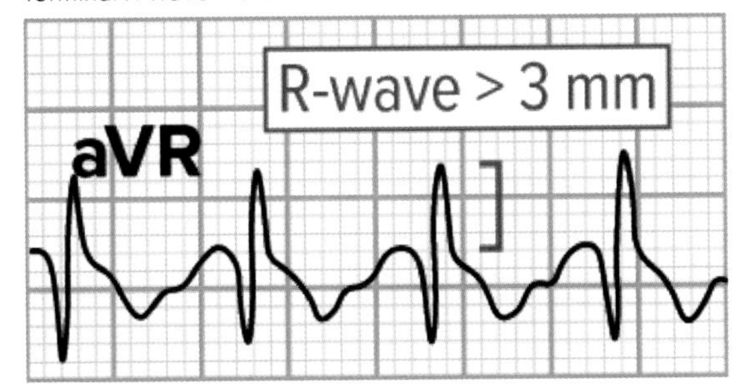

Sodium channel blocking drugs demonstrate a rate-dependent effect which means that there is an increase in the sodium channel blockade with increasing heart rates. In other words, the QRS complex duration and QT interval are more prolonged at faster ventricular rates. This effect is seen with therapeutic levels and is not a sign of toxicity. In the setting of sodium channel blocker toxicity, a prolonged QRS complex duration > 100 msec is associated with an increased risk of seizures and a prolonged QRS complex duration > 160 msec is associated with an increased risk of ventricular dysrhythmias.[1]

Tachycardia is a common finding in sodium channel blocker toxicity, but it is not caused by the sodium channel blockade. Many sodium channel blocking drugs, such as TCAs and diphenhydramine, also have anticholinergic properties, and the muscarinic effects typically result in sinus tachycardia. Other sodium channel blocking drugs, such as cocaine, have sympathomimetic properties that can cause tachycardia. These effects compete with, and predominate over, the sodium channel blocking effects of decreased pacemaker cell automaticity. This dynamic changes with severe toxicity when the sodium channel blocking effects predominate, resulting in bradycardia. When bradycardia is present, severe toxicity should be assumed and treatment should be tailored accordingly.

This patient was treated with IV sodium bicarbonate after further history was obtained and notable for the patient being on amitriptyline, a tricyclic antidepressant with sodium channel blocking properties.

Sodium Channel Blocker Toxicity Learning Points

- ECG triad of prolonged QRS complex duration, prolonged QTc interval, and right axis deviation
- ECG features include:
  - Tachycardia
  - QRS complex duration > 100 msec
  - Right axis deviation
  - Prolonged QTc interval
  - Terminal R-wave in lead aVR > 3 mm
  - R/S ratio > 0.7 in lead aVR
- Tachycardia is common
  - Due to competing muscarinic or sympathomimetic effects
  - Bradycardia is typically a sign of severe toxicity
- QRS complex duration > 100 msec is associated with toxicity
  - Mortality increases as QRS duration increases
  - Treat with sodium bicarbonate
- Sodium channel blocking drugs include:
  - Anesthetics: bupivacaine
  - Anticonvulsants: carbamazepine
  - Antidepressants: bupropion, mirtazapine, venlafaxine
  - Antiarrhythmics: Class IA (procainamide), IC (flecainide), and II (propranolol)
  - Antihistamines: diphenhydramine
  - Antimalarial drugs: chloroquine, hydroxychloroquine, quinine
  - Cocaine
  - Phenothiazines: prochlorperazine, chlorpromazine
  - Tricyclic antidepressants: amitriptyline, nortriptyline

References

1. Harrigan RA, Brady WJ. ECG abnormalities in tricyclic antidepressant ingestion. Am J Emerg Med. 1999;17(4):387-393.

NOTES:

Case 57: Presentation

A 35-year-old male presents with palpitations and chest pain.
What is your interpretation of his ECG?

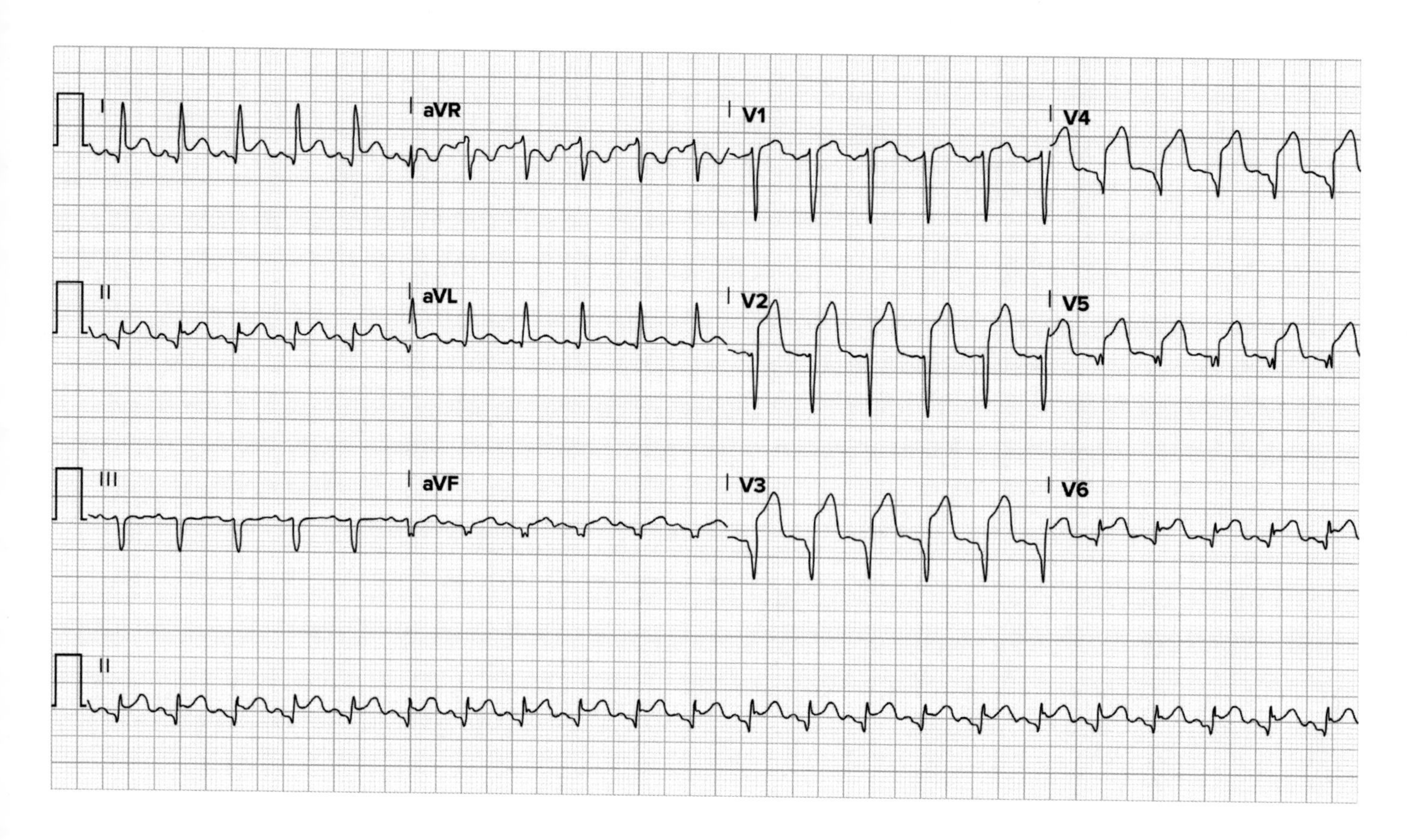

Case 57: Answer

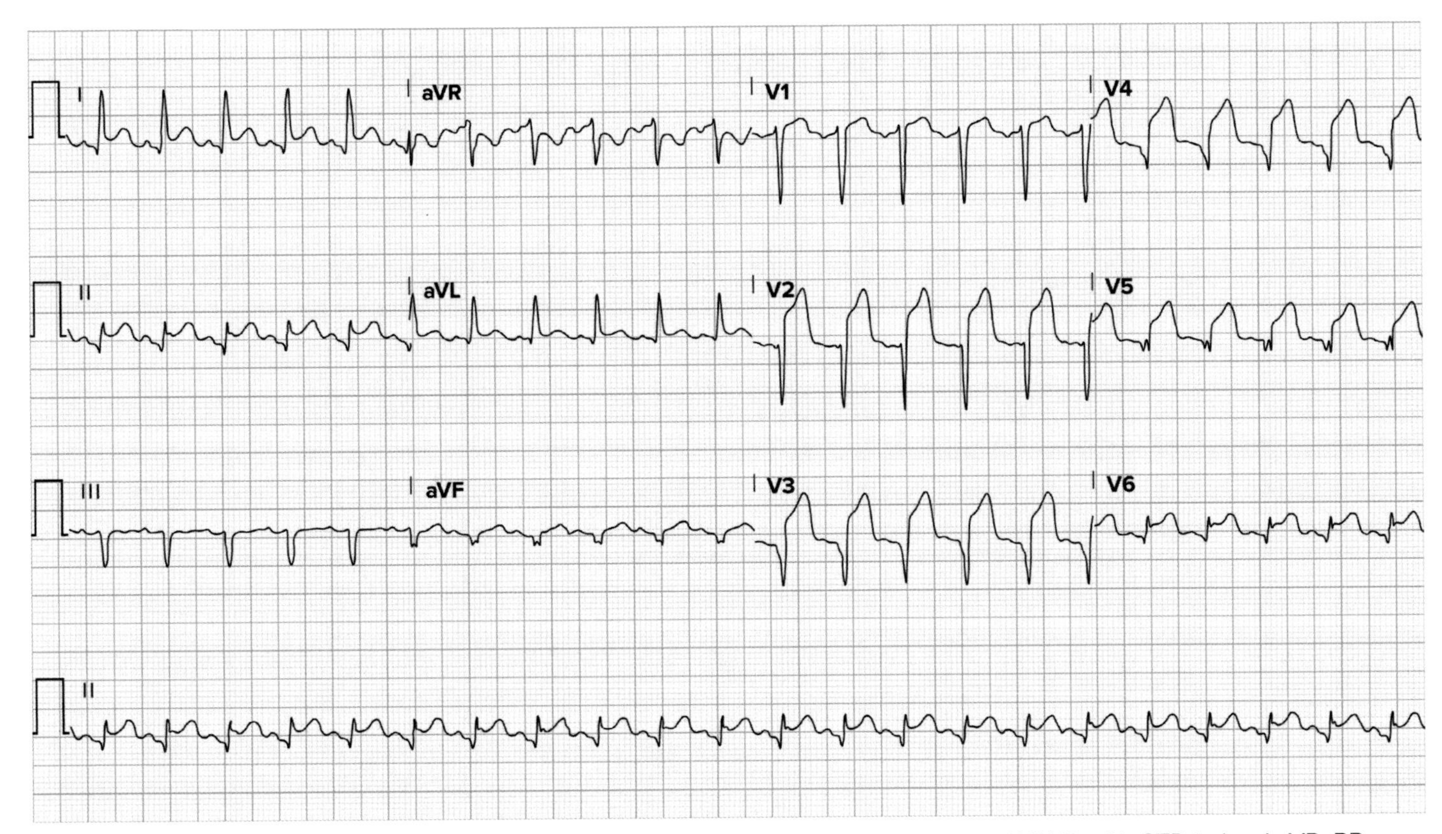

This ECG shows a sinus tachycardia at 130 bpm, normal axis, STE in leads I, aVL, II, and V1-V6 with STD in lead aVR, PR-segment elevation in lead aVR with PR-segment depression in leads I, aVL, and II, Q-waves in leads I, aVL II, and V3-V6 (V3-V4 technically have a QS complex), and poor R-wave progression.

This patient's age, presence of tachycardia, diffuse STE without reciprocal changes, and PR changes can all be seen with pericarditis, but this ECG is consistent with a very large MI, specifically an anterolateral MI. Note that reciprocal STD support, but are not required for, the ECG diagnosis of STEMI.

This ECG also show sinus tachycardia which is not a typical finding in an AMI yet can occur for a range of reasons, including compensation for developing shock, acute heart failure, severe pain/anxiety, among many other entities. In this patient, the presence of sinus tachycardia is concerning for acute heart failure and/or compensated cardiogenic shock. An extensive MI can result in significantly decreased stroke volume and the compensatory mechanism to maintain cardiac output is an increase in the HR (note that CO = SV x HR). This is critical to recognize because giving any medication that decreases preload will also reduce SV and worsen the CO and systemic perfusion.

Another finding that is less clinically relevant is the presence of poor R-wave progression (PRWP). There is no universal definition for PRWP, but a common criterion is R-wave amplitude in lead V3 ≤ 3 mm. The differential diagnosis for a PRWP is listed below in the learning points. In this case, the PRWP is due to the ischemic QS complex in lead V3.

This patient was taken to the cardiac catheterization laboratory where a 100% occlusion of the mid-LAD was successfully treated with a stent.

STEMI Learning Points

- STEMI is defined by new, or presumed new, STE at the J point in ≥ 2 anatomically contiguous leads in the absence of LVH by voltage pattern, LBBB, or ventricular-paced rhythm
  - ≥ 2.5 mm in men < 40 years old and ≥ 2 mm in men ≥ 40 years old in leads V2-V3 (or an increase of ≥ 1 mm when compared to baseline ECG)
  - ≥ 1.5 mm in women in leads V2-V3 (or an increase of ≥ 1 mm when compared to baseline ECG)
  - ≥ 1 mm in all other leads
- ST-segment is measured from the isoelectric baseline, typically the TP segment (see below)
- Reciprocal STD are not required for the diagnosis of STEMI, but their presence does increase the likelihood of the diagnosis of STEMI
  - Reciprocal STD are only present in 70% of anterior MI[1]
- Posterior MI
  - Consider whenever there is STD in leads V1-V4
  - STE ≥ 0.5 mm in posterior leads V7, V8 or V9 is diagnostic- does not require 2 contiguous leads
- Right ventricular MI
  - Consider with any inferior MI (RV MI is seen in approximately 1/3 of inferior MI)
  - STE in right precordial leads V3R and V4R ≥ 0.5 mm (≥ 1 mm for men ≤ 30 years old)
  - STE in right precordial lead V4R > 1 mm is most predictive of RV MI
  - STE in right precordial lead V4R > STE in leads V1-V3 = highly specific for RV MI
- Significant STE that does not meet the traditional distribution (ie, ≥ 2 anatomically contiguous leads) in a presentation concerning for ACS may still represent coronary artery occlusion and warrant consideration for emergent coronary reperfusion

How to Measure STE per most recent 2018 AHA Guidelines[1]

- The J point is the junction between QRS termination and ST-segment onset and is used to determine the magnitude of the ST-segment shift
- **In patients with a stable baseline, the TP segment (isoelectric interval) is a more accurate method to assess the magnitude of ST-segment shift *(see Figure 1)*,** and in distinguishing pericarditis from acute myocardial ischemia
- QRS onset should be used if TP segment does not have a stable baseline ***(see Figure 2)***
- Measurement should be made from the top of the ECG line tracing

Figure 1.
Measure STE from the TP segment if the TP segment is isoelectric (ie, horizontal)

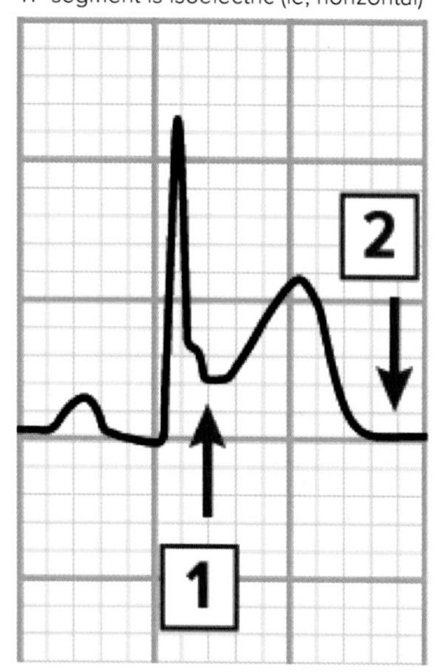

Arrow 1: onset of the ST-segment (ie, J point)
Arrow 2: TP segment

Figure 2.
Measure STE from onset of the QRS complex if the TP segment is not isoelectric (ie, not horizontal)

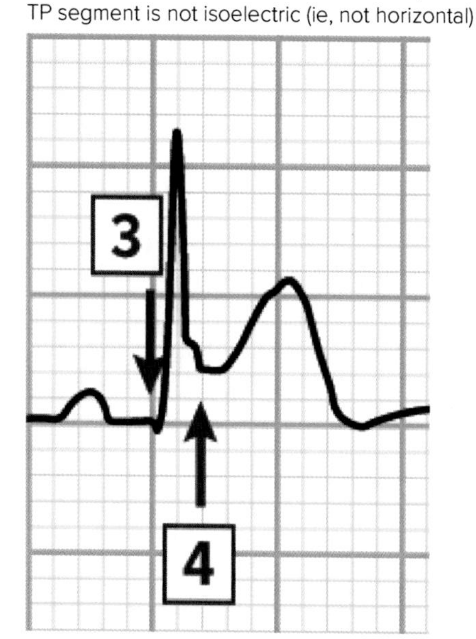

Arrow 3: initial onset of the Q-wave
Arrow 4: onset of the ST-segment (ie, J point)

Poor R-wave Progression Learning Points

- No universal definition, but common criteria include:
  - R-wave in lead V3 ≤ 3 mm
  - R-wave < 2-4 mm in lead V3 or V4
  - R-wave in lead V3 > lead V4 or lead V2 > lead V3
- Etiologies include:
  - Dilated cardiomyopathy
  - LAFB
  - LBBB
  - LVH
  - Low voltage
  - Misplaced precordial leads
  - Normal variant, especially in the elderly
  - Pre-excitation syndromes
  - Prior anterior myocardial infarction
  - RVH (eg, from COPD)

References

1. Thygesen K, Alpert JS, Jaffe AS, et al. 2018 ESC/ACC/AHA/WHF Expert Consensus Document: Fourth Universal Definition of Myocardial Infarction (2018). Circulation. 2018;138:e618-e651.

Case 58: Presentation

A 91-year-old female with history of coronary artery disease, chronic renal disease, congestive heart failure, diabetes mellitus, and pacemaker placement presents with chest pain. What is your interpretation of her ECG?

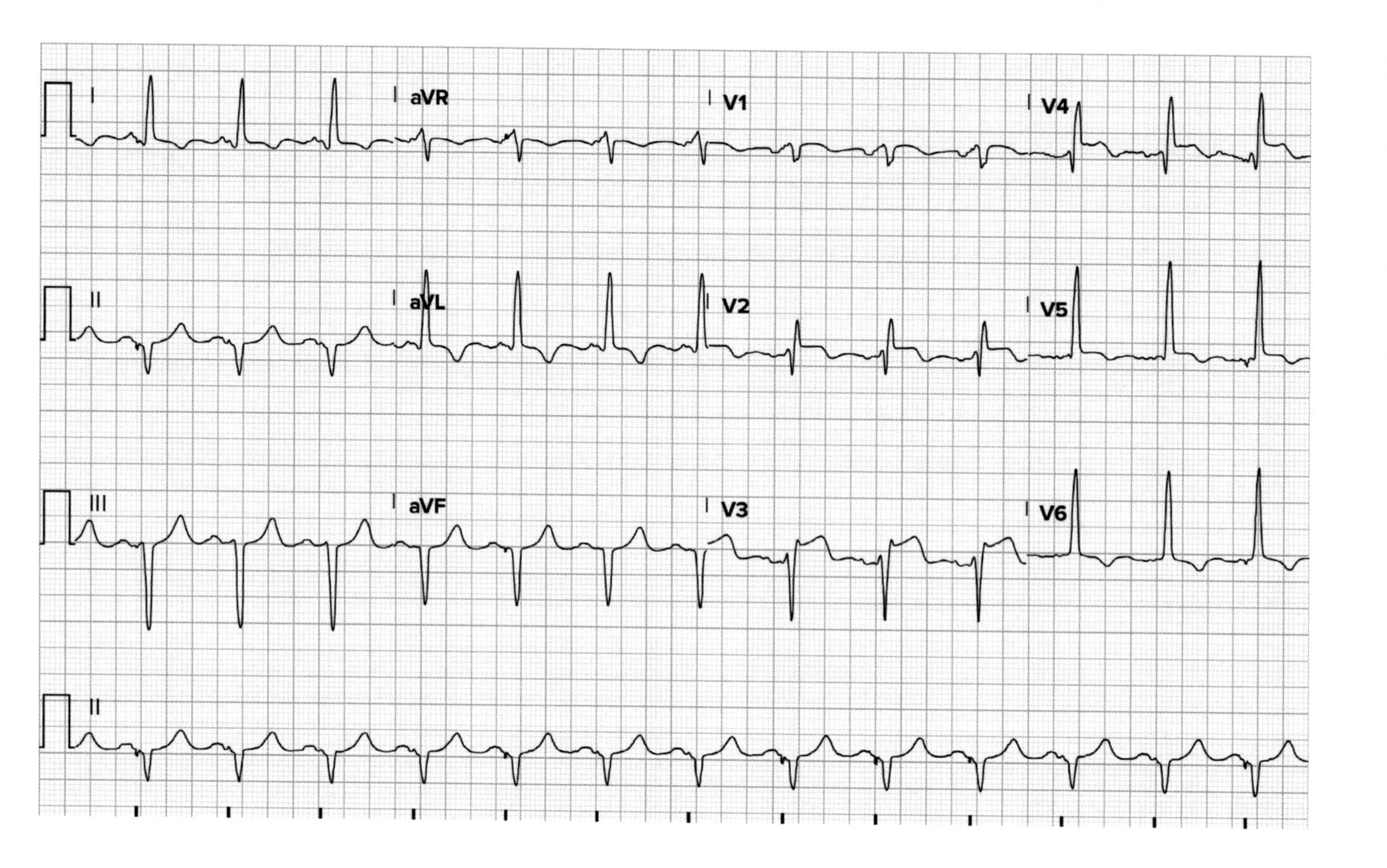

Case 58: Answer

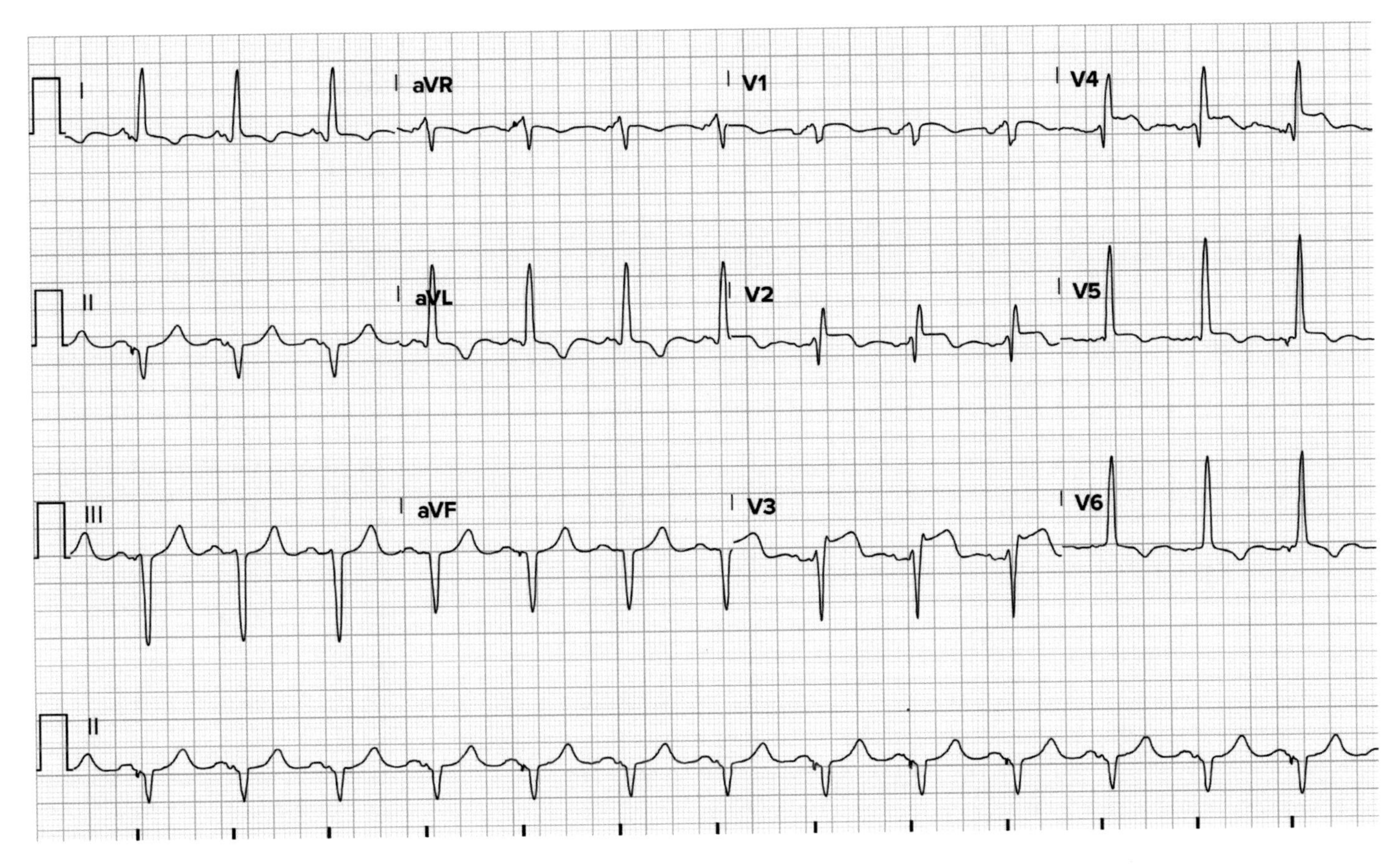

This ECG shows an atrial-sensed, biventricular-paced rhythm at 82 bpm, left axis deviation, prolonged QRS complex duration at 125 msec, STE in leads V1-V5, and discordant T-waves in leads I, aVL, II, III, aVF, and V6.

Biventricular pacing, also known as cardiac resynchronization therapy, has one atrial lead and 2 ventricular leads:

- The right atrial lead paces the right atrial appendage
- The RV lead paces the RV apex (same as with right ventricular pacing)
- The LV lead paces the surface of the posterior or lateral LV wall via the coronary sinus (ie, it is not inside the ventricle)

Ventricular Leads

The biventricular paced ECG will show 2 pacer spikes with a narrower QRS complex than compared with right ventricular pacing. The LV lead typically paces before the RV lead since it takes longer to depolarize the myocardium from the surface. The timing of the 2 ventricular pacer spikes is programmed to maximize cardiac output, so the time between the LV and RV pacer spikes is variable. ***(see Figures 1a-c)***.

Figure 1a.
Biventricular pacer spikes (from the case ECG)

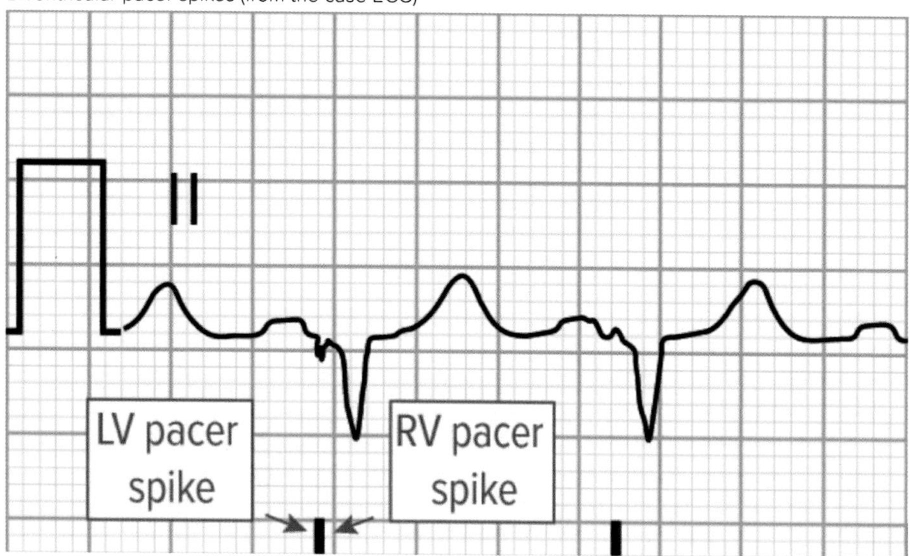

Figure 1b.
Another example of biventricular pacer spikes (from a different ECG)

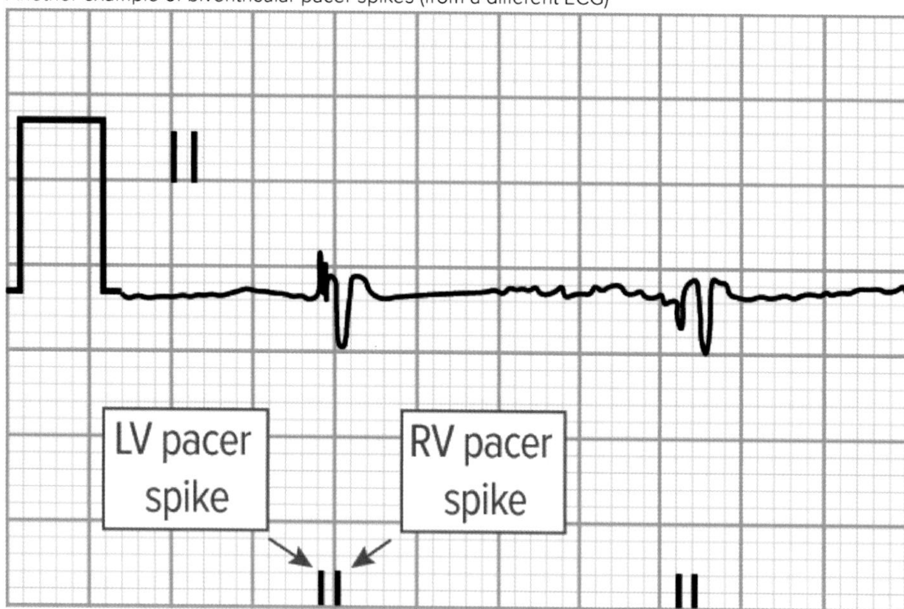

Figure 1c.
Another example of biventricular pacer spikes (from a different ECG)

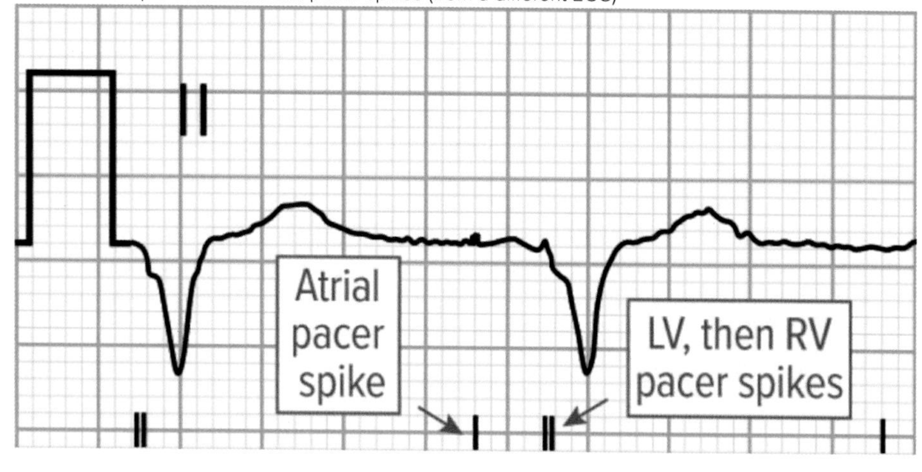

Biventricular pacing will often result in a dominant R-wave in lead V1 +/- V2 ***(see Figures 2 and 3)***.

Figure 2.
A dominant R-wave in lead V1 +/- V2 is a common finding with biventricular pacing

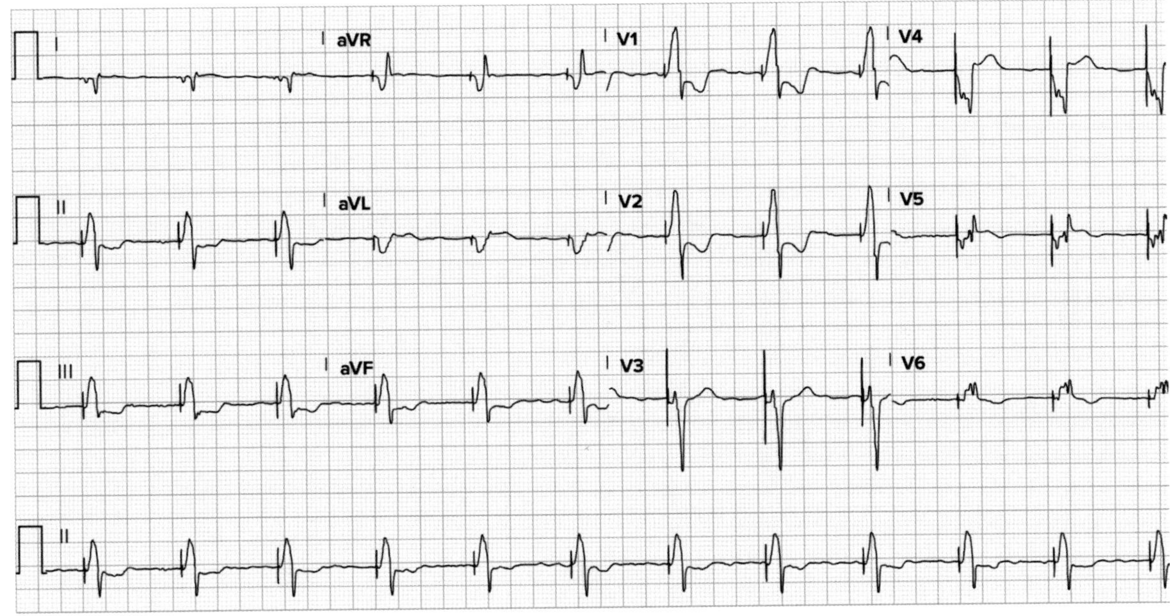

Figure 3.
A dominant R-wave in lead V1 +/- V2 is a common finding with biventricular pacing

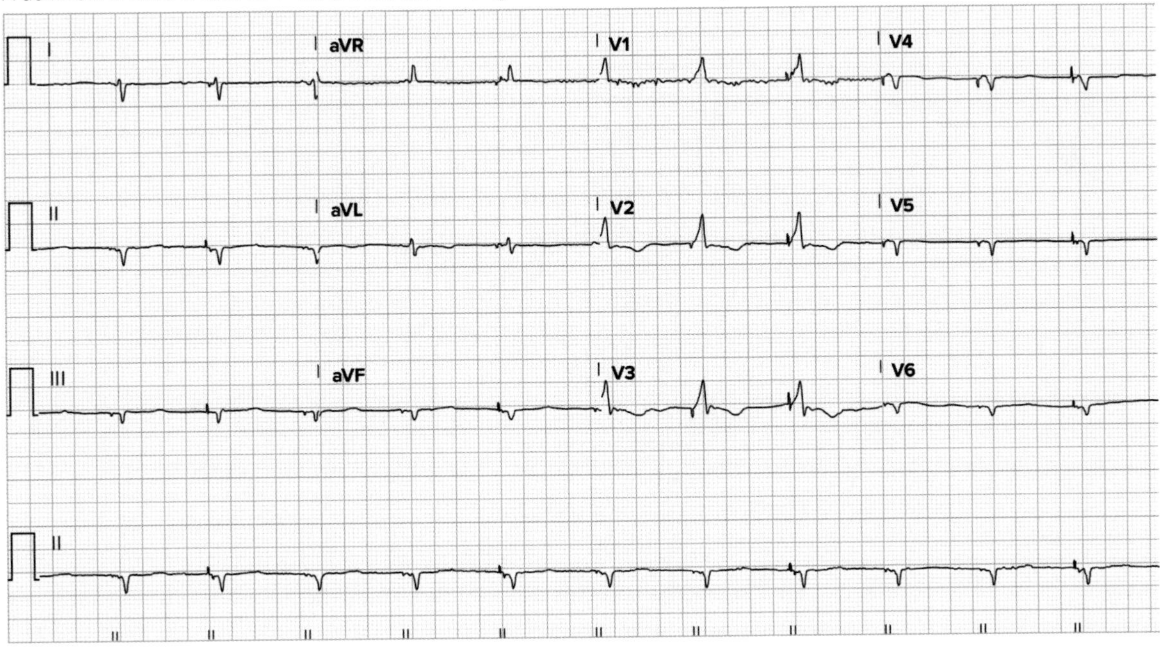

Atrial Lead

The atrial lead is programmed to sense for native atrial activity and act accordingly:

- The pacemaker senses native atrial activity, waits a preprogrammed amount of time, then paces the ventricles ***(see Figures 4 and 5)***
- The pacemaker paces the atria if no native atrial activity is detected during a preprogrammed amount of time, waits another preprogrammed amount of time, then paces the ventricles ***(see Figure 6)***

Figure 4.
The lead II rhythm strip from the case ECG shows an atrial-sensed, ventricular-paced rhythm

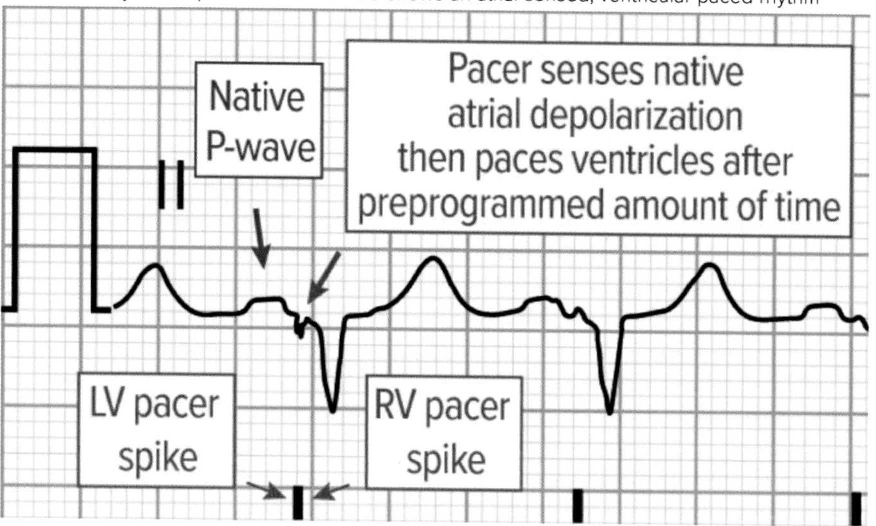

Figure 5.
Another example of an atrial-sensed, ventricular-paced rhythm (from a different ECG)

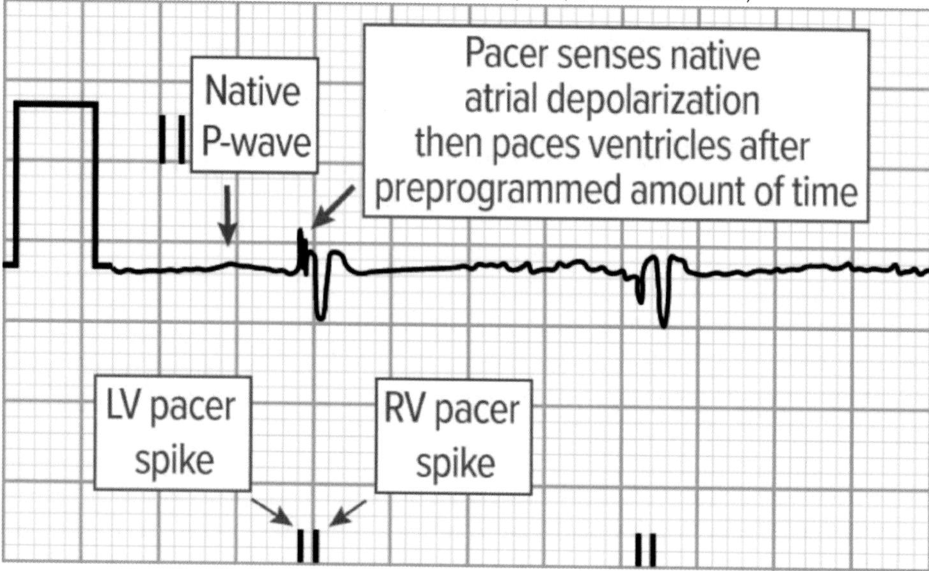

Figure 6.
An example of A-V sequential pacing (from a different ECG)

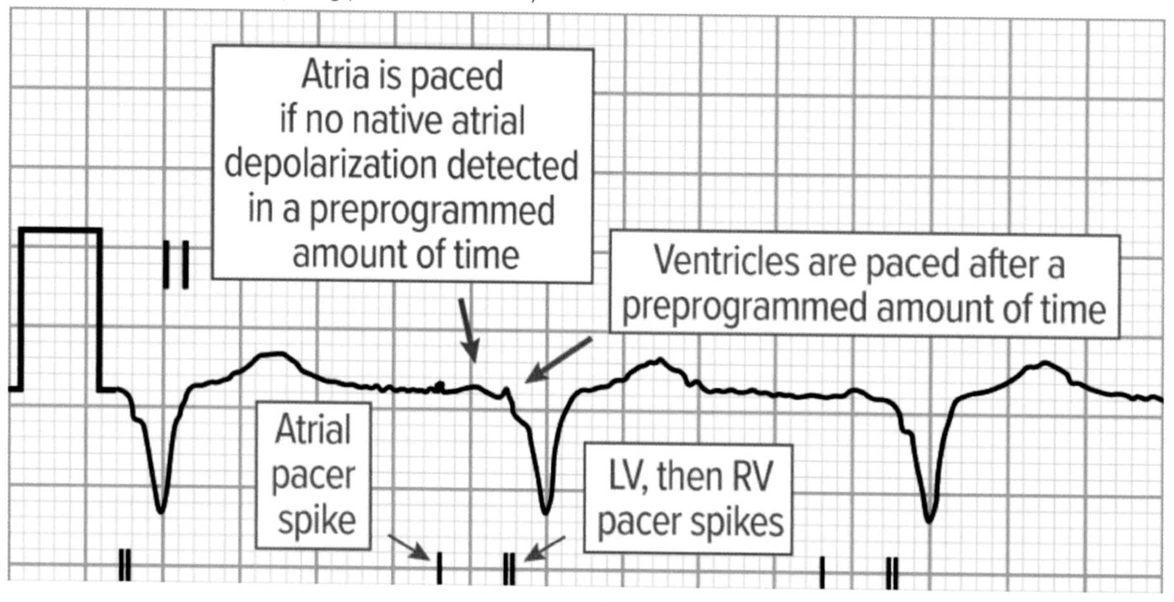

The concerning finding in this ECG is the STE in leads V1-V4 and introduces the question "how does the clinician evaluate for an AMI in the setting of biventricular pacing?" This ECG meets criteria for a STEMI using either traditional or Sgarbossa criteria:

- Traditional STEMI criteria: STE in contiguous leads V3 (≥ 1.5 mm for women) and V4 (≥ 1 mm)
- Sgarbossa criteria: concordant STE ≥ 1 mm in lead V4

Unfortunately, Sgarbossa criteria only apply to right ventricular-paced rhythms and not biventricular-paced rhythms, and the AHA guidelines do not currently include STEMI criteria for biventricular pacing. Thus, there are no evidence-based nor guideline-based recommendation on how to interpret this ECG with respect to AMI diagnosis. This patient had multiple chronic conditions which made her a poor candidate for cardiac catheterization and her symptoms were well controlled medically, so she chose to be admitted for palliative care.

Pacemaker Learning Points

- Pacer spikes are usually visible on the ECG, either at the bottom of the ECG and/or preceding the P-wave and/or QRS complex
  - Atrial pacing: spikes immediately precede P-waves
  - Ventricular pacing: spikes immediately precede QRS complexes
  - Dual chamber pacing: spikes immediately precede both P-waves and QRS complexes
  - Biventricular pacing: 2 spikes immediately precede QRS complexes
- Atrial pacing
  - Pacemaker lead usually implanted in the right atrial appendage
  - Results in P-waves with normal morphology
- Right ventricular pacing
  - Pacemaker lead usually implanted in the RV apex
  - Results in a LBBB pattern in the limb leads and anteroseptal precordial leads
  - The major difference between an intrinsic LBBB and a right ventricular-paced rhythm is that the QRS complex will almost always be negatively oriented in leads V5-V6 with a right ventricular-paced rhythm
- Biventricular pacing
  - Two pacemaker leads usually implanted in the RV apex and the surface of the posterior or lateral LV
  - Typically results in a narrower QRS complex than with right ventricular pacing
  - Dominant R-wave in lead V1 +/- V2 is common
- AICD will have a thick coil that differentiates it from a pacemaker

AMI in Right Ventricular-Paced Rhythms Learning Points

- In general, evaluate a paced ECG for ischemia as you would a LBBB, using Sgarbossa criteria
  - Discordant STE ≥ 5 mm- 99% specificity[1] (note that this study had no cases with STE > 1 mm)
  - Concordant STE ≥ 1 mm- 94% specificity[2]
  - At the time of publication, there are no published studies on the use of the Modified Sgarbossa criteria in ventricular-paced rhythms

References

1. Maloy KR, Bhat R, Davis J, Reed K, Morrissey R. Sgarbossa Criteria Are Highly Specific for Acute Myocardial Infarction with Pacemakers. West J Emerg Med. 2010;11(4):354-357.
2. Sgarbossa EB, Pinski SL, Gates KB, Wagner GS, The GUSTO-1 Investigators. Early electrocardiographic diagnosis of acute myocardial infarction in the presence of ventricular

Case 59: Presentation

A 55-year-old male with history of ESRD presents with nausea and SOB. What is your interpretation of his ECG?

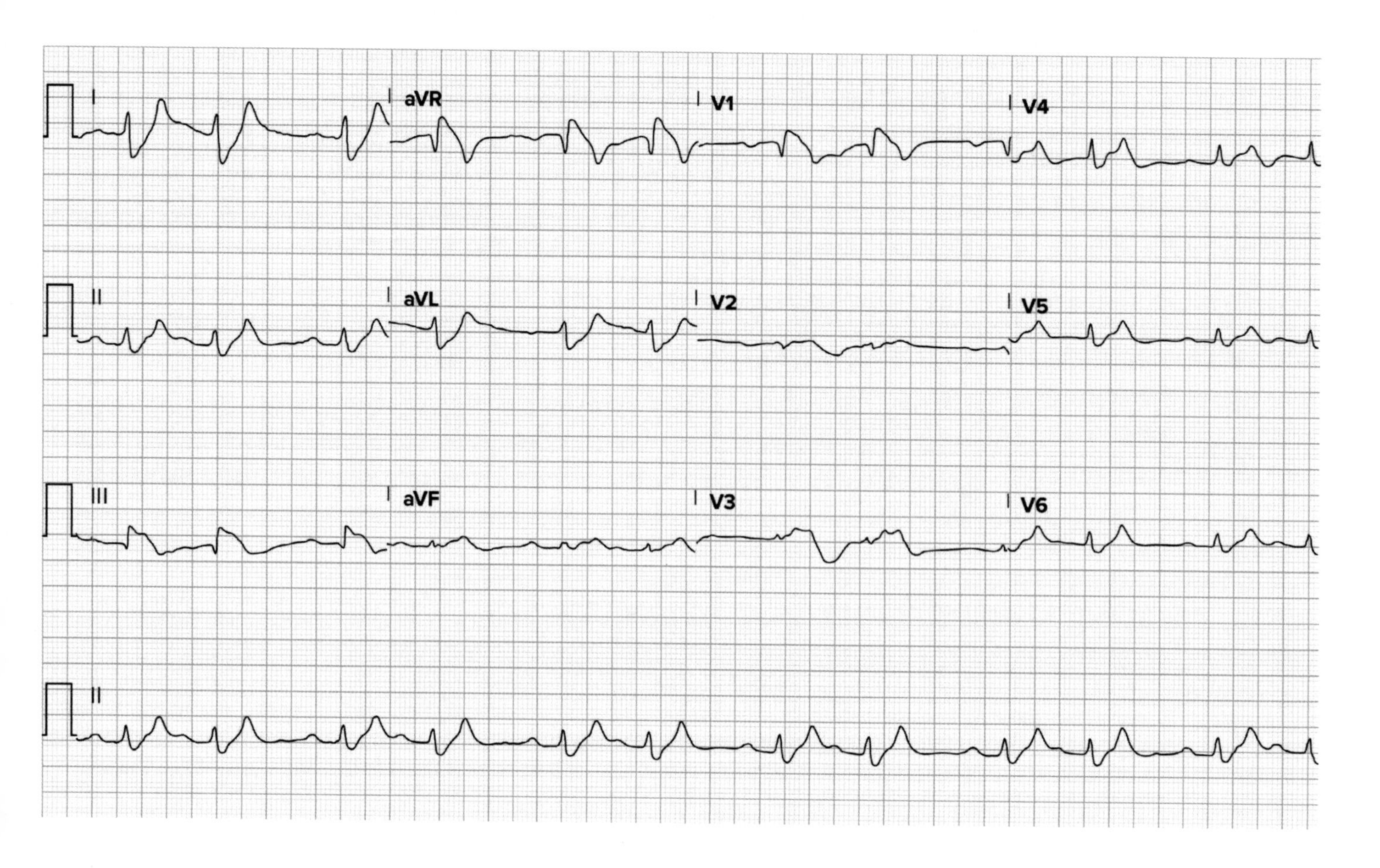

Case 59: Answer

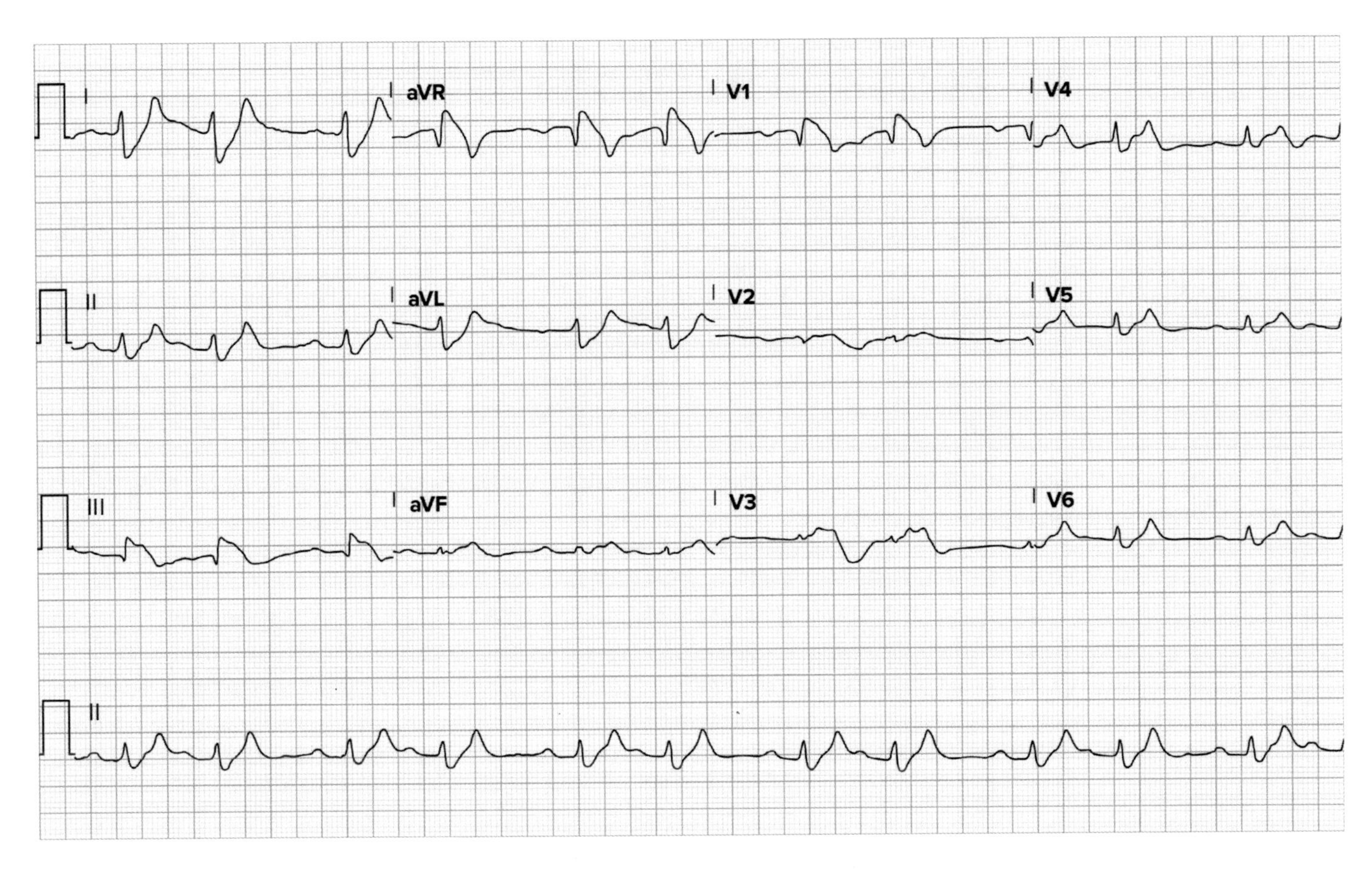

This ECG shows a 2nd degree type I (Wenckebach) sinoatrial (SA) block with an average ventricular rate of 70 bpm, right axis deviation, and a prolonged QRS complex duration of approximately 200 msec with a RBBB-like morphology. The apparent STE in leads III, aVR, and V1 with STD in leads I and aVL are due to the very wide QRS. This constellation of findings, including prolonged QRS complex duration with bizarre morphology and multiple conduction abnormalities, is most consistent with hyperkalemia.

The differential diagnosis for an irregular wide complex rhythm with normal ventricular rates includes:

- Atrial fibrillation (rate controlled) with aberrant conduction
- Atrial flutter with variable block (rate controlled) and aberrant conduction
- Atrial tachycardia with variable block (rate controlled) and aberrant conduction
- Wandering atrial pacemaker with aberrant conduction
- 2nd degree AV block Mobitz types I and II with aberrant conduction
- Variable high-degree AV block (eg, 3:1, 4:1, etc.) with aberrant conduction
- 2nd degree sinoatrial block with aberrant conduction
- Sinus arrhythmia with aberrant conduction
- NSR or accelerated junctional rhythm with aberrant conduction and irregular pattern of PAC, PJC, and/or PVC
- NSR accelerated junctional rhythm with aberrant conduction and regular patterns of PAC, PJC, and/or PVC (bigeminy, trigeminy, etc.)
  - Causes of aberrant conduction include fixed or rate-related BBB, metabolic abnormalities, sodium channel blocker toxicity, ventricular-paced rhythm, and ventricular pre-excitation (eg, WPW)

The key to correctly interpreting this ECG is recognizing the extremely prolonged QRS complex duration which is best measured in lead II ***(see Figure 1)***. A QRS complex duration > 200 msec, especially in conjunction with a bizarre QRS complex morphology, should prompt consideration of hyperkalemia.

Figure 1.
The lead II rhythm strip shows an extremely prolonged QRS complex duration concerning for hyperkalemia

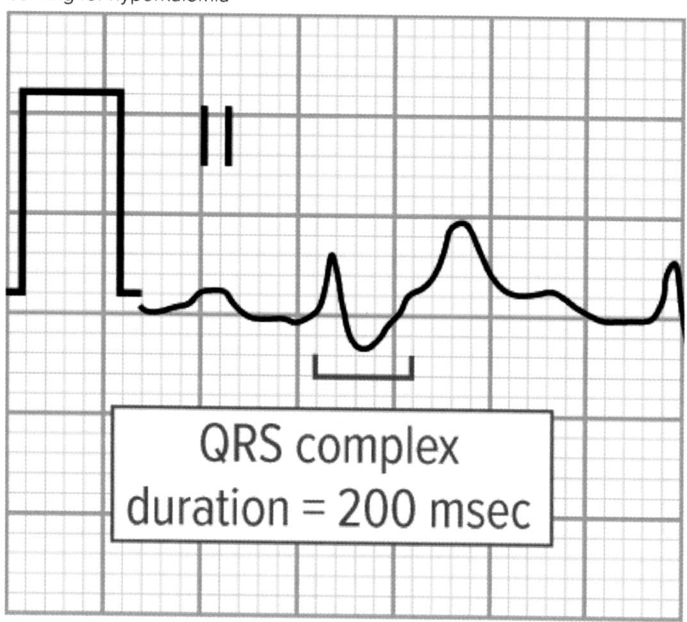

The rhythm in this ECG shows a repeating pattern of 2 P-QRS-T complexes followed by a pause with a slightly increasing PR interval that resets after the pause ***(see Figure 2)***.

Figure 2.
The repeating pattern of 2 P-QRS-T complexes with progressively lengthening PR intervals best seen in the 3rd and 4th P-QRS-T complexes in the lead II rhythm strip

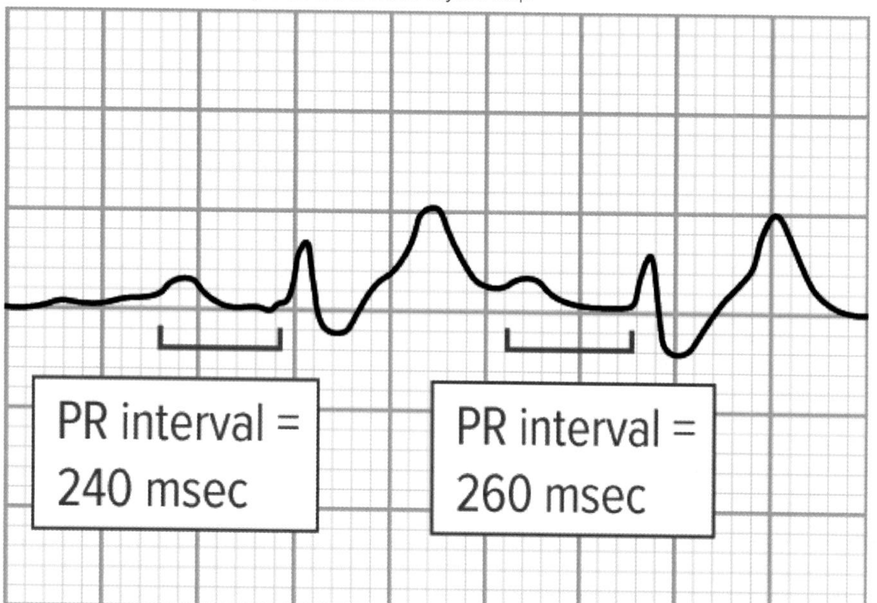

There are no P-waves followed by a missing (ie, dropped) QRS complex, which rules out a 2nd degree AV block. The P-wave morphologies, best seen preceding the 11th and 12th QRS complexes in the lead II rhythm strip, are consistent ***(see Figure 3)*** which rules out atrial bigeminy (ie, normal sinus beat followed by a PAC). PACs will demonstrate a non-sinus P-wave followed by a normal QRS complex (ie, morphology consistent with sinus QRS-T complexes).

Figure 3.
Consistent P-wave morphologies, best seen preceding the 11th and 12th QRS complexes in the lead II rhythm strip, rules out atrial bigeminy

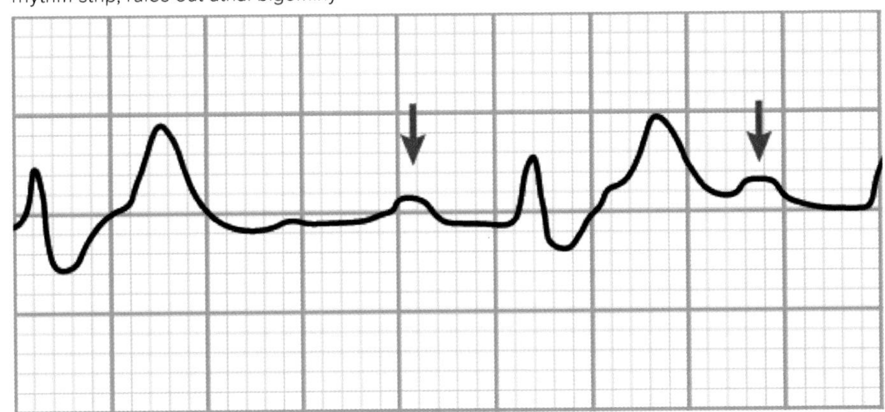

The likely etiology of this rhythm is 2nd degree type I (Wenckebach) sinoatrial (SA) block, also called a sinoatrial node exit block. In a SA block, the SA node generates an electrical impulse that does not conduct to the atria. This phenomenon will result in a missing P-wave and subsequently a missing QRS-T complex. Just as with AV blocks, there are 1st, 2nd, and 3rd degree SA blocks, but only 2nd degree can be seen on a 12-lead ECG.

Wenckebach conduction, also called Wenckebach periodicity or phenomenon, describes a conduction abnormality where there is a progressively increasing conduction delay followed by blocked conduction. In a 2nd degree type I AV block, this results in progressively longer conduction time from the atria to the ventricle, which manifests as a progressively lengthening PR interval, followed by a missing QRS complex. In a 2nd degree type I SA block, there is a progressively longer conduction time from the SA node to the atria followed by a missing P-QRS-T complex (which will look like a pause on the ECG).

What makes a 2nd degree type I SA block difficult to detect is that there is an absence of an entire P-QRS-T complex which can easily be misinterpreted as a sinus pause. A distinguishing feature of this block that can help differentiate it from a sinus pause is that it produces groups of beats that get progressively closer together before a missing P-QRS-T complex.

In general, a 2nd degree type I SA block will have consistent PR intervals, which is not seen in this ECG. A possible explanation is that there is a concurrent 2nd degree type I AV block as the PR interval increases then resets after the pause. Since the conduction block in the SA node is due to hyperkalemia and not a structural cause (eg, fibrosis), it is not unreasonable to assume that the hyperkalemia could also cause a similar conduction abnormality in the AV node.

The patient's labs were notable for a hyperkalemia of 8.1 mEq/L. He was treated immediately with calcium then emergently dialyzed in the ED.

Hyperkalemia Learning Points

- ECG is specific but not sensitive for hyperkalemia
- ECG changes are not always sequential/progressive and include:
  - Tall, narrow, peaked T-waves (best seen in precordial leads)
  - P-wave flattening and PR interval prolongation
  - Prolonged QRS complex duration, ranging from minimal to maximal
  - Conduction abnormalities (AV blocks, fascicular and bundle branch blocks)
  - Bradycardia
  - Sino-ventricular rhythm (loss of P-waves, extremely widened QRS) with normal or slow rate
  - Ventricular dysrhythmias
- Can cause STE (common in leads V1-V2 and aVR) that mimics STEMI or Brugada pattern
- Can occur simultaneously with hyperacute T-waves and obscure early changes seen in an anterior or anteroseptal AMI
- The "syphilis of ECG abnormalities," meaning that a broad range of abnormalities can be encountered with hyperkalemia[1]

References

1. Mattu A. ECG Weekly.

Case 60: Presentation

A 70-year-old male with COPD presents with SOB and chest tightness. Notable vital signs include oxygen saturation of 84% on room air. What is your interpretation of his ECG?

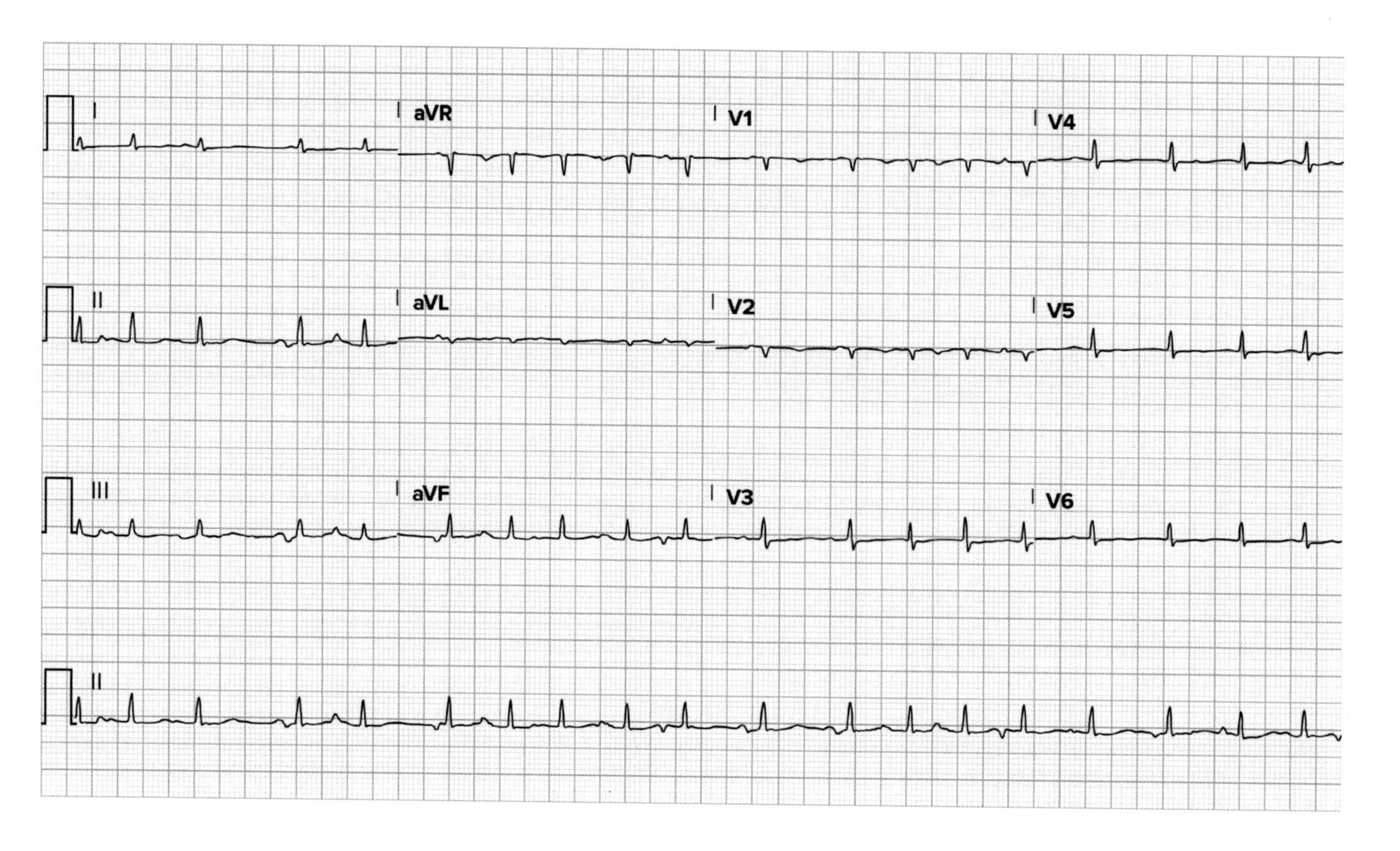

Case 60: Answer

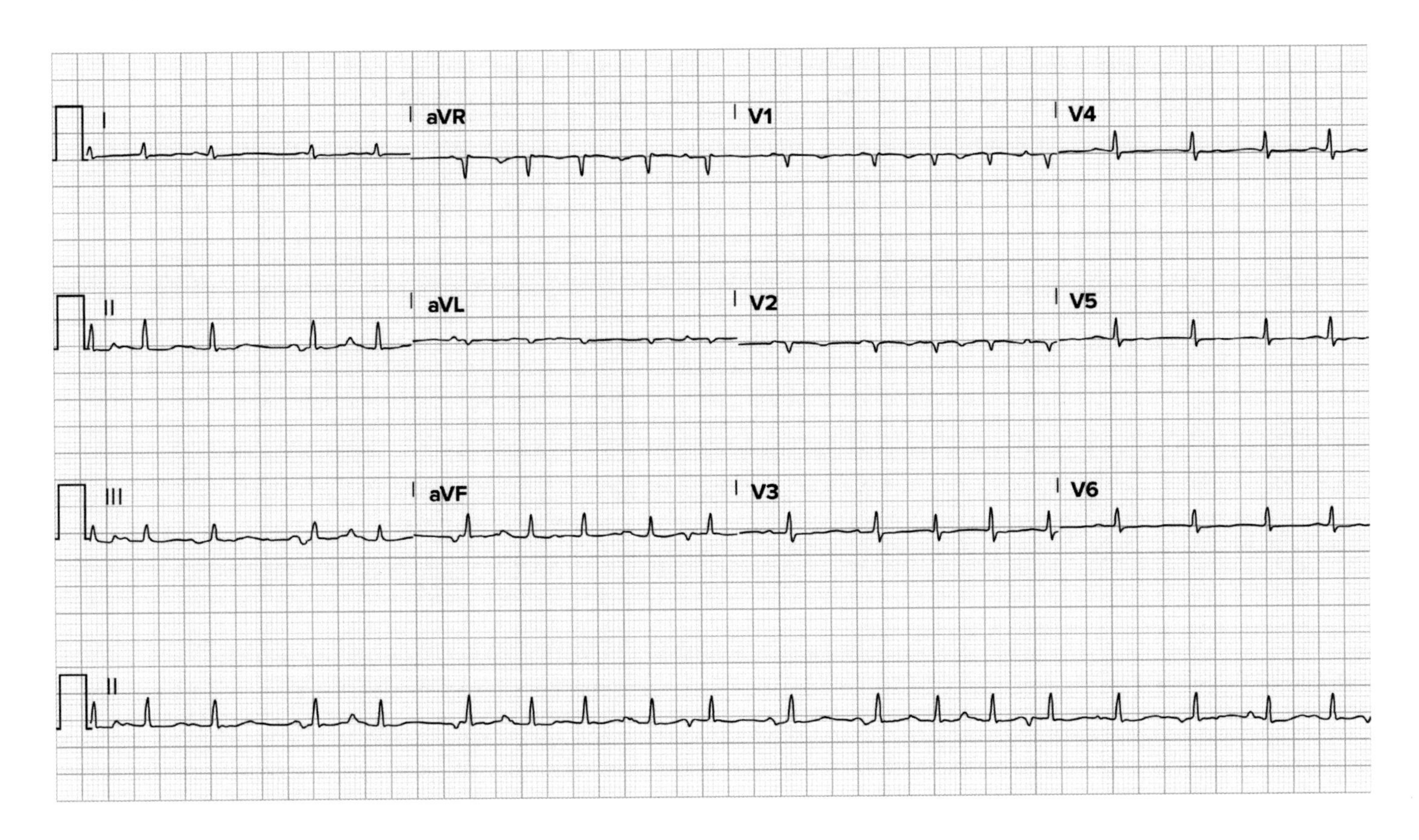

This ECG shows an irregular narrow complex tachycardia with an average ventricular rate of 110 bpm, variable P-wave morphologies and PR intervals, normal axis, and normal QRS complex duration with uniform morphology, consistent with multifocal atrial tachycardia (MAT).

The differential diagnosis for an irregular narrow-complex tachycardia includes:

- Atrial fibrillation
- Atrial flutter with variable block
- Atrial tachycardia with variable block
- Multifocal atrial tachycardia
- Sinus tachycardia with irregular pattern of PAC, PJC, and/or PVC
- Sinus tachycardia with regular patterns of PAC, PJC, and/or PVC (bigeminy, trigeminy, etc.)

The defining characteristic of MAT is an irregular rhythm with the presence of ≥ 3 different P-wave morphologies in a single lead with variable PR intervals. This is best seen in the lead II rhythm strip ***(see Figure 1)***.

Figure 1.
The lead II rhythm strip shows 3 different P-wave morphologies with 3 different PR intervals

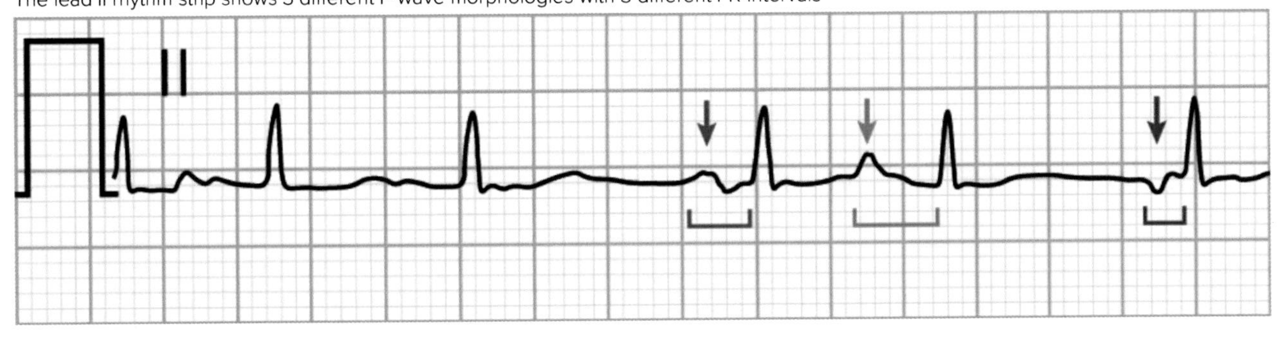

The classic teaching is that MAT is precipitated by an acute exacerbation of a chronic respiratory or cardiac disease, often a COPD exacerbation. Treatment should be focused on the underlying respiratory or cardiac pathology and not the dysrhythmia.

This ECG also shows low voltage, often defined as QRS complex amplitude < 5 mm in the limb leads or < 10 mm in the precordial leads. Regarding the low voltage criteria, some sources note "and" instead of "or" (ie, requiring both limb and precordial lead involvement). In this ECG, the low voltage criterion is met in the limb leads, but not in the precordial leads as the voltage of the first QRS complex in lead V2 is a little greater than 10 mm. The finding of low voltage, regardless of whether it is present in both the limb and precordial leads, should prompt an evaluation for the underlying cause. For this patient's ECG, the likely etiology is COPD.

The differential diagnosis for low voltage includes:

- Normal variant
- Cardiac etiologies:
  - Hypothyroidism, severe
  - Hypovolemia
  - Infiltrative cardiomyopathies
  - Myocarditis
  - Myocardial infarction
- Extracardiac etiologies:
  - Acute respiratory distress syndrome
  - Anasarca
  - Chronic obstructive pulmonary disease
  - Constrictive pericarditis
  - Obesity
  - Pericardial effusion
  - Pleural effusion
  - Pneumomediastinum
  - Pneumonia
  - Pneumopericardium
  - Pneumothorax
  - Pulmonary edema
  - Subcutaneous emphysema

This patient's workup was notable for a positive COVID-19 test, and he was admitted to the internal medicine service for further treatment.

MAT Learning Points

- Irregular tachycardia with ≥ 3 different P-wave morphologies in a single lead with variable PR intervals
  - Variable PP and RR intervals
  - QRS complexes are uniform in appearance
- Rate is typically between 101-180 bpm
  - If atrial rate ≤ 100 bpm, called multifocal atrial rhythm or wandering atrial pacemaker
- Typically seen with acute exacerbation of chronic cardiopulmonary disease

Low Voltage Learning Points

- QRS complex amplitude < 5 mm in the limb leads or < 10 mm in the precordial leads
- Low voltage + electrical alternans = pericardial effusion until proven otherwise

NOTES:

Case 61: Presentation

A 63-year-old female with history of prior CAD with cardiac stents presents with chest pain. What is your interpretation of her ECG?

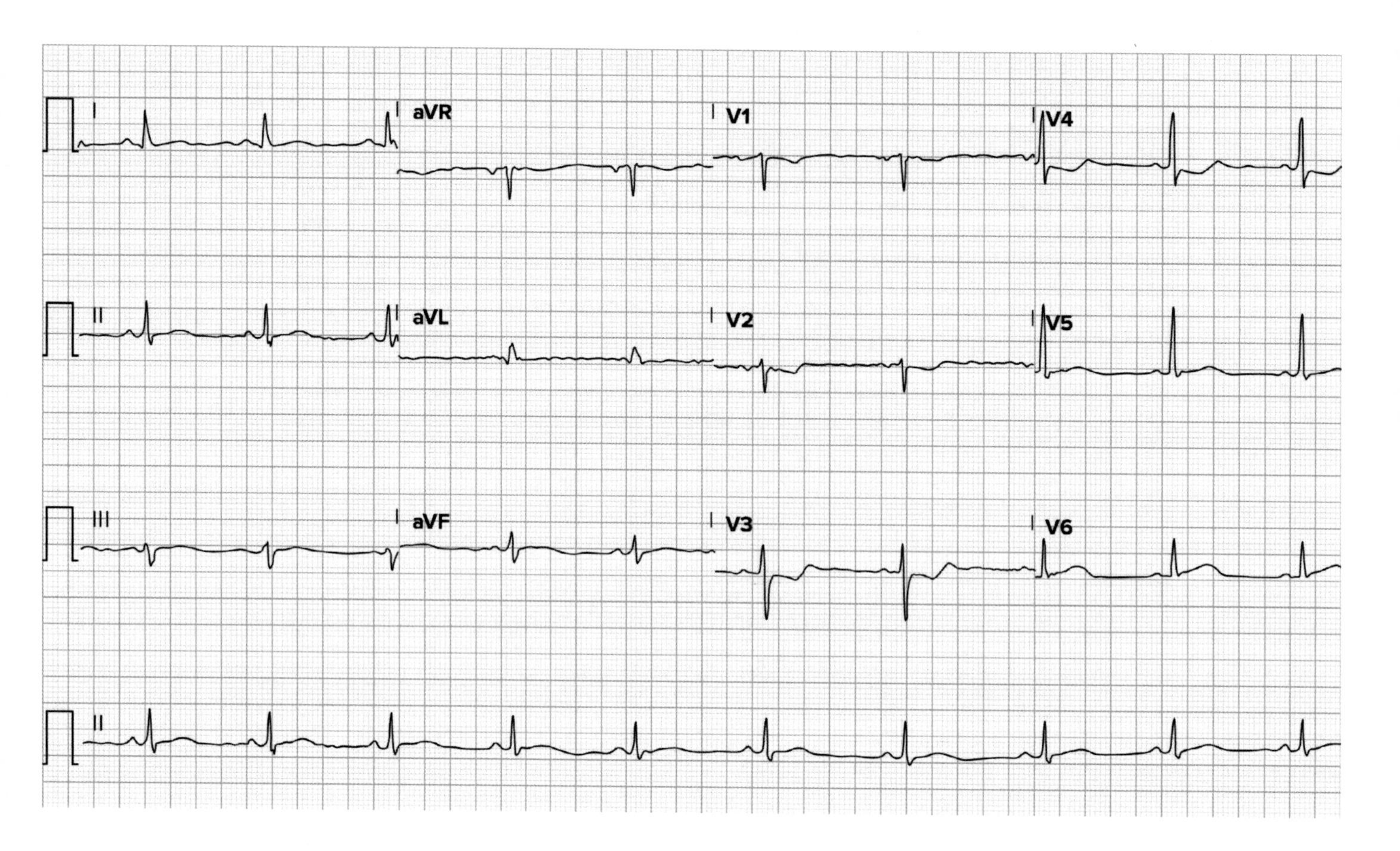

Case 61: Answer

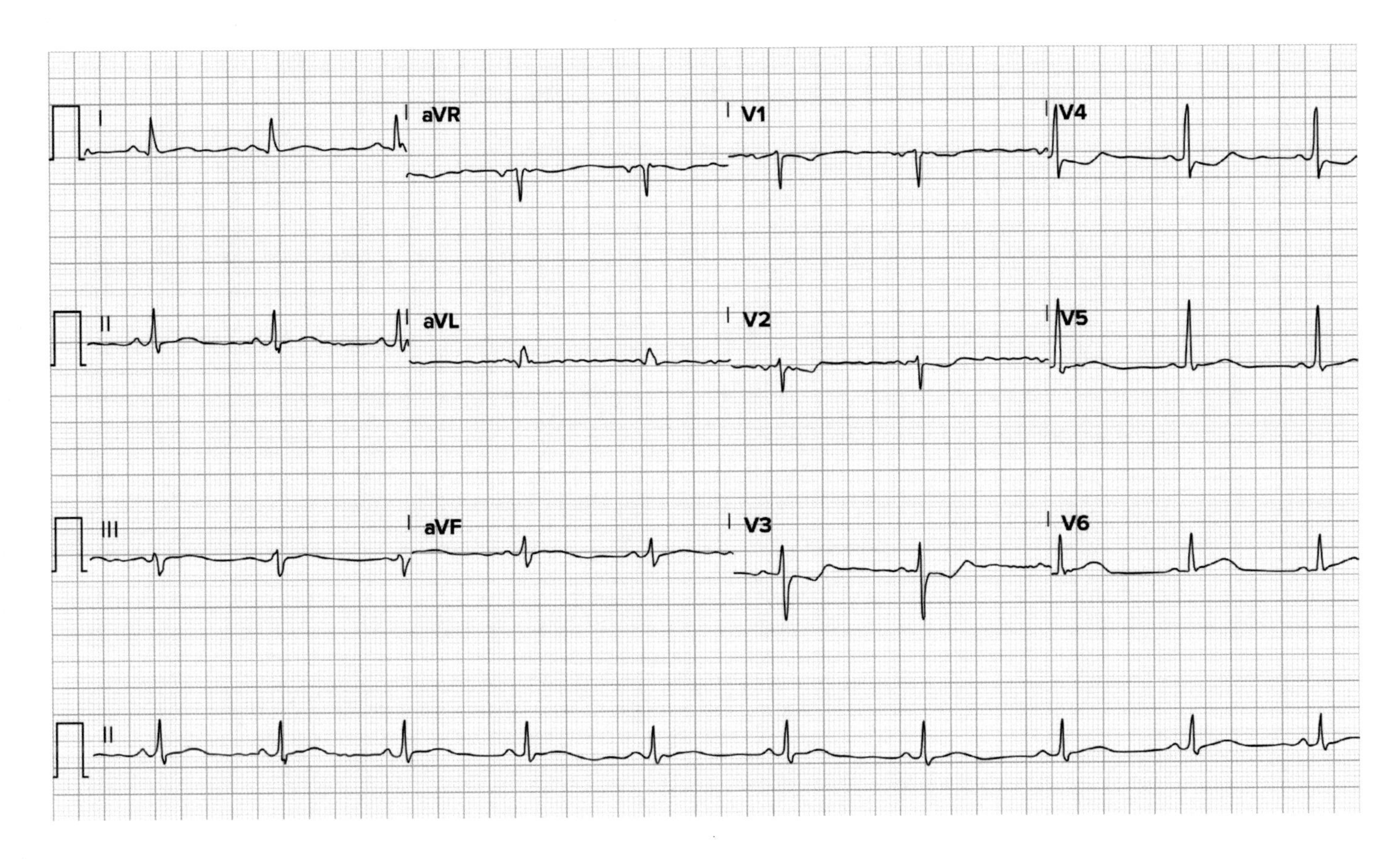

This ECG shows a normal sinus rhythm with ventricular rate of 60 bpm, normal axis, normal intervals, and subtle STD in leads V2-V4.

ACS symptoms with STD in leads V1, V2, V3, and/or V4 should prompt consideration of a posterior MI. A repeat ECG with posterior leads ***(see Figure 1)*** shows a normal sinus rhythm with a ventricular rate of 60 bpm, normal axis, STD in leads V2-V3, and STE in leads V7-V9. The STE in posterior leads V7-V9 is consistent with an isolated posterior MI.

Figure 1.
Repeat ECG with posterior leads V7-V9

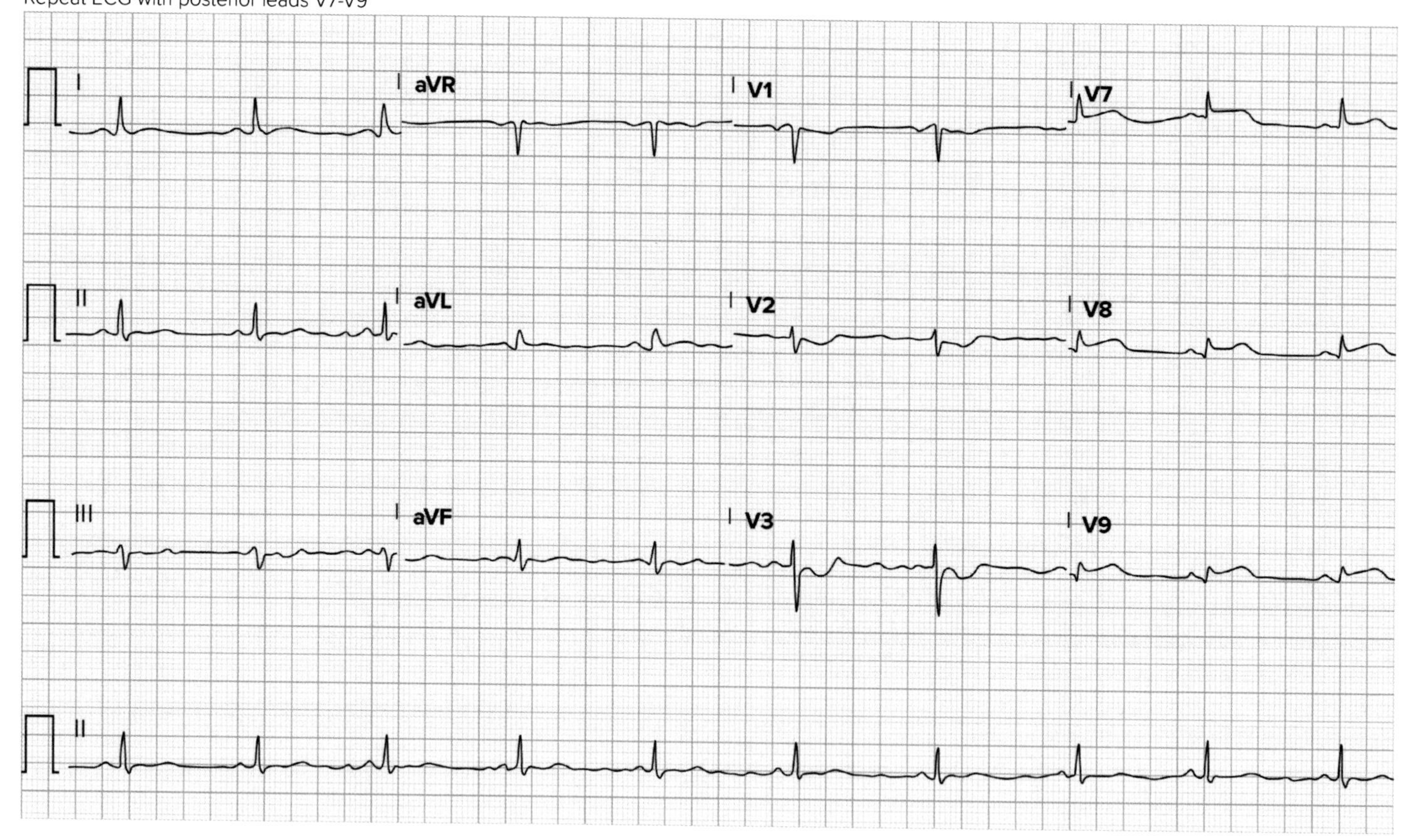

Isolated posterior, also called inferobasilar, MI are an easily missed diagnosis as they do not show STE with the standard 12-lead placement. Posterior MI are typically seen with a concurrent inferior or lateral MI, but an estimated 5% of MIs are isolated posterior MI (ie, in the absence of a concurrent AMI of the anterior, inferior, and/or lateral walls).

The key to interpreting the initial ECG is the STD in leads V2-V4. This finding, especially when seen with concurrent prominent R-waves and/or upright T-waves in these leads, is concerning for a posterior MI. The use of posterior leads is recommended but not mandated for the diagnosis of an isolated posterior MI, so local practice patterns typically dictate whether a posterior ECG is required for activation of the cardiac catheterization lab. If there is any diagnostic uncertainty about STD in leads V1-V4, it is recommended to record an ECG using posterior leads.[1] For most 12-lead ECG machines, this involves moving leads V4-V6 to the left posterior chest wall of the patient and renaming them V7-V9 ***(see Figure 2)***.

Figure 2.
Placement of posterior leads V7-V9

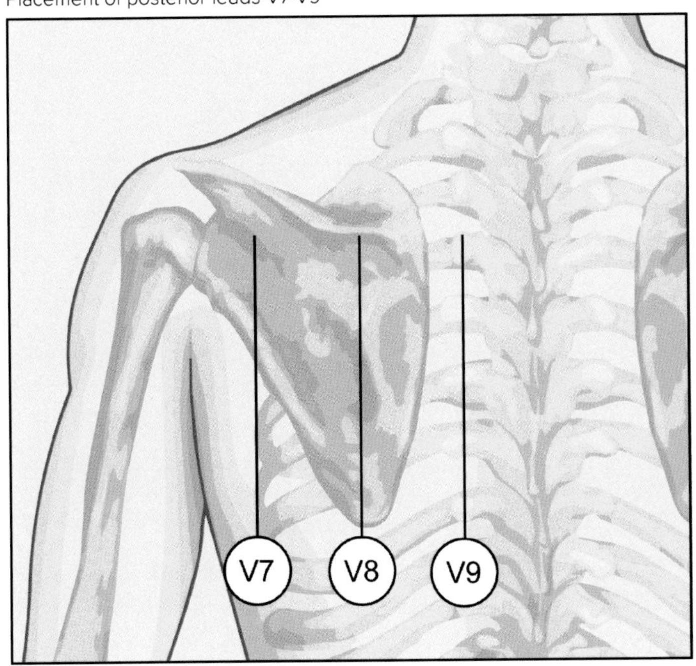

The diagnostic criteria for a posterior MI[1] differ from traditional STEMI criteria in two important ways:

- There only needs to be STE in 1 posterior lead
- STE only needs to be ≥ 0.5 mm (except for men < 40 years old, for whom the cutoff is ≥ 1 mm)

This patient was taken to the catheterization laboratory where a 100% occlusion of the left circumflex artery was successfully treated with a stent.

Posterior MI Learning Points

- Consider whenever there is STD in leads V1-V4, especially if there are concurrent prominent R-waves and/or upright T-waves in these leads
- Use posterior leads V7-V9 to evaluate for posterior MI if there is diagnostic uncertainty regarding STD in leads V1-V4
  - V7: left posterior axillary line at the 5th intercostal space
  - V8: left midscapular line at the 5th intercostal space
  - V9: left paraspinal border at the 5th intercostal space
- STE ≥ 0.5 mm (≥ 1 mm for men < 40 years old) in posterior leads V7, V8, or V9 is diagnostic
  - Does not require 2 contiguous leads

References

1. Thygesen K, Alpert JS, Jaffe AS, et al. 2018 ESC/ACC/AHA/WHF Expert Consensus Document: Fourth Universal Definition of Myocardial Infarction (2018). Circulation. 2018;138:e618-e651.

Case 62: Presentation

A 36-year-old male presents with nausea, vomiting, tremulousness, and palpitations due to alcohol withdrawal. What is your interpretation of his ECG?

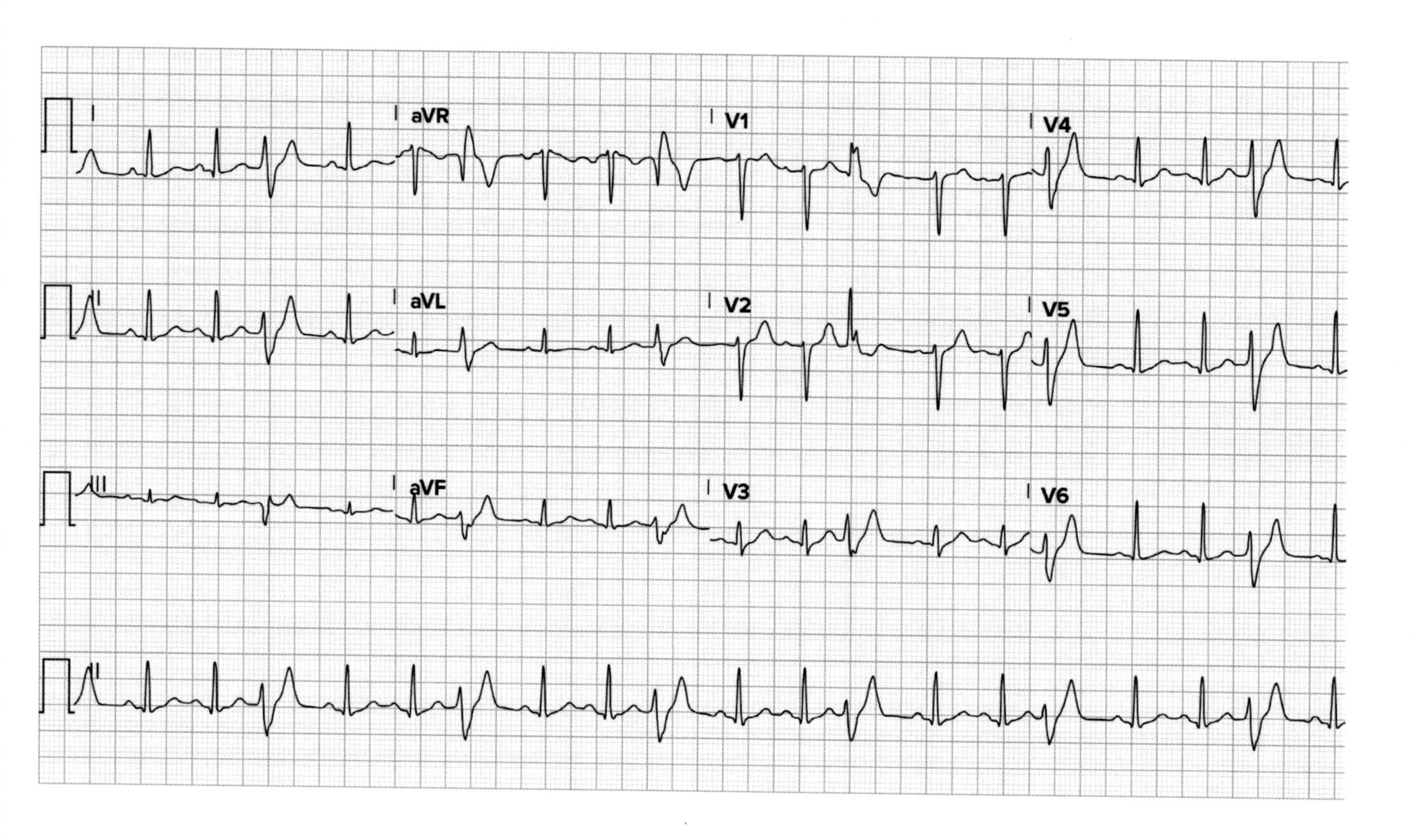

Case 62: Answer

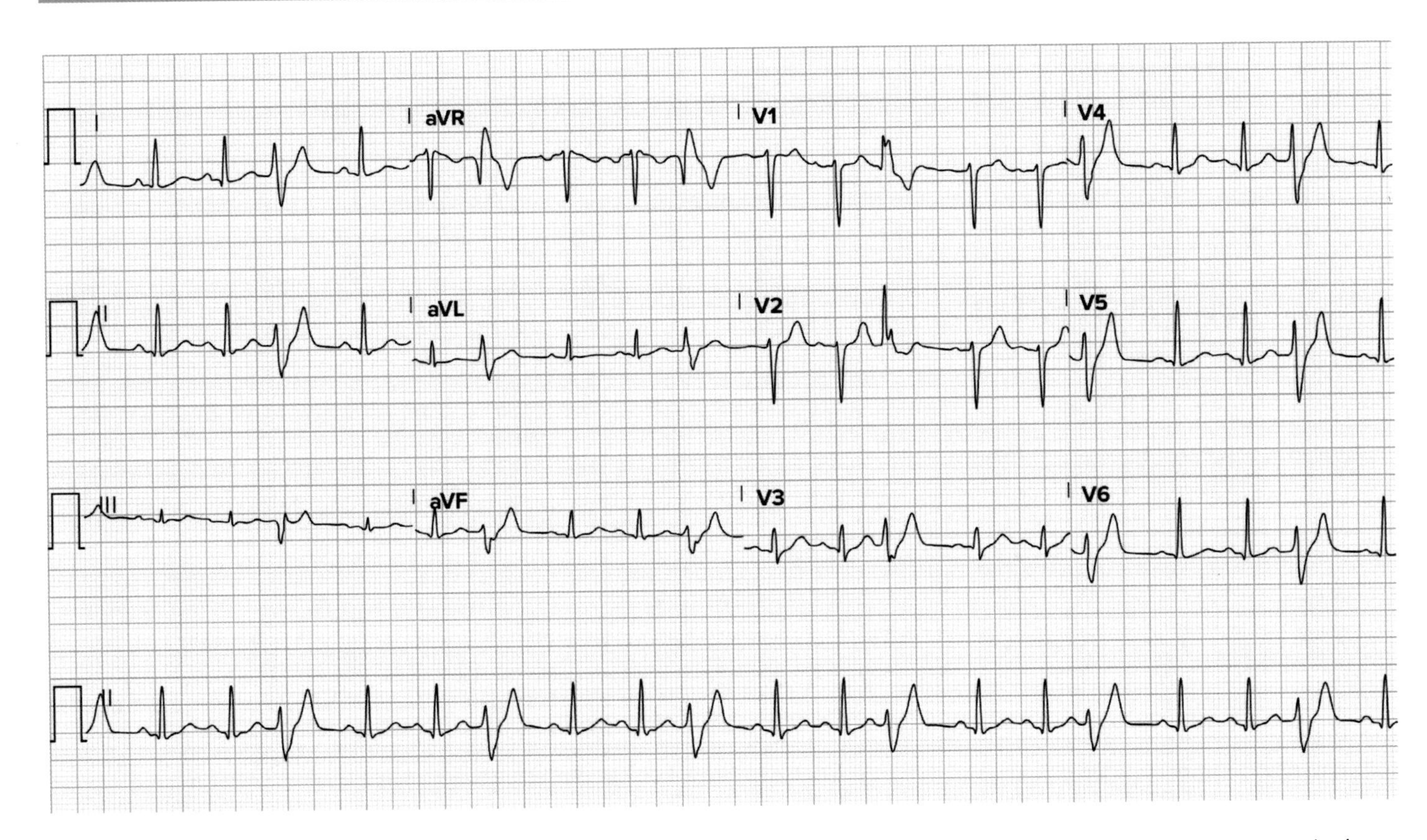

This ECG shows a sinus tachycardia with a ventricular rate of 115 bpm and ventricular trigeminy with premature ventricular complexes (PVCs).

The differential diagnosis for an irregular narrow-complex tachycardia includes:

- Atrial fibrillation
- Atrial flutter with variable block
- Atrial tachycardia with variable block
- Multifocal atrial tachycardia (MAT)
- Sinus tachycardia with irregular pattern of PAC, PJC, and/or PVC
- Sinus tachycardia with regular patterns of PAC, PJC, and/or PVC (bigeminy, trigeminy, etc.)

Ventricular trigeminy is the pattern of a PVC every 3rd beat ***(see Figure 1)***. A PVC is a wide- complex (≥ 120 msec) premature beat from a ventricular focus with no preceding P-wave. It is also called a ventricular premature beat (VPB).

Figure 1.
The lead II rhythm strip shows a pattern of 2 sinus beats followed by a PVC, consistent with ventricular trigeminy

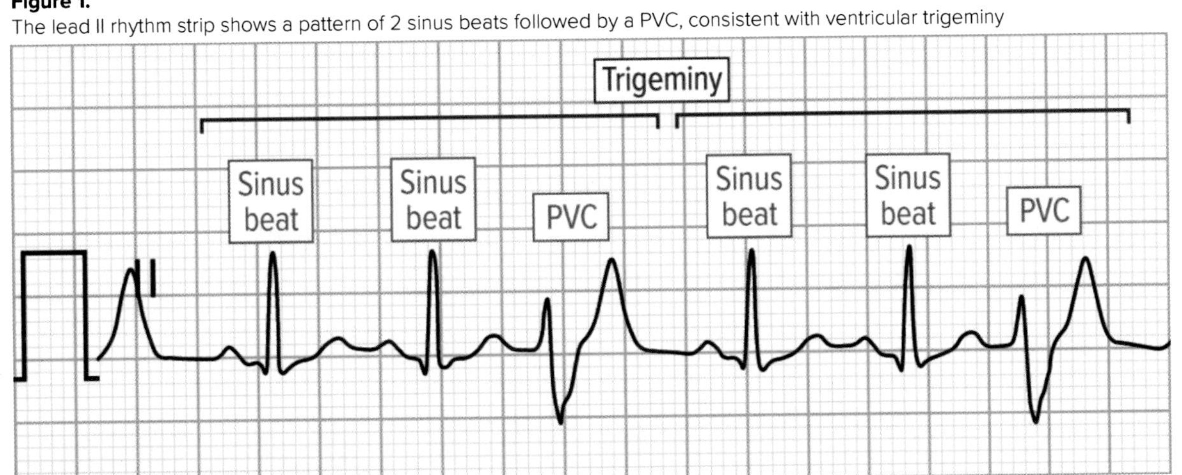

The two types of PVCs are named based on the location of the ventricular focus:

- Premature complexes originating from the left ventricle produce a RBBB-like pattern and are more likely to precipitate ventricular fibrillation
- Premature complexes originating from the right ventricle produce a LBBB-like pattern and are commonly seen in normal hearts

Left ventricular PVCs will often have an RSr' pattern in lead V1 (ie, the first peak is taller than the second peak, ***see Figure 2***) and an rS pattern in lead V6 (ie, the S-wave is bigger than the R-wave, ***see Figure 3***).

Figure 2.
Rsr' pattern in lead V1 frequently seen with left ventricular PVCs

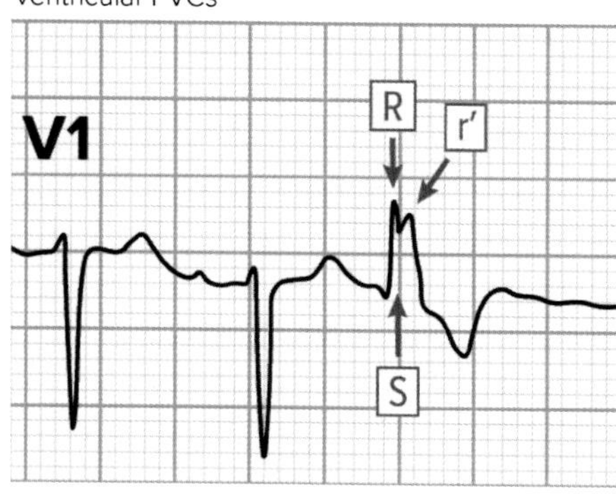

Figure 3.
rS pattern in lead V6 frequently seen with left ventricular PVCs

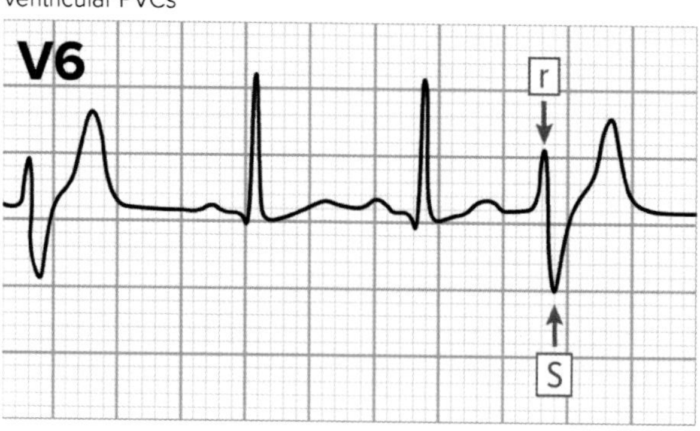

Classic teaching is that ventricular fibrillation is precipitated by PVCs that occur early in the cardiac cycle such that they occur on the T-wave of the preceding beat (ie, R-on-T, ***see Figure 4***), but ventricular fibrillation can also be triggered by PVCs late in the cardiac cycle. The highest risk of ventricular fibrillation from PVCs is in the early stages of a myocardial infarction, in the presence of hypokalemia, or with a prolonged QTc interval.

Figure 4.
R-on-T PVC- the R-wave of the PVC occurs at the same time as the T-wave of the preceding QRS complex (from a different ECG)

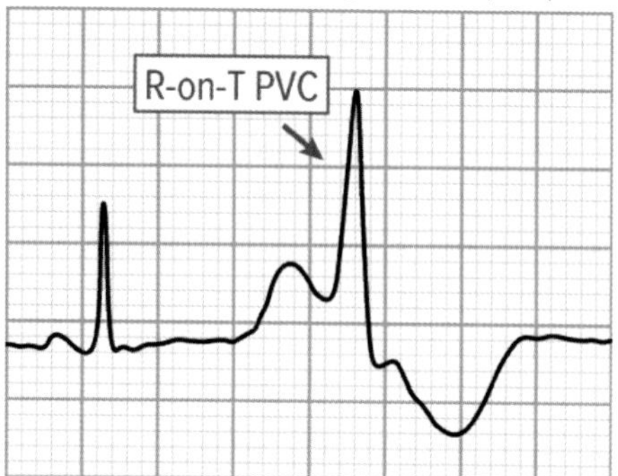

This patient was found to have a mild hypokalemia and hypomagnesemia, both of which were corrected in the ED. He required large doses of IV benzodiazepines to treat his alcohol withdrawal symptoms and was admitted to the internal medicine service.

PVC Learning Points

- Wide-complex (≥ 120 msec) premature beat from a ventricular focus with no preceding P-wave
  - Unifocal: arising from a single ectopic focus, so each PVC is identical in any single lead
  - Multifocal: arising from ≥ 2 ectopic foci, so multiple PVC morphologies in any single lead
  - Usually followed by compensatory pause
- Patterns include:
  - Bigeminy: every other beat is a PVC
  - Trigeminy: every 3rd beat is a PVC
  - Quadrigeminy: every 4th beat is a PVC
  - Couplet: two consecutive PVCs
  - Triplet: three consecutive PVCs
- Clinical significance includes:
  - Right ventricular PVCs: LBBB-like morphology, not necessarily pathologic
  - Left ventricular PVCs: RBBB-like morphology, usually pathologic, more likely to precipitate ventricular fibrillation
  - R-on-T PVC: PVC falls on T-wave of normal beat and can precipitate ventricular fibrillation

Case 63: Presentation

A 64-year-old female with no known cardiac history presents with palpitations and lightheadedness. What is your interpretation of her ECG?

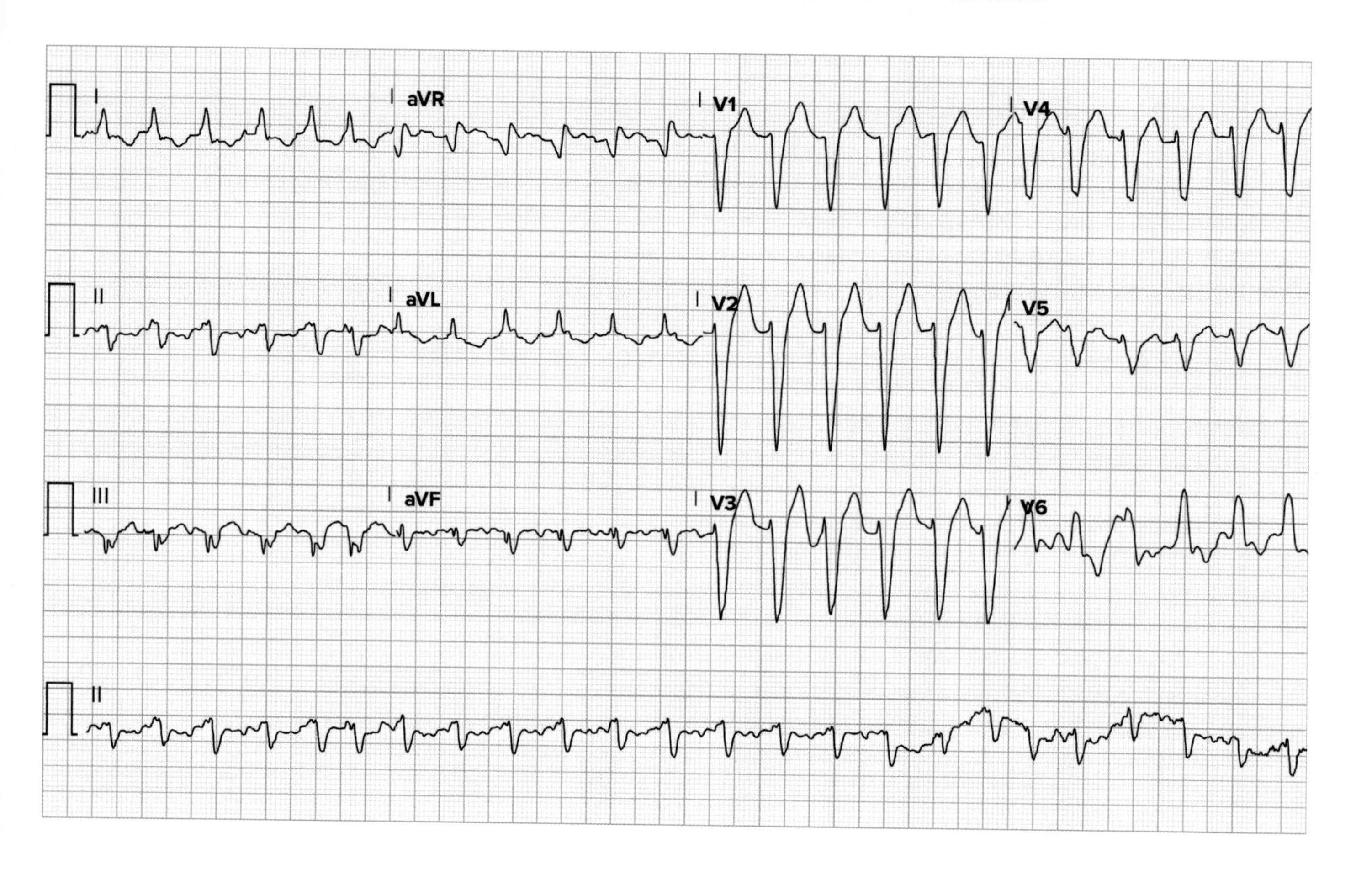

Case 63: Answer

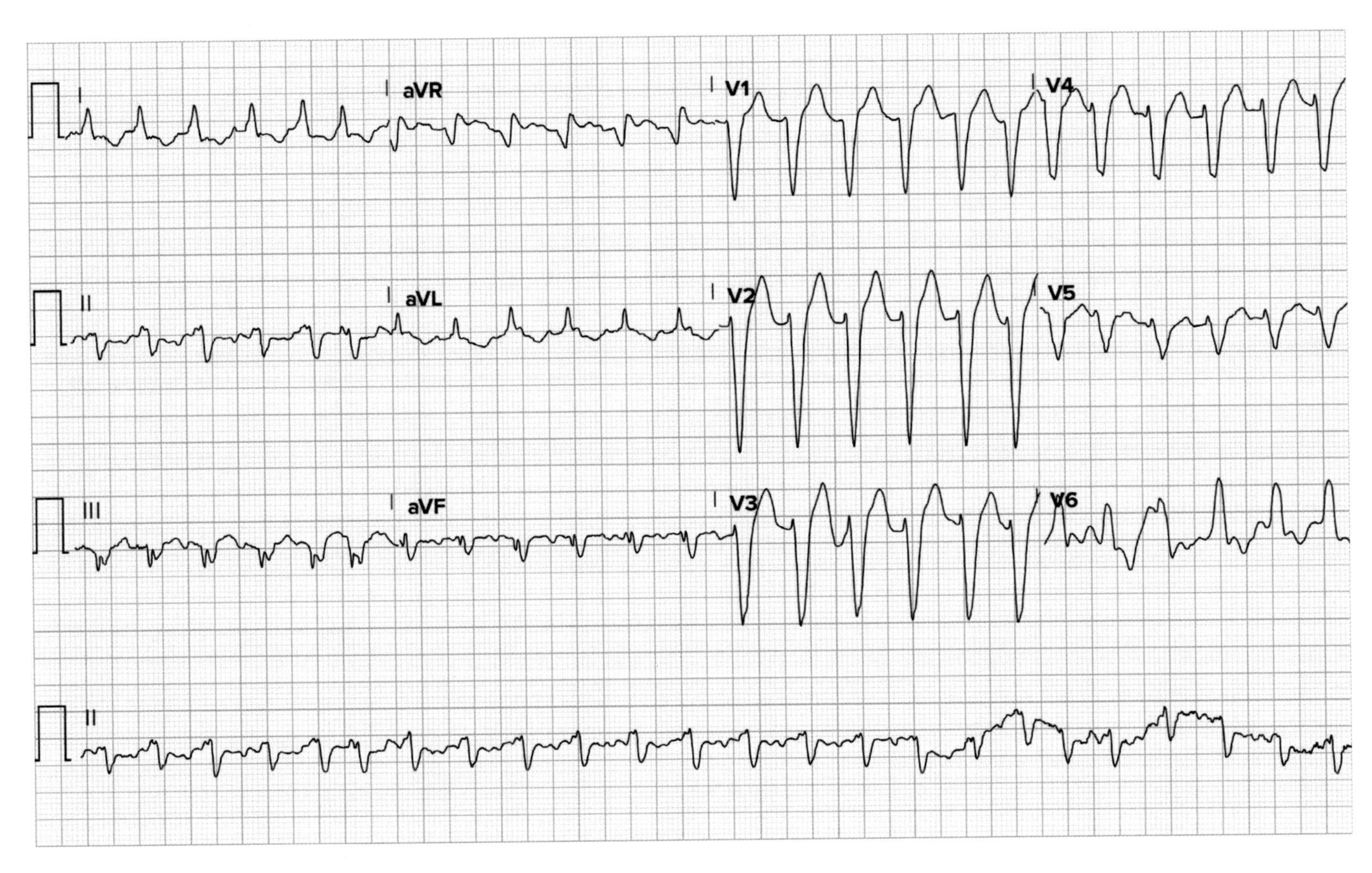

This ECG shows an irregularly irregular wide complex tachycardia with an average ventricular rate of 144 bpm and no P-waves, left axis deviation, and a prolonged QRS complex duration with a LBBB.

The differential diagnosis for an irregular WCT includes:

- Ventricular fibrillation
- Polymorphic ventricular tachycardia (including torsades de pointes)
- MAT with aberrant conduction
- Atrial flutter with variable block and aberrant conduction
- Atrial fibrillation with aberrant conduction
  - Causes of aberrant conduction include fixed or rate-related BBB, metabolic abnormalities, sodium channel blocker toxicity, ventricular-paced rhythm, and ventricular pre-excitation (eg, WPW)

The consistent QRS complex morphology rules out polymorphic VT and ventricular fibrillation, and the absence of P-waves rules out MAT. The variability in the ventricular rate is random and does not fit the whole number ratios expected with atrial flutter with variable block. The absence of P-waves and the irregularly irregular rhythm is consistent with atrial fibrillation.

The cause of the prolonged QRS complex duration in this ECG is a LBBB. This patient had no prior ECGs for comparison, so it may be rate-related (ie, it should resolve with rate control) or fixed (ie, it will persist regardless of rate). Rate-related bundle branch blocks happen when one of the bundles is still in its refractory period when the impulse is conducting to the ventricles. The common form is tachycardia-dependent BBB but there is also bradycardia-dependent BBB.

The characteristic findings in a LBBB include:

- QRS complex duration ≥ 120 msec
- Dominant S-wave in leads V1, V2, and frequently V3 ***(see Figure 1)***
- Broad and notched or slurred R-wave in leads I, aVL, V5, and V6 ***(see Figures 2 and 3)***
- Absent Q-waves in leads I, V5, and V6 (can see small Q-wave in lead aVL)

- R-wave peak time > 60 msec in leads V5 and V6 but normal in leads V1-V3 ***(see Figure 3)***
- Axis usually normal or leftward
- ST segments follow the "Rule of Appropriate Discordance"
  - ST-segment deviation in the opposite direction from the QRS complex ***(see Figures 1, 2 and 3)***

Figure 1.

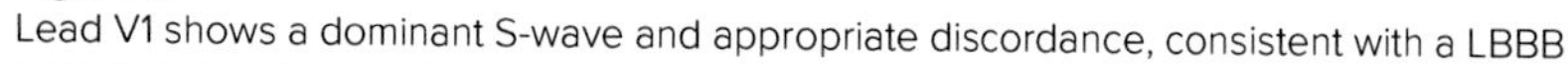
Lead V1 shows a dominant S-wave and appropriate discordance, consistent with a LBBB

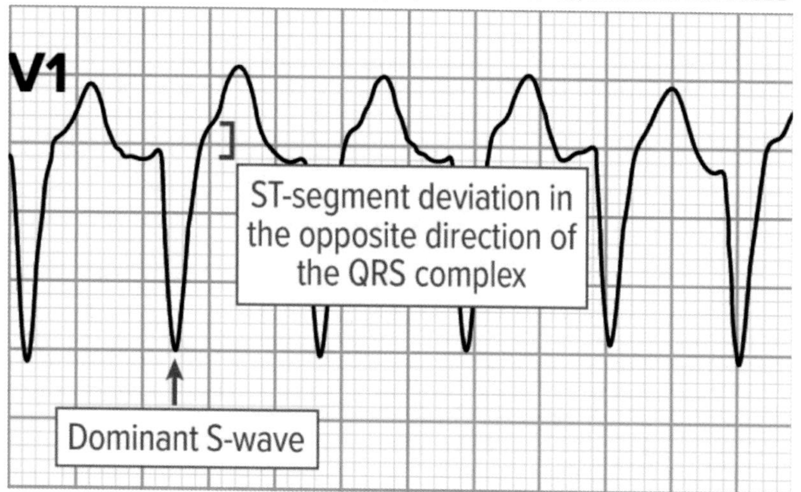

Figure 2.

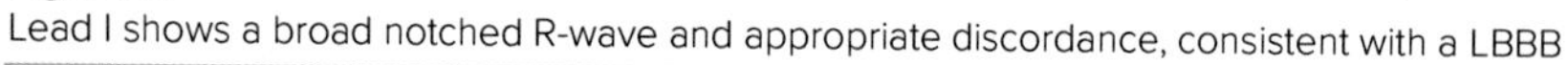
Lead I shows a broad notched R-wave and appropriate discordance, consistent with a LBBB

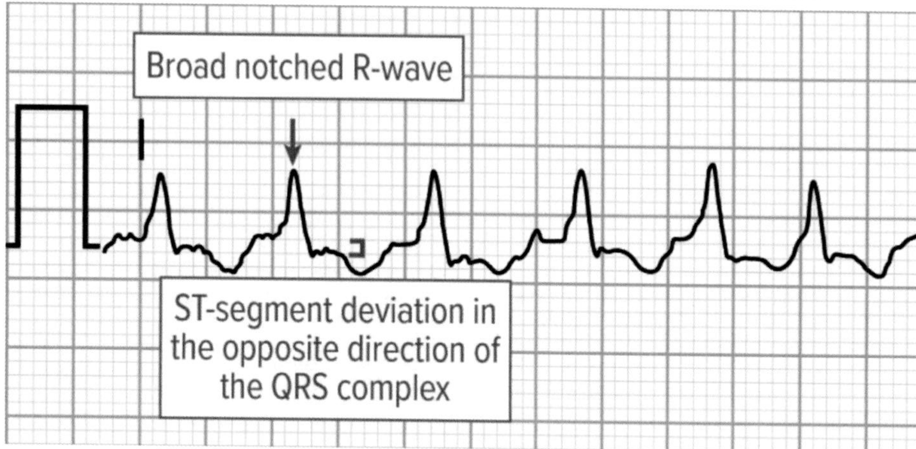

Figure 3.
Lead V6 shows a broad slurred R-wave, R-wave peak time > 60 msec, and appropriate discordance, consistent with a LBBB

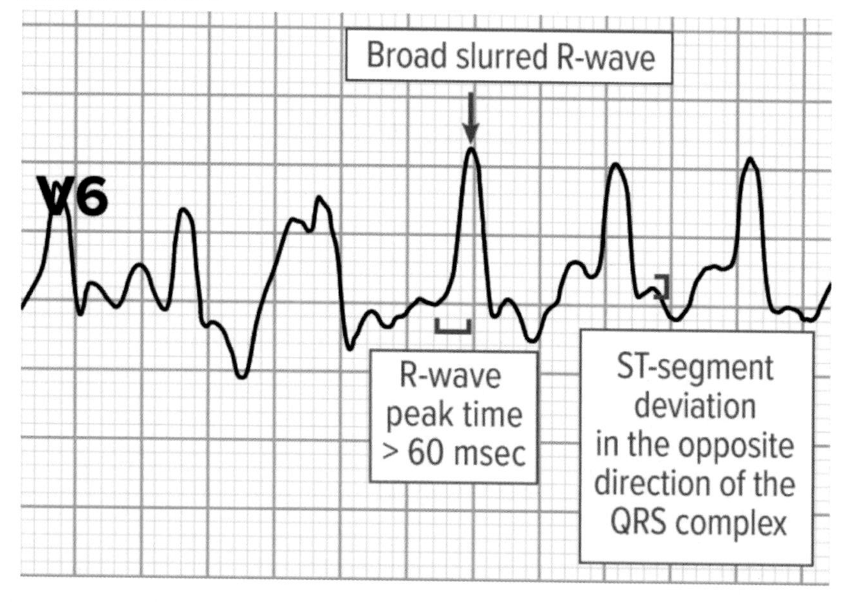

A defining feature of a LBBB is the "rule of appropriate discordance" which describes the relationship between the direction of the QRS complex and its ST-segment. In other words, if the main vector of the QRS complex points up, there will be STD, and if the main vector of the QRS complex points down, there will STE. These repolarization abnormalities confound the ECG's ability to detect AMI and other ACS findings, so interpretation of the ECG with a LBBB in a presentation suggestive of ACS requires using the Sgarbossa criteria to diagnose an AMI.

The Sgarbossa criteria are based on the underlying principle that concordance and excessive discordance in a LBBB are abnormal. The criteria assign a point value for any concordant STE ***(see Figures 4a and 4b)*** or excessively discordant STE ***(see Figure 4c)***. A score ≥ 3 is 98% specific for an AMI, so the presence of criteria A or B are considered diagnostic of an AMI. Criterion C is only assigned 2 points, so the presence of just criterion C is not diagnostic of an AMI.

Figure 4a.
Sgarbossa criterion A- concordant STE ≥ 1 mm in ≥ 1 lead (5 points = diagnostic of AMI)

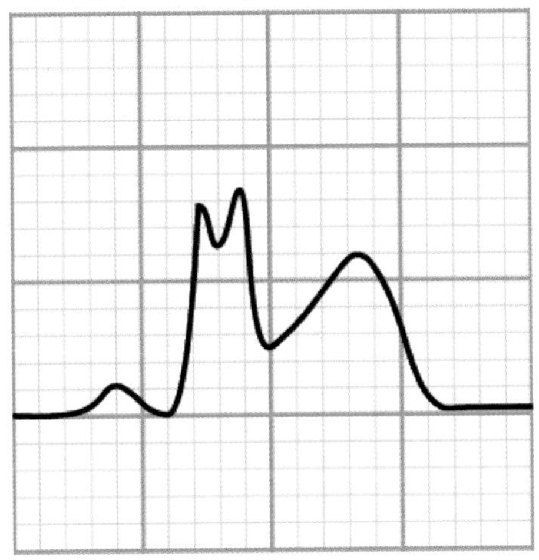

Figure 4b.
Sgarbossa criterion B- STD ≥ 1 mm in leads V1 or V2 or V3 (3 points = diagnostic of AMI)

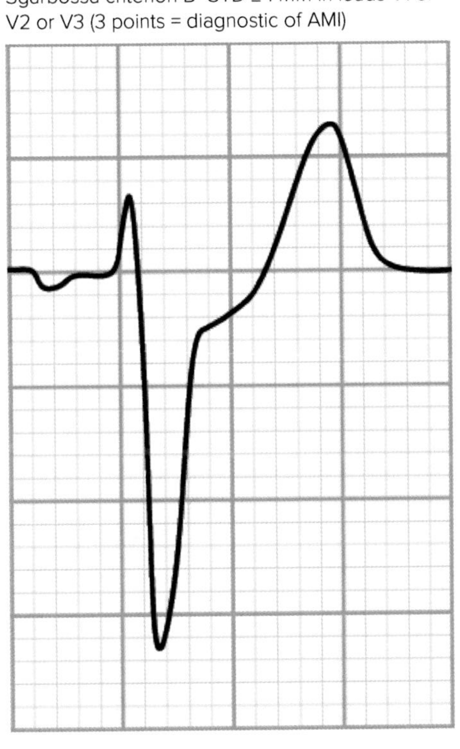

Figure 4c.
Sgarbossa criterion C- discordant STE ≥ 5 mm in ≥ 1 lead (2 points = not diagnostic of AMI)

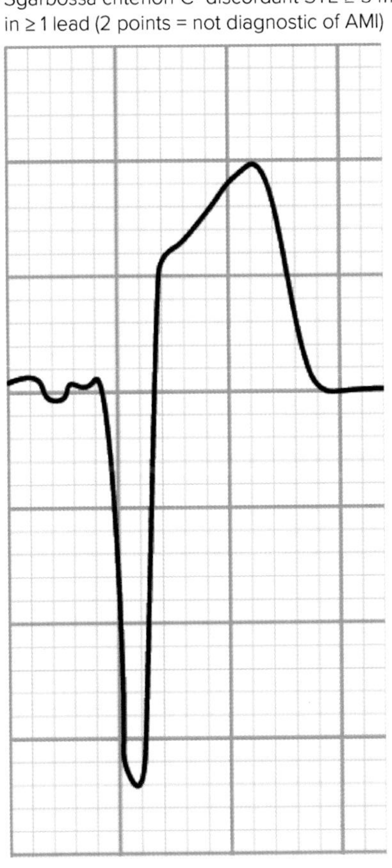

The Modified Sgarbossa criteria includes Sgarbossa criteria A and B with a variation of criterion C. Instead of using a fixed cutoff of 5 mm for discordant STE, it uses a ratio of the STE height to the S-wave depth ***(see Figure 5)***. An STE/S ratio ≥ 0.25 in ≥ 1 lead is considered diagnostic of an AMI. This means that more than 5 mm of STE is permissible if there is a large S-wave, and less than 5 mm of STE may be diagnostic if the accompanying S-wave is small. The Modified Sgarbossa criteria are not mandated in the current AHA/ACC STEMI guidelines.

This patient had an unremarkable ED workup and due to the uncertainty regarding the onset of new atrial fibrillation, the patient was treated with nodal blockers for rate control. The patient ultimately required a diltiazem drip and was admitted to the cardiology service.

Figure 5.
Modified Sgarbossa criterion C- STE/S ratio ≥ 0.25 in ≥ 1 lead (diagnostic of AMI but not mandated in current AHA/ACC STEMI guidelines)

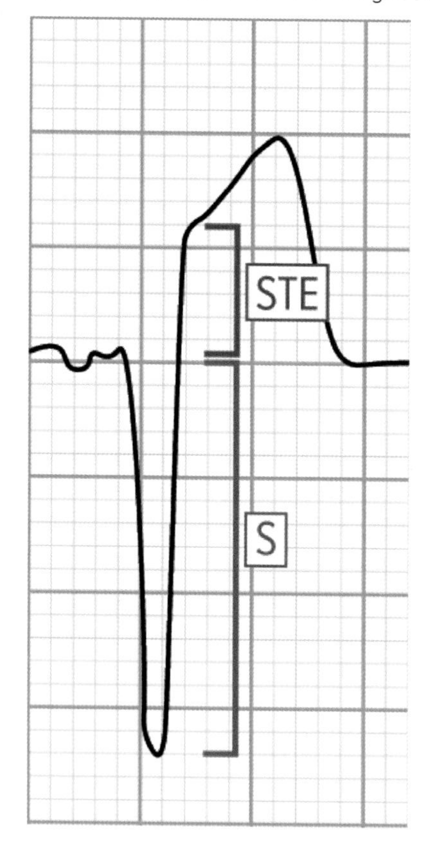

Atrial Fibrillation Learning Points

- Irregularly irregular rhythm with absence of any organized atrial activity
- ECG typically shows the absence of distinct repeating P-waves with:
  - Atrial depolarization rate typically > 300 bpm
  - Ventricular rates typically 100-200 bpm
  - Irregular RR interval when AV conduction is present (ie, there is no concurrent 3rd degree AV block)
- Untreated atrial fibrillation with ventricular rate < 100 bpm suggests significant AV node disease
- Consider atrial fibrillation with concurrent WPW if some QRS complexes are wide with variable morphologies and the ventricular rate is very rapid (eg, > 220 bpm)
  - The safest treatment for atrial fibrillation with suspected or confirmed WPW is IV procainamide or electrical cardioversion

LBBB Learning Points

- Ventricular depolarization from right to left (opposite of normal)
- ST segments follow the "Rule of Appropriate Discordance"
  - ST-segment deviation in the opposite direction from the QRS complex
- Confounds ECG's ability to detect AMI and other ACS findings
  - If ACS suspected, must use the Sgarbossa criteria to diagnose AMI
  - A presumed new LBBB in itself is no longer considered a STEMI equivalent, but is a high risk finding in ACS, so if AMI is suspected, urgent reperfusion therapy should be considered

Sgarbossa Criteria Learning Points

- Used to evaluate for STEMI in the presence of LBBB
- Based on "Rule of Appropriate Discordance"
  - In the absence of AMI, LBBB will have ST-segment deviation in the opposite direction from the QRS complex
  - Concordance and excessive discordance in LBBB are abnormal
- Concordant STE ≥ 1 mm in ≥ 1 lead or STD ≥ 1 mm in lead V1, V2, or V3 is considered diagnostic of AMI
- Modified Sgarbossa criteria
  - For discordant STE, a ratio of STE to S-wave depth ≥ 0.25 in ≥ 1 lead is considered diagnostic of AMI
  - Not mandated in current AHA/ACC STEMI guidelines

NOTES:

Case 64: Presentation

A 69-year-old female with history of pacemaker placement presents with fevers and productive cough. What is your interpretation of her ECG?

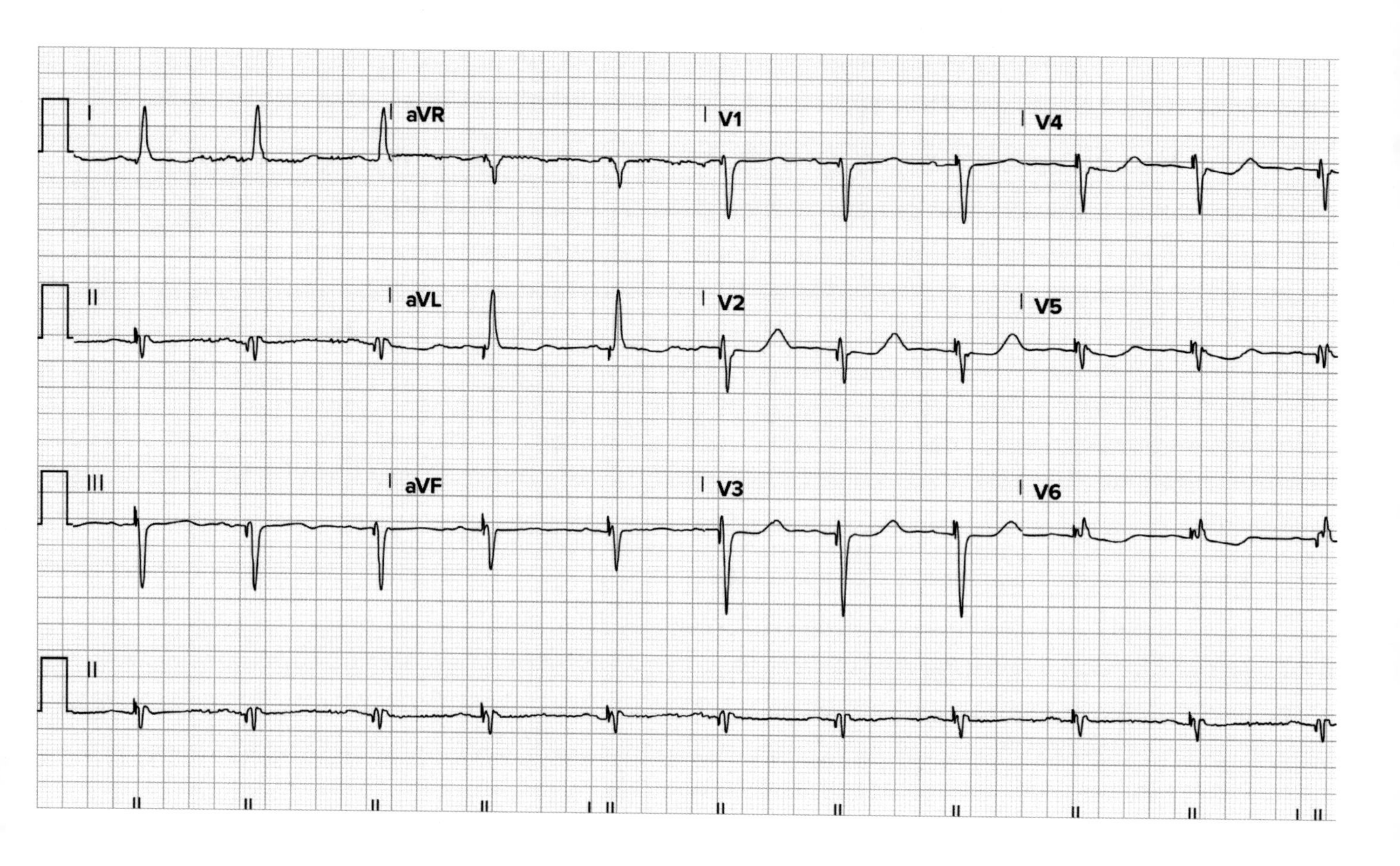

Case 64: Answer

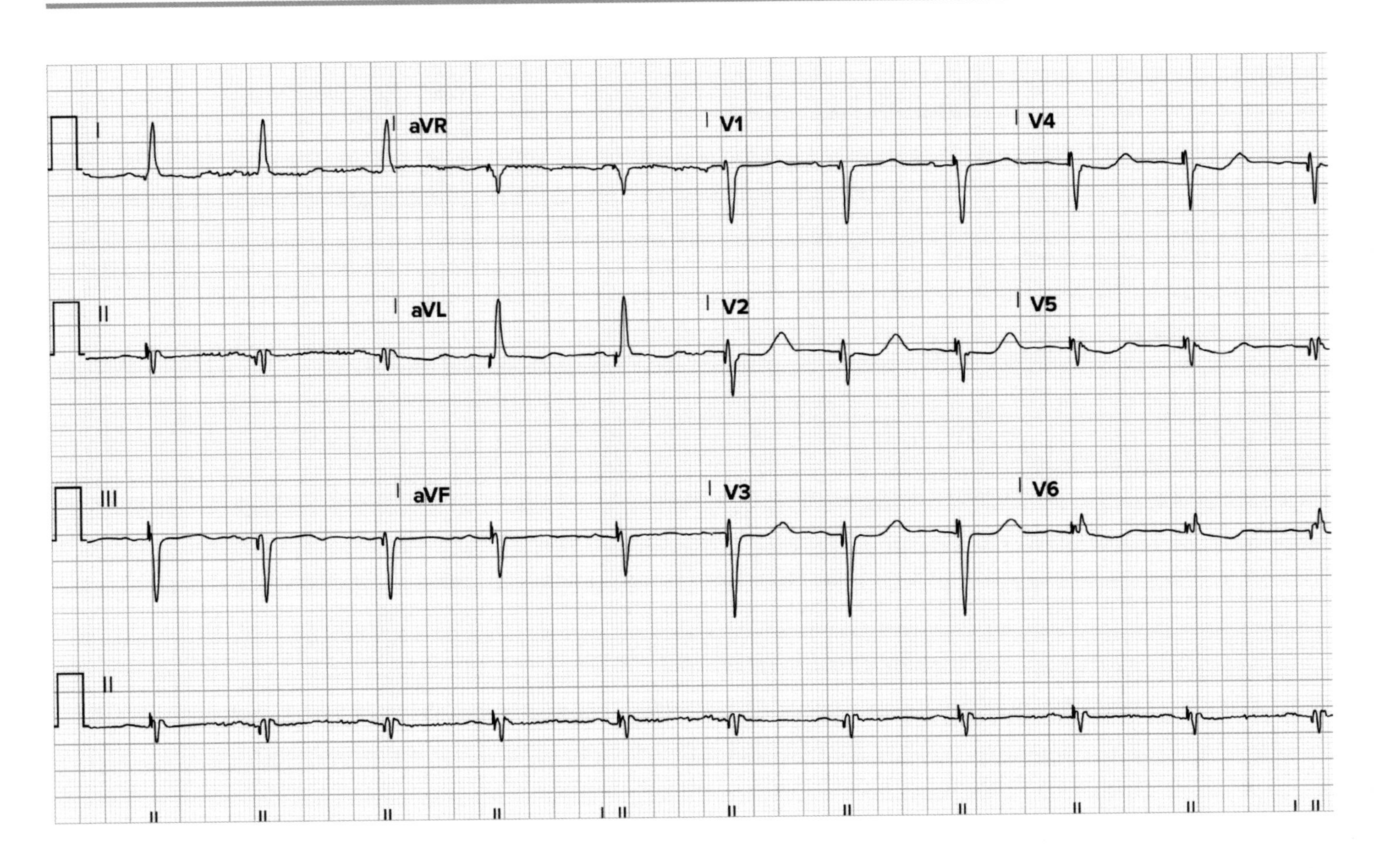

This ECG shows an atrial-sensed, biventricular-paced rhythm at a rate of 65 bpm, left axis deviation, prolonged PR interval, prolonged QRS duration at 140 msec with a LBBB morphology, STD in leads V2-V6, and failure to sense in beats 5 and 11.

Biventricular pacing, also known as cardiac resynchronization therapy, has one atrial lead and 2 ventricular leads:

- The right atrial lead paces the right atrial appendage (same as with right ventricular pacing)
- The RV lead paces the RV apex (same as with right ventricular pacing)
- The LV lead paces the surface of the posterior or lateral LV wall via the coronary sinus (ie, it is not inside the ventricle)

The biventricular-paced ECG will show 2 pacer spikes with a narrower QRS complex than with right ventricular pacing ***(see Figure 1)***. Since the LV lead is located outside of the ventricle, the pacemaker is typically programmed such that the LV lead will pace before the RV lead since it takes longer to depolarize the myocardium from the surface. There will often be a dominant R-wave in lead V1 +/- V2.

This pacemaker is programmed to sense native atrial activity, and if it does not detect native ventricular activity after a set amount of time, it will pace the ventricles ***(see Figure 1).***

Figure 1.
Atrial-sensed, biventricular-paced rhythm

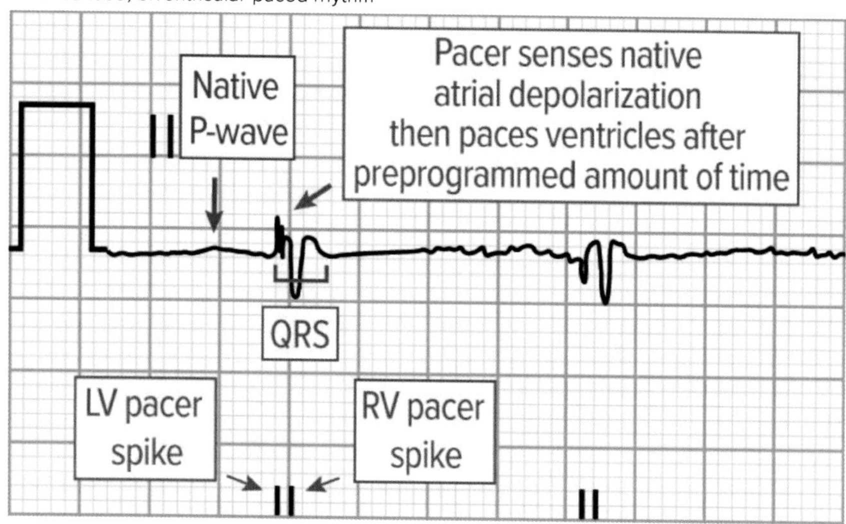

Biventricular pacers also have an atrial lead, which means they are dual chamber (ie, atria and ventricle) as well as biventricular, and are programmed to pace the atria if it does not detect native atrial activity in a programmed amount of time. If it does detect native atrial activity, it will not pace the atria.

This ECG also show failure to sense. The defining feature of failure to sense is asynchronous pacing. The pacemaker fails to detect native cardiac activity and inappropriately paces, often leading to a pacer spike during or after the P-wave or QRS complex. In this ECG, the pacemaker fails to detect the native P-wave before the 5th and 11th QRS complexes so it triggers an atrial pacer spike. The pacer spike occurs after the atria have already started to depolarize and results a pacer spike within the P-wave ***(see Figure 2)***. This is called asynchronous pacing. With normal pacing, the pacer spike should always immediately precede the P-wave or QRS complex.

Figure 2.
The lead II rhythm strip shows an atrial pacer spike within the P-wave, consistent with failure to sense

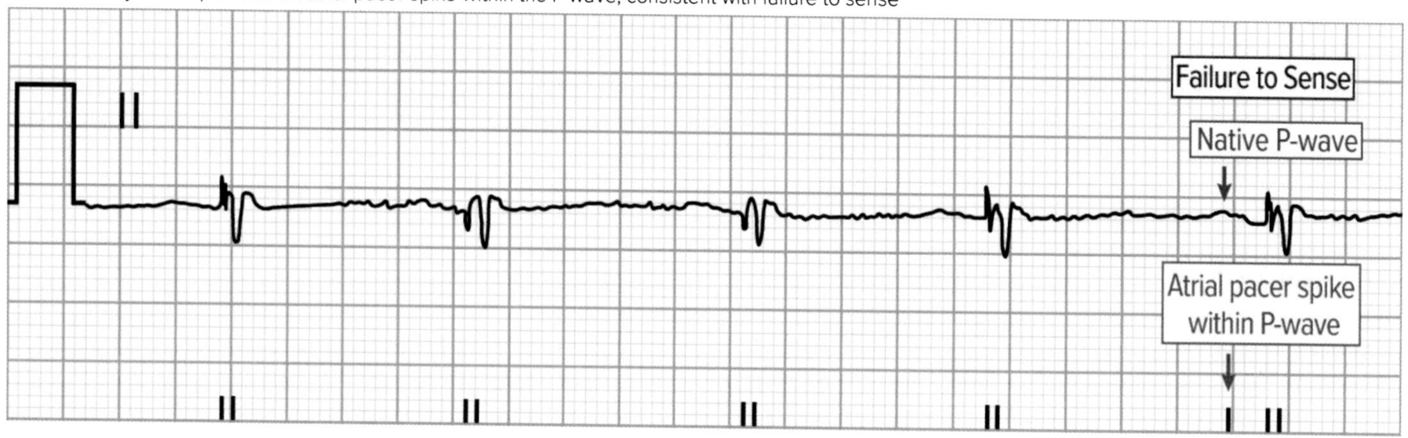

Common causes of failure to sense include lead insulation break, new intrinsic bundle branch block, electrolyte abnormalities (especially hyperkalemia)., and Class IC antidysrhythmics (eg, flecainide). Treatment is based on correcting the underlying etiology (eg, calcium for hyperkalemia) or reprogramming the pacer.

This patient was diagnosed with pneumonia and admitted to the internal medicine service for IV antibiotics. The pacer was interrogated during her admission and reprogrammed to prevent the failure to sense seen on her ECG. The etiology of the scooped STD in leads V2-V6 is likely due to the repolarization pattern inherent to the pacing as they were seen on prior ECGs and the patient was not on digoxin.

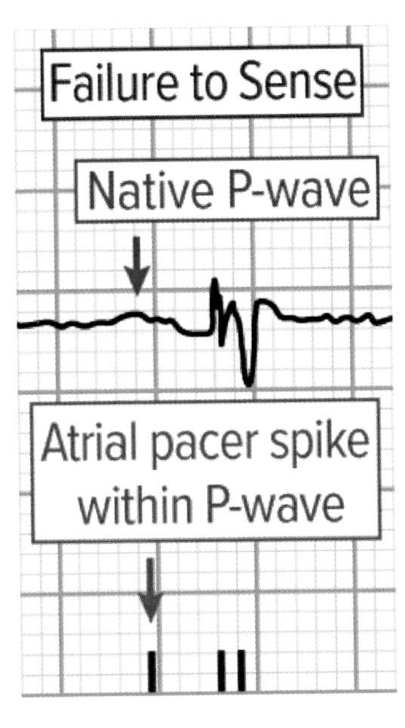

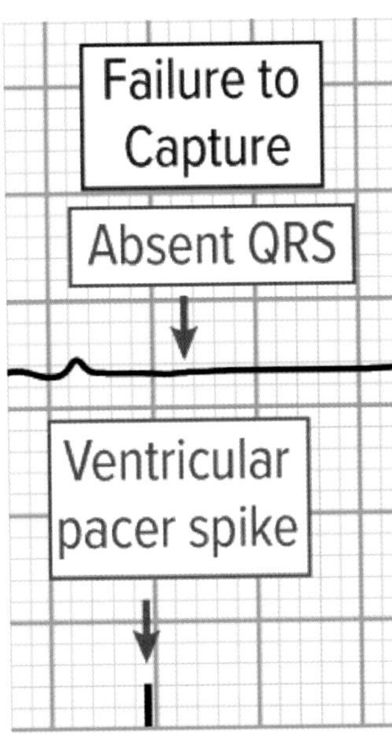

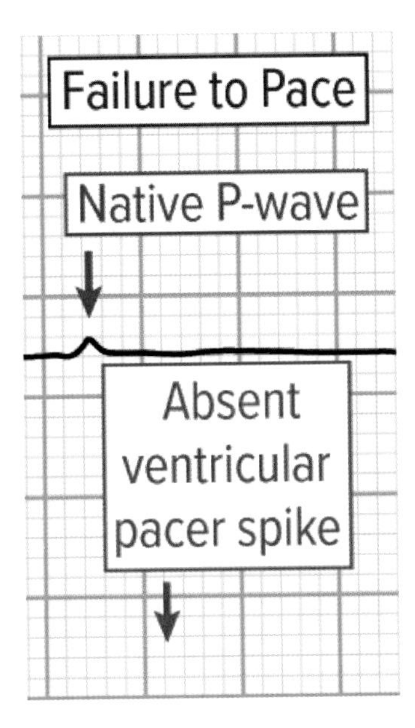

Pacemaker Learning Points

- Pacer spikes are usually visible on the ECG, either at the bottom of the ECG and/or preceding the P-wave and/or QRS complex
  - Atrial pacing: spikes immediately precede P-waves
  - Ventricular pacing: spikes immediately precede QRS complexes
  - Dual chamber pacing: spikes immediately precede both P-waves and QRS complexes
  - Biventricular pacing: 2 spikes immediately precede QRS complexes
- Atrial pacing
  - Pacemaker lead usually implanted in the right atrial appendage
  - Results in P-waves with normal morphology
- Right ventricular pacing
  - Pacemaker lead usually implanted in the RV apex
  - Results in a LBBB pattern in the limb leads and anteroseptal precordial leads
  - The major difference between an intrinsic LBBB and a right ventricular-paced rhythm is that the QRS complex will almost always be negatively oriented in leads V5-V6 with a right ventricular-paced rhythm
- Biventricular pacing
  - Two pacemaker leads usually implanted in the RV apex and the surface of the posterior or lateral LV
  - Typically results in a narrower QRS complex than with right ventricular pacing
  - Dominant R-wave in lead V1 +/- V2 is common
- AICD will have a thick coil that differentiates it from a pacemaker

Failure to Sense Learning Points

- Pacemaker fails to sense native cardiac activity → asynchronous pacing ***(see figure)***
  - Sensing refers to the pacer's ability to recognize native cardiac beats
- ECG shows pacer spikes before, after, or within P-waves and/or QRS complexes
- Causes include lead insulation break, new intrinsic bundle branch block, electrolyte abnormalities, and Class IC antidysrhythmics (eg, flecainide)

Failure to Capture Learning Points

- Delivery of pacing stimulus without subsequent myocardial depolarization ***(see figure)***
- ECG shows absence of depolarization after pacer spikes
- Causes include functional (eg, electrode displacement, wire fracture) and pathologic (eg, electrolyte disturbances, AMI)

Failure to Pace Learning Points

- Paced stimulus is not generated when expected ***(see figure)***
- ECG shows decreased or absent pacemaker function
- Causes include oversensing, lead fracture or insulation defect
  - Oversensing: pacing inhibited by non-cardiac activity (eg, skeletal muscle activity) inappropriately recognized as native cardiac activity

Case 65: Presentation

A 57-year-old female presents with generalized weakness and fatigue.
What is your interpretation of her ECG?

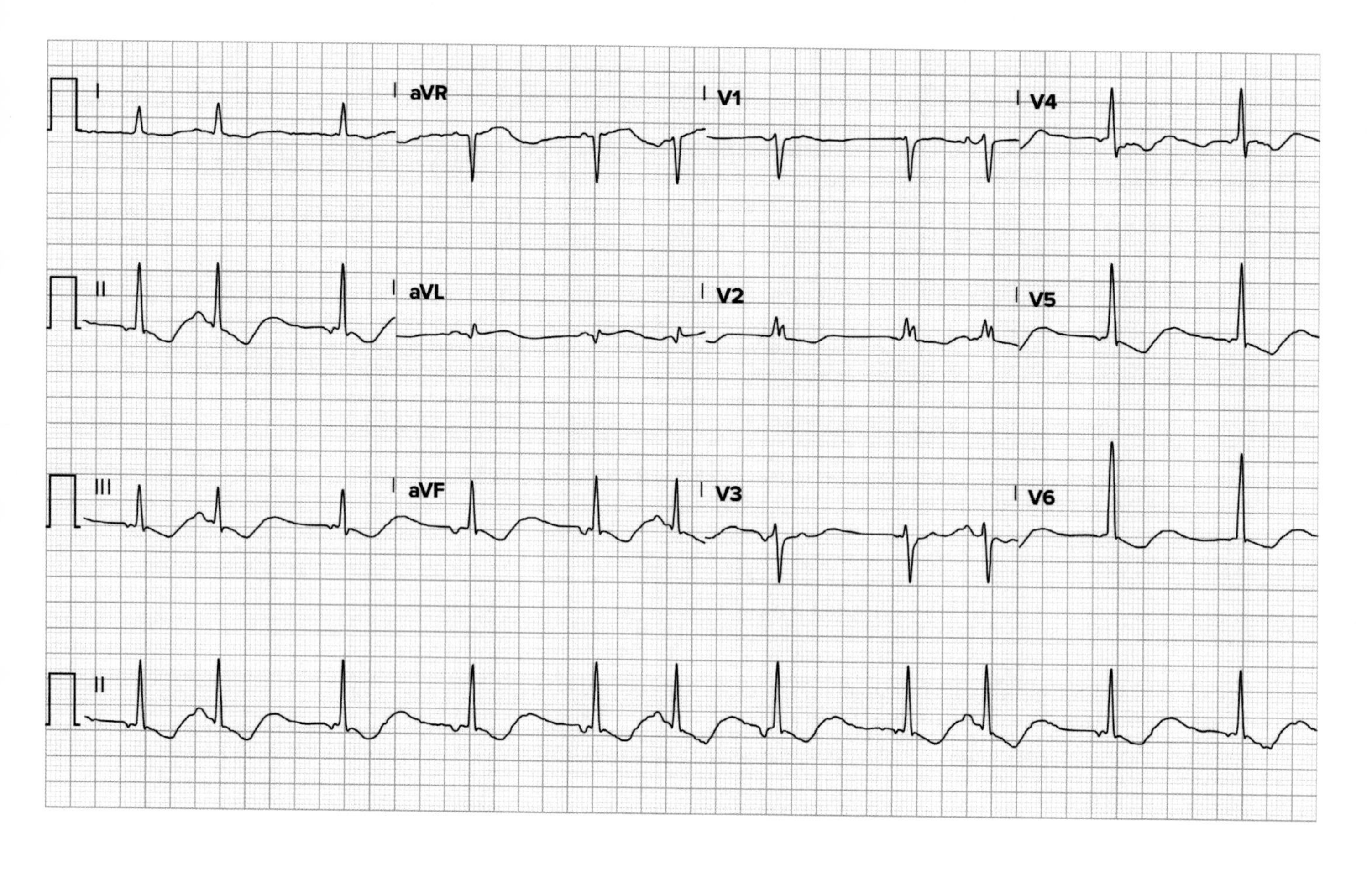

Case 65: Answer

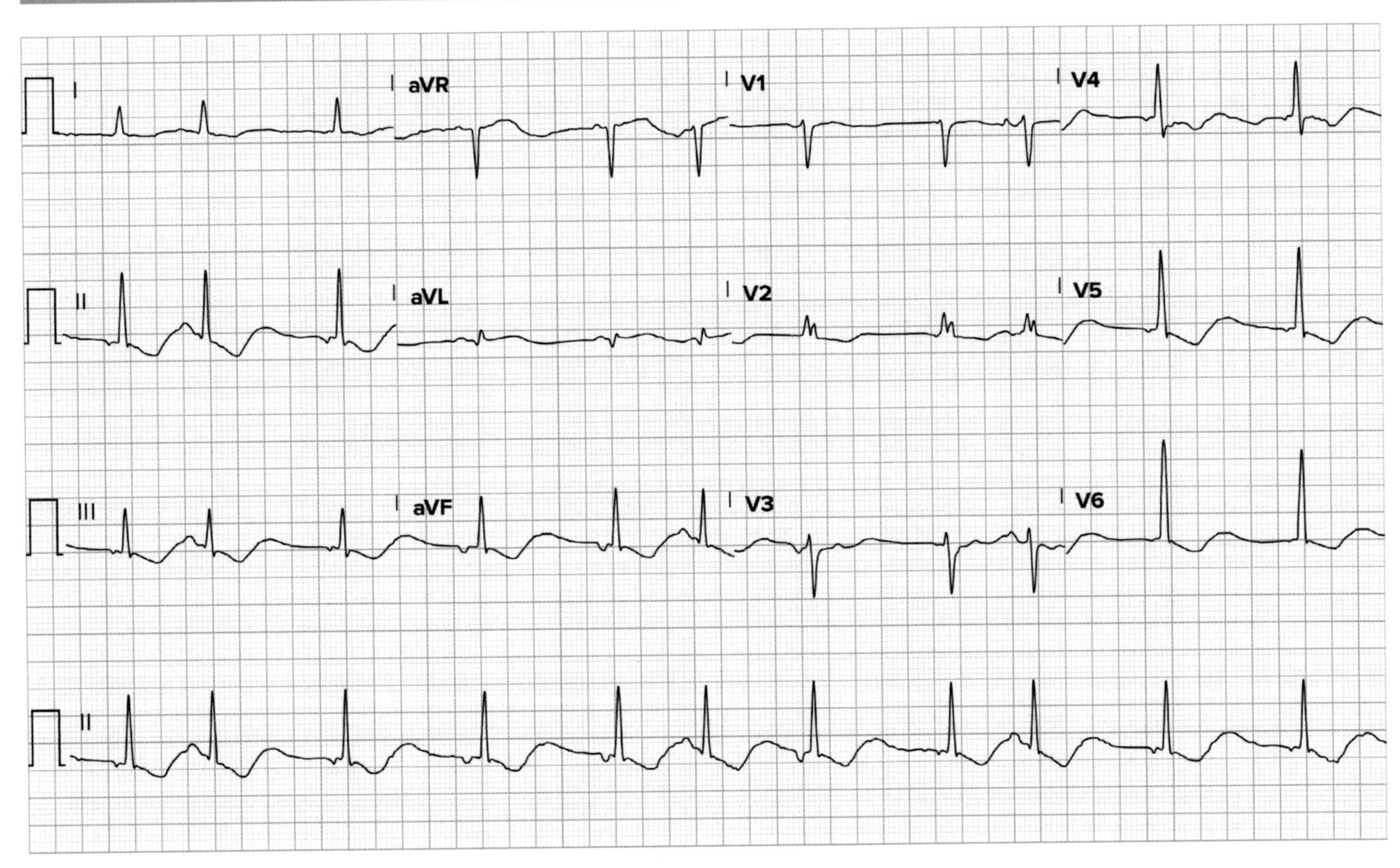

This ECG shows an irregular narrow complex rhythm an average ventricular rate of 66 bpm, variable P-wave morphologies and PR intervals, STE in lead aVL, inferolateral TWI and STD, U-waves best seen in leads II, III, aVF, and V3-V6. Although the QTc interval is normal when measured in lead aVL (where there is no U-wave), the QU interval (i.e., the QT interval that includes the U-wave) is long which is associated with a high risk for ventricular dysrhythmias, in particular torsades de pointes.

The differential diagnosis for an irregular narrow complex rhythm with normal ventricular rates includes:

- Atrial fibrillation (rate controlled)
- Atrial flutter with variable block (rate controlled)
- Atrial tachycardia with variable block (rate controlled)
- Wandering atrial pacemaker (also called multifocal atrial rhythm)
- 2nd degree AV block Mobitz types I and II
- Variable high-grade AV block (eg, 3:1, 4:1, etc.)
- 2nd degree sinoatrial block
- Sinus arrhythmia
- NSR or accelerated junctional rhythm with irregular pattern of PAC, PJC, and/ or PVC
- NSR accelerated junctional rhythm with regular patterns of PAC, PJC, and/ or PVC (bigeminy, trigeminy, etc.)

The key finding that significantly narrows the differential diagnosis for the rhythm in this ECG is the presence of 3 different P-wave morphologies that precede QRS complexes that all have the same morphology ***(see Figures 1 and 2)***. The "blue" (1st, 3rd, 8th, 10th, and 11th P-QRS-T complexes) and "red" (4th, 5th, and 7th P-QRS-T complexes) P-waves are both inverted in lead II which means that they are not sinus (see Learning Points at end of case). With the exception of beat 4, they also have PR intervals < 120 msec which can be seen with either an ectopic atrial rhythm near the AV node or a junctional rhythm with retrograde P-waves. The "green" P-waves (2nd, 6th, and 9th P-QRS-T complexes) are upright in lead II with a normal PR interval (ie, 120-200 msec), but is impossible to tell if these are sinus P-waves without a prior ECG for comparison.

Figure 1.
The lead II rhythm strip shows both sinus P-waves (green boxes) and non-sinus P-waves (red and blue boxes)

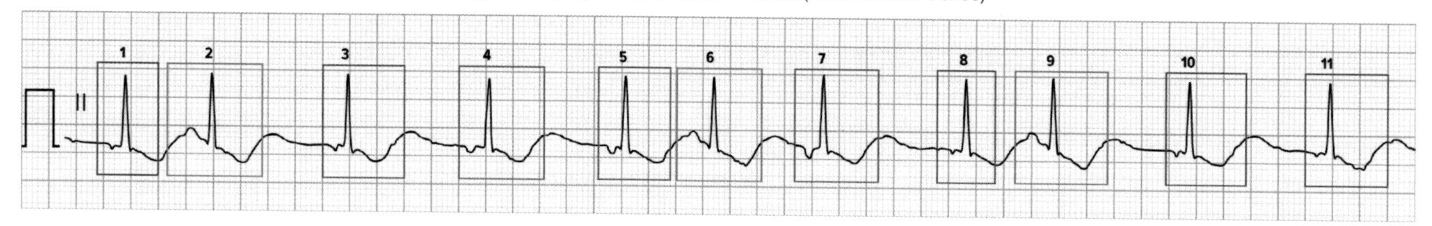

Figure 2.
The lead II rhythm strip shows 3 different P-wave morphologies (blue, green, and red boxes)

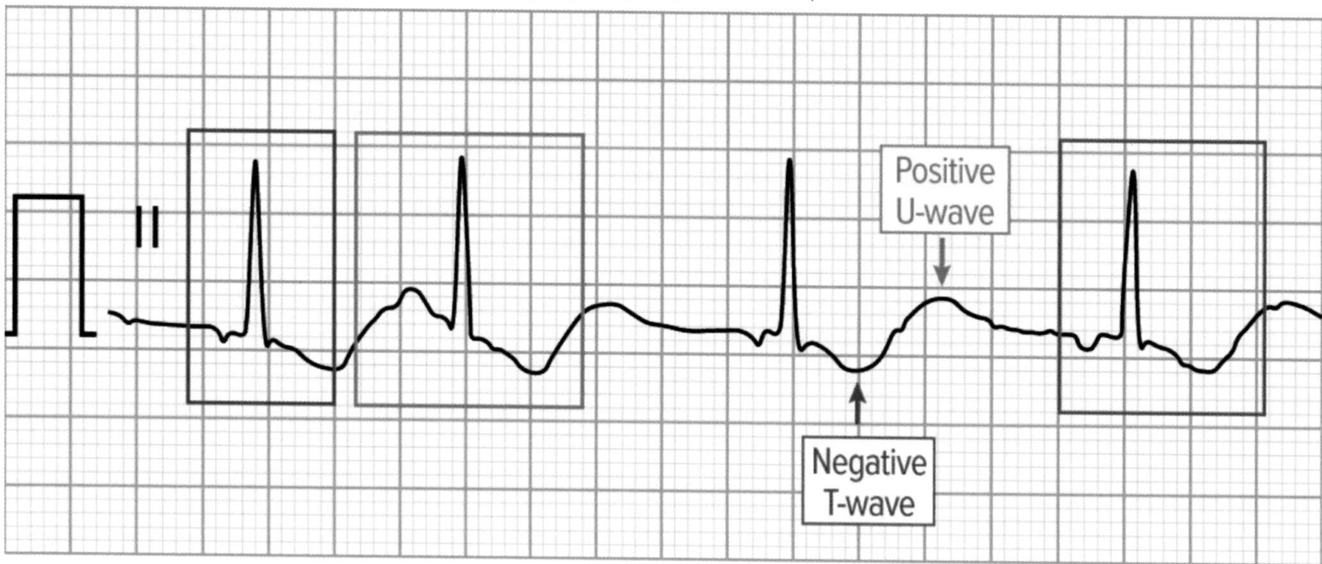

Without an electrophysiology study, it is impossible to determine the exact rhythm in this ECG. Two rhythm diagnosis possibilities include:

1. Wandering atrial pacemaker (WAP), also called multifocal atrial rhythm, which is MAT at a slower rate (≤ 100 bpm). While this ECG meets the P-wave criteria for WAP (≥ 3 different P-wave morphologies in a single lead with variable PR intervals), it does not appear irregularly irregular. P-QRS-T complexes 2-5, 7-8, and 8-11 are regular with RR intervals between 1000-1040 msec.
2. Accelerated junctional rhythm with PACs. The “blue” and “red” P-QRS-T complexes are junctional with 2 different retrograde conduction paths in the atria and the “green” P-QRS-t complexes are PACs from a supraventricular focus. However, beat 4 has a PR interval > 120 msec which is not typical for a retrograde P-wave associated with a junctional rhythm.

The ECG also shows the triad of TWI, STD, and U-waves that can be seen with severe hypokalemia. This can create a “reverse Wellens” pattern of a downward deflection followed by an upward deflection following the QRS complex ***(see Figure 3)***. This pattern has also been named “NikEleKam T-waves” by Amal Mattu (it’s a combination of his kids’ names). The U-waves often fuse with the T-waves, so the QT interval should be measured in a lead without U waves, typically lead aVL or aVR.

Figure 3.
"Reverse Wellens" pattern seen with hypokalemia

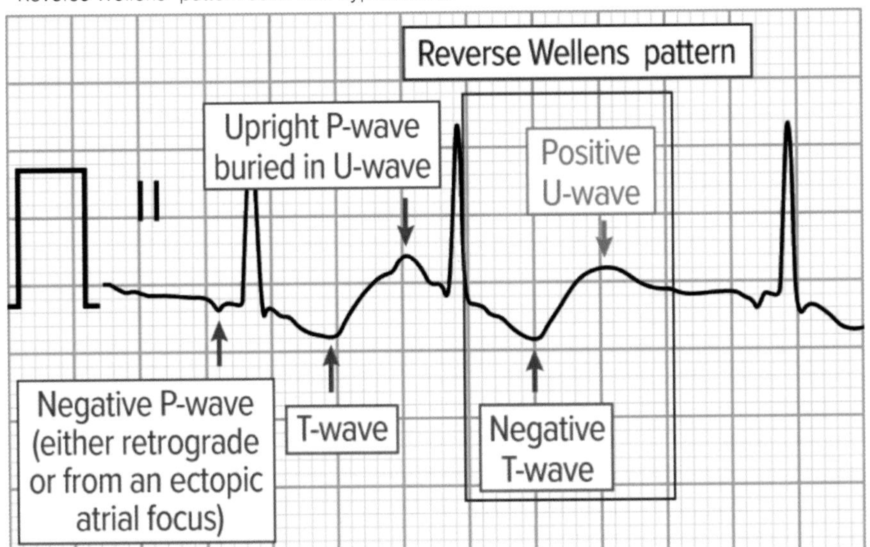

This patient's workup was notable for a serum potassium level of 1.4 mEq/L. This patient was treated with IV and oral potassium and admitted to the internal medicine service. The etiology of the STE in lead aVL is unclear but likely secondary to the severe hypokalemia, and not ischemia, as it resolved after the hypokalemia was corrected.

Normal P-wave and T-wave Learning Points

- Normal P-wave and T-wave morphologies[1] in normal sinus rhythm in the absence of conduction abnormalities, ischemia, structural abnormalities, etc., include:

I P: always upright T: always upright	**aVR** P: always inverted T: always inverted	**V1** P: usually biphasic (+/-) but can be entirely upright or inverted T: upright or inverted	**V4** P: upright T: almost always upright
II P: always upright T: always upright	**aVL** P: upright, inverted, or biphasic (-/+) T: upright or inverted	**V2** P: usually biphasic (+/-) but can be entirely upright (entirely inverted is rare) T: usually upright	**V5** P: upright T: always upright
III P: upright, inverted, or biphasic (+/-) T: upright or inverted	**aVF** P: usually upright but can be flat or biphasic T: usually upright	**V3** P: upright T: usually upright	**V6** P: upright T: always upright

- Inverted, flat, or positive-negative biphasic T-waves in lead V1 (less so in leads V2-V3) can be normal
- Positive-negative biphasic T-waves in leads V1-V3 can be abnormal or a normal variant
- T-wave amplitude is typically < 6 mm in limb leads and < 10 mm in precordial leads

Hypokalemia Learning Points

- ECG changes seen in hypokalemia include:
  - T-wave flattening or inversion
  - U waves
  - Slight STD
  - STE in lead aVR
  - Increased P-wave amplitude and duration
  - PR interval prolongation
  - QTc interval prolongation
  - Increased ectopy (eg, premature beats) and tachydysrhythmias

U Wave Learning Points

- U-waves are typically low-amplitude deflections that follow the T-wave, best seen in the anterior precordial leads at slower heart rates
- Clinical significance not fully understood
  - Can see U-waves larger than T-waves with moderate to severe hypokalemia
  - Inverted U-waves in leads V2-V5 is abnormal (seen with ischemia and hypertension)
- When measuring the QT interval, exclude U-waves or measure in a lead without U-waves (usually leads aVR or aVL)

MAT Learning Points

- Irregular tachycardia with ≥ 3 different P-wave morphologies in a single lead with variable PR intervals
  - Variable PP and RR intervals
  - QRS complexes are uniform in appearance
- Rate is typically between 101-180 bpm
  - If atrial rate ≤ 100 bpm, called multifocal atrial rhythm or wandering atrial pacemaker
- Typically seen with acute exacerbation of chronic cardiopulmonary disease

Ectopic Atrial Rhythm Learning Points

- Ectopic focus from the atria other than the SA node
- ECG shows ventricular rate 60-100 bpm with normal QRS complex duration unless concurrent conduction abnormality (eg, bundle branch block)
- P-waves with have different morphology/axis than sinus P-waves
- PR interval typically normal at 120-200 msec but can be < 120 msec if the focus is near the AV node

Junctional Rhythm Learning Points

- Ectopic focus from AV node or proximal Purkinje system
  - Also called AV junctional rhythm, nodal rhythm, nodal escape rhythm, junctional escape rhythm, AV nodal rhythm
- ECG shows ventricular rate of 40-60 bpm with normal QRS complex duration unless concurrent conduction abnormality (eg, bundle branch block)
- May have retrograde P-waves that precede (with PR interval < 120 msec) or follow QRS complex, typically best seen in the inferior leads
- Variations include:
  - Junctional Bradycardia: ventricular rate < 40 bpm
  - Accelerated Junctional Rhythm: ventricular rate 61–100 bpm
  - Junctional Tachycardia: ventricular rate > 100 bpm

References

1. Knilans T, Surawicz B. Chou's Electrocardiography in Clinical Practice. Philadelphia, PA: Elsevier. 2020.
2. Berberian, JG. Normal P-waves and T-waves. In: Berberian JG, Brady WJ, Mattu A. EMRA EKG Guide, 2nd ed. Emergency Medicine Residents' Association. Dallas, TX:2022:1.

NOTES:

Case 66: Presentation

A 50-year-old male with history of hypertension presents to the ED due to an irregular heartbeat. What is your interpretation of his ECG?

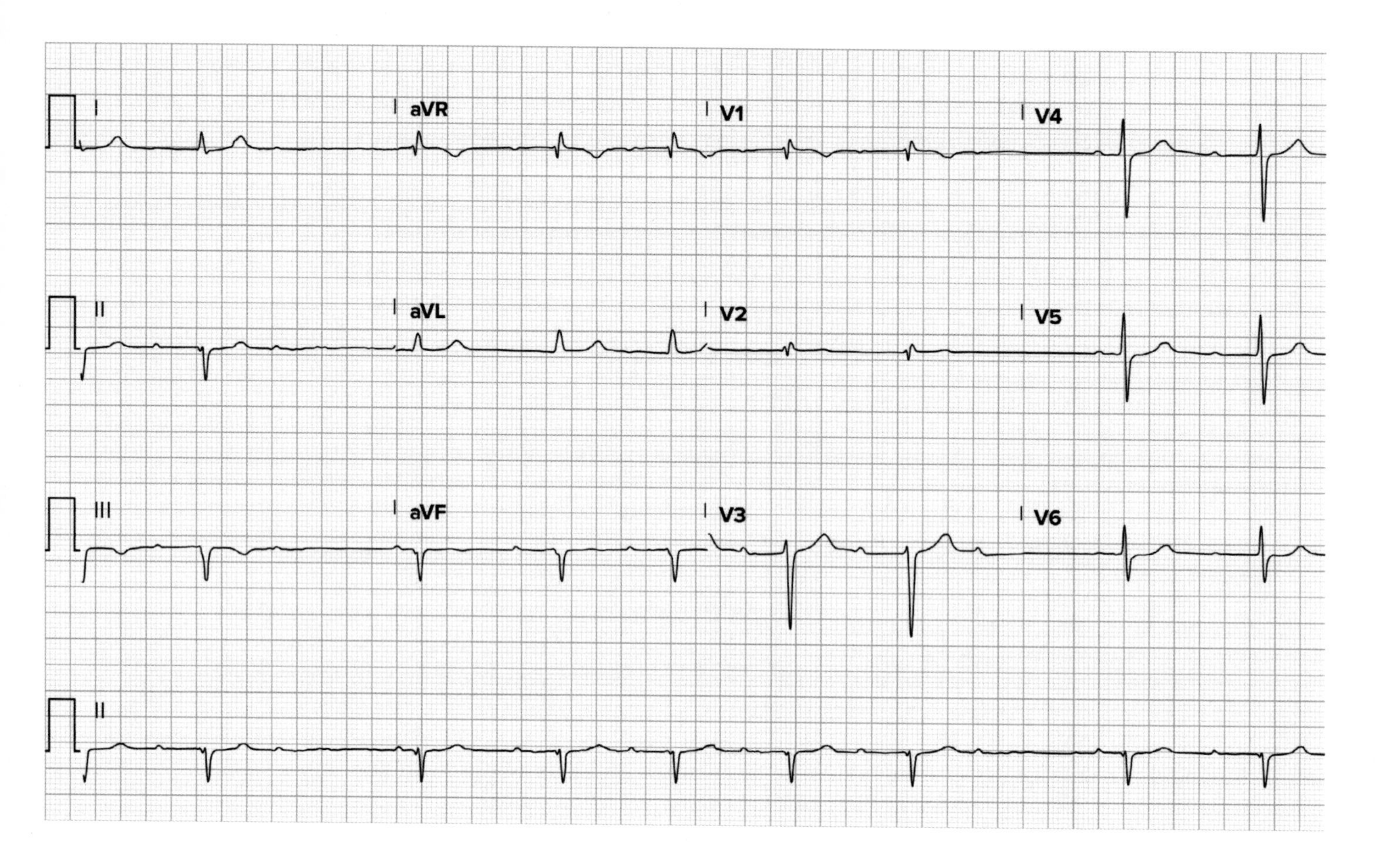

Case 66: Answer

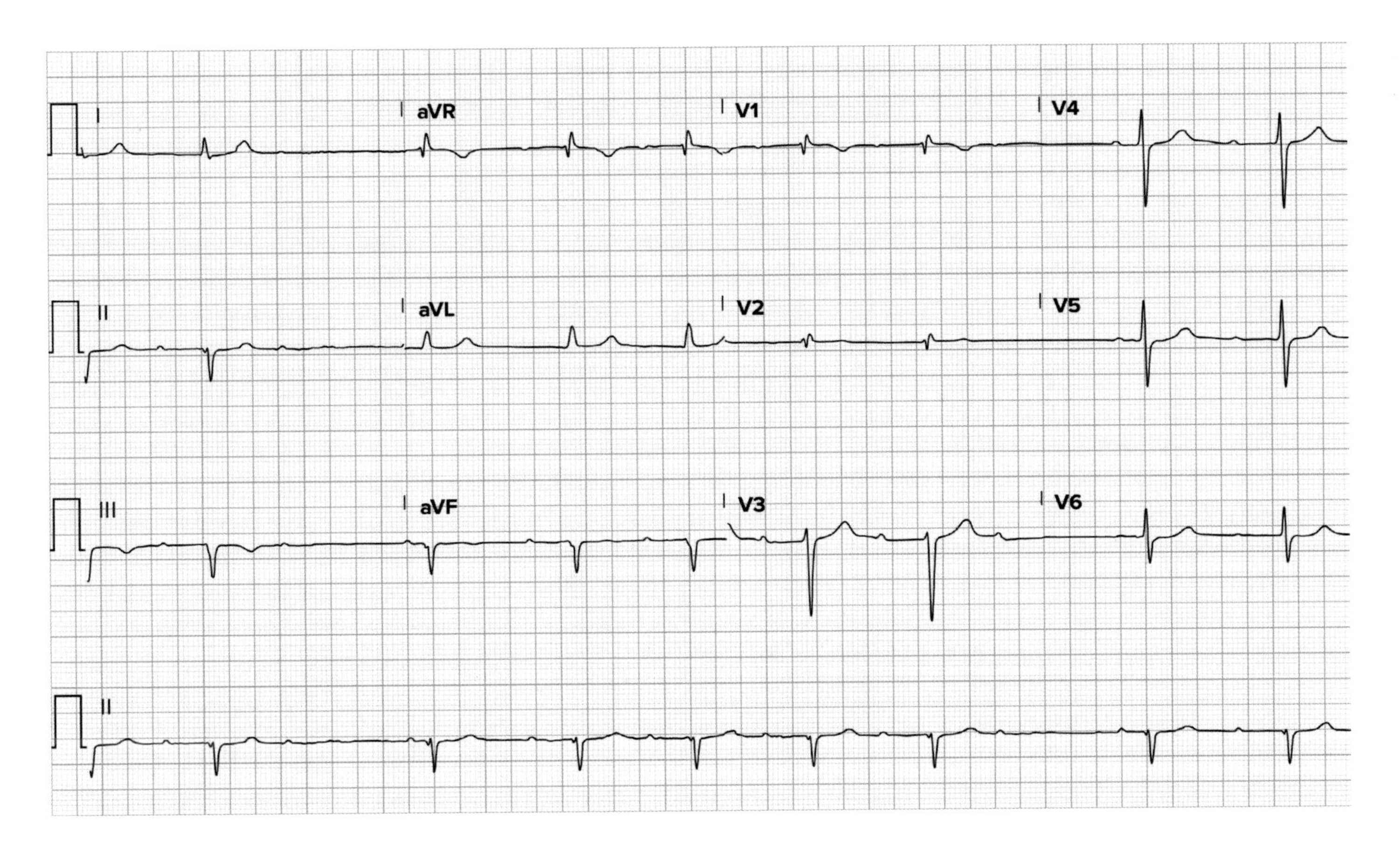

This ECG shows a Mobitz type I 2nd degree AV block with an average ventricular rate of 48 bpm, left axis deviation, normal intervals, and Q-waves in the inferior leads consistent with a prior MI.

The differential diagnosis for an irregular narrow complex rhythm with bradycardic ventricular rates includes:

- Atrial fibrillation (rate controlled)
- Atrial flutter with variable block (rate controlled)
- Atrial tachycardia with variable block (rate controlled)
- Wandering atrial pacemaker
- 2nd degree AV block Mobitz types I and II
- Variable high-grade AV block (eg, 3:1, 4:1, etc.)
- 2nd degree sinoatrial block
- Sinus arrhythmia
- Sinus bradycardia, junctional rhythm, or junctional bradycardia with irregular pattern of PAC, PJC, and/or PVC
- Sinus bradycardia, junctional rhythm, or junctional bradycardia with regular patterns of PAC, PJC, and/or PVC (bigeminy, trigeminy, etc.)

Mobitz type I AV conduction, also called Wenckebach conduction, is due to intermittent failure of conduction at the AV node. This most often occurs due to excessive vagal tone. The distinguishing feature of Mobitz type I conduction is progressive increase in the PR interval and decreasing RR interval followed by a non-conducted P-wave (ie, a P-wave without accompanying QRS complex) ***(see Figure 1).*** The PR interval resets after the non-conducted P-wave so that the PR interval after the non-conducted P-wave is shorter than the PR interval preceding the non-conducted P-wave. The biggest increase in the PR interval typically happens between the 1st and 2nd beats of each cycle (as seen in this ECG).

Figure 1.
The 2nd - 6th P-QRS-T complexes in the lead II rhythm strip show a progressively increasing PR interval followed by a non-conducted P-wave, consistent with a Mobitz type I 2nd degree AV block

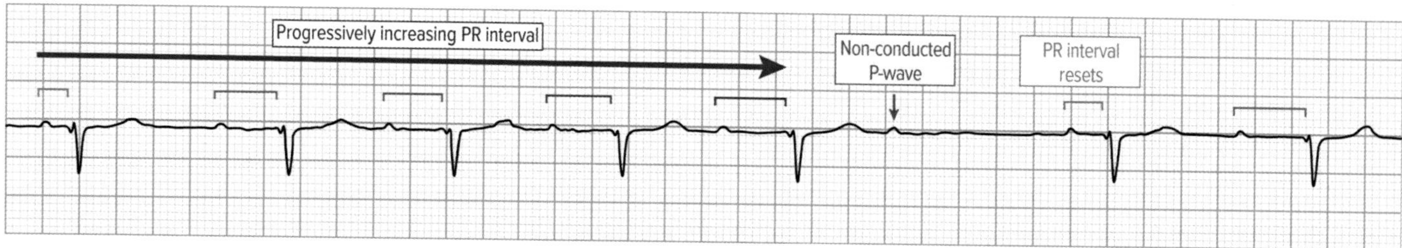

It is essential to differentiate Mobitz type I conduction from Mobitz type II conduction, as the former is typically transient with a more benign course while the latter has a high risk of progressing to a 3rd degree AV block, frequently produces hemodynamic compromise, and is associated with worse outcomes if not treated. The QRS complex duration is typically not useful in differentiating between a Mobitz type I and a Mobitz type II, as a Mobitz type I can have a prolonged QRS complex duration if there is aberrant conduction (eg, an intrinsic bundle branch block) and a Mobitz type II can have a narrow QRS complex (ie, duration < 110 msec) if the block is in the AV node. The key to distinguishing between the two is to compare the RR interval that includes the non-conducted P-wave to the PP interval.

In a Mobitz type I AV block, the RR interval that includes the non-conducted P-wave will be less than twice the PP interval. This is evident is the lead II rhythm strip from the case ECG ***(see Figure 2)*** where the RR interval that includes the non-conducted P-wave (1700 msec) is less than twice the PP interval (1880 msec).

Figure 2.
In a Mobitz type I AV block, the RR interval that includes the non-conducted P-wave is less than twice the PP interval

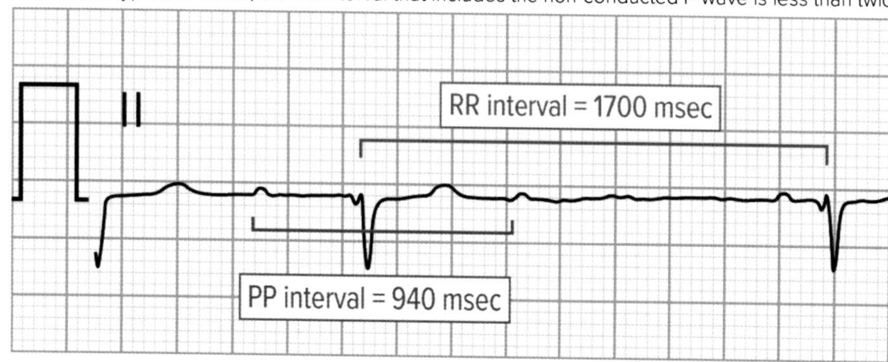

In a Mobitz type II AV block, the RR interval that includes the non-conducted P-wave will equal exactly twice the PP interval. In the example below from a different ECG ***(see Figure 3)***, the RR interval that includes the non-conducted P-wave (1440 msec) is equal to exactly twice the PP interval (1440 msec).

Figure 3.
In a Mobitz type II AV block, the RR interval that includes the non-conducted P-wave is equal to exactly twice the PP interval (from a different ECG)

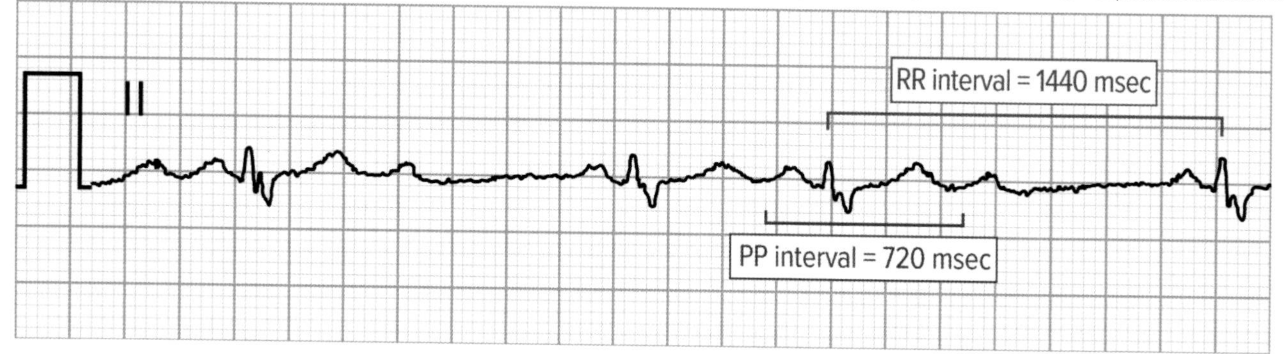

This patient had an unremarkable ED workup and the Mobitz type I AV block resolved when his heart rate increased with ambulation. He was seen in the ED by cardiology who suspected that a recent increase in his antihypertension medication metoprolol was a contributing factor.

Mobitz type I AV Block Learning Points

- Progressively increasing PR interval and decreasing RR interval until a non-conducted P-wave occurs (ie, P-wave without accompanying QRS complex)
  - PR interval immediately after non-conducted P-wave is shorter than PR interval preceding non-conducted P-wave
  - RR interval that includes non-conducted P-wave < twice the PP interval
- Can be normal variant and usually does not produce hemodynamic compromise
  - Typically associated with excess vagal tone and therefore usually responds to atropine when acute treatment is needed
  - Can lead to a more advanced AV block if associated with a pathologic etiology
  - Can be seen with inferior MI

Mobitz type II AV Block Learning Points

- Constant PR interval in conducted beats
  - Described as ratio of P-waves to QRS complexes
  - Typically an infranodal block resulting in a prolonged QRS complex duration
  - RR interval that includes non-conducted P-wave = twice the PP interval
- Never a normal variant and frequently produces hemodynamic compromise
  - High risk of progressing to a 3rd degree AV block
  - Atropine is unlikely to lead to clinical improvement and may lead to a high-grade AV block

High-grade (or advanced) AV Block Learning Points

- 2nd degree AV block with ≥ 2 sequential non-conducted P-waves
  - Most commonly a variant of a Mobitz type II but can be associated with a Mobitz type I
  - PP and RR intervals should have a whole number ratio
- Named as ratio of P-waves to QRS complexes
- Can be seen after anterior MI or with significant pathology of the conduction pathway
- High risk of progressing to a 3rd degree AV block

Case 67: Presentation

A 90-year-old female presents with exertional fatigue and near syncope.
What is your interpretation of her ECG?

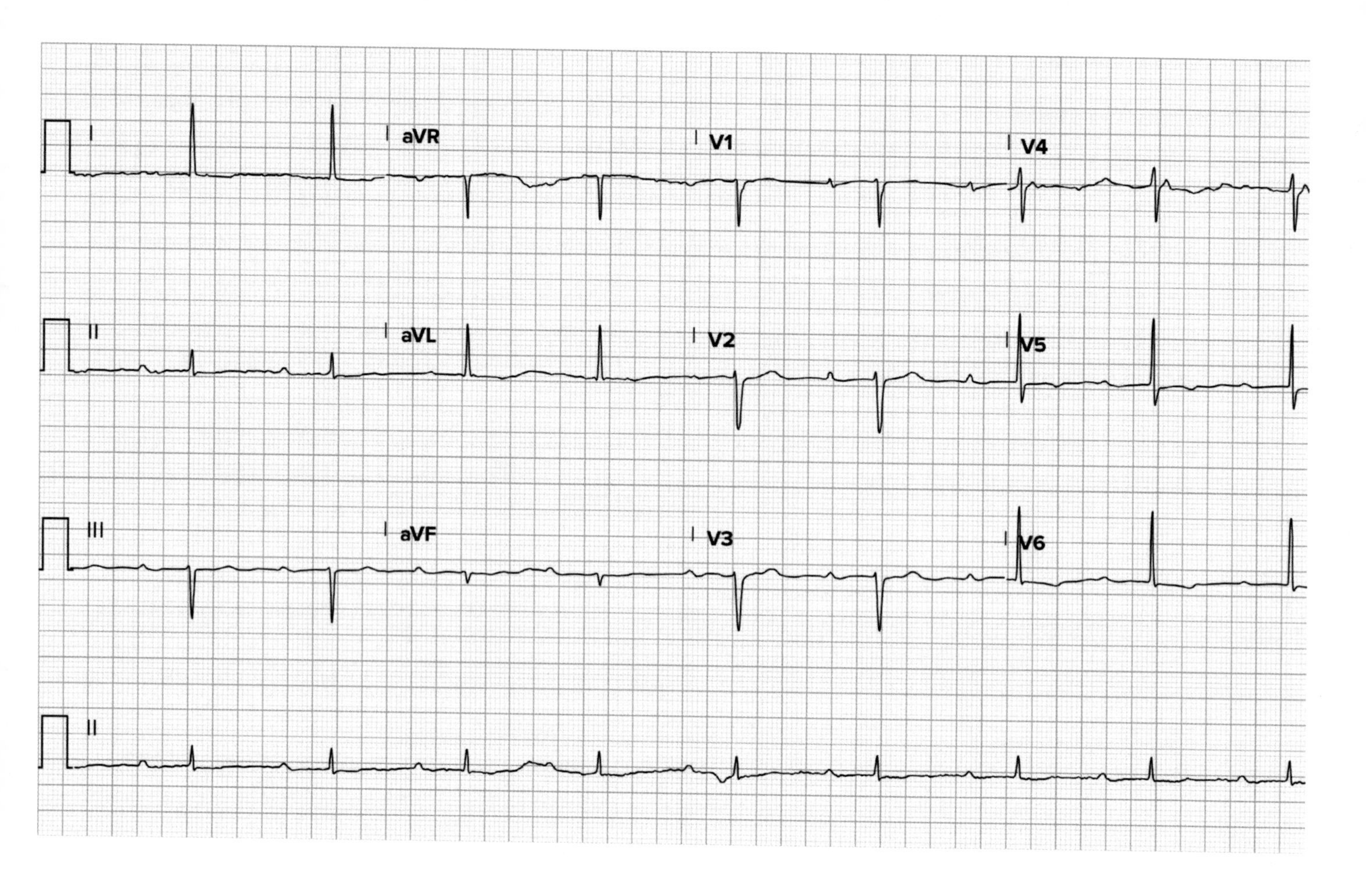

Case 67: Answer

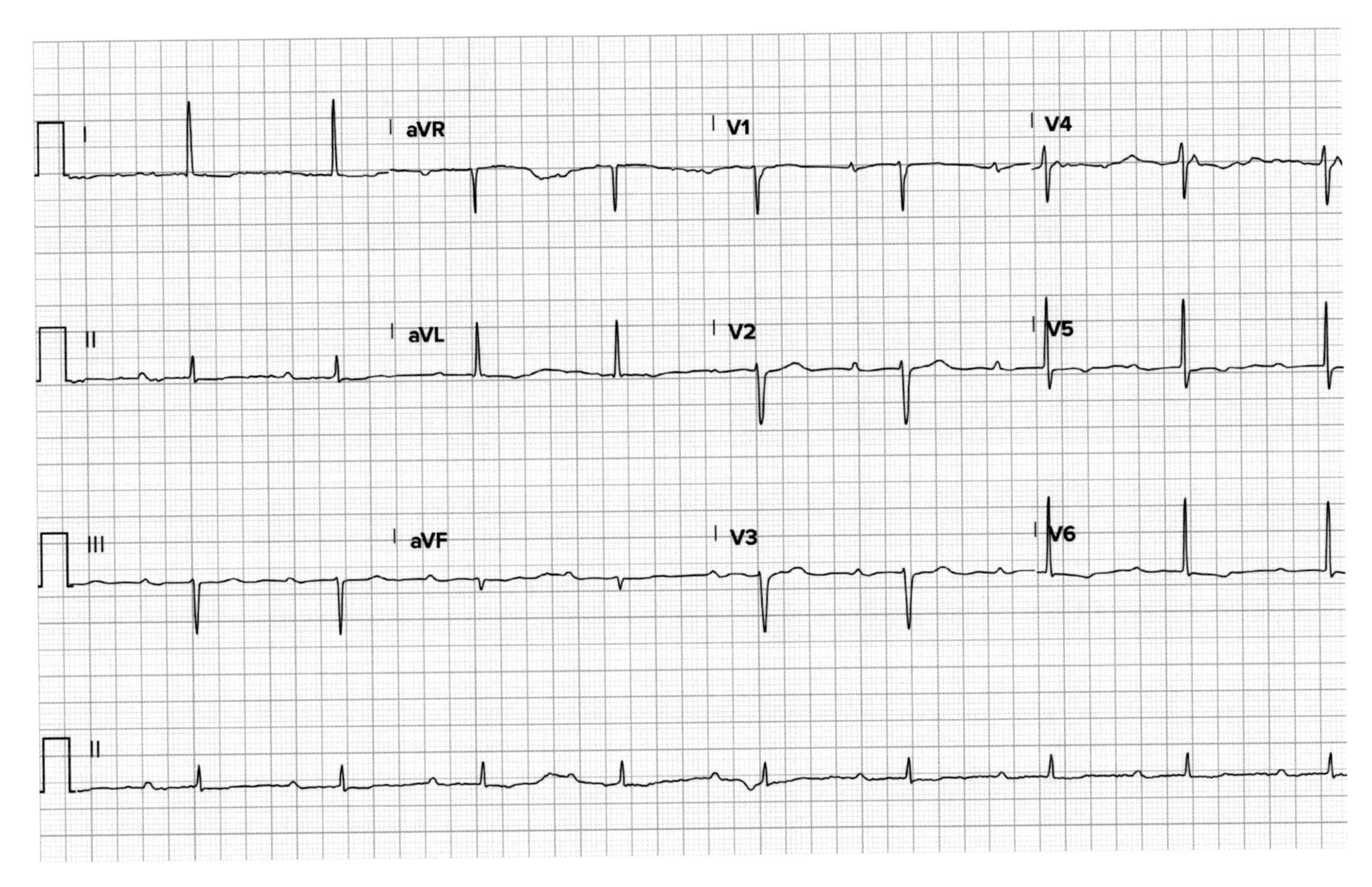

This ECG shows sinus bradycardia with a ventricular rate of 55 bpm, normal axis, first degree AV block, and findings suggestive of LVH (eg, poor R-wave progression, TWI in leads V5-V6, and meeting Cornell voltage criteria). There is some intermittent baseline artifact best seen in the lead II rhythm strip preceding the 4th and 5th P-QRS-T complexes. Note that while LVH is an echocardiographic diagnosis, it is important to recognize the associated strain pattern on ECG which can mimic ischemia.

The clinically significant finding in this ECG is the 1st degree AV block. The PR interval is 397 msec which is severely prolonged. This leads to AV dyssynchrony and subsequent loss of atrial kick and cardiac output. Symptoms are usually worse with activities that require increased cardiac output. This syndrome was first seen in dual chamber pacemakers, so it was called pacemaker syndrome. When seen in patients without pacemakers, it is commonly called "pseudo-pacemaker syndrome" or "AV dyssynchrony syndrome." The treatment for patients with a pacemaker is reprogramming to better sync the timing of the atrial and ventricular contraction. For patients without a pacemaker, the treatment is often pacemaker placement to artificially improve AV synchrony.

This patient had an unremarkable workup in the ED. She had an appropriate increase in her heart rate with ambulation, which rules out inappropriate sinus bradycardia, a type of sick sinus syndrome when there is persistent bradycardia that is unable to meet physiologic demands. She was admitted to the cardiology service for evaluation for pacemaker placement.

1st Degree AV Block Learning Points

- Due to conduction delay typically at AV node
- ECG shows a prolonged PR interval (> 200 msec) that remains constant
  - Normal PR interval is 120-220 msec
  - Every P-wave followed by a QRS complex and every QRS complex is preceded by a P-wave with normal (ie, sinus) P-wave and QRS complex morphology

- Usually benign and can be normal variant
  - Can lead to a more advanced AV block if associated with a pathologic etiology
  - Associated with increased long-term risk for worsening conduction abnormalities and atrial fibrillation
  - Symptomatic (syncope, near syncope, fatigue) patients with PR interval > 300 msec, commonly called "pseudo-pacemaker syndrome," may benefit from evaluation for pacemaker

NOTES:

Case 68: Presentation

A 52-year-old male presents to the emergency department with chest pain.
What is your interpretation of his ECG

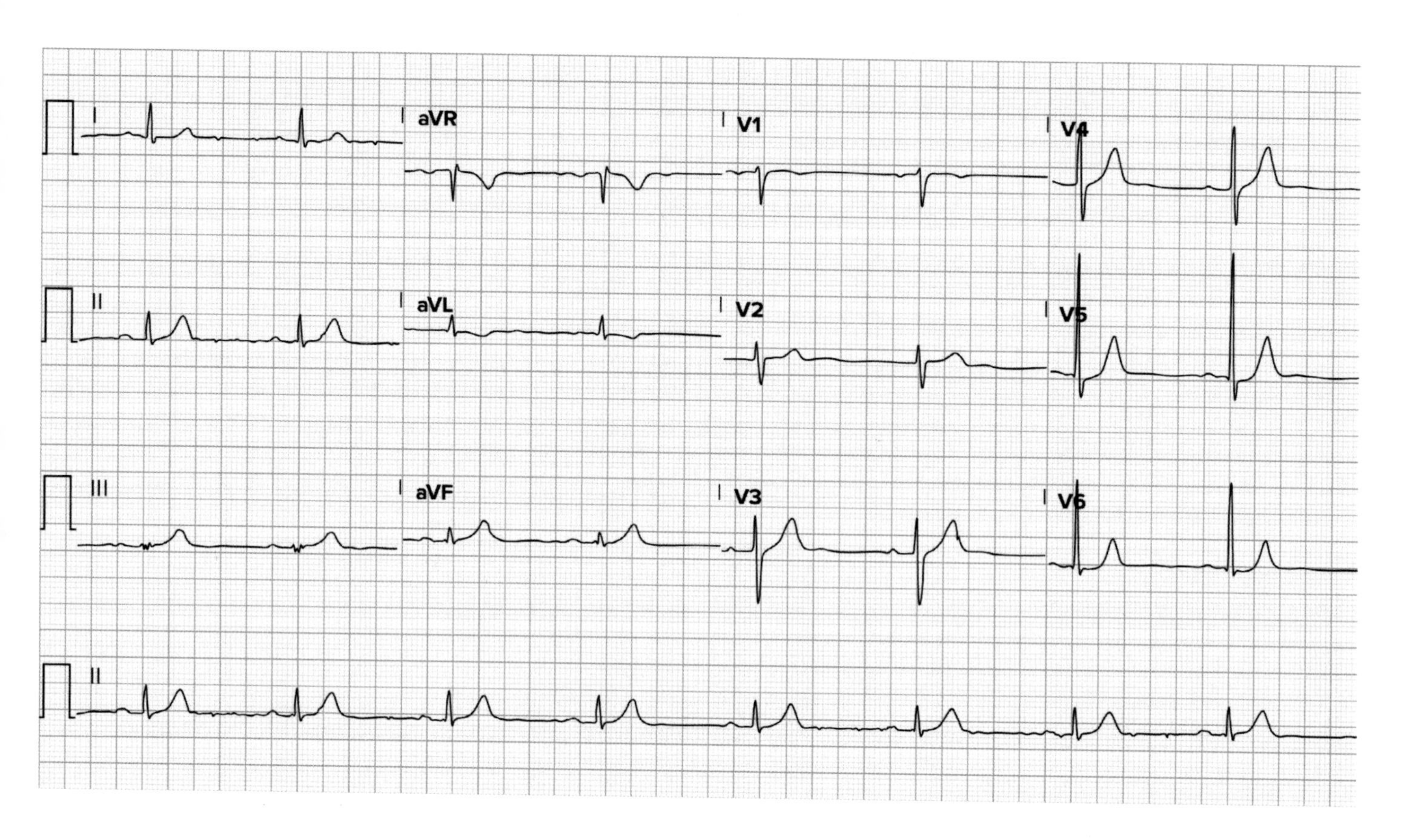

Case 68: Answer

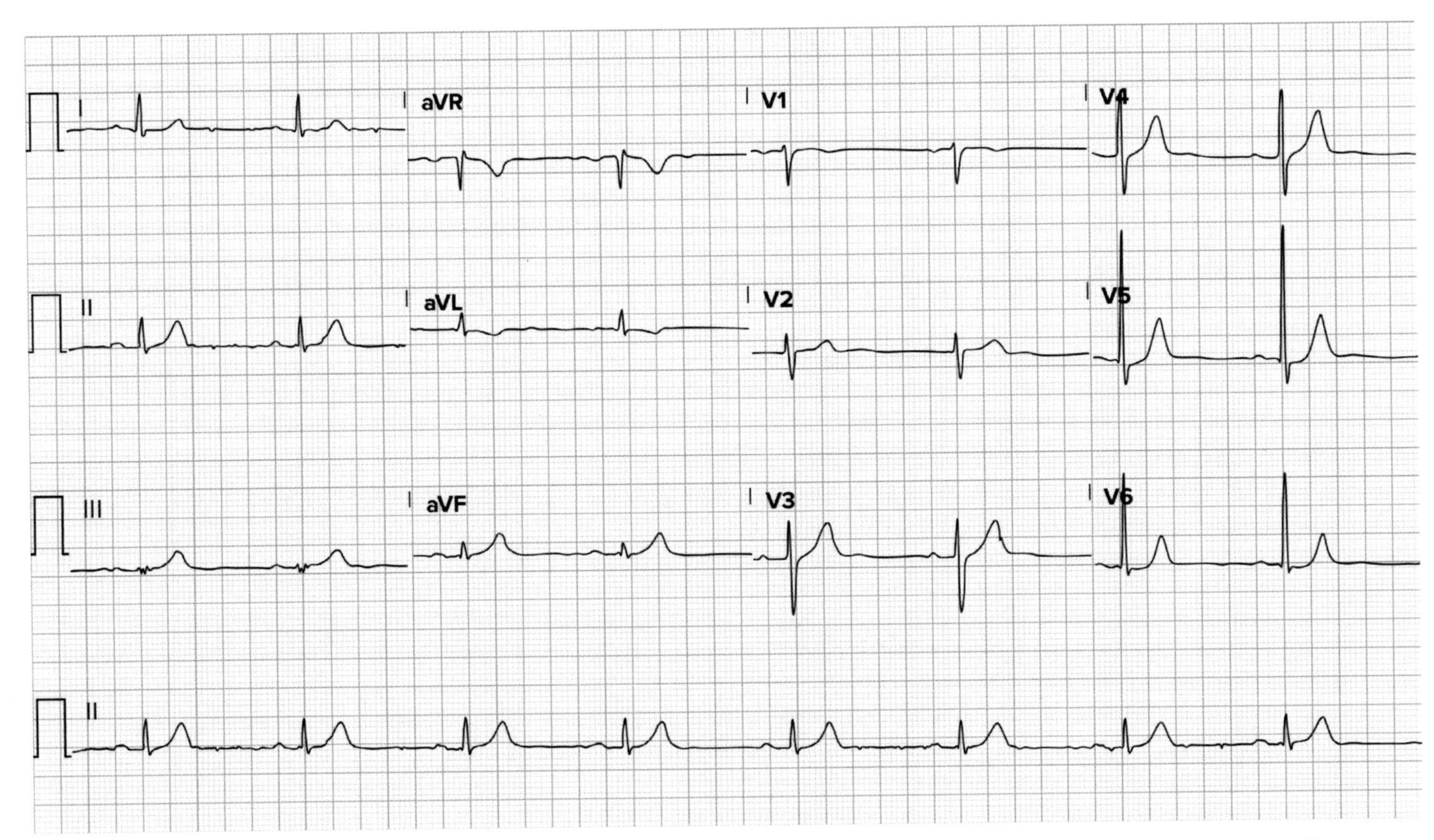

This ECG shows sinus bradycardia with a ventricular rate of 49 bpm, normal intervals, T-wave inversions in lead aVL, hyperacute T-waves in the inferior leads, and slight STD in leads V5-V6. In a patient presenting with chest pain, these findings are concerning for ischemia and/or impending infarction.

The differential diagnosis for prominent upright T-waves includes:	The differential diagnosis for TWI includes:
• Acute ischemia	• Acute ischemia (early reciprocal changes)
• Benign early repolarization/normal variant STE	• Bundle branch blocks
• Bundle branch blocks	• Cardiomyopathy (eg, Takotsubo, HCM)
• Hyperkalemia	• CNS injury
• LVH	• Digitalis effect
• Ventricular rhythms (paced or intrinsic) or ectopy	• Intra-abdominal disorders
	• Juvenile T-wave pattern
	• LVH
	• Metabolic abnormalities
	• Pericarditis
	• Pre-excitation syndromes
	• Pulmonary embolism
	• Reperfusion (eg, Wellens syndrome)
	• Toxicologic abnormalities
	• Ventricular rhythms (paced or intrinsic) or ectopy

There is no universally accepted definition for hyperacute T-waves, but they are generally described as broad based and disproportionately tall ***(see Figures 1-3)***. Hyperacute T-waves can be an early ECG finding in an ischemic event, preceding STE and/or STD. There is no consensus on whether the height of the T-wave should be compared to the amplitude of the preceding R-wave or the entire QRS complex. In this ECG it doesn't matter since the amplitude of the R-wave is almost the same as that of the entire QRS complex. Note that the hyperacute T-waves in this ECG are not visually impressive, but when considered in light of the relatively smaller amplitude QRS complexes, they are hyperacute.

The isolated TWI in lead aVL, when new from prior, is associated with both impending inferior wall MI and mid-LAD lesions. It has a high specificity for mid-LAD lesions, and in the setting of an inferior MI has a high sensitivity, specificity, and PPV for right ventricular involvement and a higher morbidity and mortality.

Figure 1.

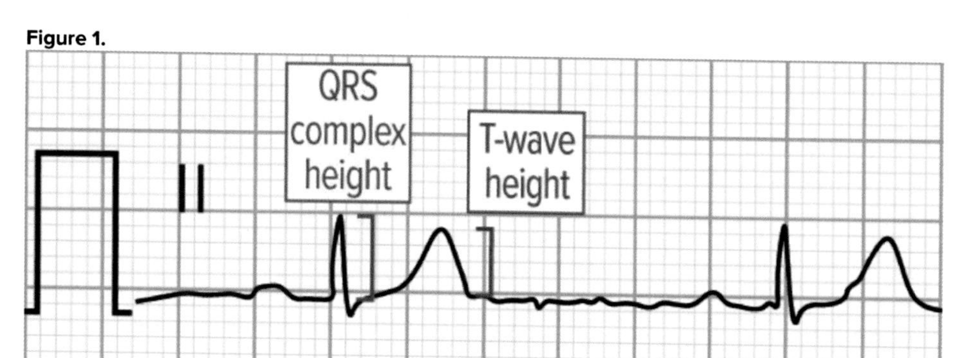

Figure 2.

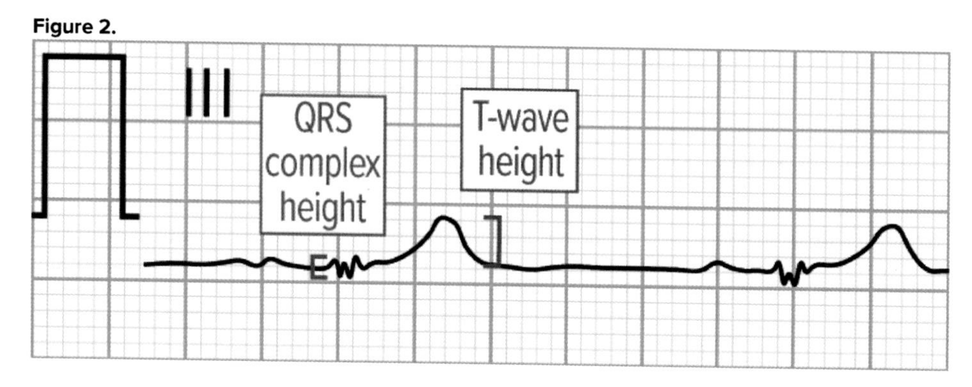

Figure 3.

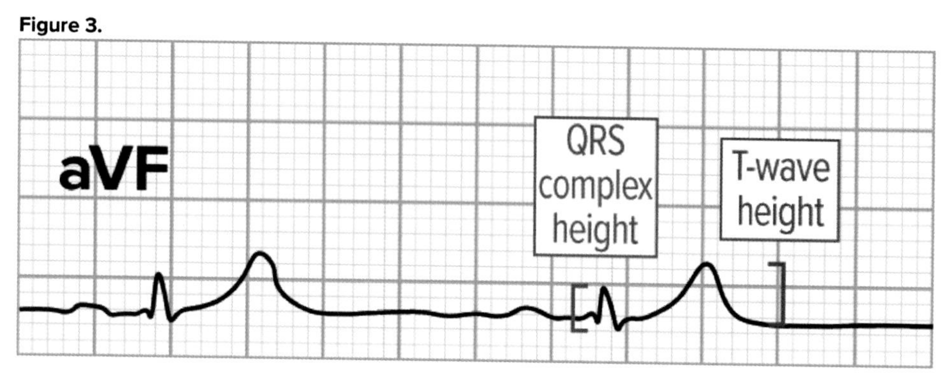

Normal P-wave and T-wave Learning Points

- Normal P-wave and T-wave morphologies[1] in normal sinus rhythm in the absence of conduction abnormalities, ischemia, structural abnormalities, etc., include:

I P: always upright T: always upright	**aVR** P: always inverted T: always inverted	**V1** P: usually biphasic (+/-) but can be entirely upright or inverted T: upright or inverted	**V4** P: upright T: almost always upright
II P: always upright T: always upright	**aVL** P: upright, inverted, or biphasic (-/+) T: upright or inverted	**V2** P: usually biphasic (+/-) but can be entirely upright (entirely inverted is rare) T: usually upright	**V5** P: upright T: always upright
III P: upright, inverted, or biphasic (+/-) T: upright or inverted	**aVF** P: usually upright but can be flat or biphasic T: usually upright	**V3** P: upright T: usually upright	**V6** P: upright T: always upright

- Inverted, flat, or positive-negative biphasic T-waves in lead V1 (less so in leads V2-V3) can be normal
- Positive-negative biphasic T-waves in leads V1-V3 can be abnormal or a normal variant
- T-wave amplitude is typically < 6 mm in limb leads and < 10 mm in precordial leads

Figure 4.
Hyperacute T-waves

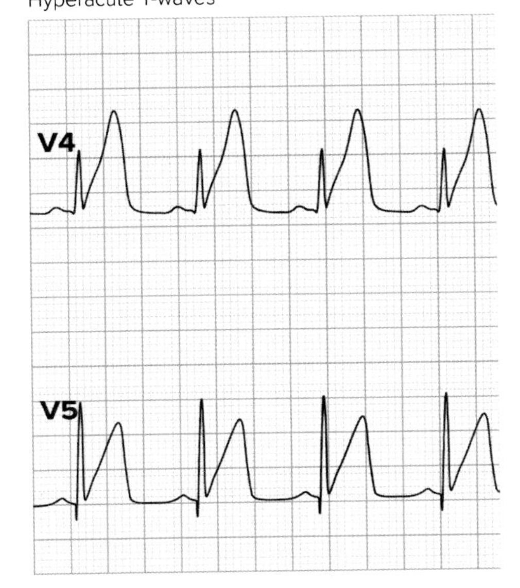

T-wave Inversions Learning Points

- Ischemic TWI:
  - New from prior TWI ≥ 1 mm in ≥ 2 contiguous leads with prominent R-wave or R/S ratio > 1
- TWI in lead aVL:
  - Can be seen in inferior MI before inferior STE and has high sensitivity/ specificity/positive predictive value for RV AMI
  - When in doubt, obtain serial ECGs

Hyperacute T-waves Learning Points

- There is no universally accepted definition of hyperacute T-waves (ie, no absolute specific amplitude), but the general characteristics include ***(see Figure 4)***:
  - Broad based and disproportionately tall
  - Asymmetric morphology with more gradual upslope and more abrupt return to the baseline
  - J point elevation is common
- Hyperacute T-waves + STD/TWI in reciprocal leads = early AMI
- When in doubt, obtain serial ECGs

References

1. Knilans T, Surawicz B. Chou's Electrocardiography in Clinical Practice. Philadelphia, PA: Elsevier. 2020.
2. Berberian, JG. Normal P-waves and T-waves. In: Berberian JG, Brady WJ, Mattu A. EMRA EKG Guide, 2nd ed. Emergency Medicine Residents' Association. Dallas, TX:2022:1.

Case 69: Presentation

A 51-year-old male with no known cardiac history presents with palpitations and lightheadedness. What is your interpretation of his ECG?

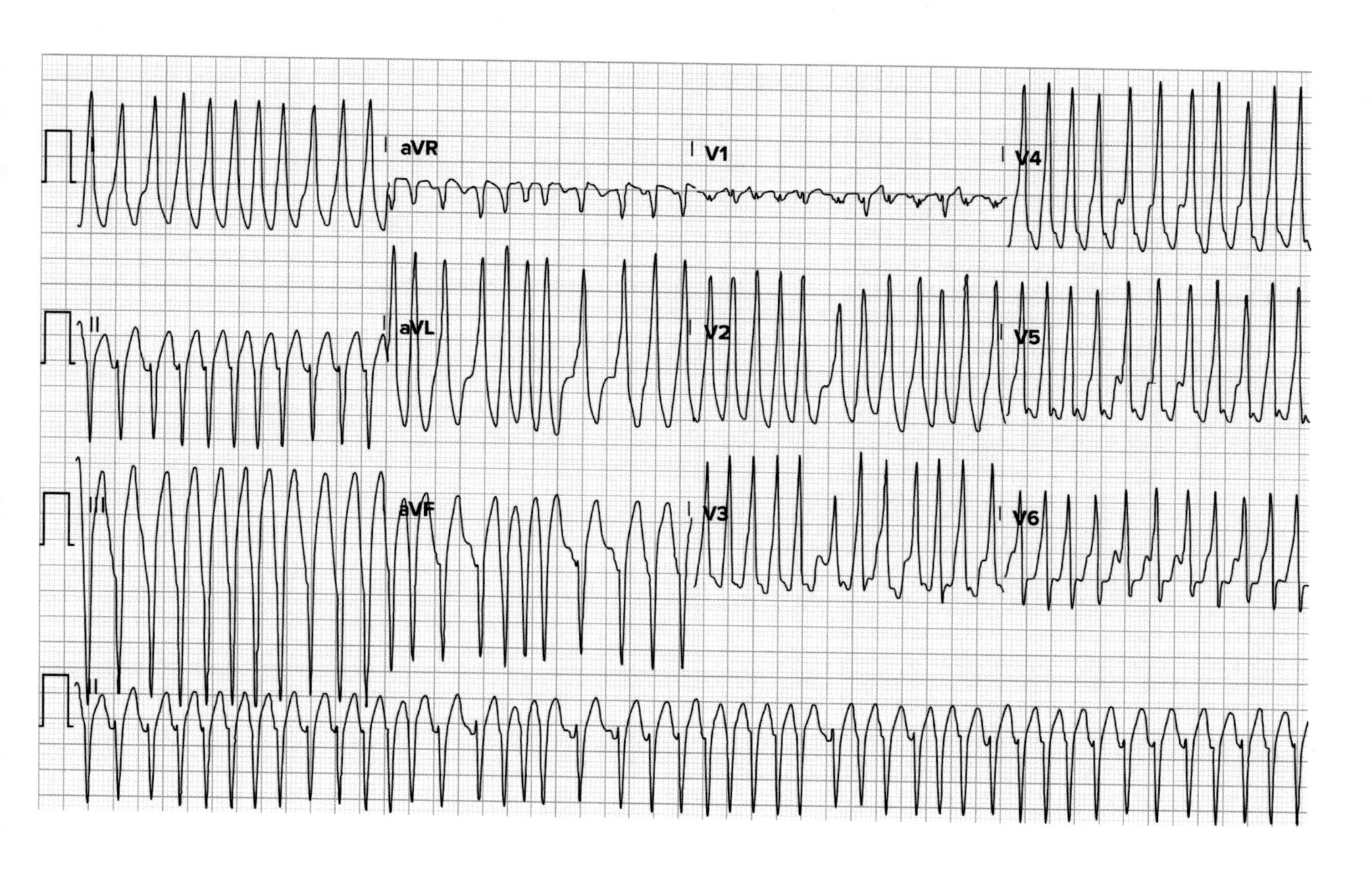

Case 69: Answer

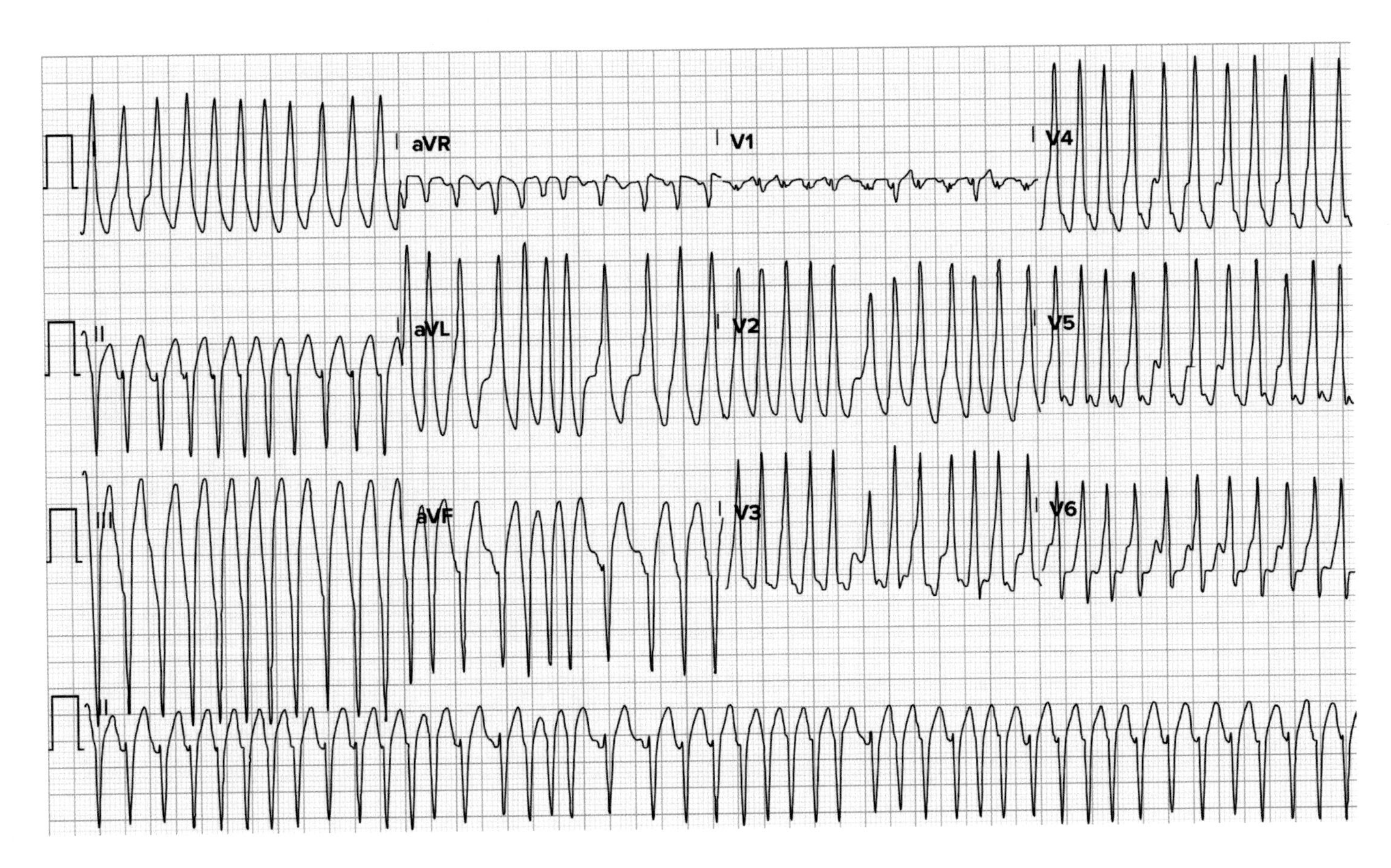

This ECG shows an irregular wide complex tachycardia with an average ventricular rate of 270 bpm and intermittent rates up to 375 bpm, no P-waves, left axis deviation, and prolonged QRS complex duration with beat-to-beat variation in the QRS complex morphology.

The differential diagnosis for an irregular WCT includes:

- Ventricular fibrillation
- Polymorphic ventricular tachycardia (including torsades de pointes)
- MAT with aberrant conduction
- Atrial flutter with variable block and aberrant conduction
- Atrial fibrillation with aberrant conduction
  - Causes of aberrant conduction include fixed or rate-related BBB, metabolic abnormalities, sodium channel blocker toxicity, ventricular-paced rhythm, and ventricular pre-excitation (eg, WPW)

This ECG shows the triad, as yet unnamed, of irregularly irregular rhythm, markedly changing QRS complex morphologies, and extremely fast rates up to 375 bpm in some regions ***(see Figure 1)*** that is only seen with polymorphic ventricular tachycardia and atrial fibrillation with WPW. Polymorphic ventricular tachycardia will have phasic variation (ie, happens over a number of beats) of the QRS complex polarity (ie, axis) and amplitude. Conversely, atrial fibrillation with WPW will have beat-to-beat variation in the QRS complex morphology and relatively consistent QRS polarity, as seen in this patient's ECG.

Figure 1.
Lead aVL shows an irregularly irregular rhythm with variable QRS complex morphologies and extremely fast ventricular rates (up to 375 bpm in this case), consistent with atrial fibrillation with WPW

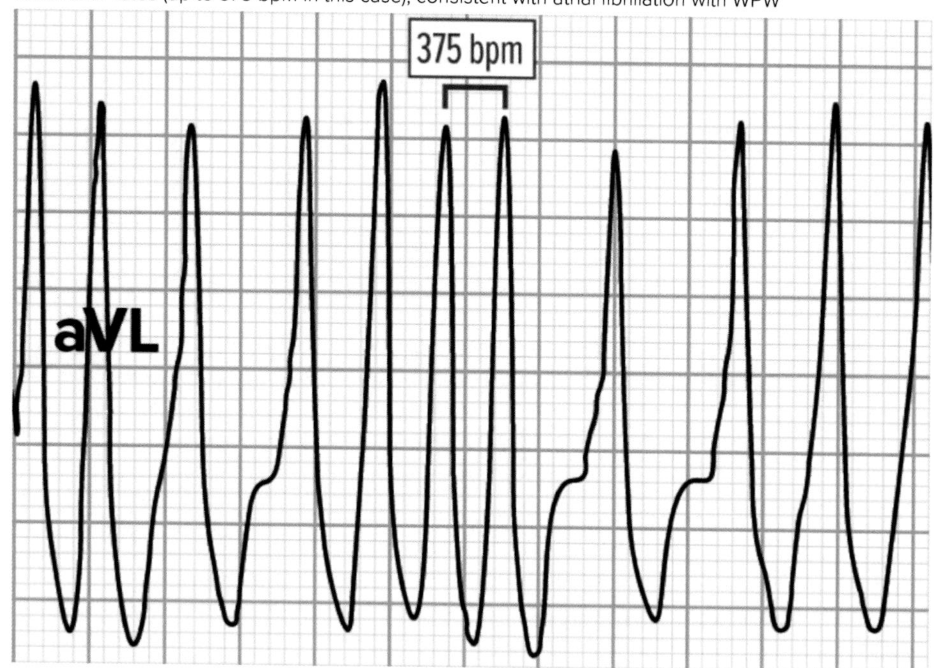

This patient was electrically cardioverted and a repeat ECG showed the characteristic short PR interval and delta waves consistent with WPW ***(see Figures 2 and 3)***. Delta waves represent pre-excitation of a portion of the ventricular myocardium via the AP. The depolarization wave resulting from this portion of pre-excited ventricular myocardium subsequently fuses with the depolarization caused by conduction via the AV node, ultimately creating the characteristic morphology of a QRS complex with a delta wave.

Figure 2.
A repeat ECG after electrical cardioversion shows delta waves and a short PR interval seen with WPW in sinus rhythm

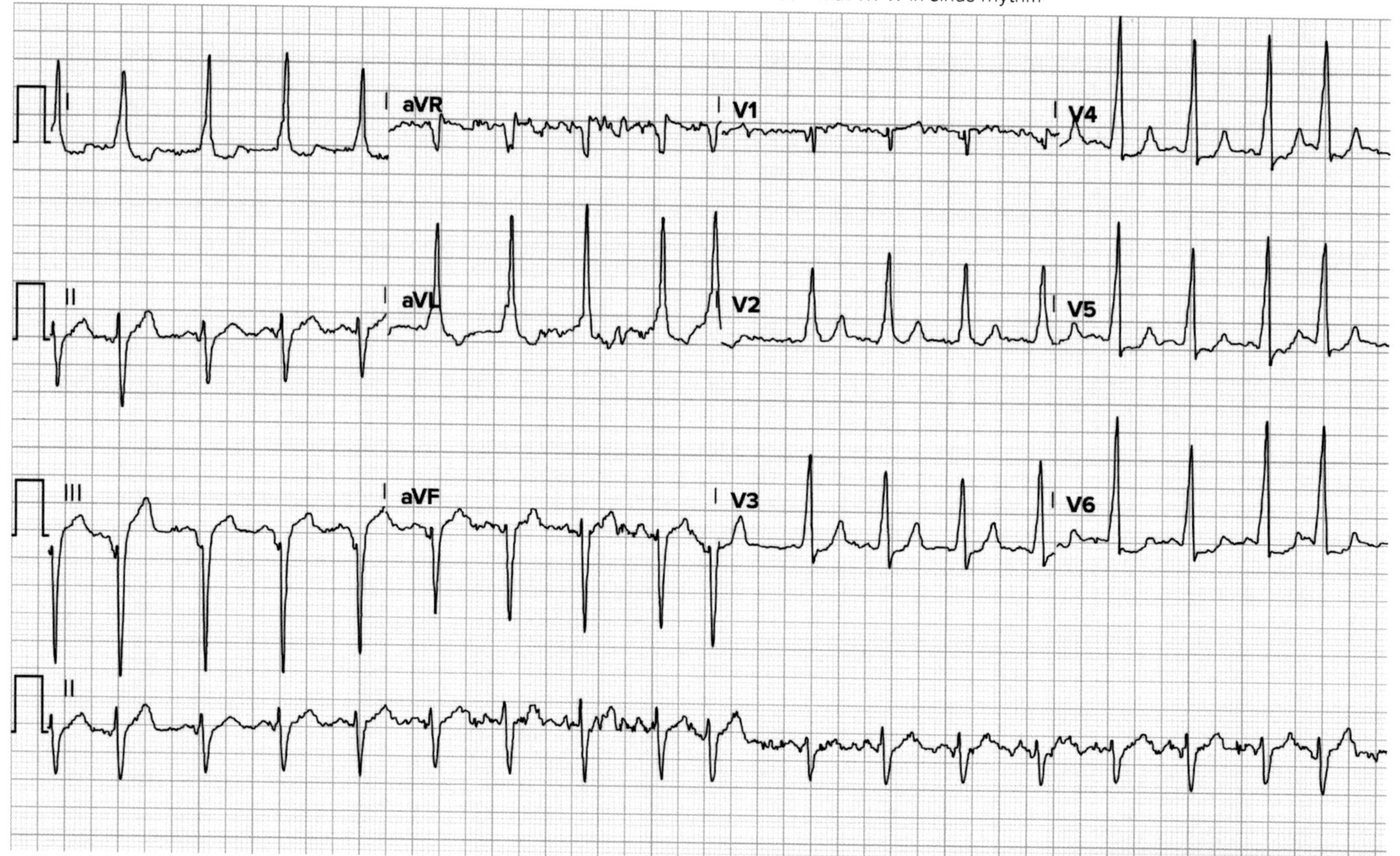

The AV node's intrinsic refractory period prevents ventricular rates from exceeding 220-240 bpm in the absence of any extrinsic factors that increase conduction velocity (eg, catecholamine surge, sympathomimetic toxicity, or hyperthyroidism), so atrial fibrillation with intermittent conduction at rates faster than 220-240 bpm should prompt concern for an AP. The danger of conduction via an AP in atrial fibrillation is due to its short refractory period relative to the AV node. This allows the AP to conduct at much faster rates than the AV node. In atrial fibrillation with WPW, the AV node acts as a brake that tempers the faster AP conduction. Without the protection provided by the AV node, conduction via the AP can lead to extremely rapid rates and related cardiovascular decompensation (eg, ventricular fibrillation). This is why AV nodal blockers should be avoided in atrial fibrillation with known or suspected WPW.

Figure 3.
Lead V5 from Figure 2 shows delta waves and short PR intervals consistent with WPW in sinus rhythm

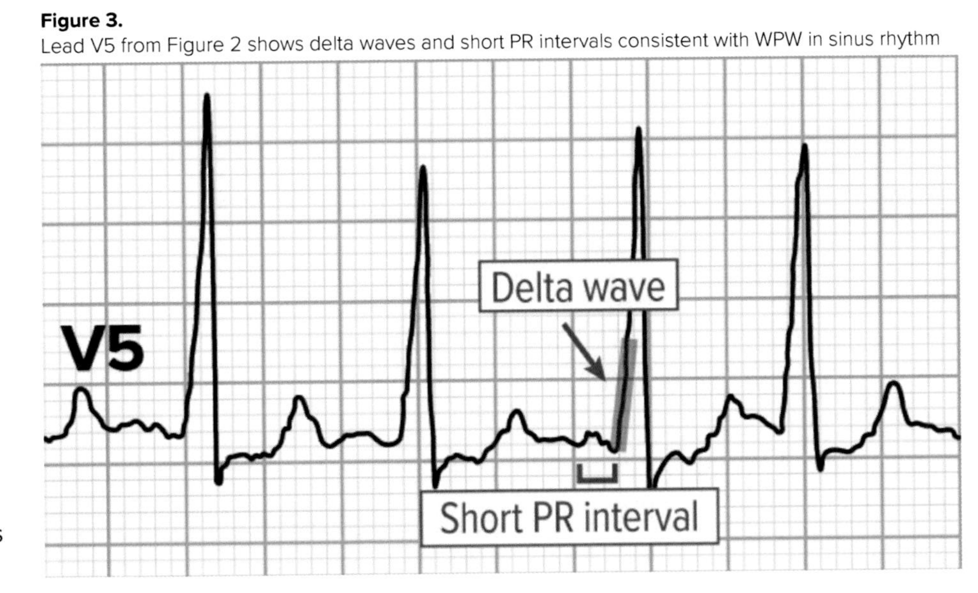

Treatment for atrial fibrillation with WPW includes electrical cardioversion (for stable or unstable patients) and IV procainamide or ibutilide for stable patients.[1] Procainamide and ibutilide reduce conduction velocity throughout the entire cardiac conduction system, including the AP and ventricle. Verapamil, diltiazem, adenosine, digoxin, lidocaine, and intravenous amiodarone should not be used.[1]

This patient was admitted to the cardiology service and found to have untreated hyperthyroidism which likely contributed to the exceptionally fast ventricular rates seen on his ECG. An electrophysiology study showed an antegrade bypass tract consistent with WPW, which was successfully ablated after the patient's hyperthyroidism was controlled.

WPW Learning Points

- Congenital condition involving abnormal conduction pathway between atria and ventricle
  - Most common dysrhythmia is orthodromic AVRT
- ECG findings seen in sinus rhythm include:
  - Shortened PR interval (< 120 msec)
  - Delta wave: slurring of initial portion of the QRS complex
  - QRS complex duration prolonged, usually > 110 msec
  - Secondary ST and T-wave changes
  - Patients with WPW can have baseline ECGs (ie, in normal sinus rhythm) with a normal PR interval, normal QRS complex duration, and/or without delta waves
- Regular rhythm tachycardias in WPW can be narrow (orthodromic conduction via AV node) or wide (antidromic conduction via accessory pathway)
  - WPW with orthodromic AVRT (most common dysrhythmia): regular NCT, treat like AVNRT (PSVT)
  - WPW with antidromic AVRT: regular WCT, treat like monomorphic VT
- WPW with atrial fibrillation
  - Rapid, irregularly irregular wide complex tachycardia with beat-to-beat variation in QRS complex morphologies
  - Treatment includes electrical cardioversion (for stable or unstable patients) and IV procainamide or ibutilide for stable patients (avoid AV nodal blocking medications)
- In wide-complex atrial fibrillation, ventricular rates > 220-240 bpm suggest anterograde conduction via an accessory pathway

References

1. January CT, Wann LS, Alpert JS, et al. 2014 AHA/ACC/ HRS guideline for the management of patients with atrial fibrillation: a report of the American College of Cardiology/American Heart Association Task Force on Practice Guidelines and the Heart Rhythm Society. J Am Coll Cardiol. 2014;64:e1–76.

Case 70: Presentation

A 61-year-old female with no past medical history presents with fever, flu-like symptoms, and palpitations. What is your interpretation of her ECG?

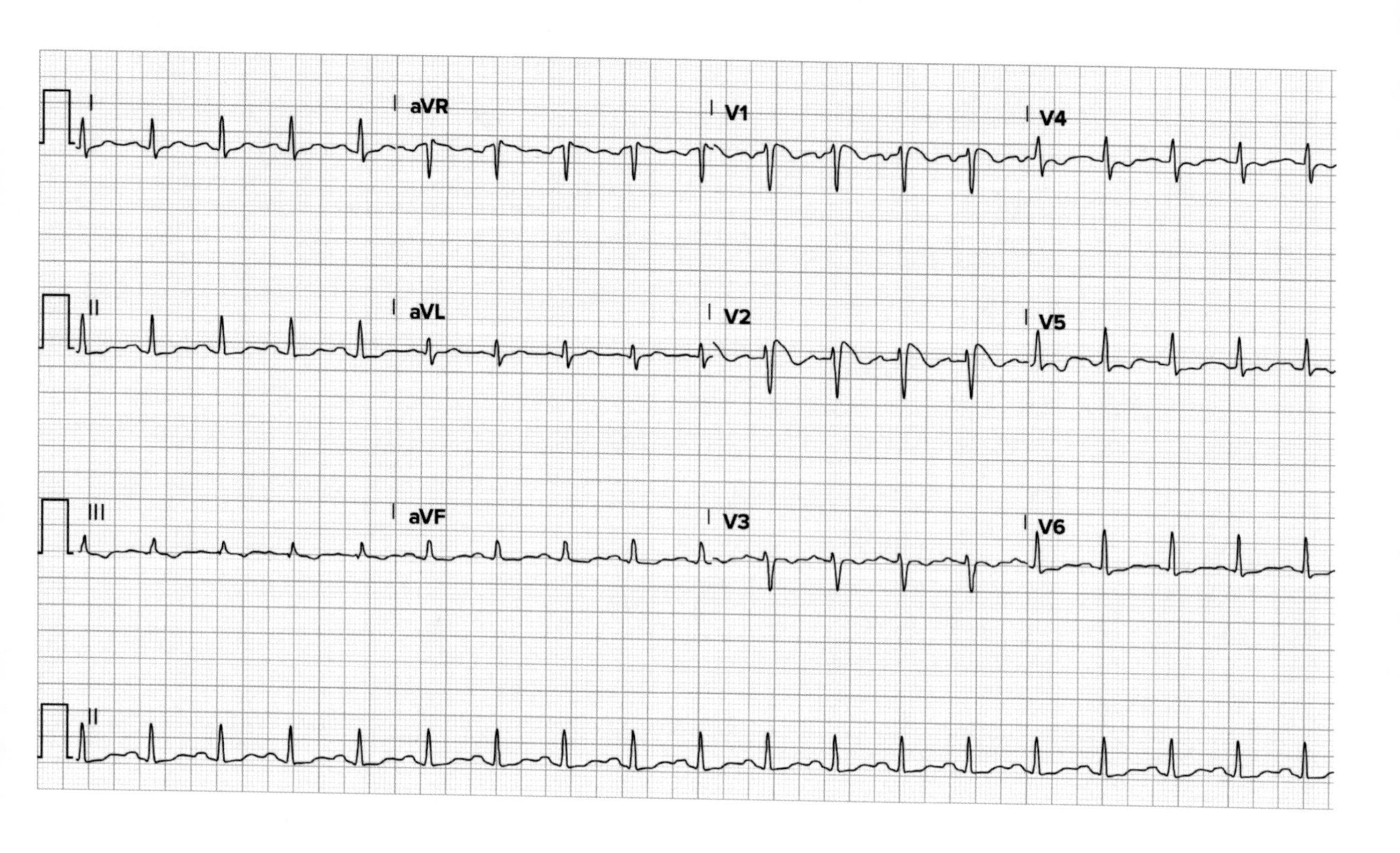

Case 70: Answer

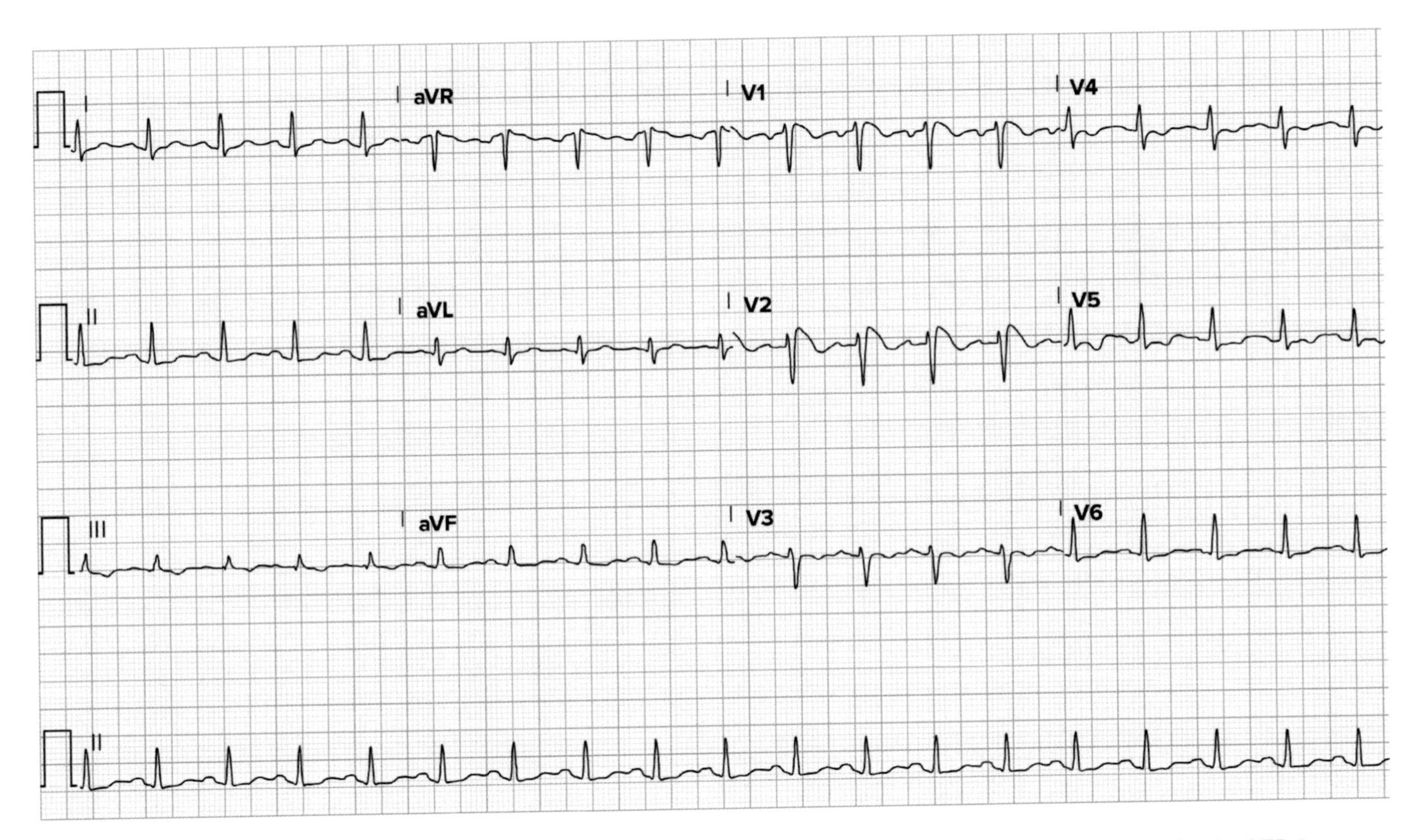

This ECG shows sinus tachycardia with a ventricular rate of 110 bpm, normal axis, normal intervals, normal axis, STD in leads I, II, and V4-V6, and coved STE > 2 mm followed by a negative T-wave in lead V2. This ECG is concerning for Brugada syndrome.

The differential diagnosis for STE in lead V1 includes:

- Acute MI (anteroseptal or right ventricular)
- Acute RV strain (eg, PE)
- Brugada syndrome
- Hyperkalemia
- LBBB
- LVH
- Sodium channel blocker toxicity
- Ventricular-paced rhythm

Brugada syndrome is a sodium channelopathy that can lead to unprovoked dysrhythmias (polymorphic ventricular tachycardia or ventricular fibrillation) and cardiac arrest. The diagnostic criteria include both ECG changes and clinical criteria (see Learning Points below). Notably, up to 40% of patients with Brugada syndrome will have normal resting ECGs.

The initial Brugada ECG criteria set forth in 2002[1] included 3 types:

- Type 1: Coved STE ≥ 2 mm followed by a negative T-wave in > 1 of leads V1-V3 ***(see Figure 1)***
- Type 2: ≥ 2 mm of saddleback shaped STE in > 1 of leads V1-V3 ***(see Figure 2)***
- Type 3: Type 1 or 2 morphology not meeting above criteria in > 1 of leads V1-V3

Figure 1.
Brugada type 1

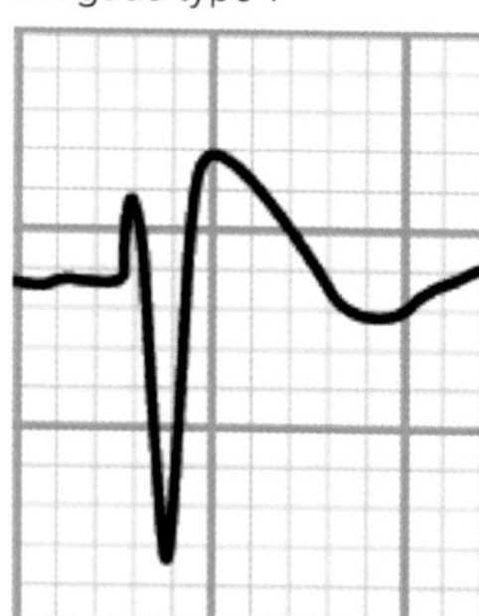

Figure 2.
Brugada type 2

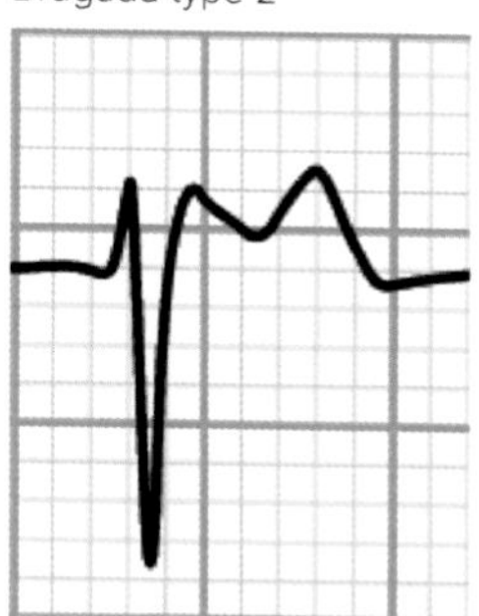

More recent 2013 guidelines[2] narrowed the definition:

> "Brugada syndrome is diagnosed in patients with ST-segment elevation with type 1 morphology ≥ 2 mm in ≥ 1 lead in the right precordial leads V1, V2, positioned in the 2nd, 3rd, or 4th intercostal space occurring either spontaneously or after provocative drug test with intravenous administration of class I antiarrhythmic drugs."

The important changes in the new definition include:

- Type 1 is the only potentially diagnostic pattern
- Type 1 only needs to be seen in one lead and can be seen in lead(s) V1/V2 when positioned higher than the traditional 4th intercostal space
- Type 2 is non-diagnostic and it is only clinically significant if the type I pattern is seen or can be provoked with sodium channel blocking antidysrhythmics
- Type 3 is no longer part of the criteria
- Lead V3 is no longer part of the criteria

There are multiple conditions that can mimic type 1 on the ECG, such as ARVC, septal hypertrophy, and pectus excavatum. Positioning leads V1 and V2 in the 2nd or 3rd intercostal space increases the sensitivity for detecting type 1 and can help differentiate it from a mimic. Conversely, inadvertent placement of leads V1 and V2 in the 2nd or 3rd intercostal spaces can produce a type 2 mimic in young athletes.

There are multiple unrelated conditions that can "unmask" a Brugada ECG pattern, notably fever and medications. The significance of this finding depends on the patient's clinical history, as the diagnostic criteria for Brugada syndrome include both ECG and clinical criteria.

This patient's ED workup was notable for a positive flu swab. A repeat ECG after her fever was treated showed resolution of the Brugada morphology seen on the initial ECG. As well, the STD seen on the initial ECG resolved once her heart rate come down. She was evaluated by Electrophysiology, who deferred any further risk stratification for Brugada syndrome given her lack of clinical criteria and variable utility and accuracy of electrophysiology studies for asymptomatic patients with fever-induced Brugada.

Brugada Syndrome Learning Points

- Sodium channelopathy that can lead to unprovoked dysrhythmias (polymorphic ventricular tachycardia or ventricular fibrillation) and cardiac arrest
- Diagnosis made from both ECG and clinical criteria (see table)
  - Type 1 is the only ECG abnormality that is potentially diagnostic
  - Type 2 is non-diagnostic but may warrant further investigation in the appropriate clinical situation
  - Type 3 is no longer considered useful in diagnosis
- Treatment is AICD placement

ECG Criteria	Clinical Criteria (must have ≥ 1):
• Complete or incomplete RBBB pattern with coved STE ≥ 2 mm followed by a negative T-wave in ≥ 1 of leads V1-V2	• Documented VF or polymorphic VT
	• Family history of sudden cardiac death at < 45 years old
	• Coved-type ECG in family members
	• Inducibility of VT with programmed electrical stimulation
	• Syncope
	• Nocturnal agonal respiration

References

1. Wilde AAM, Antzelevitch C, Borggrefe M, et al. Proposed Diagnostic Criteria for the Brugada Syndrome Consensus Report. Circulation. 2002;106(19):2514-2519.
2. Sieira J, Brugada P. The definition of the Brugada syndrome. Eur Heart J. 2017;38(40):3029-3034.

Case 71: Presentation

A 22-year-old female presents with vomiting, diarrhea, and generalized weakness and fatigue. What is your interpretation of her ECG?

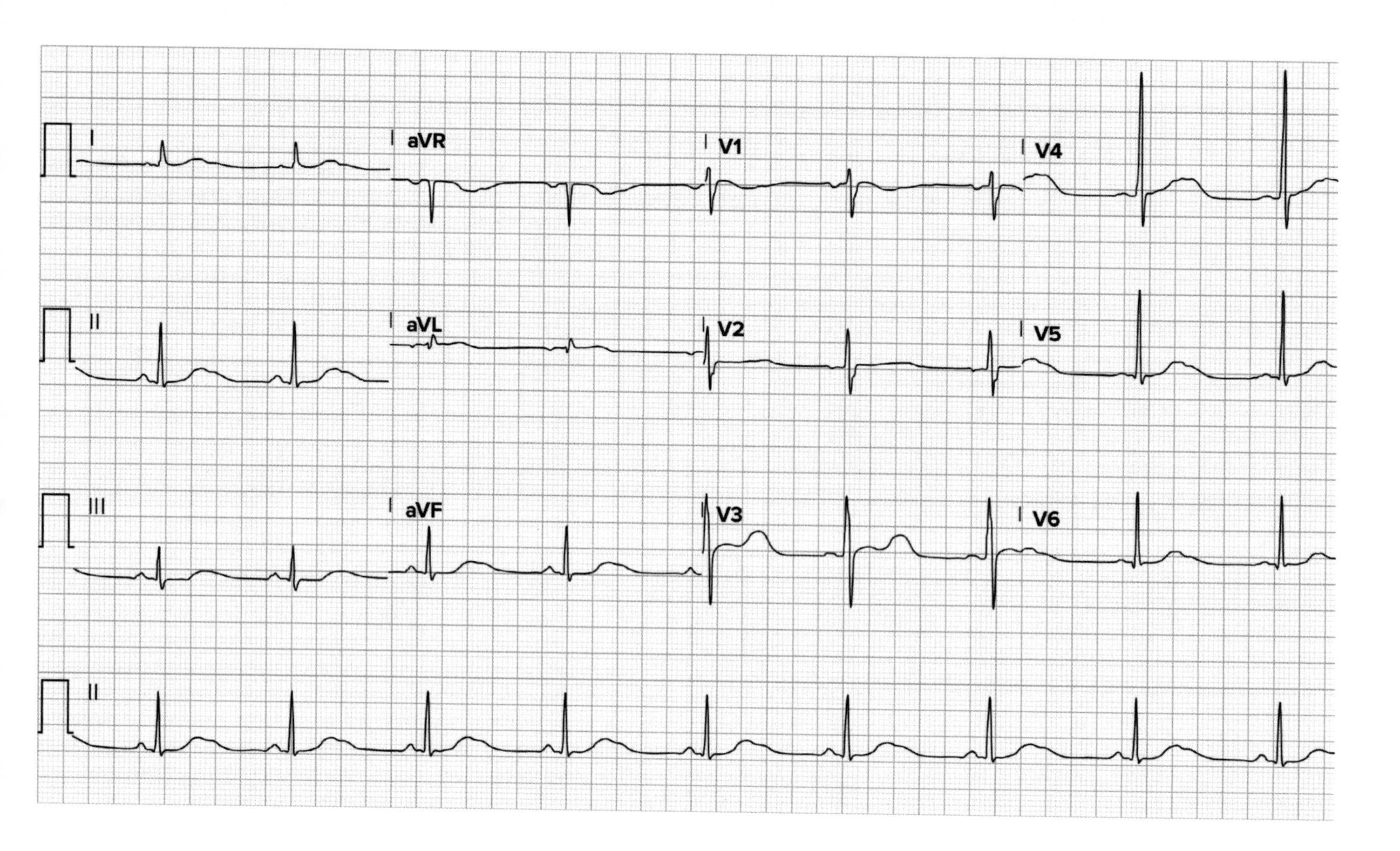

Case 71: Answer

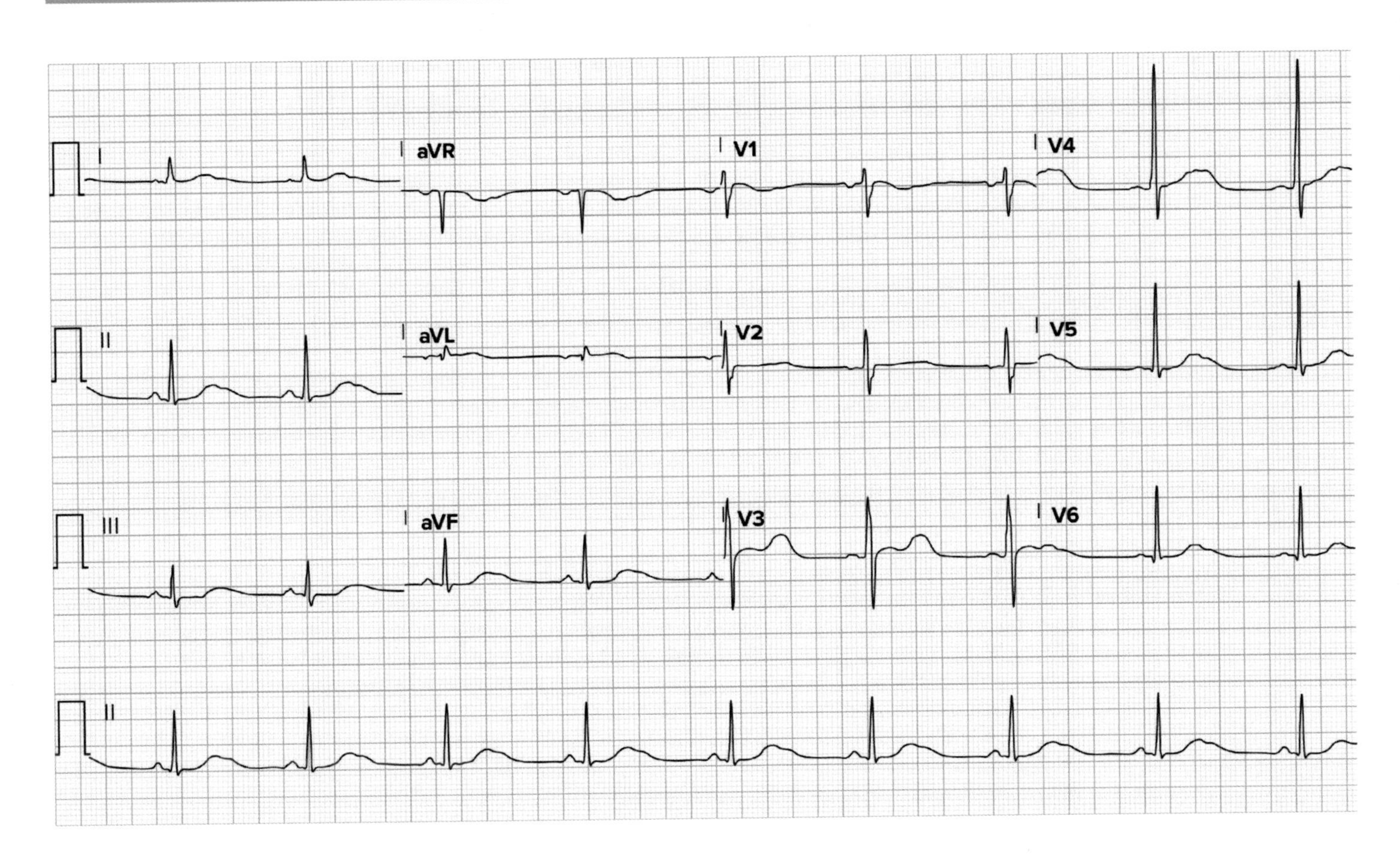

This ECG shows a sinus bradycardia at 55 bpm, normal axis, and subtle U-waves that fuse with the T-waves. Although the QTc interval is normal when measured in lead aVL (where there is no U-wave), the QU interval (ie, the QT interval that includes the U-wave) is long which is associated with a high risk for ventricular dysrhythmias, in particular torsades de pointes. Lead aVL appears to have STE relative to the TP segment but not the PR segment.

The key to interpreting this ECG is identifying the U-wave which is not immediately obvious as it fuses with the T-wave forming TU complexes ***(see Figure 1)***. This makes it difficult to measure the QTc interval, so leads without U waves, typically lead aVL and/or lead aVR, should be used ***(see Figure 2)***. In this patient's case, the QT interval measured in lead aVL, where there are no U-waves, is 380 msec (which equates to a QTc of 364 msec). In comparison, the QT interval measured in lead II, where there are U-waves, is 560 msec (which equates to a QTc of 564). There is controversy regarding whether hypokalemia truly causes a prolonged QT interval or just the appearance of a prolonged QT interval due to the presence of U-waves. Regardless, hypokalemia that produces the appearance of a prolonged QT interval, TU complexes, or significant U-waves, increases the risk for ventricular dysrhythmias, in particular torsades de pointes.

Figure 1.
The U-wave fuses with the T-wave to form a TU complex

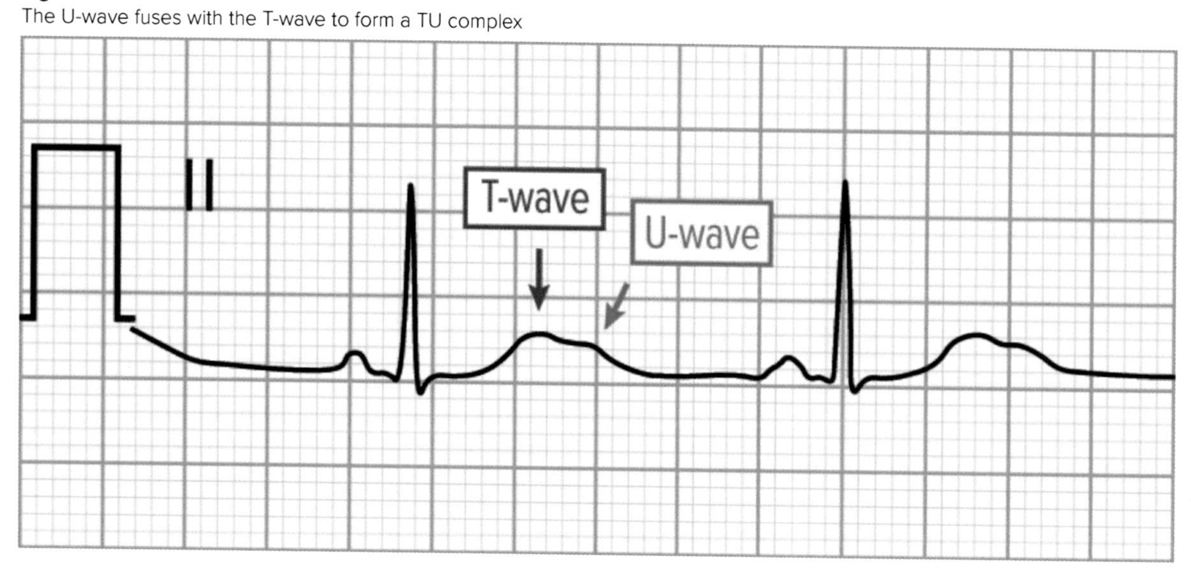

Figure 2.
The QT interval should be measured in leads without U-waves, typically lead aVL or aVR

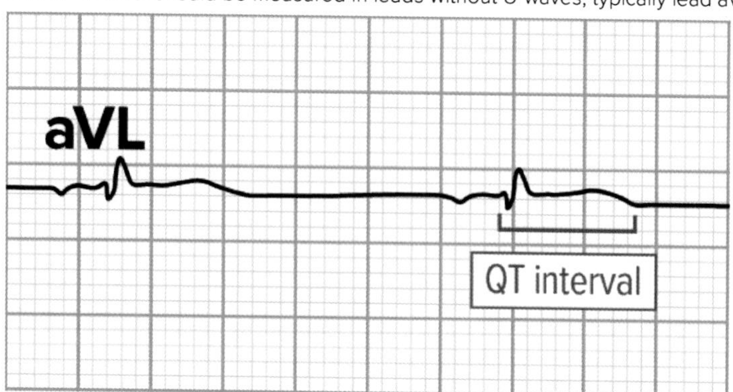

This patient's workup was notable for a serum potassium level of 1.6 mEq/L. The classic triad of ECG changes associated with hypokalemia includes TWI, STD, and U-waves, but all three findings are not always present, even with severe hypokalemia, as evidenced by this patient's ECG, which only had U-waves. This patient was treated with IV and oral potassium and admitted to the internal medicine service.

Hypokalemia Learning Points

- ECG changes seen in hypokalemia include:
  - T-wave flattening or inversion
  - U-waves
  - Slight STD
  - STE in lead aVR
  - Increased P-wave amplitude and duration
  - PR interval prolongation
  - QTc interval prolongation
  - Increased ectopy (eg, premature beats) and tachydysrhythmias

U-Wave Learning Points

- U-waves are typically low-amplitude deflections that follow the T-wave, best seen in the anterior precordial leads at slower heart rates
- Clinical significance not fully understood
  - Can see U-waves larger than T-waves with moderate to severe hypokalemia
  - Inverted U-waves in leads V2-V5 is abnormal (seen with ischemia and hypertension)
- When measuring the QT interval, exclude U-waves or measure in a lead without U-waves (usually leads aVR or aVL)

Case 72: Presentation

A 69-year-old male presents to the ED due to an abnormal outpatient pre-op ECG. He has no complaints. What is your interpretation of his ECG?

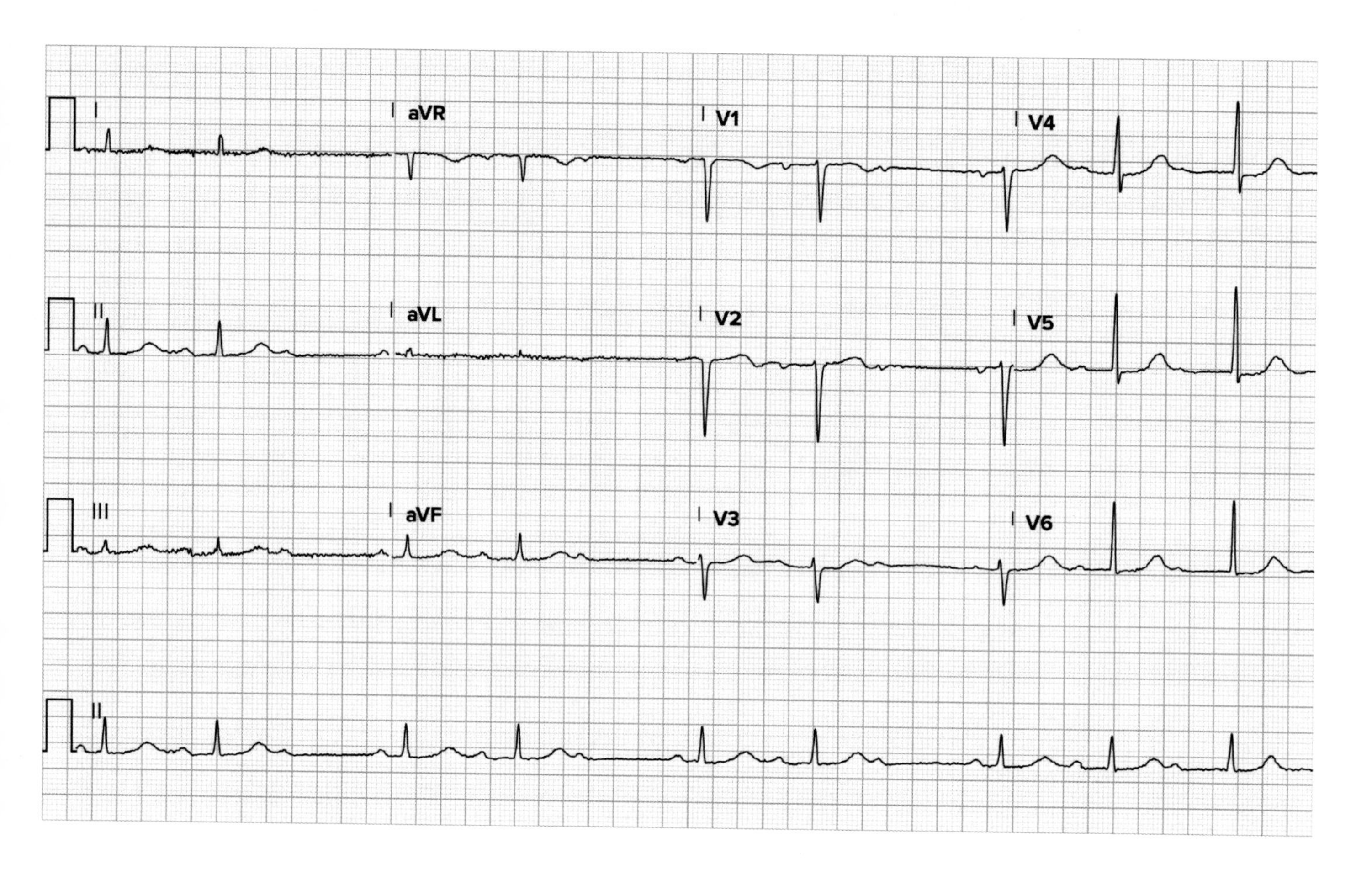

Case 72: Answer

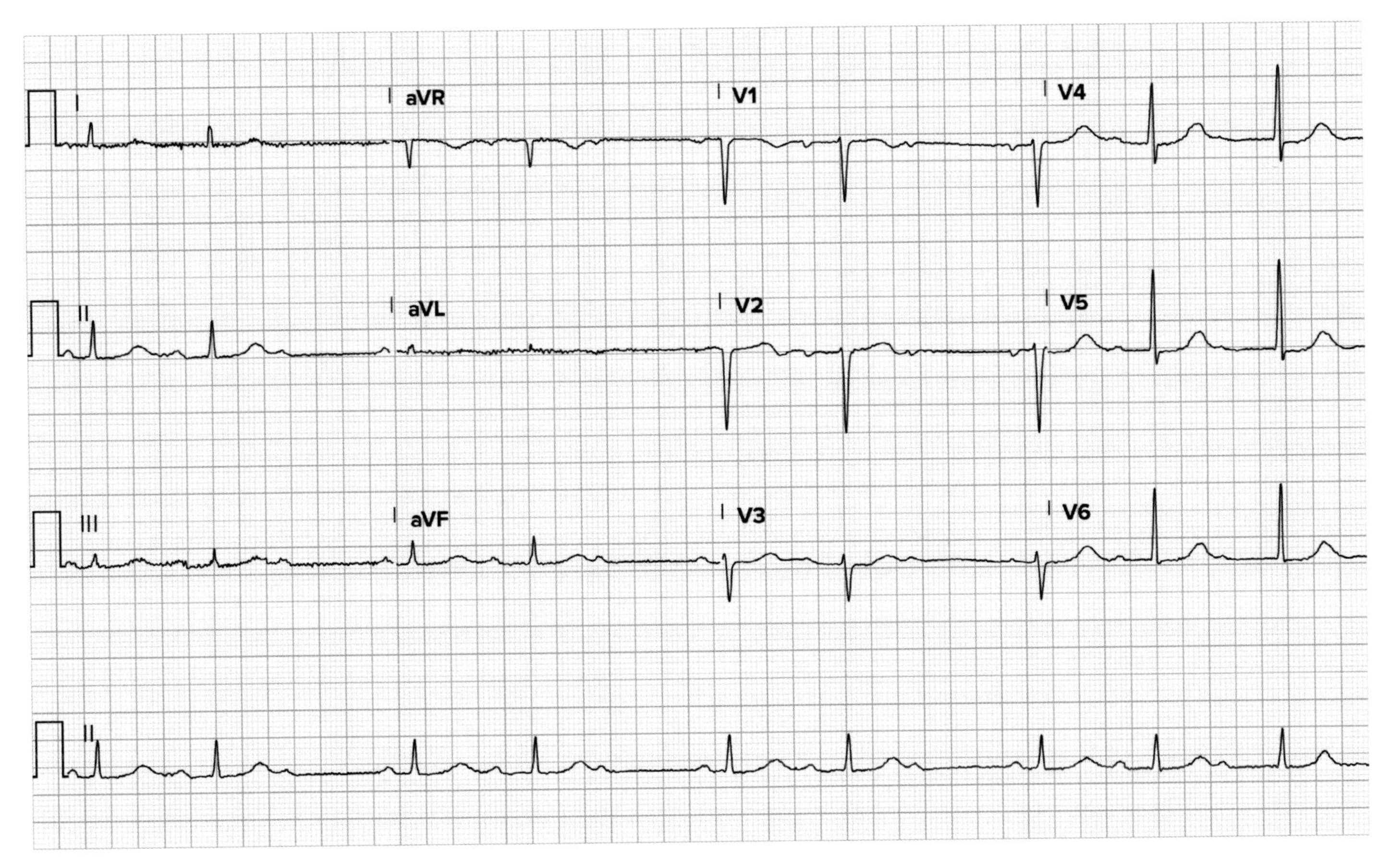

This ECG shows a Mobitz type I 2nd degree AV block with an average ventricular rate of 53 bpm, normal axis, and normal intervals.

The differential diagnosis for an irregular narrow complex rhythm with bradycardic ventricular rates includes:

- Atrial fibrillation (rate controlled)
- Atrial flutter with variable block (rate controlled)
- Atrial tachycardia with variable block (rate controlled)
- Wandering atrial pacemaker
- 2nd degree AV block Mobitz types I and II
- Variable high-grade AV block (eg, 3:1, 4:1, etc.)
- 2nd degree sinoatrial block
- Sinus arrhythmia
- Sinus bradycardia, junctional rhythm, or junctional bradycardia with irregular pattern of PAC, PJC, and/or PVC
- Sinus bradycardia, junctional rhythm, or junctional bradycardia with regular patterns of PAC, PJC, and/or PVC (bigeminy, trigeminy, etc.)

Mobitz type I AV conduction, also called Wenckebach conduction, is due to intermittent failure of conduction at the AV node. This most often occurs due to excessive vagal tone. The distinguishing feature of Mobitz type I conduction is progressive increase in the PR interval and decreasing RR interval followed by a non-conducted P-wave (i.e., a P-wave without accompanying QRS complex) ***(see Figure 1)***. The PR interval resets after the non-conducted P-wave so that the PR interval after the non-conducted P-wave is shorter than the PR interval preceding the non-conducted P-wave. The biggest increase in the PR interval typically happens between the 1st and 2nd beats of each cycle.

Figure 1.
The lead II rhythm strip shows progressively increasing PR interval followed by a non-conducted P-wave, consistent with a Mobitz type I AV block

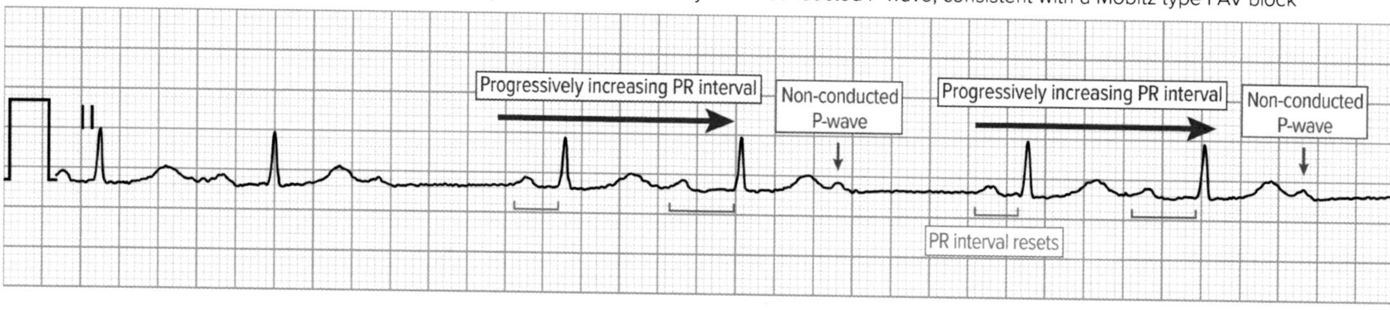

The pattern of 3:2 conduction (ie, 3 P-waves for every 2 QRS complexes) repeats three times after which the conduction ratio changes starting with the 7th P-QRS-T complex. There is a hidden P-wave in the last T-wave of the ECG that becomes apparent by marching out the P-waves ***(see Figure 2).*** It is impossible to know whether this P-wave is non-conducted (which would be consistent with 4:3 conduction) without a longer rhythm strip.

Figure 2.
Marching out the P-waves on the lead II rhythm strip helps identify a P-wave hidden in the T-wave of the 9th QRS-T complex

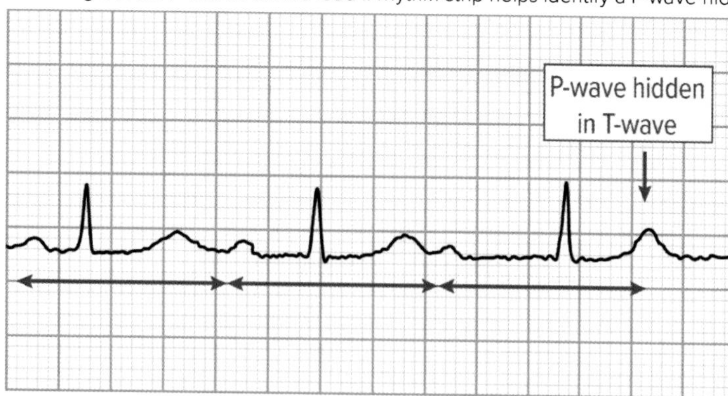

It is essential to differentiate Mobitz type I conduction from Mobitz type II conduction, as the former is typically transient with a more benign course while the latter has a high risk of progressing to a 3rd degree AV block, frequently produces hemodynamic compromise, and is associated with worse outcomes if not treated. The QRS complex duration is typically not useful in differentiating between a Mobitz type I and a Mobitz type II, as a Mobitz type I can have a prolonged QRS complex duration if there is aberrant conduction (eg, an intrinsic bundle branch block) and a Mobitz type II can have a narrow QRS complex (ie, duration < 110 msec) if the block is in the AV node. The key to distinguishing between the two is to compare the RR interval that includes the non-conducted P-wave to the PP interval.

In a Mobitz type I, the RR interval that includes the non-conducted P-wave will be less than twice the PP interval. This is evident in the lead II rhythm strip in the case ECG ***(see Figure 3)*** where the RR interval that includes the non-conducted P-wave (1520 msec) is less than twice the PP interval (1680 msec).

Figure 3.
In a Mobitz type I AV block, the RR interval that includes the non-conducted P-wave is less than twice the PP interval

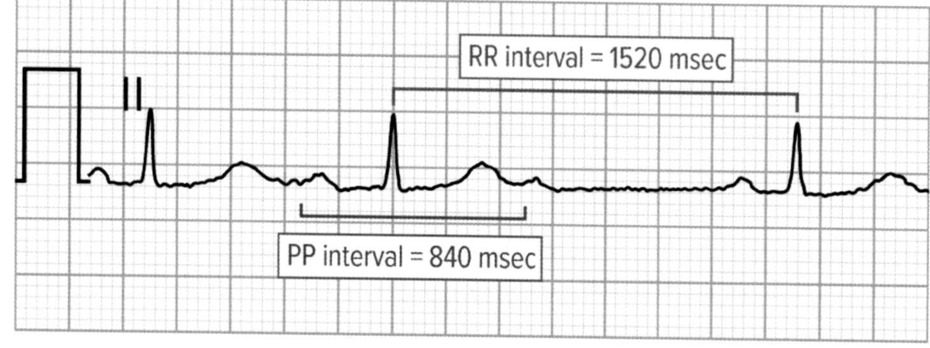

In a Mobitz type II AV block, the RR interval that includes the non-conducted P-wave will be equal to twice the PP interval. In the example below from a different ECG ***(see Figure 4)***, the RR interval that includes the non-conducted P-wave (1440 msec) is equal to exactly twice the PP interval (1440 msec).

Figure 4.
In a Mobitz type II AV block, the RR interval that includes the non-conducted P-wave is equal to exactly twice the PP interval (from a different ECG)

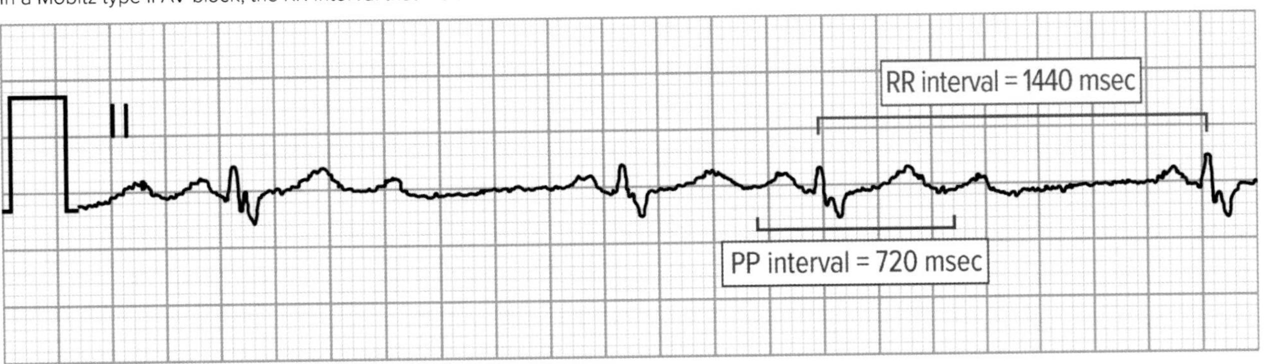

The patient had an unremarkable ED workup and was discharged with cardiology follow-up.

Mobitz type I AV Block Learning Points

- Progressively increasing PR interval and decreasing RR interval until a non-conducted P-wave occurs (ie, P-wave without accompanying QRS complex)
  - PR interval immediately after non-conducted P-wave is shorter than PR interval preceding non-conducted P-wave
  - RR interval that includes non-conducted P-wave < twice the PP interval
- Can be normal variant and usually does not produce hemodynamic compromise
  - Typically associated with excess vagal tone and therefore usually responds to atropine when acute treatment is needed
  - Can lead to a more advanced AV block if associated with a pathologic etiology
  - Can be seen with inferior MI

Mobitz type II AV Block Learning Points

- Constant PR interval in conducted beats
  - Described as ratio of P-waves to QRS complexes
  - Typically an infranodal block resulting in a prolonged QRS complex duration
  - RR interval that includes non-conducted P-wave = twice the PP interval
- Never a normal variant and frequently produces hemodynamic compromise
  - High risk of progressing to a 3rd degree AV block
  - Atropine is unlikely to lead to clinical improvement and may lead to a high-grade AV block

High-grade (or advanced) AV Block Learning Points

- 2nd degree AV block with ≥ 2 sequential non-conducted P-waves
  - Most commonly a variant of a Mobitz type II but can be associated with a Mobitz type I
  - PP and RR intervals should have a whole number ratio
- Named as ratio of P-waves to QRS complexes
- Can be seen after anterior MI or with significant pathology of the conduction pathway
- High risk of progressing to a 3rd degree AV block

Case 73: Presentation

This is the pre-op ECG of an 80-year-old female being admitted for a hip fracture. What is your interpretation of her ECG?

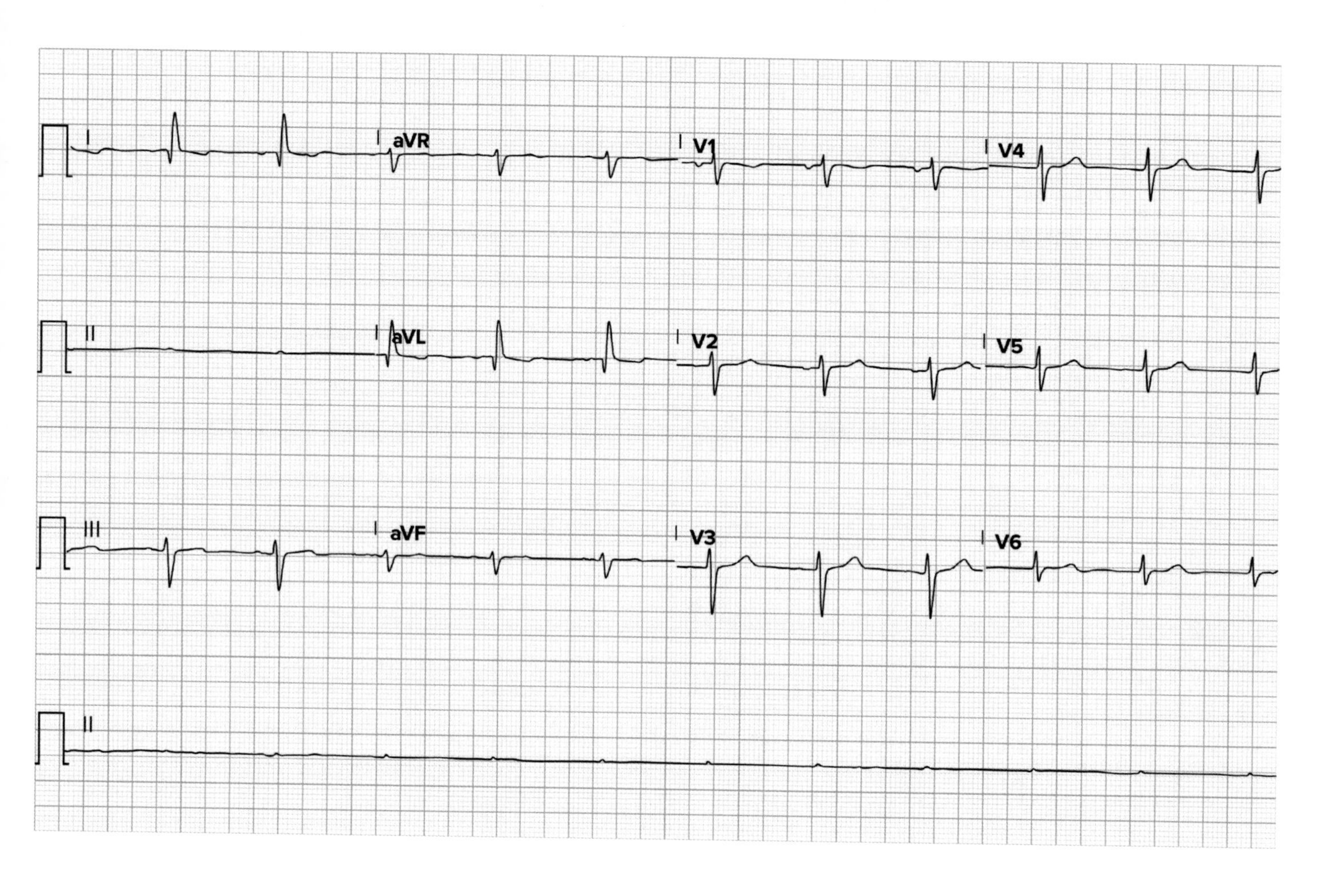

Case 73: Answer

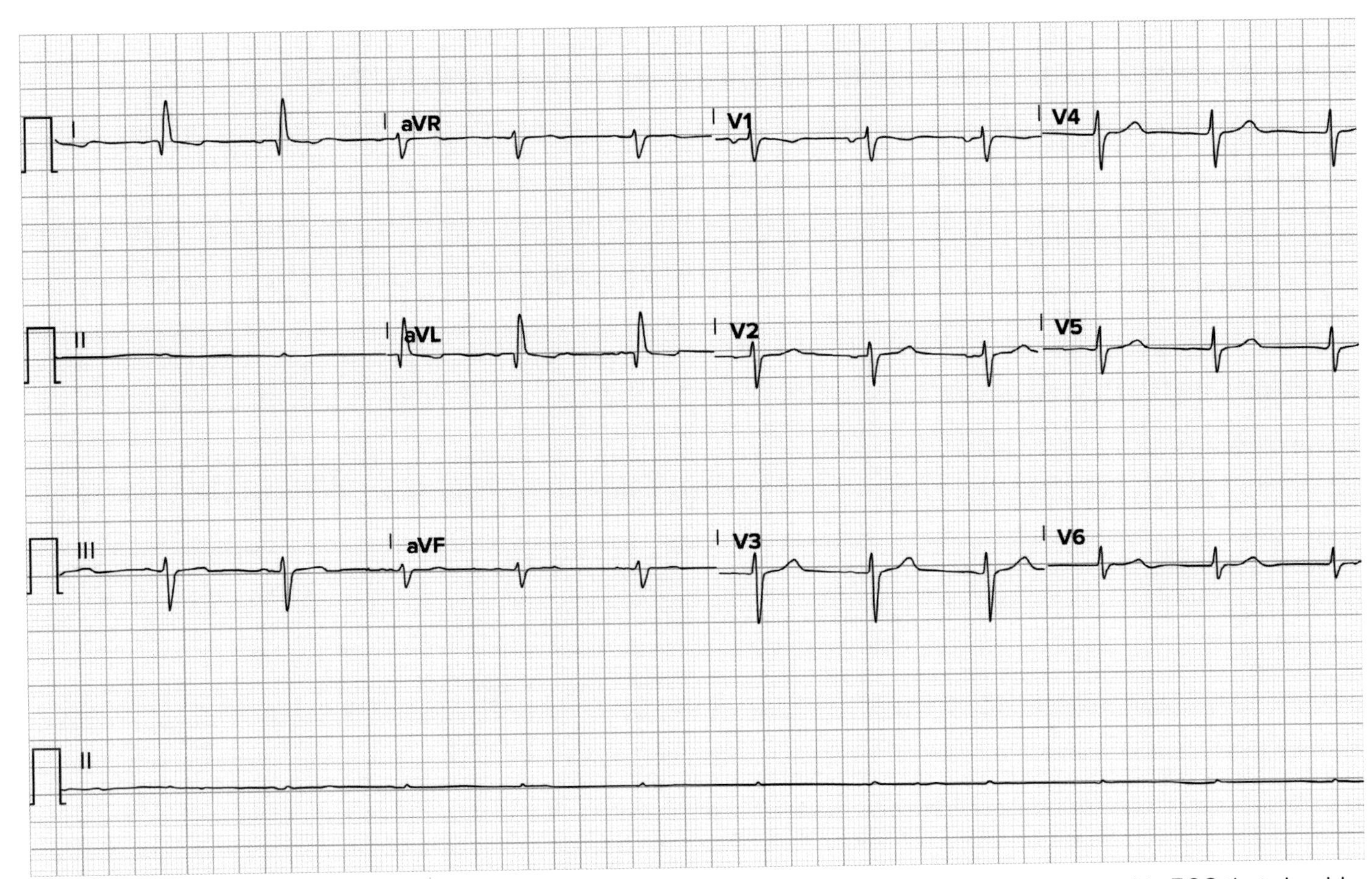

This ECG shows right arm-right leg (RA-RL) lead reversal. The most easily recognizable abnormality in this ECG that should prompt concern for RA-RL lead reversal is that lead II is almost "flatline" with barely discernible P-QRS-T complexes, often referred to as "pseudo-asystole." ***Figure 1*** shows a repeat ECG with correct lead placement.

Figure 1.
Repeat ECG with correct lead placement

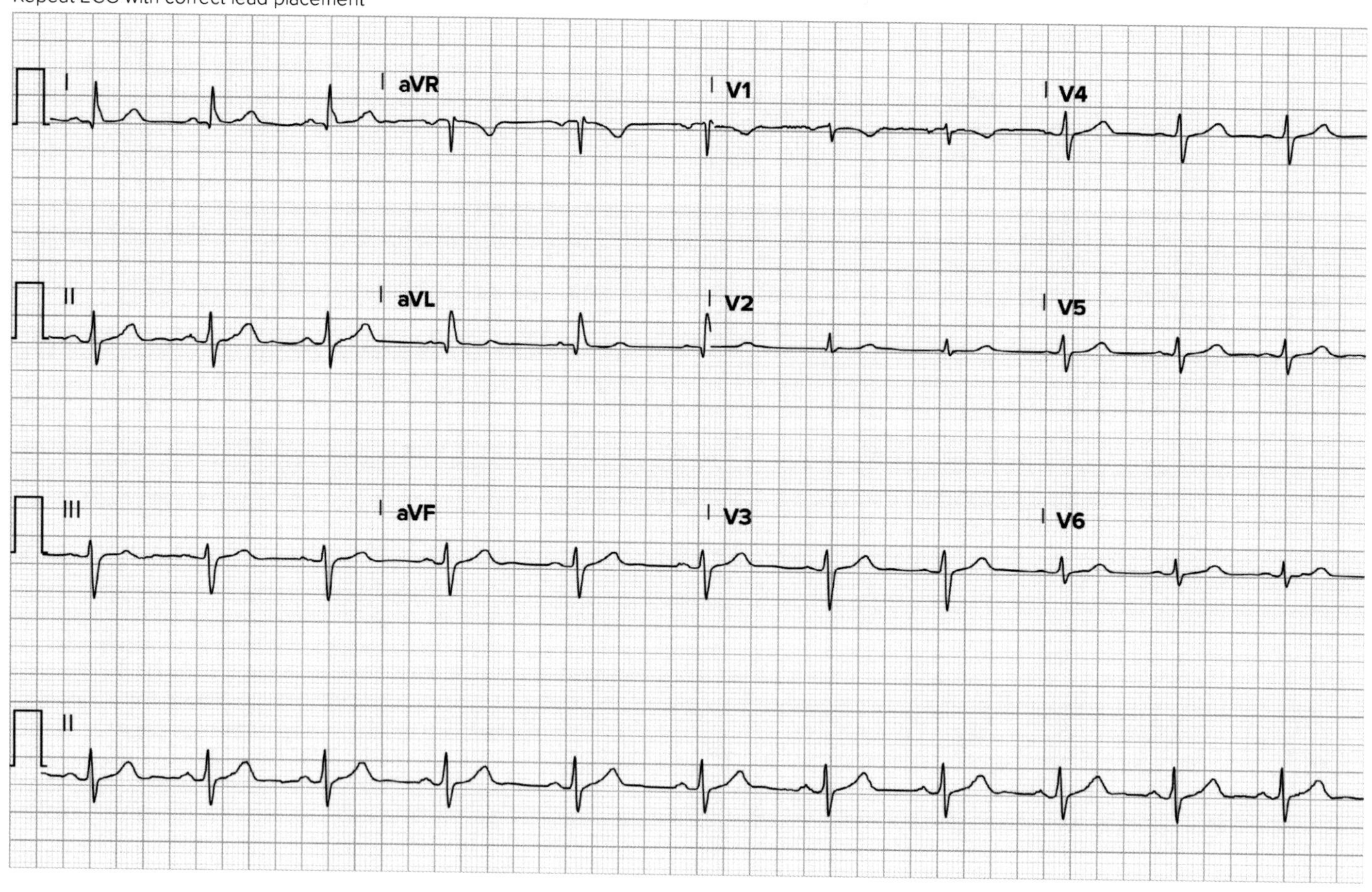

ECG findings seen with RA-RL lead reversal include *(see Figure 2)*:

1. Lead II is almost a straight line with barely discernible P-QRS-T complexes
2. P-QRS-T complexes in leads I and aVL appear as a mirror image of the P-QRS-T complexes in lead III (ie, inverted over the y-axis)
3. P-QRS-T complexes in lead aVR appear similar to those in lead aVF (including a positive P-wave)
4. Lead III is unchanged

Figure 2.
Comparison of the limb leads from the case ECG with RA-RL lead reversal with the repeat ECG with correct lead placement

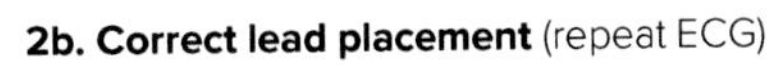

2a. RA-RL reversal (case ECG)

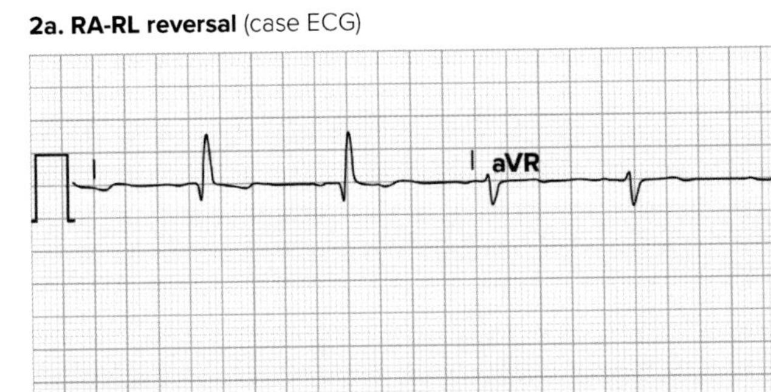

2b. Correct lead placement (repeat ECG)

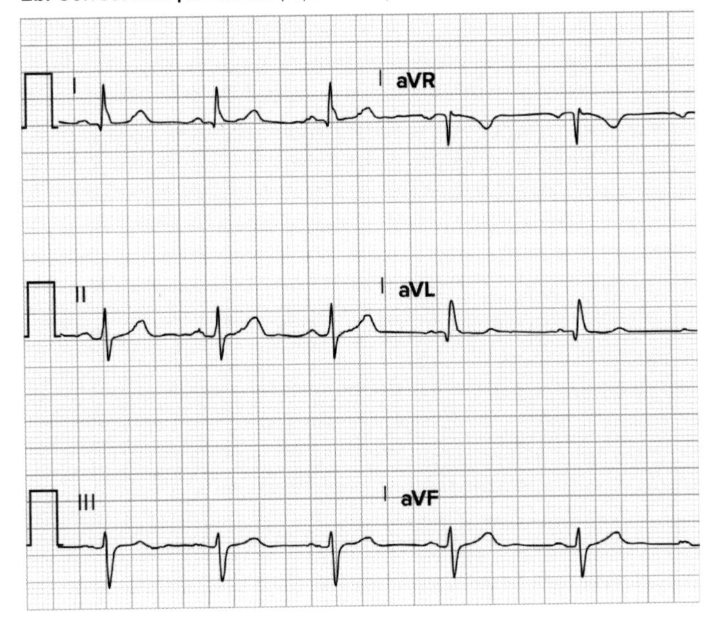

Lead Reversal Learning Points

Lead Reversal Summary

	I	II	III	aVR	aVL	aVF	V1-V6
LA-RA	Inverted	Switches with III	Switches with II	Switches with aVL	Switches with aVR	No change	No change
LA-LL	Switches with II	Switches with I	Inverted	No change	Switches with aVF	Switches with aVL	No change
LA-RL	Looks like II	Unchanged	Flatline	Looks like inverted II	Looks identical to aVF	Looks identical to aVL	No change
RA-LL	Switches with inverted III	Inverted	Switches with inverted I	Switches with aVF	No change	Switches with aVR	No change
RA-RL	Looks like inverted III	Flatline	Unchanged	Looks identical to aVF	Looks like inverted III	Looks identical to aVR	No change
LA-LL + RA-RL	Flatline	Looks like inverted III	Inverted	Looks identical to aVL	Looks identical to aVR	Looks like inverted III	No change
Dextrocardia	Inverted	Switches with III	Switches with II	Switches with aVL	Switches with aVR	No change	Dominant S-wave and poor R-wave progression

***NOTE:** RL is a ground lead, so RL-LL reversal does not result in any significant changes*

Case 74: Presentation

A 68-year-old male presents with exertional near syncope and fatigue.
What is your interpretation of his ECG?

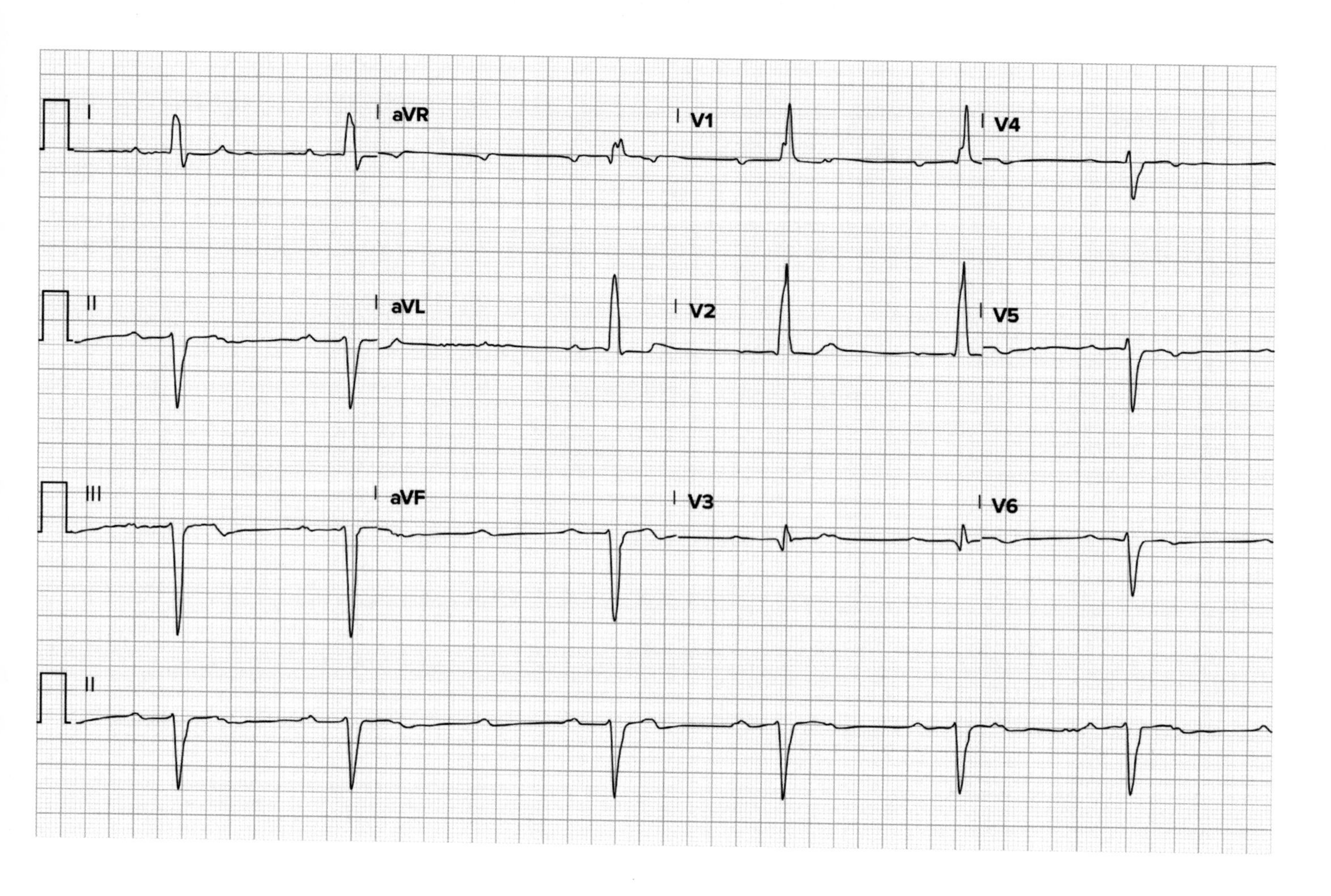

Case 74: Answer

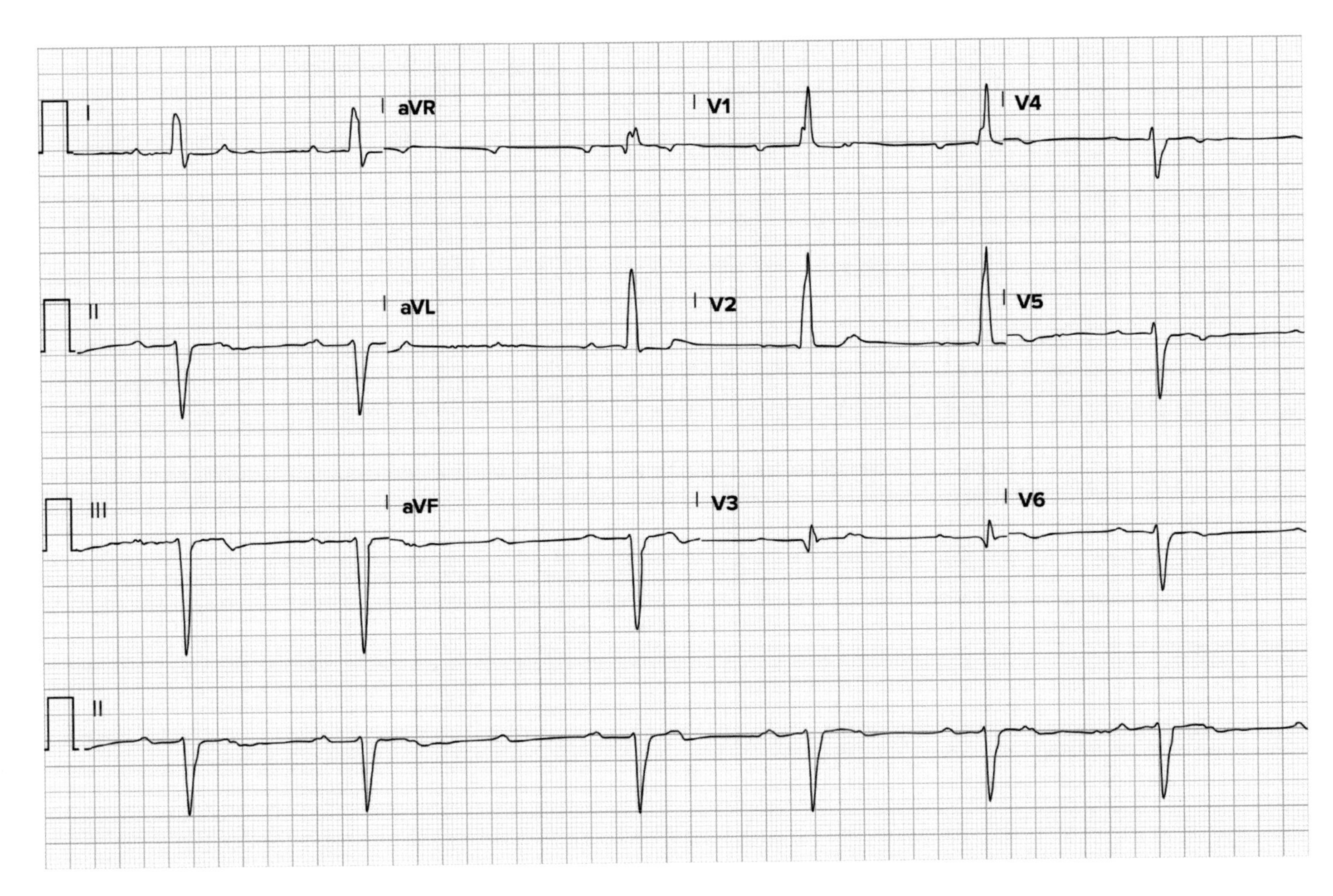

This ECG shows a high-grade AV block with 2:1 and 3:1 conduction with an average ventricular rate of 38 bpm, prolonged PR interval at 360 msec, left axis deviation, prolonged QRS complex duration with a RBBB, and a left anterior fascicular block.

The differential diagnosis for an irregular wide complex rhythm with bradycardic ventricular rates includes:

- Atrial fibrillation (rate controlled) with aberrant conduction
- Atrial flutter with variable block (rate controlled) and aberrant conduction
- Atrial tachycardia with variable block (rate controlled) and aberrant conduction
- Wandering atrial pacemaker with aberrant conduction
- 2nd degree AV block Mobitz types I and II with aberrant conduction
- Variable high-grade AV block (eg, 3:1, 4:1, etc.) with aberrant conduction
- 2nd degree sinoatrial block with aberrant conduction
- Sinus arrhythmia with aberrant conduction
- Sinus bradycardia, junctional rhythm, or junctional bradycardia with aberrant conduction and irregular pattern of PAC, PJC, and/or PVC
- Sinus bradycardia, junctional rhythm, or junctional bradycardia with aberrant conduction and regular patterns of PAC, PJC, and/or PVC (bigeminy, trigeminy, etc.)
  - Causes of aberrant conduction include fixed or rate-related BBB, metabolic abnormalities, sodium channel blocker toxicity, ventricular-paced rhythm, and ventricular pre-excitation (eg, WPW)

The key to correctly interpreting this ECG is recognizing the non-conducted P-waves buried in the T-waves. These are more easily identified by increasing the gain which will be reflected in the calibration signal box on the left side of the ECG ***(see Figure 1)***. This box represents the calibration of the recording speed (x-axis) and voltage (y-axis) of the ECG. Time is represented by the width of the rectangle and is set for 0.2 sec. Voltage is represented by the height and is set for 10 mV. Standard calibration is 25 mm/sec (ie, one small box = 0.04 sec) and 10 mm/mV (ie, one small box = 0.1 mV).

When the gain is increased 2x, the height of the calibration box will become twice as tall, so now 20 mm = 1 mV (ie, one small box = 0.05 mV) ***(see Figure 1)***.

For this ECG, the 2 consecutive P-waves that precede the 3rd QRS complex provide an easy PP interval to use to march out the P-waves ***(see Figure 1)***. Note that the PR intervals are all consistent which is expected with a high-grade AV block.

Figure 1.
The lead II rhythm strip with the gain increased 2x (note that calibration rectangle is 20 mm high) shows consistent PR intervals (brackets) and PP intervals (arrows)

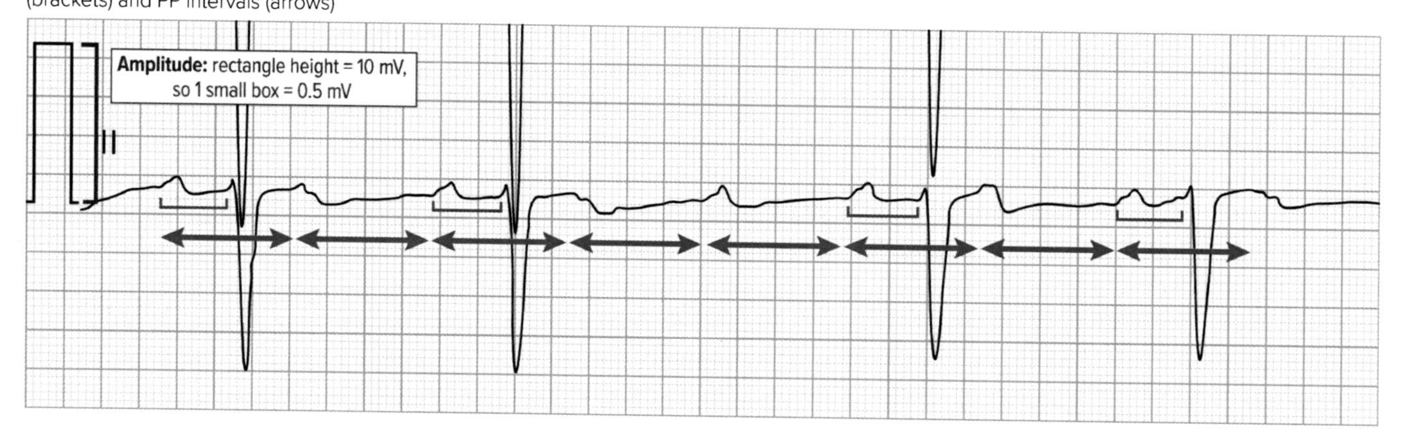

Once the buried P-waves are identified, the pattern of 2:1 and 3:1 AV blocks becomes more apparent ***(see Figure 2)***.

Figure 2.
The lead II rhythm strip with the gain increased 2x (note that calibration rectangle is 20 mm high) shows a pattern of 2:1 and 3:1 AV blocks

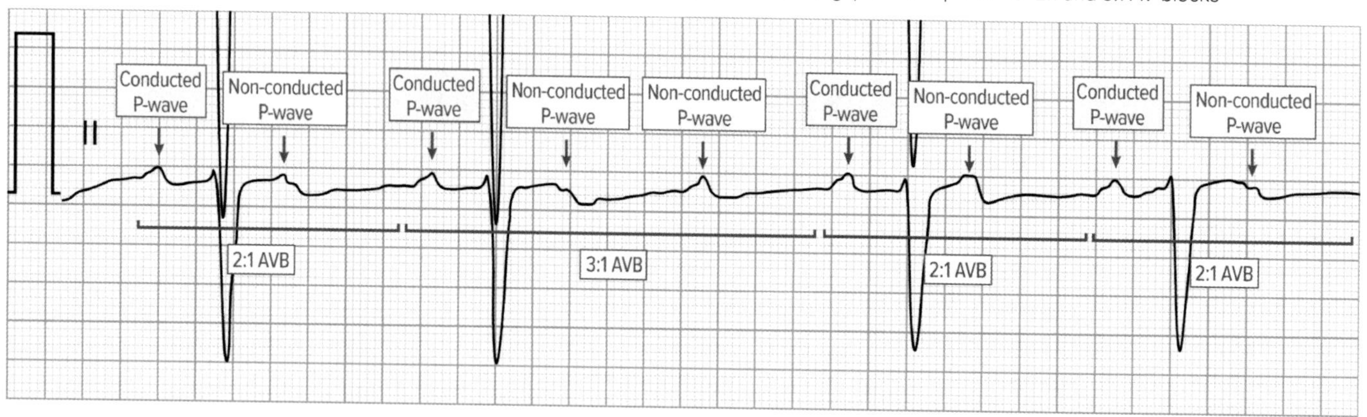

In a 2:1 AV block, there are no sequential conducting P-waves to compare PR intervals, so it is often impossible to determine if the underlying pathology is a Mobitz type I or Mobitz type II. The presence of a 3:1 AV block strongly suggests an underlying Mobitz type II, although high-grade AV blocks can be seen with an underlying Mobitz type I. The term high-grade AV block, also called advanced AV block, is used to describe when ≥ 2 sequential P-waves are not conducted. These blocks are most commonly a variant of a Mobitz type II and have a high risk of progressing to a 3rd degree AV block.

This ECG also shows a RBBB. The characteristic findings in a RBBB include:

- QRS complex duration ≥ 120 msec
- rsr', rsR', or rSR' pattern in lead V1 +/- V2
  - Variations in lead V1 include qR pattern or broad R-wave that is often notched
  - In lead V1, the initial upward deflection should always be smaller than the 2nd upward deflection
- S-wave duration > R-wave or > 40 msec in leads I and V6
- Normal R-wave peak time in leads V5 and V6 but > 50 msec in lead V1 (only required if broad R-wave +/- notch is present in lead V1)
- Repolarization abnormalities include STD and TWI in lead V1 +/- lead(s) V2-V3 if they have an rsR' pattern, so STE and/or upright T-waves in those leads are concerning for ischemia

Note that the QRS complex morphology in lead I is atypical for a RBBB as the R-wave duration is greater than the S-wave duration.

The presence of a RBBB with an axis deviation should prompt evaluation for a concurrent fascicular block. This ECG shows a LAFB *(see Figure 3)*.

The characteristic findings in a LAFB include:

- Left axis deviation between -45° and -90°
- qR complex in lead aVL +/- lead I
- rS complex in leads II, III, and aVF
- Prolonged R-wave peak time ≥ 45 msec in lead aVL
- QRS complex duration < 120 msec in the absence of a concurrent conduction delay

Figure 3.
Findings in a left anterior fascicular block include qR complexes in leads I and aVL (red box), rS complexes in leads II, III, and aVF (purple box), and left axis deviation (green arrow)

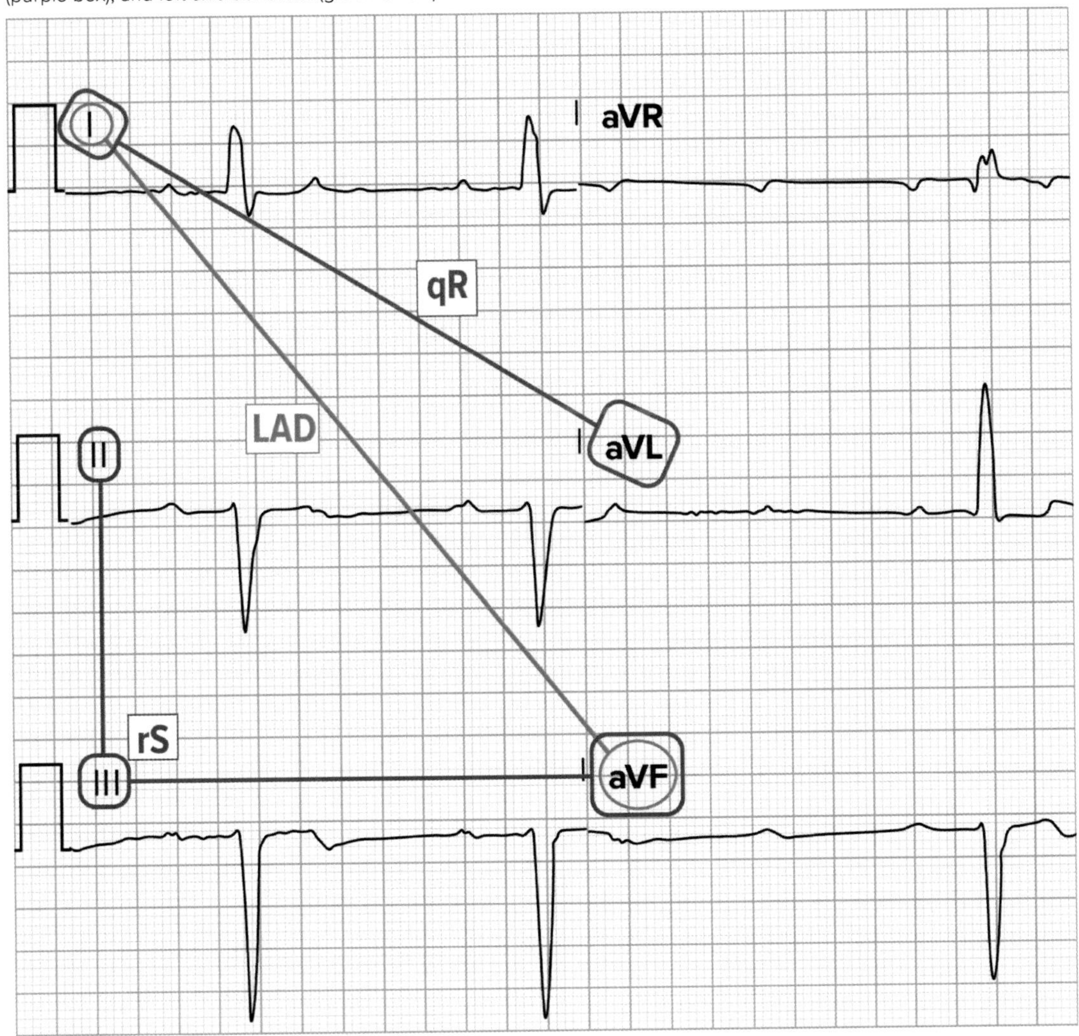

The constellation of a RBBB + fascicular block + any AV block is called a trifascicular block, which is further differentiated as complete or incomplete:

- Complete trifascicular block = 3rd degree AV block + RBBB + LAFB or LPFB
- Incomplete trifascicular block = 1st or 2nd degree AV block + RBBB + LAFB or LPFB, or RBBB + alternating LAFB/LPFB on successive ECGs

This patient had an unremarkable ED workup and was admitted to the cardiology service for evaluation for a pacemaker. While waiting for an inpatient bed, he was noted to have a regular bradycardic rhythm on telemetry so a repeat ECG was obtained *(see Figure 4)*.

Figure 4.
A repeat ECG shows a 3rd degree AV block with every other P-wave hidden in a QRS complex

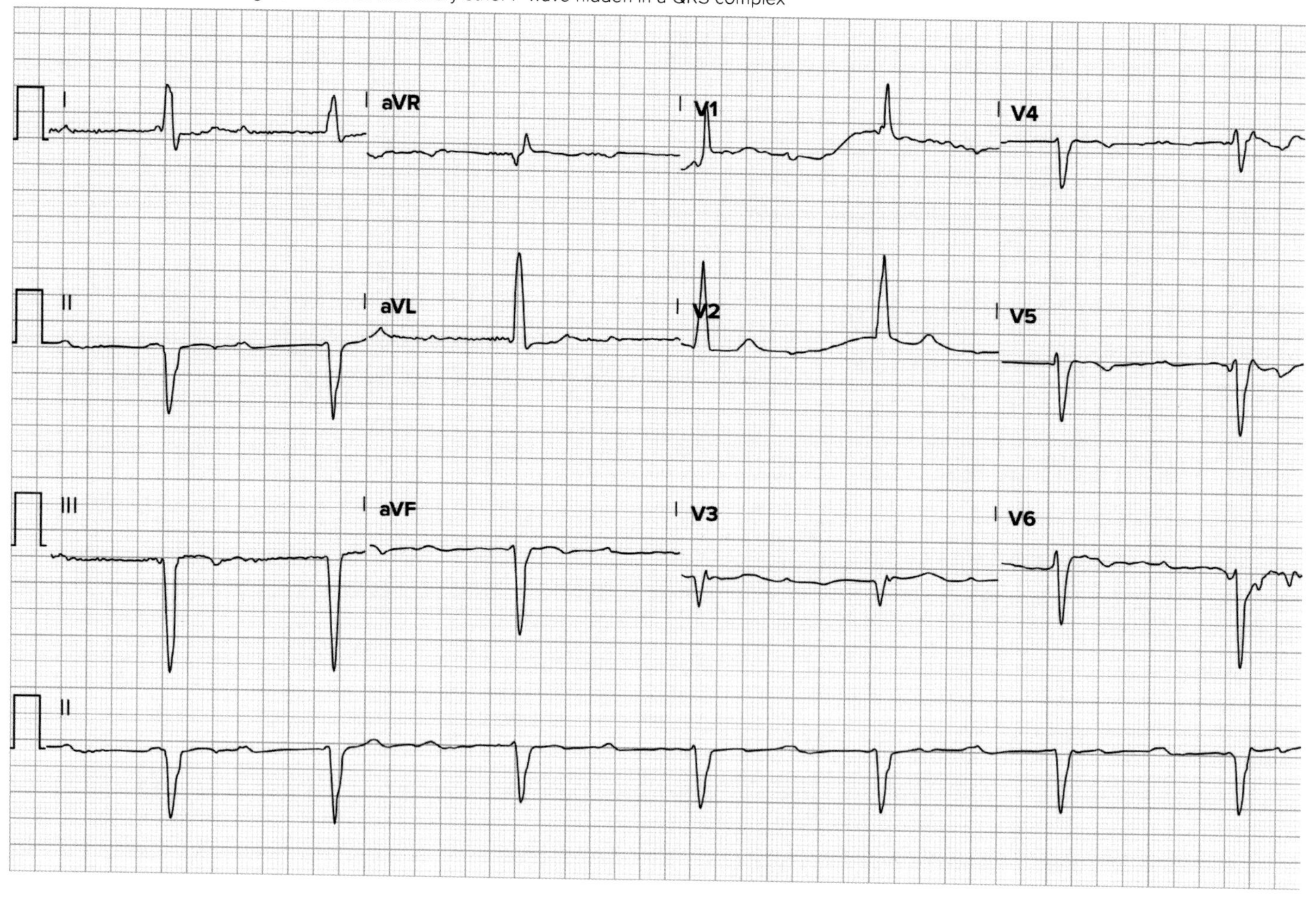

The repeat ECG shows a 3rd degree AV block with every other P-wave hidden in a QRS complex. Recognizing that the visible P-waves seen between the QRS complexes do not have consistent PR intervals and are extremely prolonged is key to avoiding misinterpreting this ECG as a sinus bradycardia with a 1st degree AV block. Another axiom for finding hidden P-waves is called the "Bix rule" (named after cardiologist Harold Bix) which states that whenever there are P-waves halfway between the QRS complexes, there are likely additional P-waves hidden within the QRS complexes.

High-grade (or advanced) AV Block Learning Points

- 2nd degree AV block with ≥ 2 sequential non-conducted P-waves
  - Most commonly a variant of a Mobitz type II but can be associated with a Mobitz type I
  - PP and RR intervals should have a whole number ratio
- Named as ratio of P-waves to QRS complexes
- Can be seen after anterior MI or with significant pathology of the conduction pathway
- High risk of progressing to a 3rd degree AV block

Fascicular Blocks Learning Points

- Complete trifascicular block
  - 3rd degree AV block + RBBB + LAFB or LPFB
  - Always gets admitted for pacemaker placement
- Incomplete trifascicular block
  - 1st or 2nd degree AV block + RBBB + LAFB or LPFB, or RBBB + alternating LAFB/LPFB on successive ECGs
  - Syncope + incomplete trifascicular block = usually requires admission for cardiac monitoring for transient 3rd degree AV block and evaluation for pacemaker placement

NOTES:

Case 75: Presentation

TA 31-year-old female with no known cardiac history presents with palpitations and lightheadedness. What is your interpretation of her ECG?

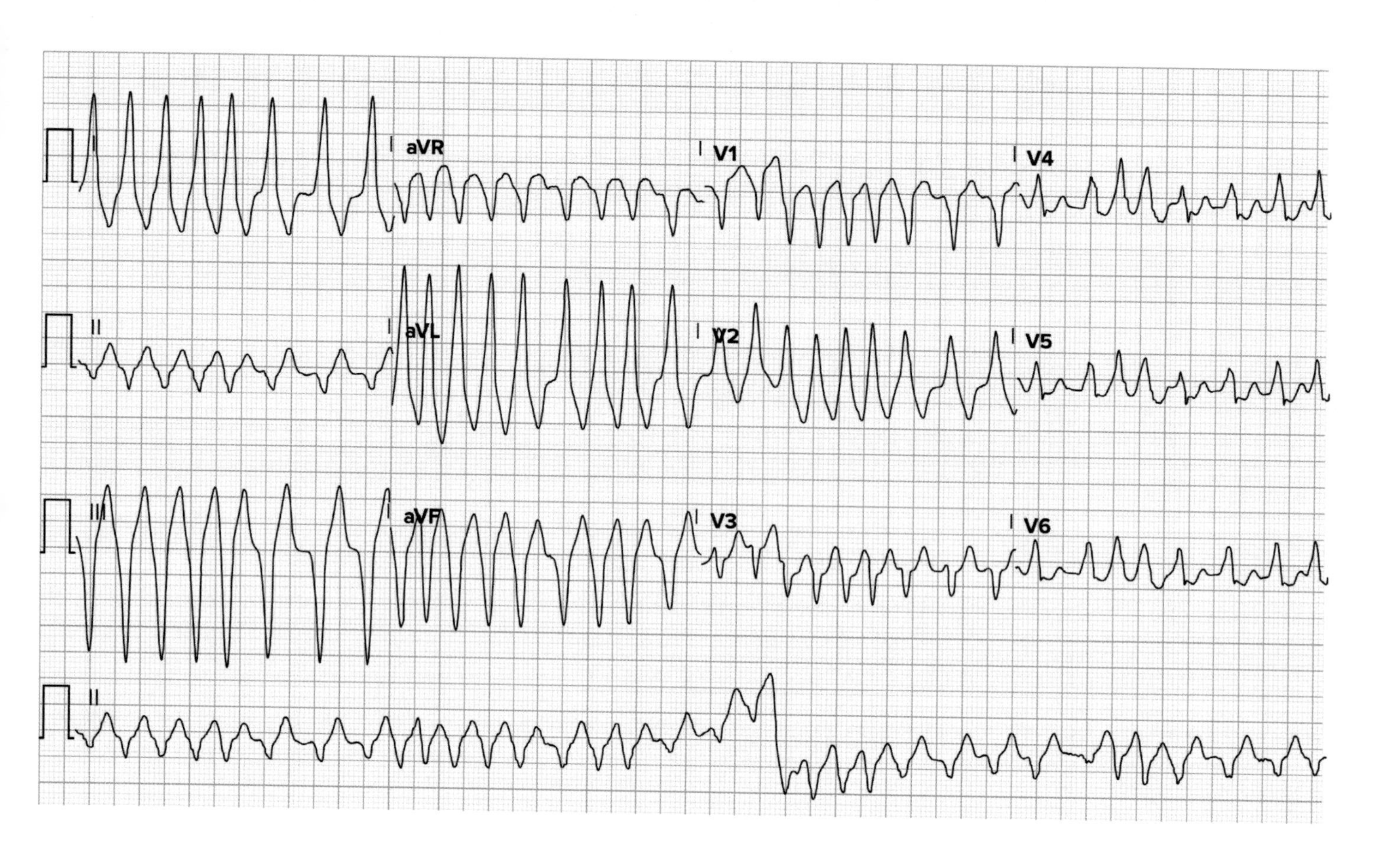

Case 75: Answer

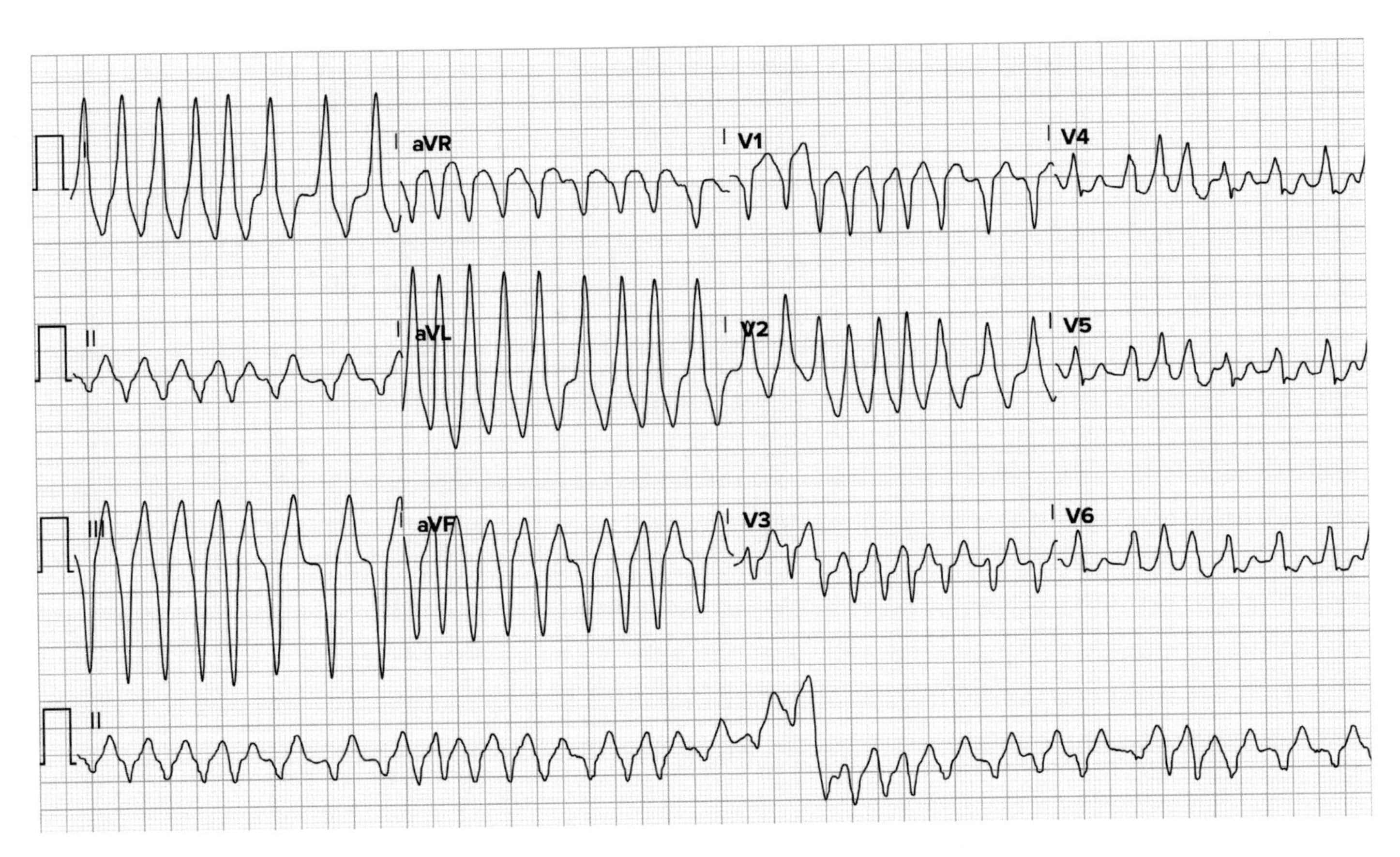

This ECG shows an irregular wide complex tachycardia with an average ventricular rate of 198 bpm and intermittent rates up to 280 bpm, no P-waves, left axis deviation, and prolonged QRS complex duration with beat-to-beat variation in the QRS complex morphology.

The differential diagnosis for an irregular WCT includes:

- Ventricular fibrillation
- Polymorphic ventricular tachycardia (including torsades de pointes)
- MAT with aberrant conduction
- Atrial flutter with variable block and aberrant conduction
- Atrial fibrillation with aberrant conduction
  - Causes of aberrant conduction include fixed or rate-related BBB, metabolic abnormalities, sodium channel blocker toxicity, ventricular-paced rhythm, and ventricular pre-excitation (eg, WPW)

This ECG shows the triad, as yet unnamed, of and irregularly irregular rhythm, markedly changing QRS complex morphologies, and extremely fast rates up to 273 bpm in some regions ***(see Figure 1)*** that is only seen with polymorphic ventricular tachycardia and atrial fibrillation with WPW. Polymorphic ventricular tachycardia will have phasic variation (ie, happens over a number of beats) of the QRS complex polarity (ie, axis) and amplitude. Conversely, atrial fibrillation with WPW will have beat-to-beat variation in the QRS complex morphology and relatively consistent QRS complex polarity, as seen in this patient's ECG.

Figure 1.
Lead V1 shows an irregularly irregular rhythm with variable QRS complex morphologies and extremely fast ventricular rates (up to 273 bpm in this case), consistent with atrial fibrillation with WPW

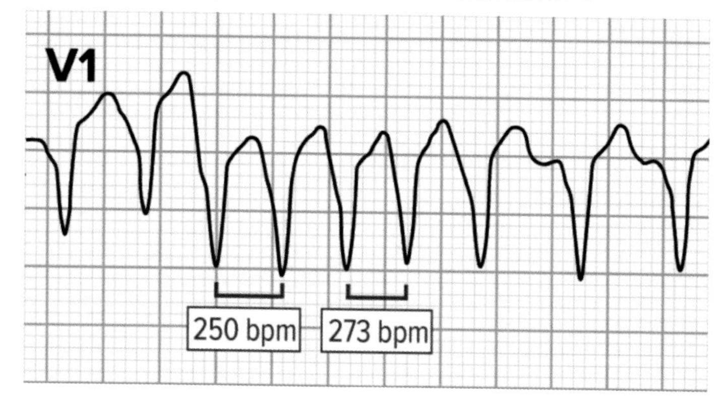

This patient was chemically cardioverted with procainamide and a repeat ECG showed the characteristic short PR interval and delta waves consistent with WPW ***(see Figures 2 and 3).*** Delta waves represent pre-excitation of a portion of the ventricular myocardium via the accessory pathway (AP). The depolarization wave resulting from this portion of pre-excited ventricular myocardium subsequently fuses with the depolarization caused by conduction via the AV node, ultimately creating the characteristic morphology of a QRS complex with a delta wave.

Figure 2.
A repeat ECG after cardioversion shows delta waves and short PR intervals seen with WPW in sinus rhythm

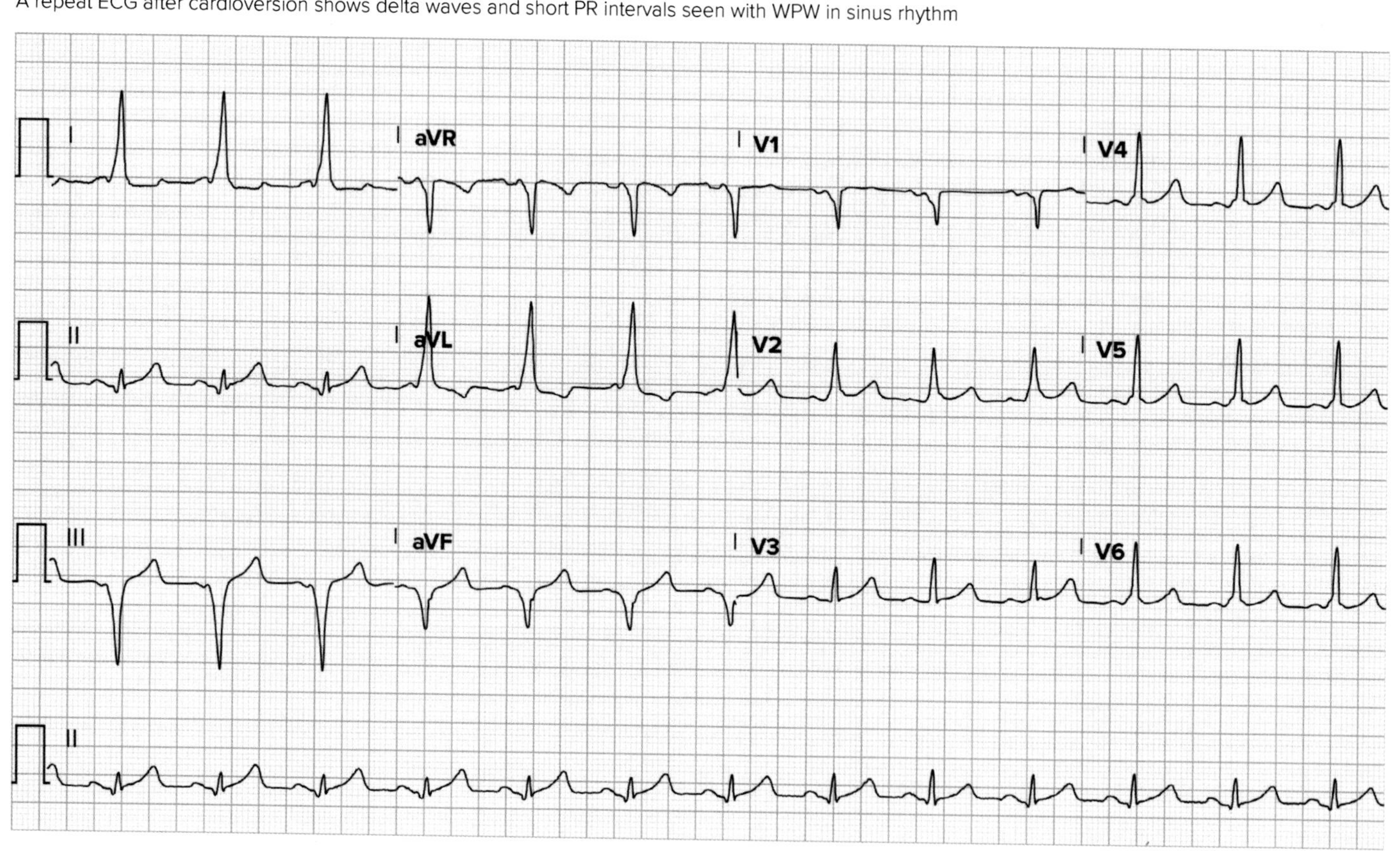

Figure 3.
Lead I from Figure 2 shows delta waves and short PR intervals seen with WPW in sinus rhythm

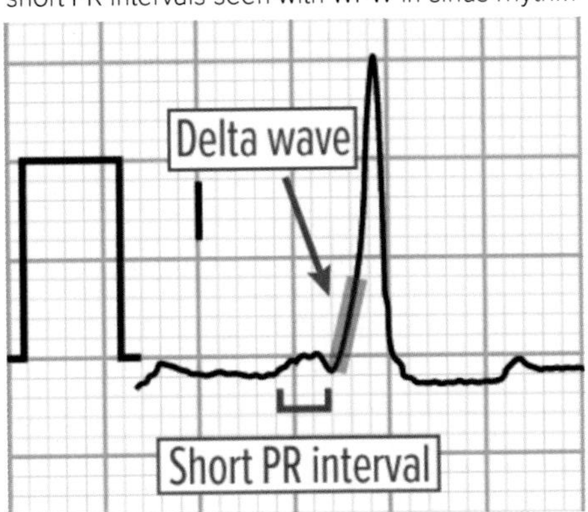

The AV node's intrinsic refractory period prevents ventricular rates from exceeding 220-240 bpm in the absence of any extrinsic factors that increase conduction velocity (eg, catecholamine surge, sympathomimetic toxicity, or hyperthyroidism), so atrial fibrillation with intermittent conduction at rates faster than 220-240 bpm should prompt concern for an AP. The danger of conduction via an AP in atrial fibrillation is due to its short refractory period relative to the AV node. This allows the AP to conduct at much faster rates than the AV node. In atrial fibrillation with WPW, the AV node acts as a brake that tempers the faster AP conduction. Without the protection provided by the AV node, conduction via the AP can lead to extremely rapid rates and related cardiovascular decompensation (eg, ventricular fibrillation). This is why AV nodal blockers should be avoided in atrial fibrillation with known or suspected WPW.

Treatment for atrial fibrillation with WPW includes electrical cardioversion (for stable or unstable patients) and IV procainamide or ibutilide for stable patients.[1] Procainamide and ibutilide reduce conduction velocity throughout the entire cardiac conduction system, including the AP and ventricles. Verapamil, diltiazem, adenosine, digoxin, lidocaine, and intravenous amiodarone should not be used.[1]

This patient was admitted to the cardiology service and an electrophysiology study showed an antegrade bypass tract, consistent with WPW, which was successfully ablated.

WPW Learning Points

- Congenital condition involving abnormal conduction pathway between atria and ventricle
  - Most common dysrhythmia is orthodromic AVRT
- ECG findings seen in sinus rhythm include:
  - Shortened PR interval (< 120 msec)
  - Delta wave: slurring of initial portion of the QRS complex
  - QRS complex duration prolonged, usually > 110 msec
  - Secondary ST and T-wave changes
  - Patients with WPW can have baseline ECGs (ie, in normal sinus rhythm) with a normal PR interval, normal QRS complex duration, and/or without delta waves
- Regular rhythm tachycardias in WPW can be narrow (orthodromic conduction via AV node) or wide (antidromic conduction via accessory pathway)
  - WPW with orthodromic AVRT (most common dysrhythmia): regular NCT, treat like AVNRT (PSVT)
  - WPW with antidromic AVRT: regular WCT, treat like monomorphic VT
- WPW with atrial fibrillation
  - Rapid, irregularly irregular wide complex tachycardia with beat-to-beat variation in QRS complex morphologies
  - Treatment includes electrical cardioversion (for stable or unstable patients) and IV procainamide or ibutilide for stable patients (avoid AV nodal blocking medications)
- In wide-complex atrial fibrillation, ventricular rates > 220-240 bpm suggest anterograde conduction via an accessory pathway

References

1. January CT, Wann LS, Alpert JS, et al. 2014 AHA/ACC/ HRS guideline for the management of patients with atrial fibrillation: a report of the American College of Cardiology/American Heart Association Task Force on Practice Guidelines and the Heart Rhythm Society. J Am Coll Cardiol. 2014;64:e1–76.

Case 76: Presentation

An 18-year-old male with no past medical history presents after a syncopal episode while eating dinner. What is your interpretation of his ECG?

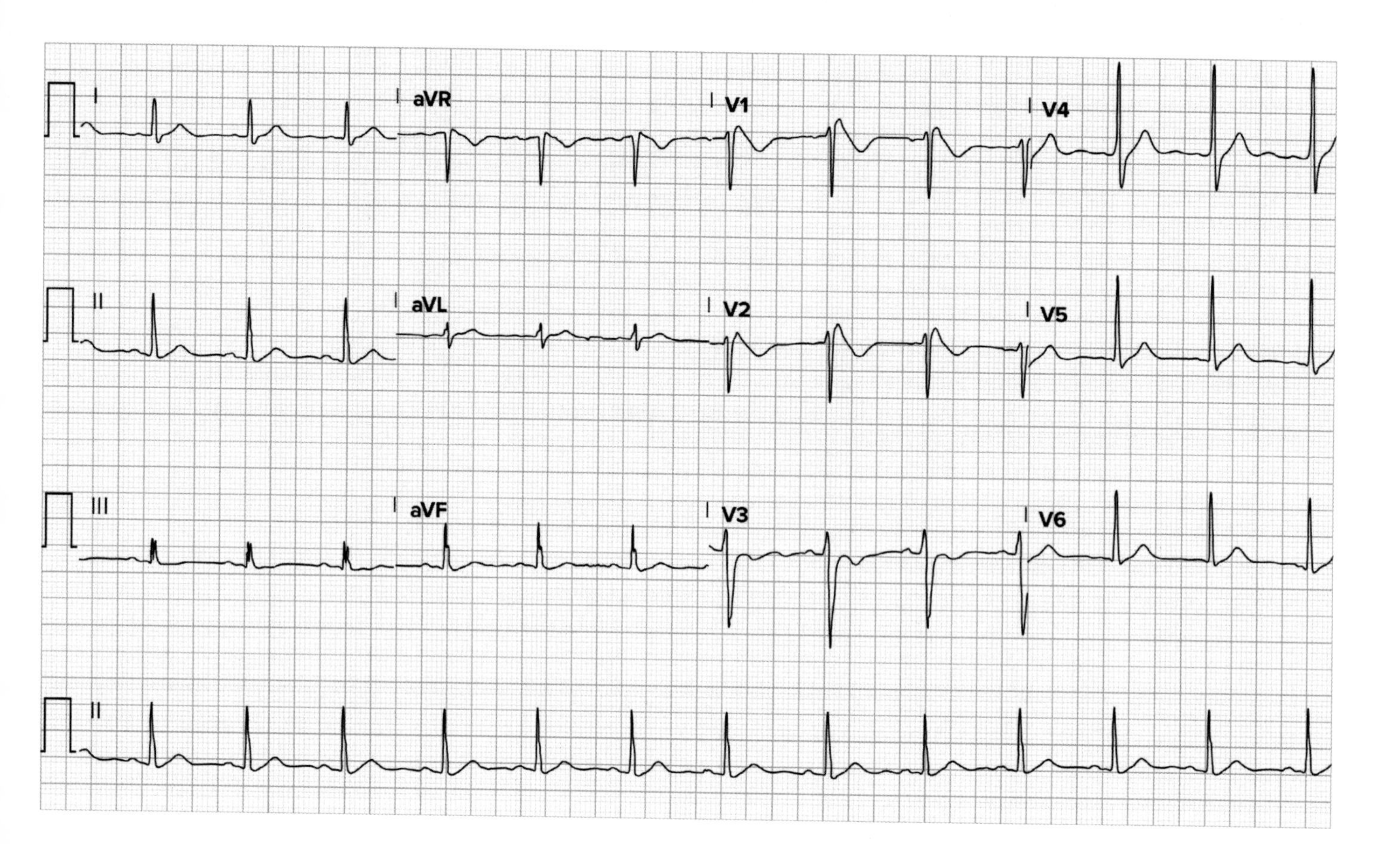

Case 76: Answer

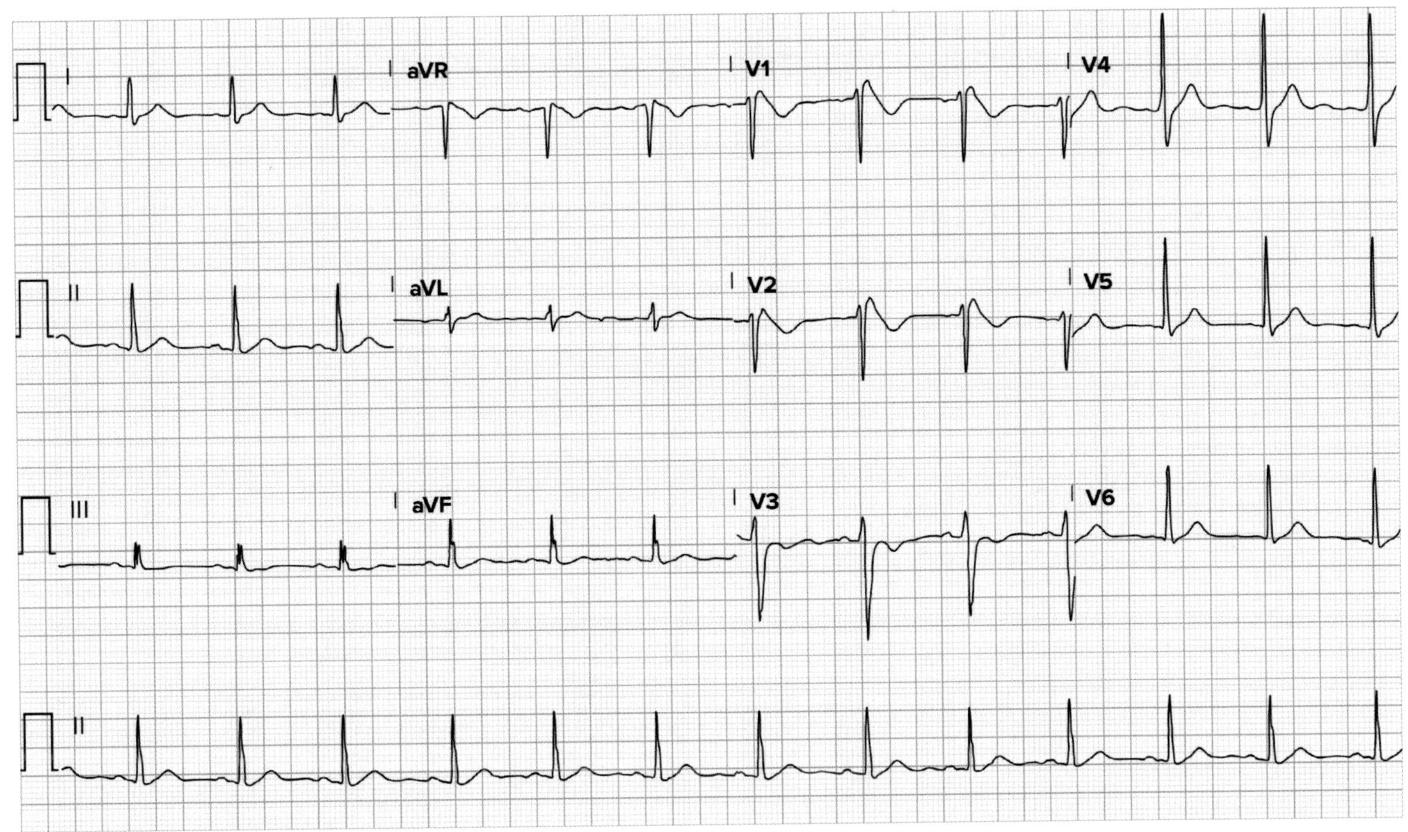

This ECG shows a normal sinus rhythm at 80 bpm, normal axis, prolonged QRS complex duration at 115 msec with an incomplete RBBB, and coved STE > 2 mm followed by a negative T-wave in leads V1-V2. This patient's history and ECG are concerning for Brugada syndrome.

ECG findings to look for in syncope patients include:

- Ischemia/infarct
- Severe bradycardia or tachycardia
- Conduction abnormalities (e.g. AV blocks)
- Low voltage +/- electrical alternans
- Syncope syndromes:
  - ARVD/ARVC
  - Brugada
  - HCM
  - QT Syndromes (long and short)
  - WPW

The differential diagnosis for STE in lead V1 includes:

- Acute MI (anteroseptal or right ventricular)
- Acute RV strain (eg, PE)
- Brugada syndrome
- Hyperkalemia
- LBBB
- LVH
- Sodium channel blocker toxicity
- Ventricular-paced rhythm

Brugada syndrome is a sodium channelopathy that can lead to unprovoked dysrhythmias (polymorphic ventricular tachycardia or ventricular fibrillation) and cardiac arrest. The diagnostic criteria include both ECG changes and clinical criteria (see Learning Points, to follow). Notably, up to 40% of patients with Brugada syndrome will have normal resting ECGs.

The initial Brugada ECG criteria set forth in 2002[1] included 3 types:

- Type 1: Coved STE ≥ 2 mm followed by a negative T-wave in > 1 of leads V1-V3 ***(see Figure 1)***
- Type 2: ≥ 2 mm of saddleback shaped STE in > 1 of leads V1-V3 ***(see Figure 2)***
- Type 3: Type 1 or 2 morphology not meeting above criteria in > 1 of leads V1-V3

Figure 1.
Brugada type 1

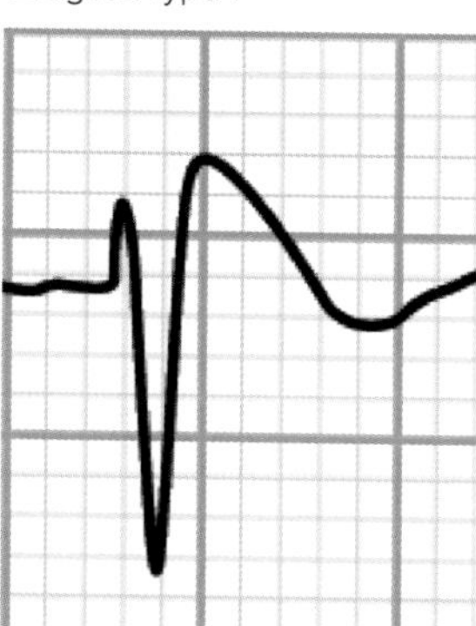

Figure 2.
Brugada type 2

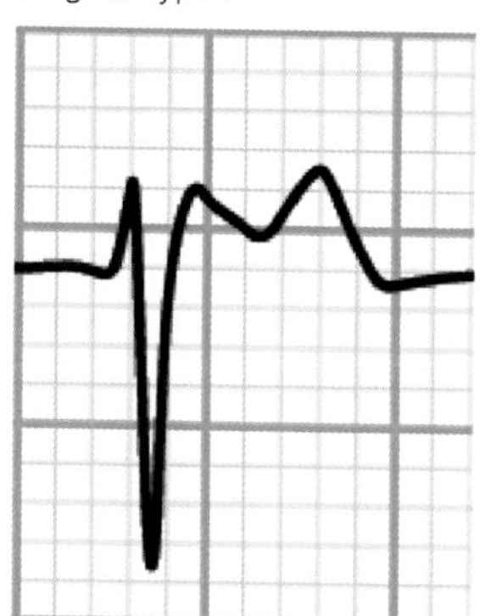

More recent 2013 guidelines[2] narrowed the definition:

> *"Brugada syndrome is diagnosed in patients with ST-segment elevation with type 1 morphology ≥ 2mm in ≥ 1 lead in the right precordial leads V1, V2, positioned in the 2nd, 3rd, or 4th intercostal space occurring either spontaneously or after provocative drug test with intravenous administration of class I antiarrhythmic drugs."*

The important changes in the new definition include:

1. Type 1 is the only potentially diagnostic pattern
2. Type 1 only needs to be seen in one lead and can be seen in lead(s) V1/V2 when positioned higher than the traditional 4th intercostal space
3. Type 2 is non-diagnostic and it is only clinically significant if the type I pattern is seen or can be provoked with sodium channel blocking antidysrhythmics
4. Type 3 is no longer part of the criteria
5. Lead V3 is no longer part of the criteria

There are multiple conditions which can mimic type 1 on the ECG, such as ARVC, septal hypertrophy, and pectus excavatum. Positioning leads V1 and V2 in the 2nd or 3rd intercostal space increases the sensitivity for detecting type 1 and can help differentiate it from a mimic. Conversely, inadvertent placement of leads V1 and V2 in the 2nd or 3rd intercostal spaces can produce a type 2 mimic in young athletes.

There are multiple unrelated conditions that can unmask a Brugada ECG pattern, notably fever and medications. The significance of this finding depends on the patient's clinical history as the diagnostic criteria for Brugada syndrome include both ECG and clinical criteria.

This patient had an unremarkable ED workup and was admitted to the cardiology service. He was evaluated by Electrophysiology and was discharged after AICD placement.

Brugada Syndrome Learning Points

- Sodium channelopathy that can lead to unprovoked dysrhythmias (polymorphic ventricular tachycardia or ventricular fibrillation) and cardiac arrest
- Diagnosis made from both ECG and clinical criteria (see table)
  - Type 1 is the only ECG abnormality that is potentially diagnostic
  - Type 2 is non-diagnostic but may warrant further investigation in the appropriate clinical situation
  - Type 3 is no longer considered useful in diagnosis
- Treatment is AICD placement

ECG Criteria	Clinical Criteria (must have ≥ 1):
• Complete or incomplete RBBB pattern with coved STE ≥ 2 mm followed by a negative T-wave in ≥ 1 of leads V1-V2	• Documented VF or polymorphic VT
	• Family history of sudden cardiac death at < 45 years old
	• Coved-type ECG in family members
	• Inducibility of VT with programmed electrical stimulation
	• Syncope
	• Nocturnal agonal respiration

References

1. Wilde AAM, Antzelevitch C, Borggrefe M, et al. Proposed Diagnostic Criteria for the Brugada Syndrome Consensus Report. Circulation. 2002;106(19):2514-2519.
2. Sieira J, Brugada P. The definition of the Brugada syndrome. Eur Heart J. 2017;38(40):3029-3034.

Case 77: Presentation

A 75-year-old female presents due to syncope. Her prior ECG was normal.
What is your interpretation of her ECG?

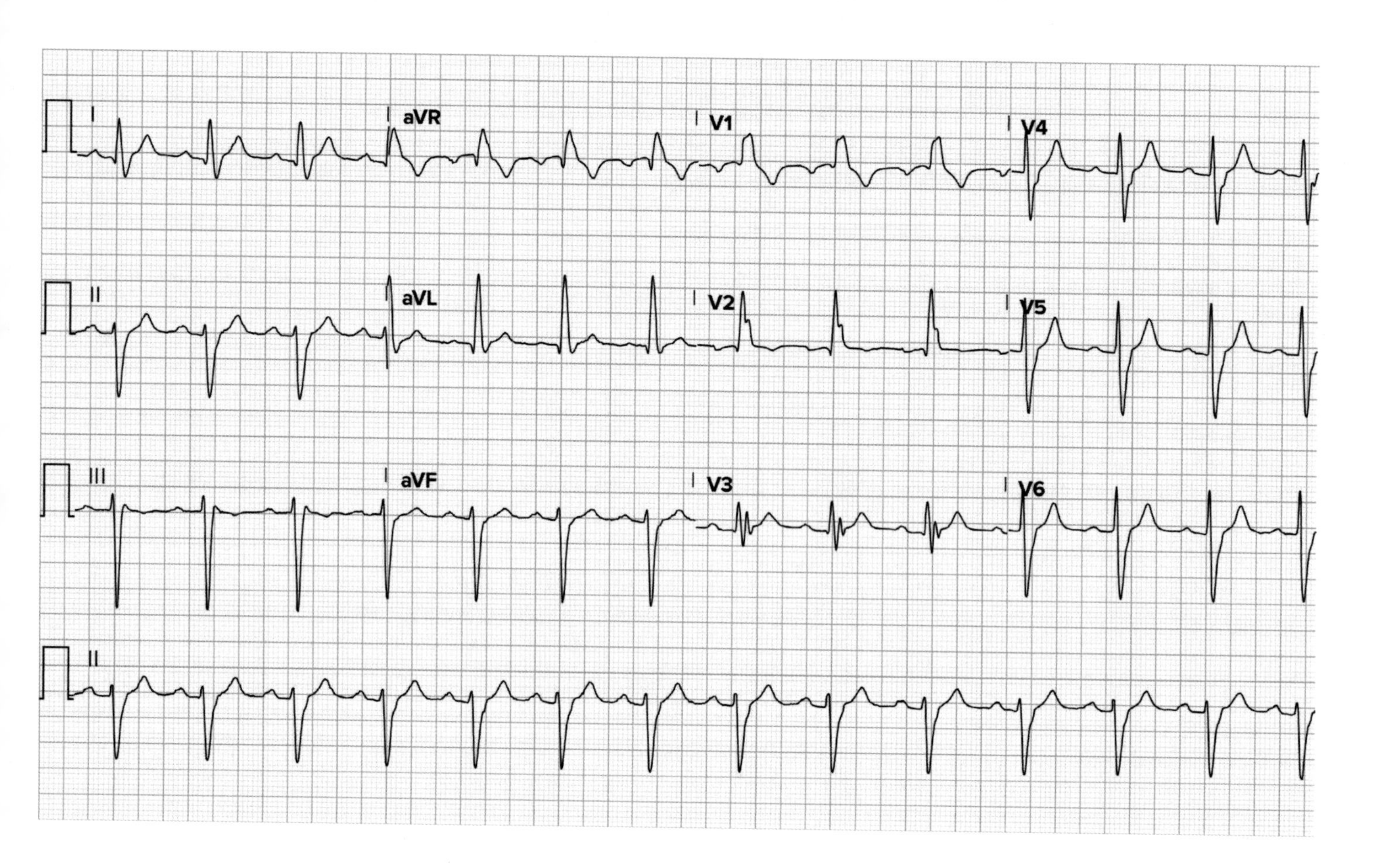

Case 77: Answer

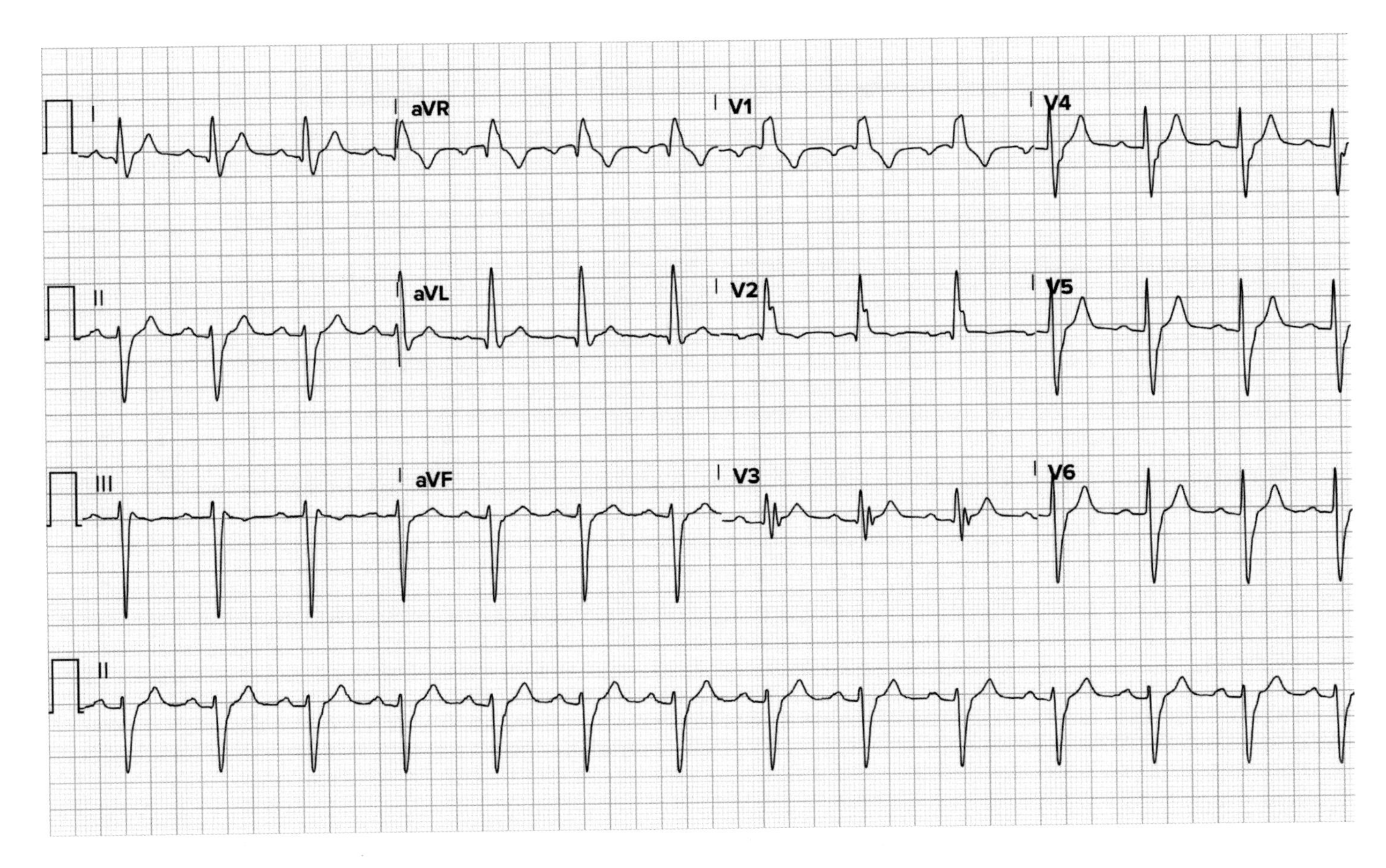

This ECG shows a normal sinus rhythm with a ventricular rate of 80 bpm, 1st degree AV block, left axis deviation, prolonged QRS complex duration with a RBBB, and a LAFB. There are TWI and STD in lead V1 which are expected in a RBBB.

ECG findings to look for in syncope patients include:

- Ischemia/infarct
- Severe bradycardia or tachycardia
- Conduction abnormalities (eg, AV blocks)
- Low voltage +/- electrical alternans
- Syncope syndromes:
  - ARVD/ARVC
  - Brugada
  - HCM
  - QT syndromes (long and short)
  - WPW

The key to accurately interpreting this ECG is recognizing the multiple conduction abnormalities. The presence of a RBBB with an axis deviation should prompt evaluation for a concurrent fascicular block. When there is also a concurrent AV block, this constellation of conduction abnormalities is sometimes called a trifascicular block. These are further categorized as complete or incomplete:

- Complete trifascicular block = 3rd degree AV block + RBBB + LAFB or LPFB
- Incomplete trifascicular block = 1st or 2nd degree AV block + RBBB + LAFB or LPFB, or RBBB + alternating LAFB/LPFB on successive ECGs

The presence of a new trifascicular block in the setting of syncope may warrant admission for cardiac monitoring as these patients can have transient episodes of 3rd degree AV block. This patient's ECG shows a 1st degree AV block, RBBB, and LAFB, consistent with an incomplete trifascicular block, which means the left posterior fascicle is the only part of the cardiac conduction system that doesn't have a conduction delay.

The characteristic findings in a RBBB include:

- QRS complex duration ≥ 120 msec
- rsr', rsR', or rSR' pattern in lead V1 +/- V2
  - Variations in lead V1 include qR pattern or broad R-wave that is often notched (***see Figure 1***)
  - In lead V1, the initial upward deflection should always be smaller than the 2nd upward deflection
- S-wave duration > R-wave or > 40 msec in leads I and V6 (***see Figures 2 and 3***)
- Normal R-wave peak time in leads V5 and V6 but > 50 msec in lead V1 (only required if broad R-wave +/- notch is present in lead V1)
- Repolarization abnormalities include STD and TWI in lead V1 +/- lead(s) V2-V3 if they have an rsR' pattern, so STE and/or upright T-waves in those leads are concerning for ischemia

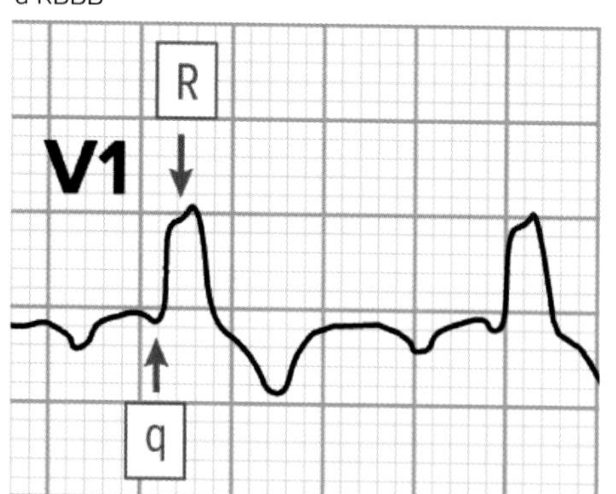

Figure 1.
qR pattern in lead V1, consistent with a RBBB

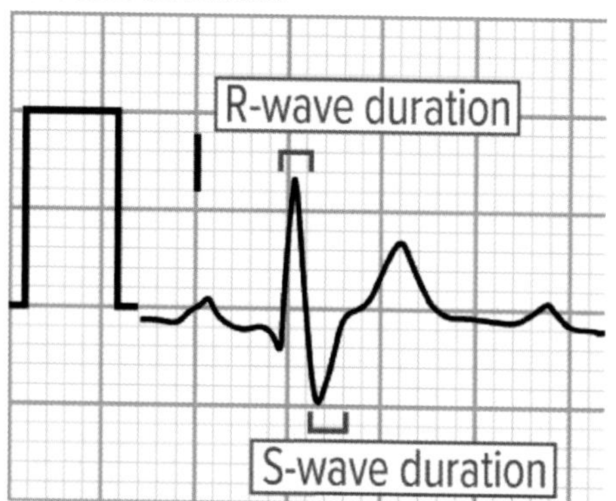

Figure 2.
S-wave duration > R-wave duration in lead I, consistent with a RBBB

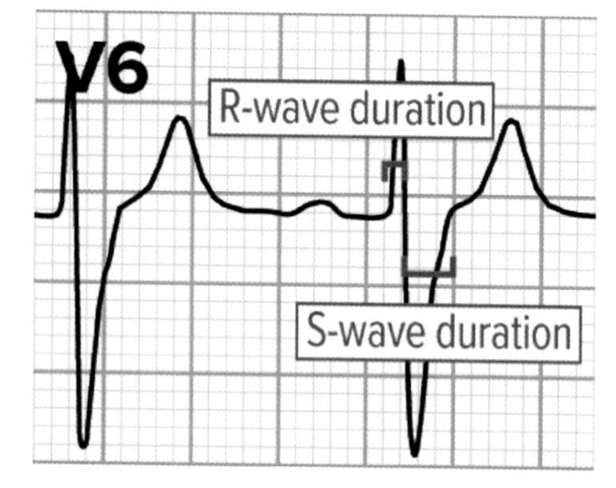

Figure 3.
S-wave duration > R-wave duration in lead V6, consistent with a RBBB

A RBBB will typically have STD and TWI in lead V1, and if leads V2-V3 have an rsR' pattern present, they will also typically have STD and TWI. Consequently, upright T-waves or STE in those leads with an rsR' pattern is concerning for ischemia, and even isoelectric or minimally elevated ST-segments can be a subtle indicator of early AMI. Otherwise, the presence of a RBBB does not confound the ECG evaluation of ACS as does a LBBB.

The characteristic findings in a LAFB include (***see Figure 4***):

- Left axis deviation between -45° and -90°
- qR complex in lead aVL +/- lead I
- rS complex in leads II, III, and aVF
- Prolonged R-wave peak time ≥ 45 msec in lead aVL
- QRS complex duration < 120 msec in the absence of a concurrent conduction delay

Figure 4.
Findings in a left anterior fascicular block include qR complexes in leads I and aVL (red), rS complexes in leads II, III, and aVF (purple), and left axis deviation (green)

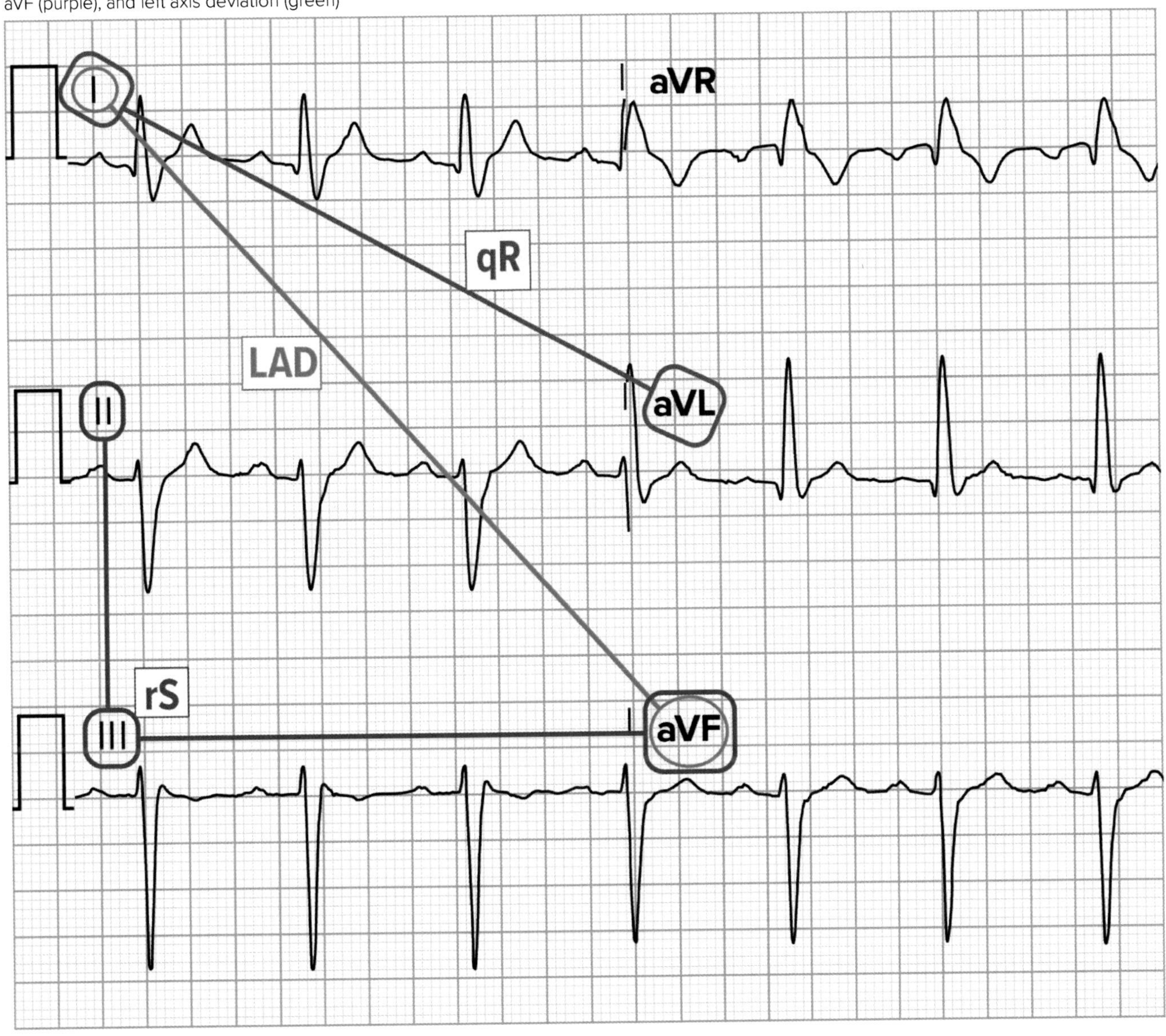

The patient had an unremarkable ED workup and was admitted to the cardiology service due to syncope in the setting of multiple new conduction abnormalities.

RBBB Learning Points

- Delayed conduction through right ventricle with normal left ventricular conduction
- In lead V1, the initial upward deflection should always be smaller than the 2nd upward deflection
- Repolarization abnormalities include STD and TWI in lead V1 +/- lead(s) V2-V3 if they have an rsR' pattern, so STE and/or upright T-waves in those leads are concerning for ischemia
  - Otherwise, the presence of a RBBB does not confound the ECG evaluation of ACS as does a LBBB
- RBBB with axis deviation should prompt evaluation for a concurrent LAFB or LPFB

Fascicular Blocks Learning Points

- Complete trifascicular block
  - 3rd degree AV block + RBBB + LAFB or LPFB
  - Always gets admitted for pacemaker placement
- Incomplete trifascicular block
  - 1st or 2nd degree AV block + RBBB + LAFB or LPFB, or RBBB + alternating LAFB/LPFB on successive ECGs
  - Syncope + incomplete trifascicular block = usually requires admission for cardiac monitoring for transient 3rd degree AV block and evaluation for pacemaker placement

Case 78: Presentation

A 73-year-old male presents to the ED after accidentally taking too much metoprolol. What is your interpretation of his ECG?

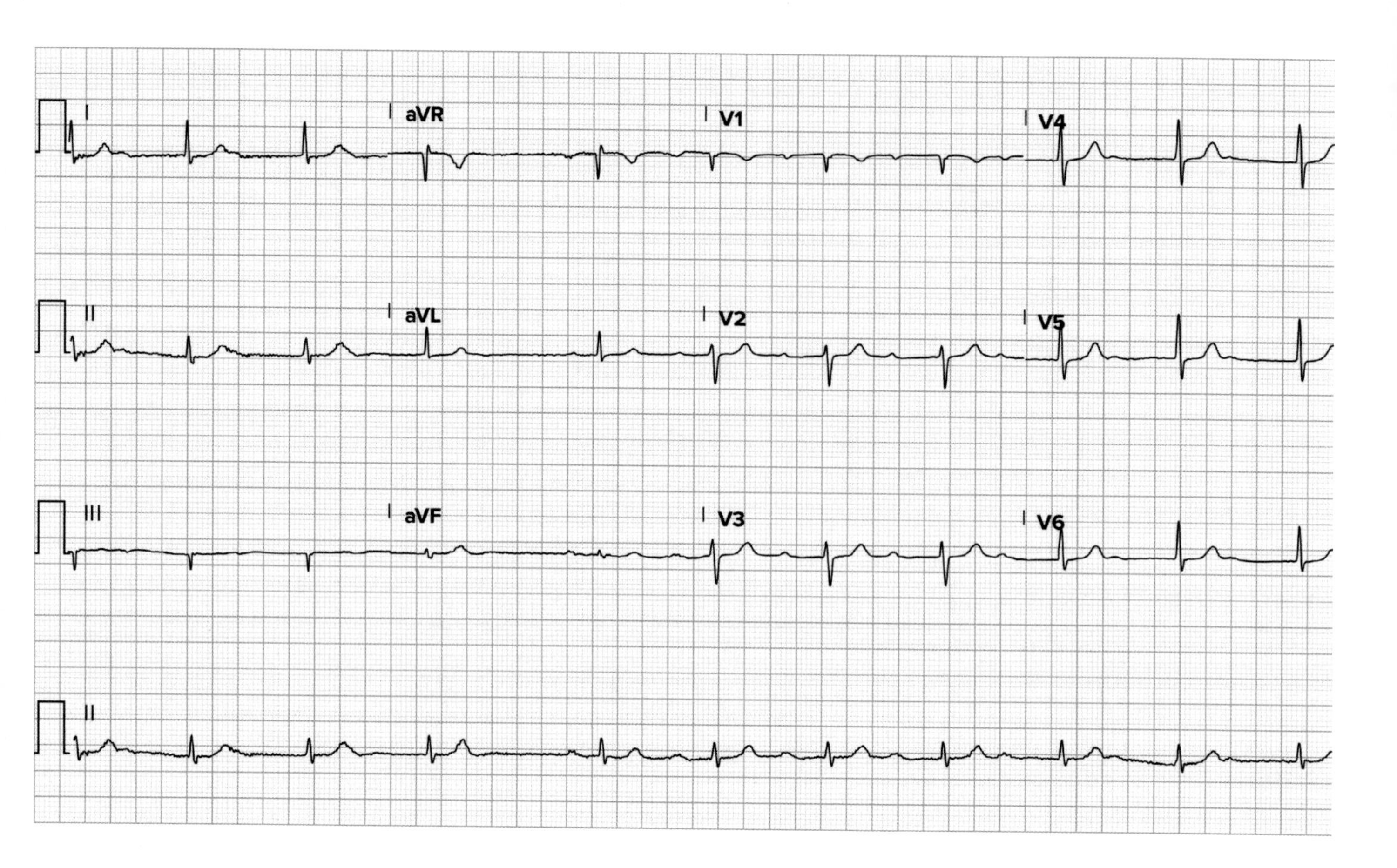

Case 78: Answer

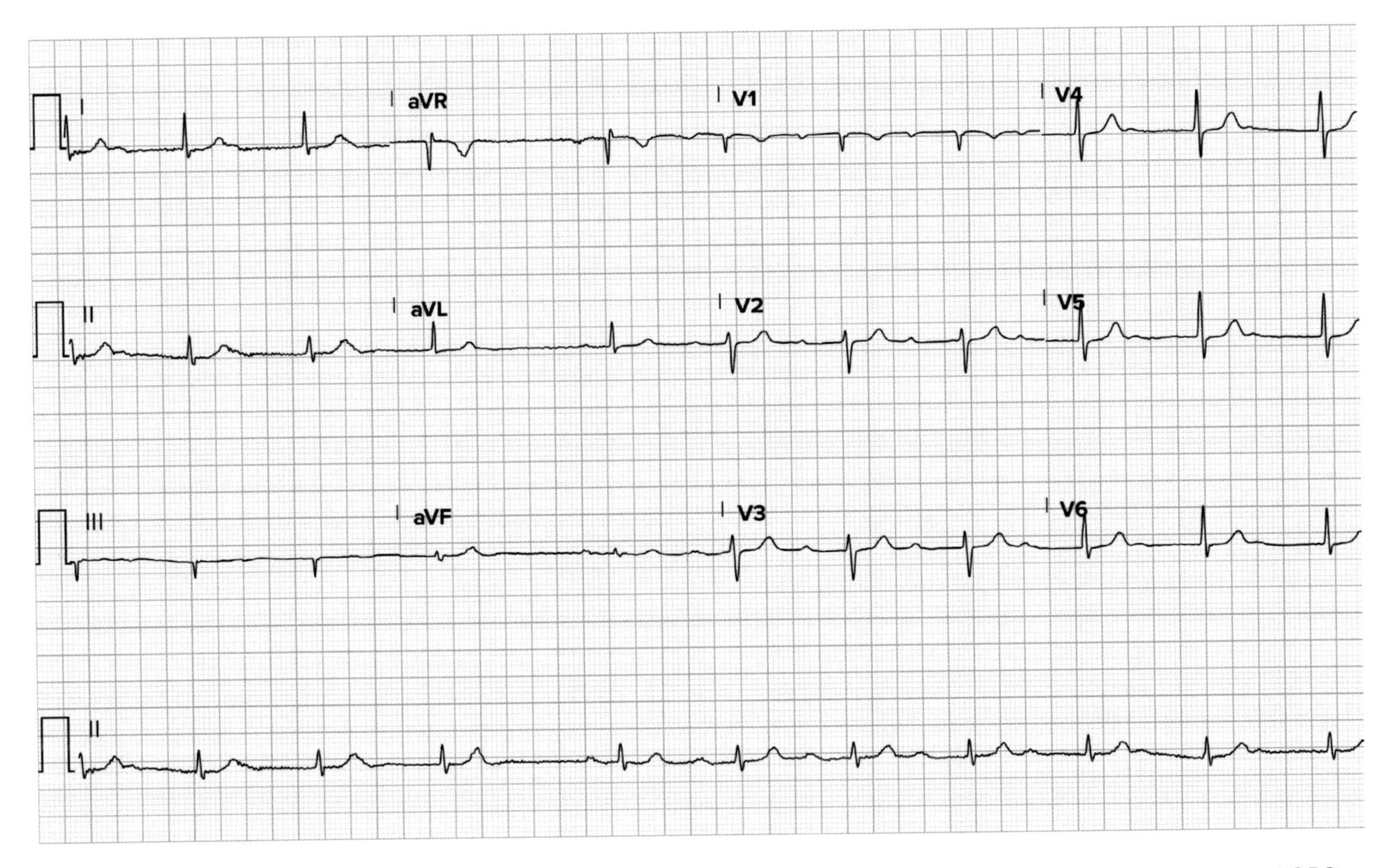

This ECG shows a Mobitz type I 2nd degree AV block with an average ventricular rate of 60 bpm, normal axis, normal QRS duration, and normal QTc interval.

The differential diagnosis for an irregular narrow complex rhythm with normal ventricular rates includes:

- Atrial fibrillation (rate controlled)
- Atrial flutter with variable block (rate controlled)
- Atrial tachycardia with variable block (rate controlled)
- Wandering atrial pacemaker (also called multifocal atrial rhythm)
- 2nd degree AV block Mobitz types I and II
- Variable high-grade AV block (eg, 3:1, 4:1, etc.)
- 2nd degree sinoatrial block
- Sinus arrhythmia
- NSR or accelerated junctional rhythm with irregular pattern of PAC, PJC, and/or PVC
- NSR or accelerated junctional rhythm with regular pattern of PAC, PJC, and/or PVC (bigeminy, trigeminy, etc.)

What makes this ECG tricky is that there are multiple P-waves buried or hidden within the T-waves as well as very long PR intervals. The key to interpreting this ECG is recognizing the increasing PR intervals that are followed by a non-conducted P-wave ***(see Figure 1)***.

Figure 1.
The lead II rhythm strip shows a progressively increasing PR interval followed by a non-conducted P-wave, consistent with a Mobitz type I AV block

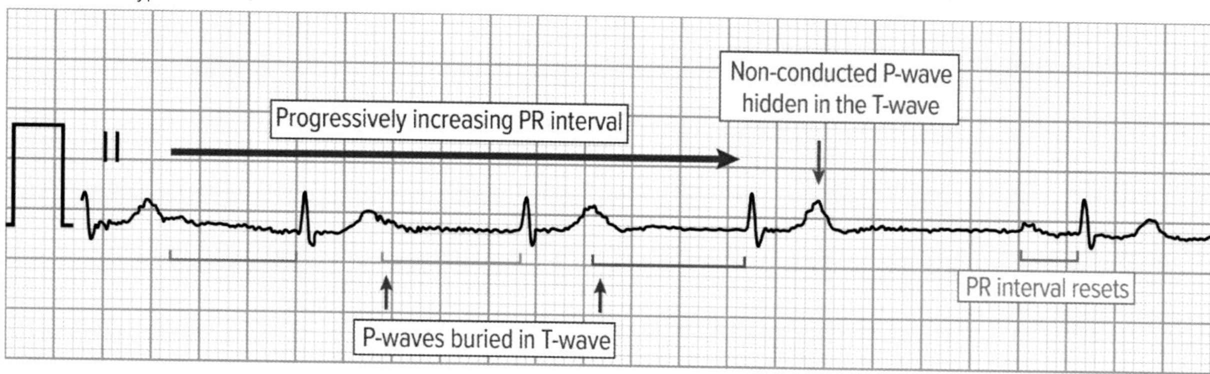

Mobitz type I conduction, also called Wenckebach conduction, is due to intermittent failure of conduction at the AV node. This most often occurs due to excessive vagal tone. The distinguishing feature of Mobitz type I conduction is progressively increasing PR interval and decreasing RR interval followed by a non-conducted P-wave (ie, a P-wave without accompanying QRS complex). The PR interval resets after the non-conducted P-wave so that the PR interval after the non-conducted P-wave is shorter than the PR interval preceding the non-conducted P-wave. The biggest increase in the PR interval typically happens between the 1st and 2nd beats of each cycle (as seen in this ECG).

It is essential to differentiate Mobitz type I conduction from Mobitz type II conduction, as the former is typically transient with a more benign course while the latter has a high risk of progressing to a 3rd degree AV block, frequently produces hemodynamic compromise, and is associated with worse outcomes if not treated. The QRS complex duration is typically not useful in differentiating between a Mobitz type I and a Mobitz type II, as a Mobitz type I can have a prolonged QRS complex duration if there is aberrant conduction (eg, an intrinsic bundle branch block) and a Mobitz type II can have a narrow QRS complex (ie, duration < 110 msec) if the block is in the AV node. The key to distinguishing between the two is to compare the RR interval that includes the non-conducted P-wave to the PP interval.

In a Mobitz type I AV block, the RR interval that includes the non-conducted P-wave will be less than twice the PP interval. This is evident in the lead II rhythm strip of the case ECG ***(see Figure 2)*** where the RR interval that includes the non-conducted P-wave (1360 msec) is less than twice the PP interval (1600 msec).

Figure 2.
In a Mobitz type I AV block, the RR interval that includes the non-conducted P-wave is less than twice the PP interval

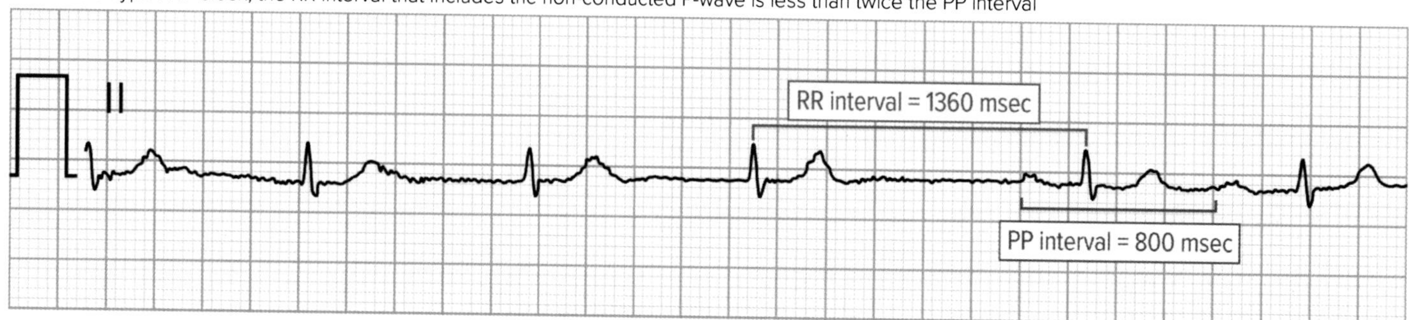

In a Mobitz type II AV block, the RR interval that includes the non-conducted P-wave will be equal to twice the PP interval. In the example below from a different ECG ***(see Figure 3)***, the RR interval that includes the non-conducted P-wave is 1440 msec which is equal to exactly twice the PP interval (1440 msec).

Figure 3.
In a Mobitz type II AV block, the RR interval that includes the non-conducted P-wave is equal to exactly twice the PP interval (from a different ECG)

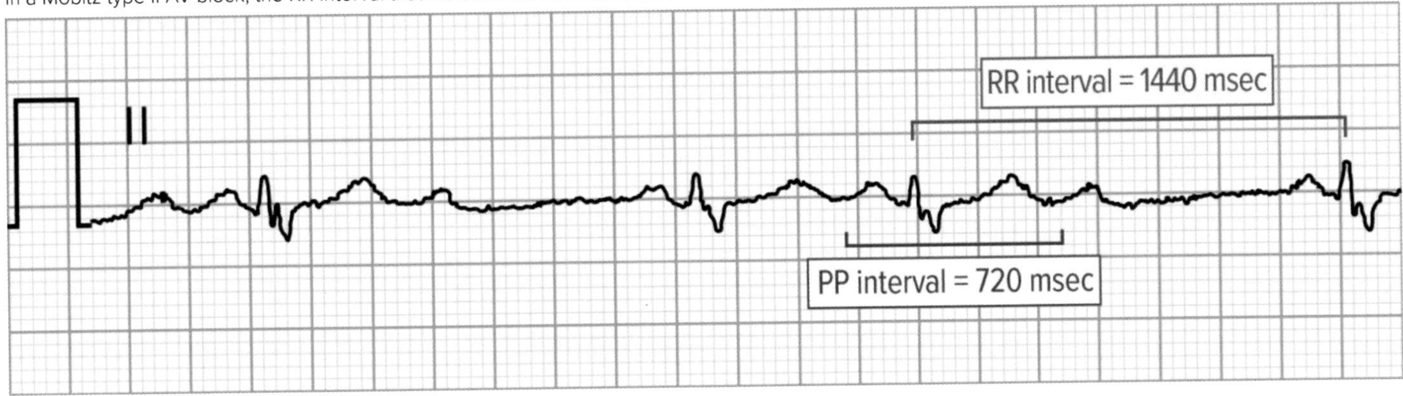

Another key finding in this ECG is the long PR intervals. The shortest PR interval in this ECG is 240 msec and occurs immediately after the non-conducted P-wave. The PR interval for the last two P-QRS-T complexes in this ECG are 520 msec and 560 msec ***(see Figure 4)***. This is a very long PR interval and can lead to AV dyssynchrony and subsequent loss of atrial kick and cardiac output as well as transient AV dissociation. The common teaching is that a Mobitz type I is usually benign, but it can also be ominous as in this case when it is associated with profoundly prolonged PR intervals.

Figure 4.
The lead II rhythm strip shows severely prolonged PR intervals preceding the 10th and 11th P-QRS-T complexes

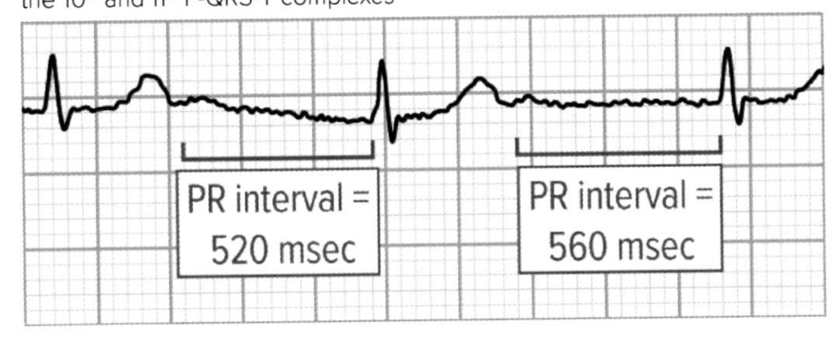

This patient had an unremarkable ED workup and the suspected etiology of the Mobitz type I was beta-blocker toxicity. He was admitted to the cardiology service for telemetry monitoring and converted back to normal sinus rhythm after his beta-blocker was withheld.

Mobitz type I AV Block Learning Points

- Progressively increasing PR interval and decreasing RR interval until a non-conducted P-wave occurs (ie, P-wave without accompanying QRS complex)
  - PR interval immediately after non-conducted P-wave is shorter than PR interval preceding non-conducted P-wave
  - RR interval that includes non-conducted P-wave < twice the PP interval
- Can be normal variant and usually does not produce hemodynamic compromise
  - Typically associated with excess vagal tone and therefore usually responds to atropine when acute treatment is needed
  - Can lead to a more advanced AV block if associated with a pathologic etiology
  - Can be seen with inferior MI

Mobitz type II AV Block Learning Points

- Constant PR interval in conducted beats
  - Described as ratio of P-waves to QRS complexes
  - Typically an infranodal block resulting in a prolonged QRS complex duration
  - RR interval that includes non-conducted P-wave = twice the PP interval
- Never a normal variant and frequently produces hemodynamic compromise
  - High risk of progressing to a 3rd degree AV block
  - Atropine is unlikely to lead to clinical improvement and may lead to a high-grade AV block

High-grade (or advanced) AV Block Learning Points

- 2nd degree AV block with ≥ 2 sequential non-conducted P-waves
  - Most commonly a variant of a Mobitz type II but can be associated with a Mobitz type I
  - PP and RR intervals should have a whole number ratio
- Named as ratio of P-waves to QRS complexes
- Can be seen after anterior MI or with significant pathology of the conduction pathway
- High risk of progressing to a 3rd degree AV block

Case 79: Presentation

An 81-year-old male presents with chest pain. What is your interpretation of his ECG?

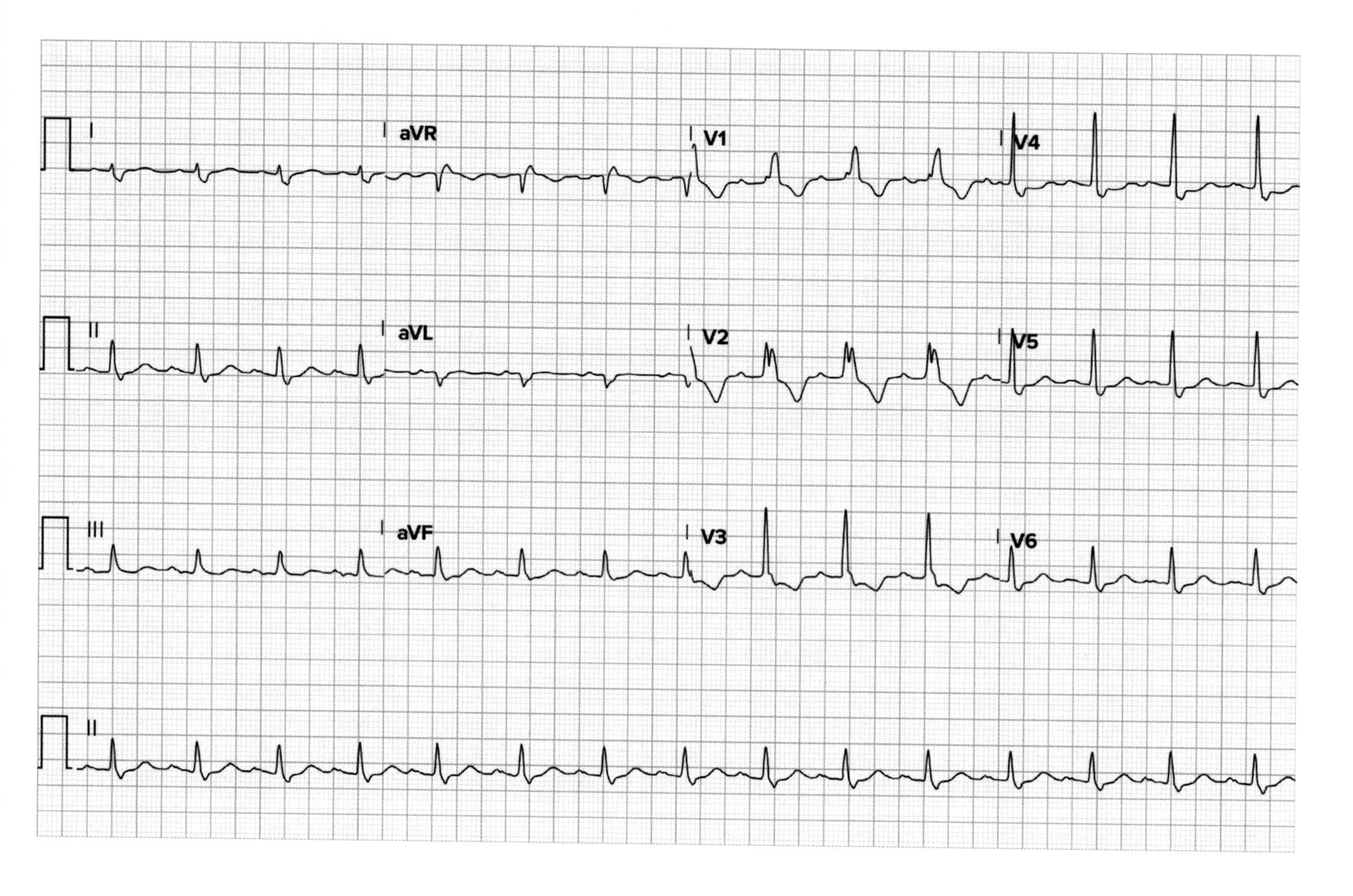

Case 79: Answer

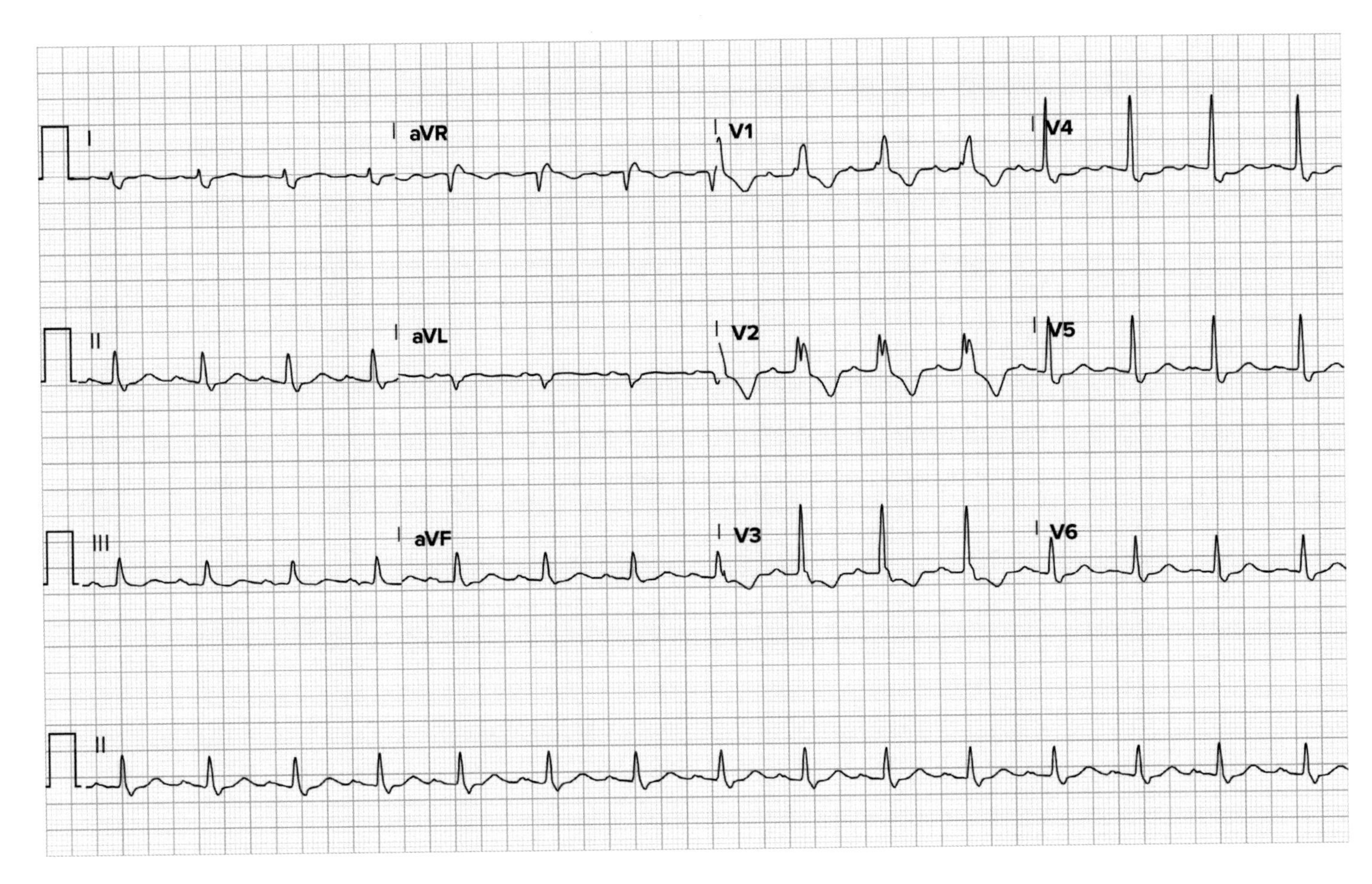

This ECG shows a normal sinus rhythm with a ventricular rate of 90 bpm, 1st degree AV block, normal axis, and prolonged QRS complex duration with a RBBB. There are TWI and STD most evident in leads V1-V3 which are expected repolarization abnormalities in a RBBB.

The characteristic findings in a RBBB include:

- QRS complex duration ≥ 120 msec
- rsr', rsR', or rSR' pattern in lead V1 +/- V2 ***(see Figure 1)***
  - Variations in lead V1 include qR pattern or broad R-wave that is often notched
  - In lead V1, the initial upward deflection should always be smaller than the 2nd upward deflection ***(see Figure 1)***
- S-wave duration > R-wave or > 40 msec in leads I and V6 ***(see Figures 2 and 3)***
- Normal R-wave peak time in leads V5 and V6 but > 50 msec in lead V1 (only required if broad R-wave +/- notch is present in lead V1)
- Repolarization abnormalities include STD and TWI in lead V1 +/- lead(s) V2-V3 if they have an rsR' pattern, so STE and/or upright T-waves in those leads are concerning for ischemia

Figure 1.
rSR' pattern in lead V1, consistent with a RBBB

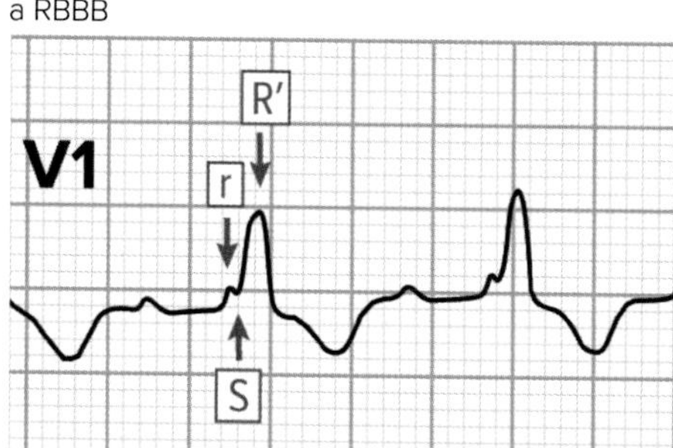

Figure 2.
S-wave duration > R-wave duration in lead I, consistent with a RBBB

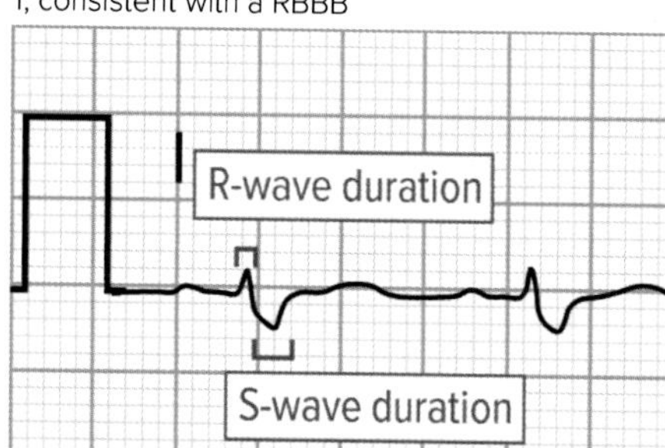

Figure 3.
S-wave duration > R-wave duration in lead V6, consistent with a RBBB

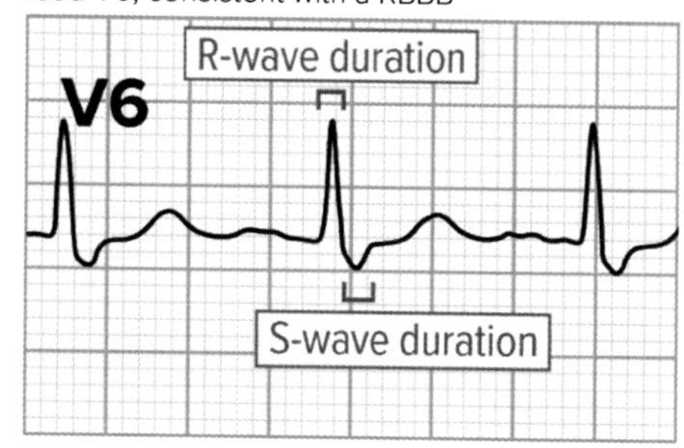

A RBBB will typically have STD and TWI in lead V1, and if leads V2-V3 have an rsR' pattern present, they will also typically have STD and TWI. Consequently, upright T-waves or STE in those leads with an rsR' pattern is concerning for ischemia, and even isoelectric or minimally elevated ST-segments can be a subtle indicator of early AMI. Otherwise, the presence of a RBBB does not confound the ECG evaluation of ACS as does a LBBB.

RBBB Learning Points

- Delayed conduction through right ventricle with normal left ventricular conduction
- In lead V1, the initial upward deflection should always be smaller than the 2nd upward deflection
- Repolarization abnormalities include STD and TWI in lead V1 +/- lead(s) V2-V3 if they have an rsR' pattern, so STE and/or upright T-waves in those leads are concerning for ischemia
  - Otherwise, the presence of a RBBB does not confound the ECG evaluation of ACS as does a LBBB
- RBBB with axis deviation should prompt evaluation for a concurrent LAFB or LPFB

NOTES:

Case 80: Presentation

An 84-year-old male with history of congestive heart failure with EF of 25% and AICD placement presents with fatigue and exertional near-syncope. His prior ECGs do not show a paced rhythm. What is your interpretation of his ECG?

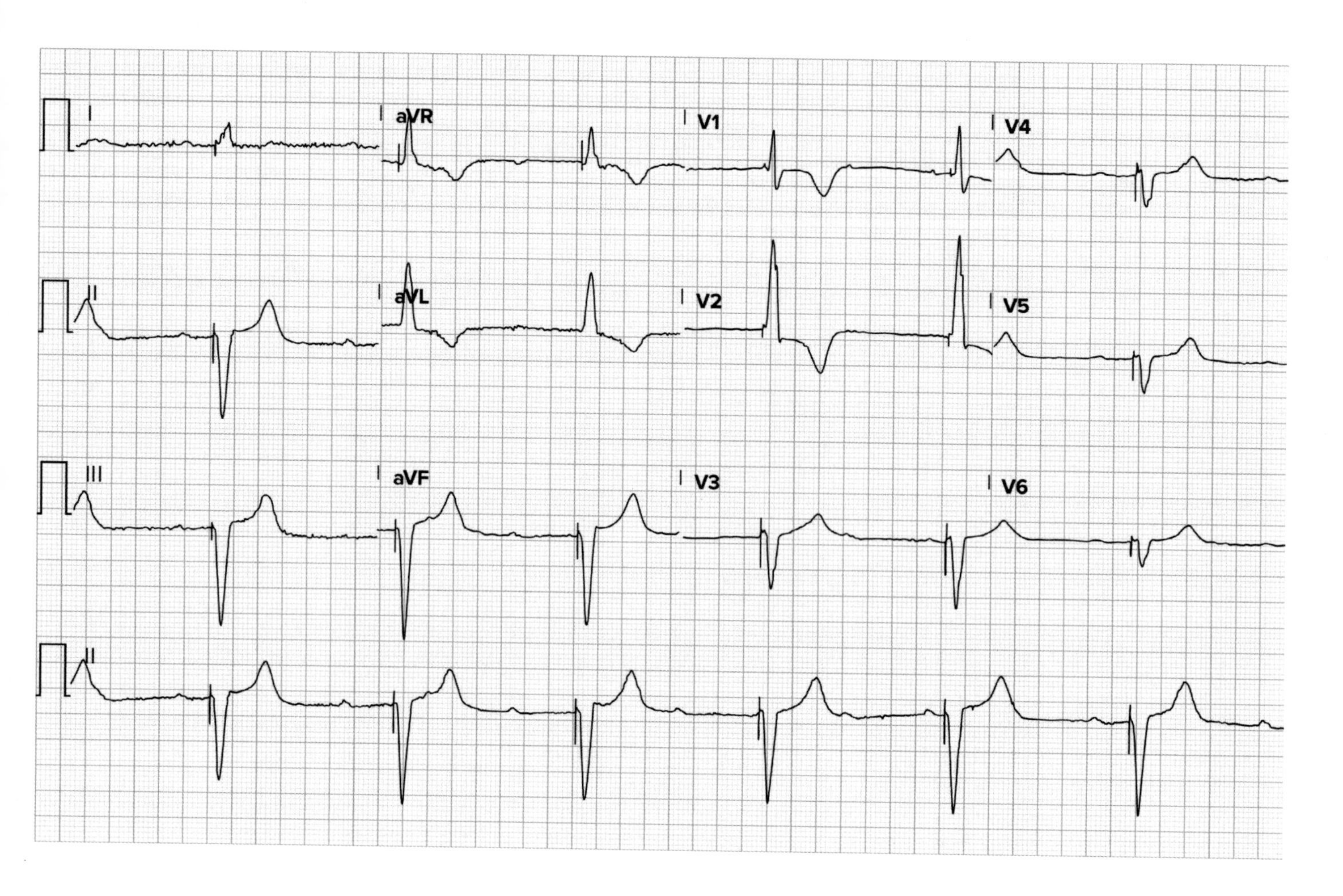

Case 80: Answer

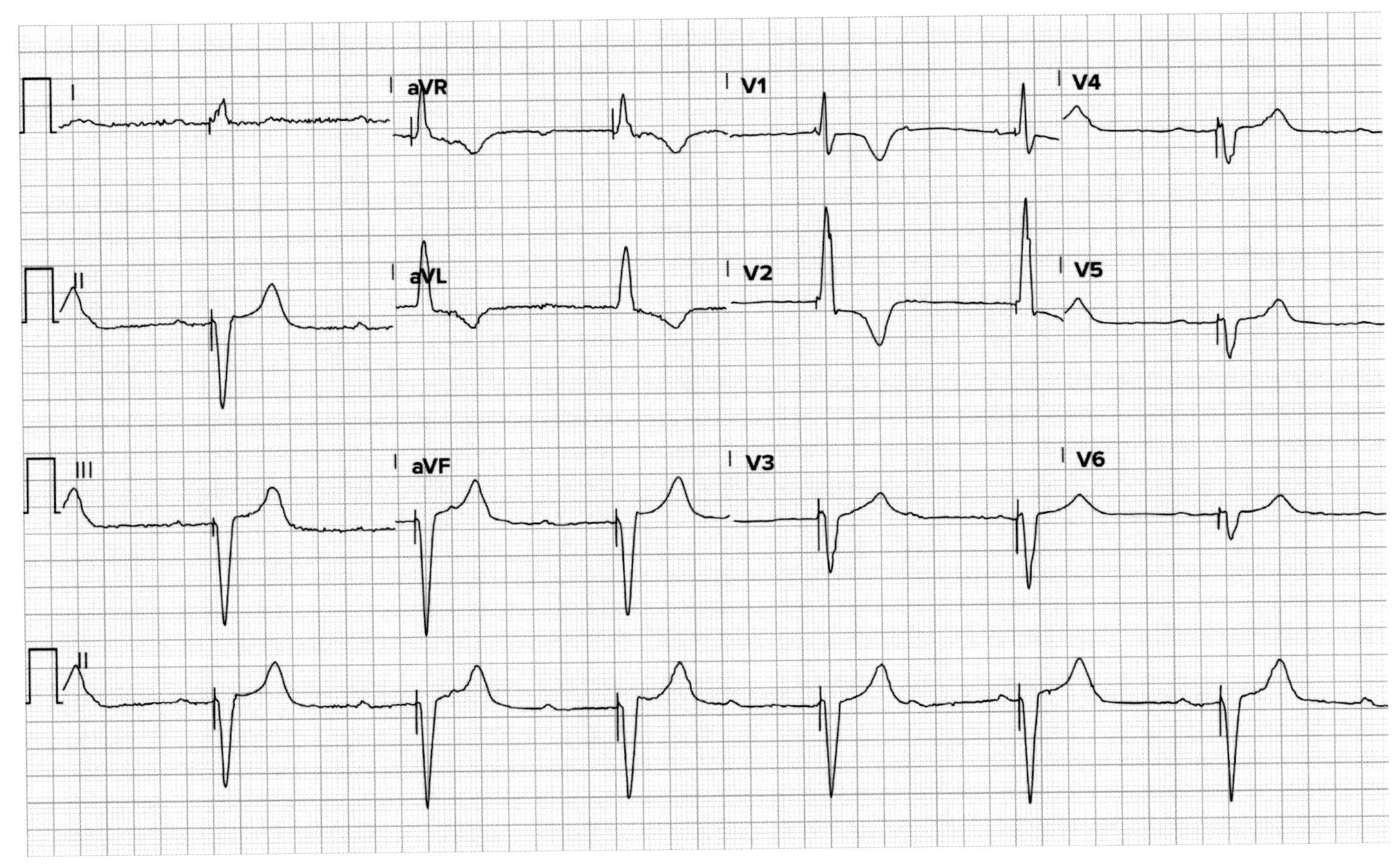

This ECG shows a ventricular-paced rhythm at a rate of 40 bpm with an underlying 3rd degree AV block, left axis deviation, prolonged QRS complex duration of 140 msec, and a dominant R-wave with TWI in leads V1-V2.

The initial 4 beats of this ECG show a progressively longer PR interval with a missing QRS complex after the 4th beat. This could be mistaken for a Mobitz type I 2nd degree AV block, but there are two findings that suggest otherwise:

1. The ventricular rhythm is regular which rules out a Mobitz type I 2nd degree AV block (unless there is 2:1 conduction, which is not seen)
2. The PR interval before the 4th beat is 680 msec which is extremely long and unlikely to result in normal conduction and subsequent ventricular depolarization

The key to correctly interpreting this ECG is recognizing the P-waves buried or hidden in the QRS-T complexes ***(see Figure 1).*** This is best done by marching out the 2 P-waves seen between the 4th and 5th QRS complexes.

Figure 1.
The lead II rhythm strip with purple arrows showing the PP interval, blue arrows pointing to the easily identifiable P-waves, and red arrows pointing to the P-waves buried or hidden in QRS-T complexes

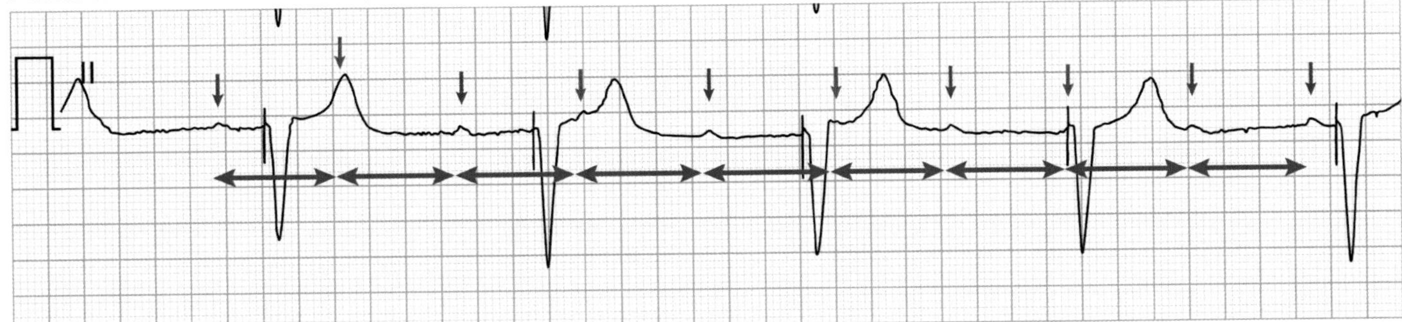

The QRS morphology in leads V1-V2 is atypical for a right ventricular-paced rhythm. Pacing in the RV creates a pattern consistent with a LBBB in leads V1-V2 so it would be expected that there would be a dominant S-wave. There are a couple of possibilities for the RBBB pattern in leads V1-V2 seen in this ECG:

1. Leads V1-V2 are placed too high on the chest (eg, 2nd intercostal space) which can be confirmed by repeating the ECG after ensuring appropriate placement of these leads in the 4th intercostal space
2. The RV lead was accidentally placed in the middle cardiac vein which can be confirmed on a chest X-ray with PA and lateral views

The clinically significant finding in this ECG is the very slow ventricular rate. An AICD can produce ventricular pacing at a fixed programmed rate, but unless there is an atrial lead, it lacks the capacity to synchronize with the atria. The combination of the lack of an atrial kick, the fixed slow rate, and a baseline poor EF will result in a significantly impaired cardiac output which is the likely cause of the patient's symptoms.

This patient was seen by Electrophysiology in the ED and had significant improvement of his symptoms after the fixed ventricular rate was increased to 70 bpm. He was admitted to the cardiology service for placement of a biventricular pacemaker/AICD. Biventricular pacing, also called cardiac resynchronization therapy, includes both RV and LV leads along with a right atrial lead (which means it is also dual chamber). This improves cardiac output by synchronizing the atrial kick and coordinating the ventricular contractions.

Pacemaker Learning Points

- Pacer spikes are usually visible on the ECG, either at the bottom of the ECG and/or preceding the P-wave and/or QRS complex
  - Atrial pacing: spikes immediately precede P-waves
  - Ventricular pacing: spikes immediately precede QRS complexes
  - Dual chamber pacing: spikes immediately precede both P-waves and QRS complexes
  - Biventricular pacing: 2 spikes immediately precede QRS complexes
- Atrial pacing
  - Pacemaker lead usually implanted in the right atrial appendage
  - Results in P-waves with normal morphology
- Right ventricular pacing
  - Pacemaker lead usually implanted in the RV apex
  - Results in a LBBB pattern in the limb leads and anteroseptal precordial leads
  - The major difference between an intrinsic LBBB and a right ventricular-paced rhythm is that the QRS complex will almost always be negatively oriented in leads V5-V6 with a right ventricular-paced rhythm
- Biventricular pacing
  - Two pacemaker leads usually implanted in the RV apex and the surface of the posterior or lateral LV
  - Typically results in a narrower QRS complex than with right ventricular pacing
  - Dominant R-wave in lead V1 +/- V2 is common
- AICD will have a thick coil that differentiates it from a pacemaker

3rd Degree AV Block Learning Points

- A 3rd degree AV block, or complete heart block, is defined by the absence of conduction through the AV node leading to complete AV dissociation
  - P-waves "march out" (ie, constant PP interval) and do not conduct to produce a QRS complex
  - PR intervals are variable
  - Atrial rate > ventricular rate
  - Ventricular rhythm is usually junctional or ventricular escape rhythm
- All patients require admission and evaluation for pacemaker placement

NOTES:

Case 81: Presentation

A 24-year-old male with no known cardiac history presents with palpitations and lightheadedness. What is your interpretation of his ECG?

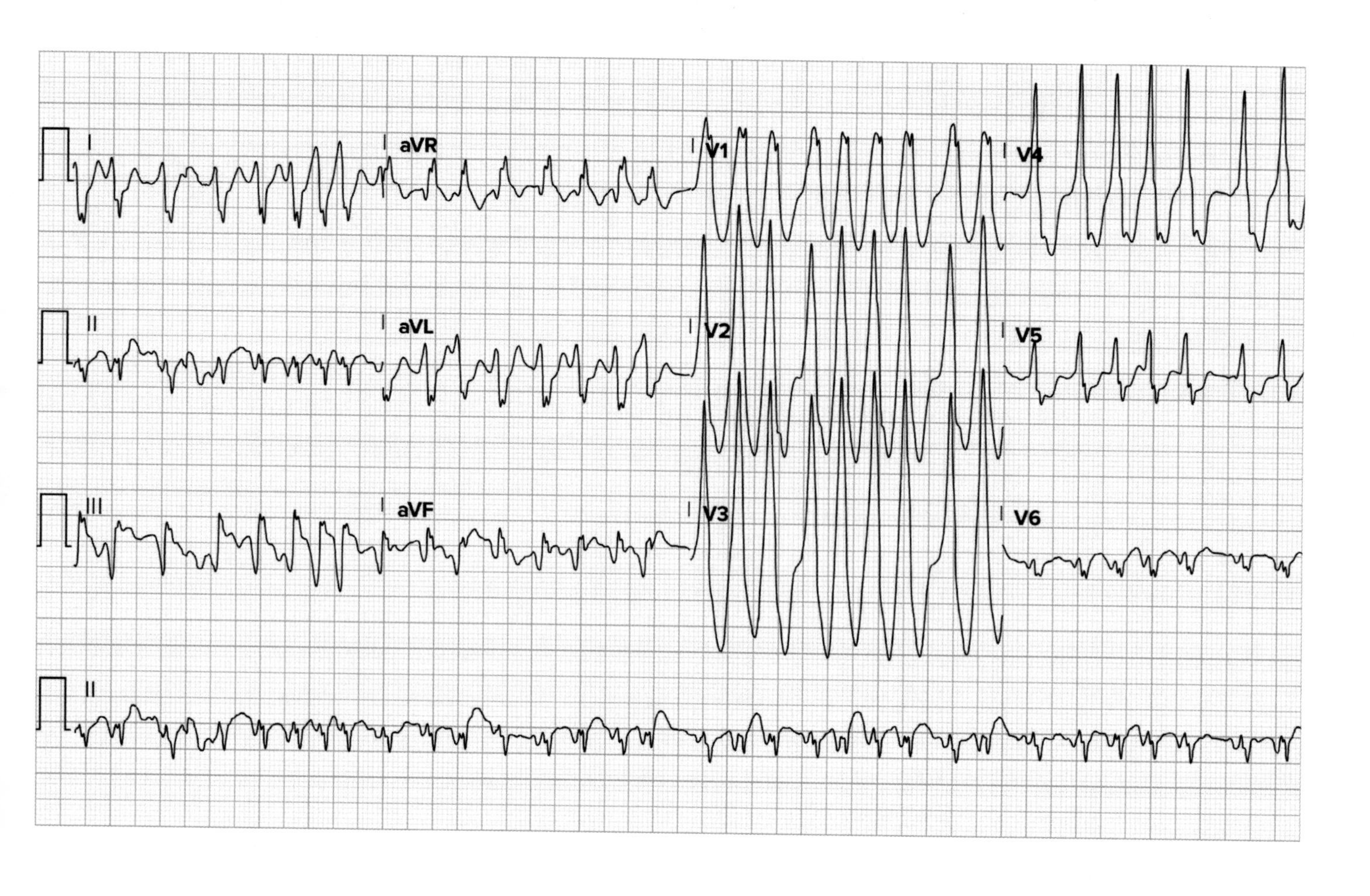

Case 81: Answer

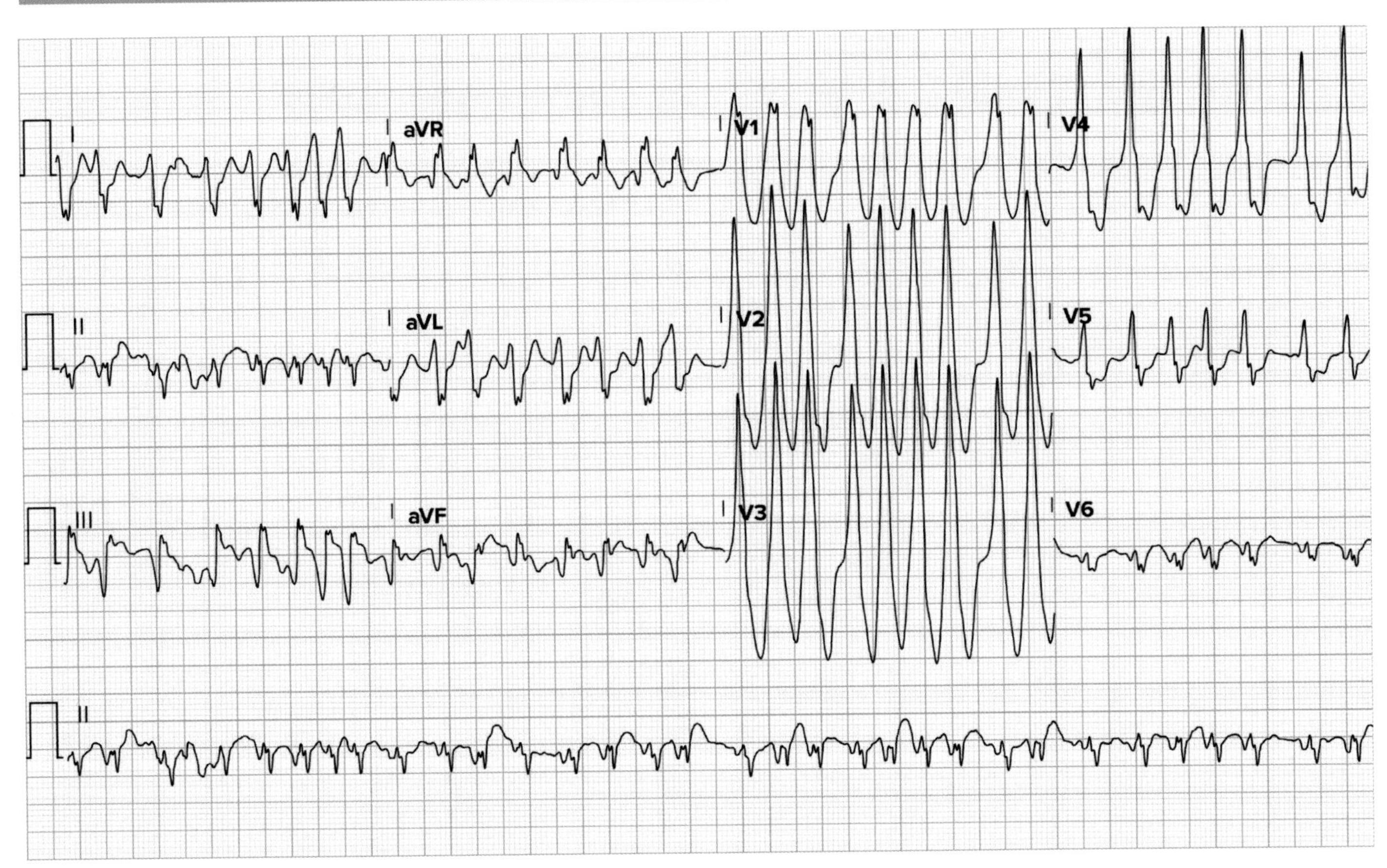

This ECG shows an irregular wide complex tachycardia with an average ventricular rate of 186 bpm and intermittent rates up to 332 bpm, no P-waves, extreme/northwest axis deviation, and prolonged QRS complex duration with beat-to-beat variation in the QRS complex morphology.

The differential diagnosis for an irregular WCT includes:

- Ventricular fibrillation
- Polymorphic ventricular tachycardia (including torsades de pointes)
- MAT with aberrant conduction
- Atrial flutter with variable block and aberrant conduction
- Atrial fibrillation with aberrant conduction
  - Causes of aberrant conduction include fixed or rate-related BBB, metabolic abnormalities, sodium channel blocker toxicity, ventricular-paced rhythm, and ventricular pre-excitation (eg, WPW)

This ECG shows the triad, as yet unnamed, of an irregularly irregular rhythm, markedly changing QRS complex morphologies, and extremely fast rates up to 333 bpm in some regions ***(see Figure 1)*** that is only seen with polymorphic ventricular tachycardia and atrial fibrillation with WPW. Polymorphic ventricular tachycardia will have phasic variation (ie, happens over a number of beats) of the QRS complex polarity (ie, axis) and amplitude. Conversely, atrial fibrillation with WPW will have beat-to-beat variation in the QRS complex morphology and relatively consistent QRS complex polarity, as seen in this patient's ECG.

Figure 1.
The lead II rhythm strip shows an irregularly irregular rhythm with variable QRS complex morphologies and extremely fast ventricular rates (up to 333 bpm in this case), consistent with atrial fibrillation with WPW

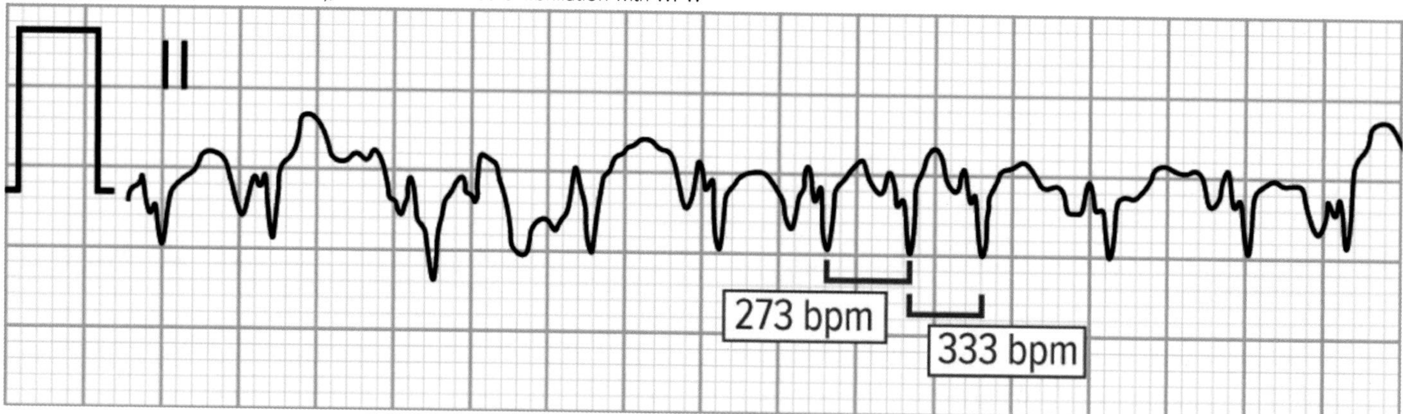

This patient was electrically cardioverted after which a repeat ECG was obtained *(see Figure 2)*. The repeat ECG shows normal sinus rhythm with a ventricular rate of 77 bpm, normal axis, normal QRS complex duration, and shortened PR interval and delta waves in leads V3-V4.

Figure 2.
A repeat ECG after electrical cardioversion shows shortened PR interval and delta waves in leads V3-V4

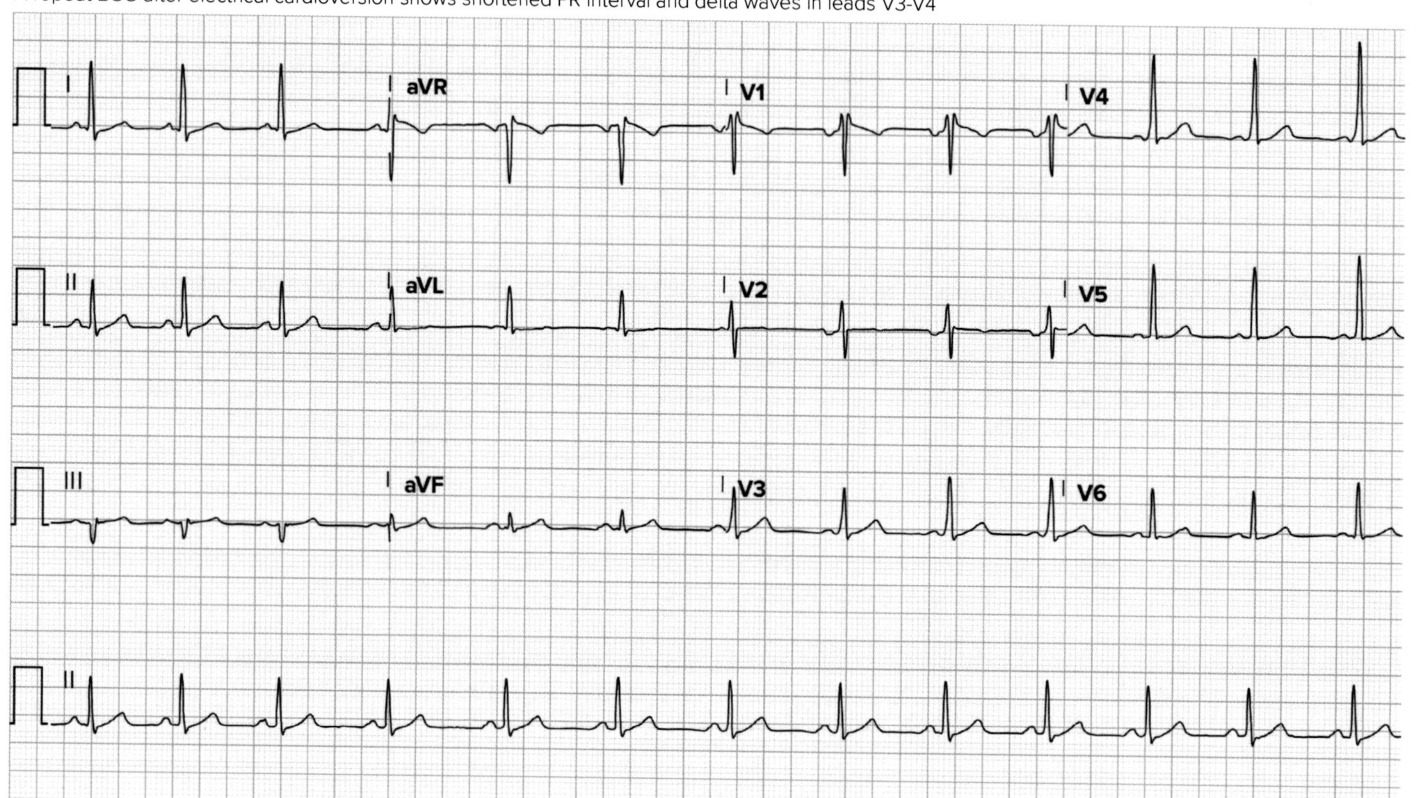

The repeat ECG demonstrates that patients with WPW can have baseline ECGs (ie, in normal sinus rhythm) that only show findings consistent with ventricular pre-excitation in one or two leads, and when present, may not show all 3 findings associated with ventricular pre-excitation (ie, shortened PR interval, prolonged QRS complex duration, and delta wave) ***(see Figures 3-6)***. In fact, patients with WPW can have ECGs in normal sinus rhythm without any findings that suggest ventricular pre-excitation. Accordingly, it is important to examine all 12 leads for findings that suggest ventricular pre-excitation, and the absence of these findings does not rule out WPW if there is high clinical suspicion. For example, the presenting ECG in this case (atrial fibrillation with beat-to-beat variation in the QRS complex morphology and extremely fast rates) is diagnostic of WPW regardless of whether the baseline ECG shows findings suggestive of ventricular pre-excitation.

Figure 3.
Lead V3 from the repeat ECG shows a shortened PR interval and delta wave but a normal QRS complex duration

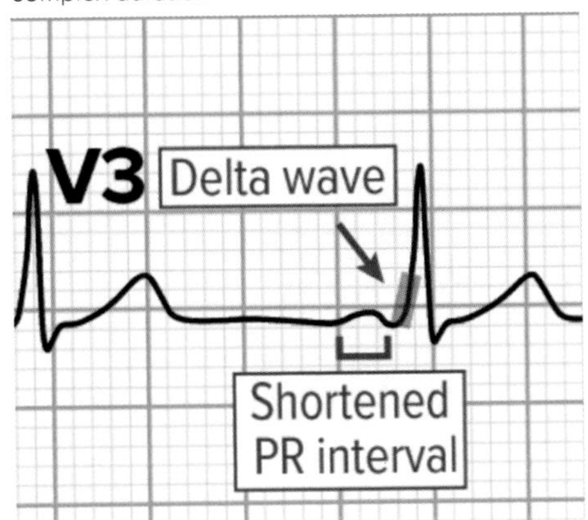

Figure 4.
Lead V4 from the repeat ECG shows a shortened PR interval and delta wave but a normal QRS complex duration

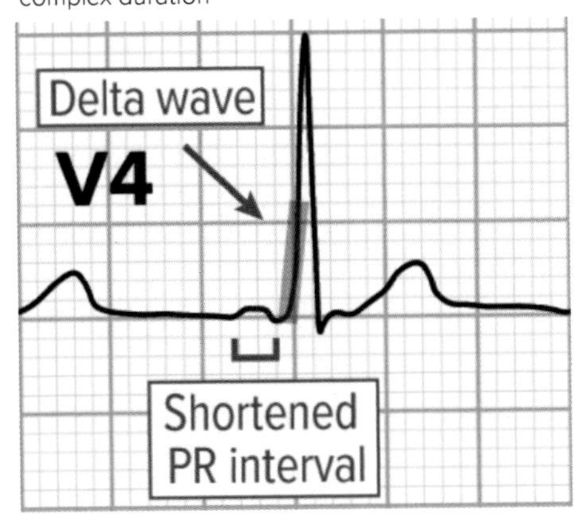

Figure 5.
Lead V5 from the repeat ECG shows no signs of ventricular pre-excitation (ie, normal PR interval, normal QRS complex duration, and no delta wave)

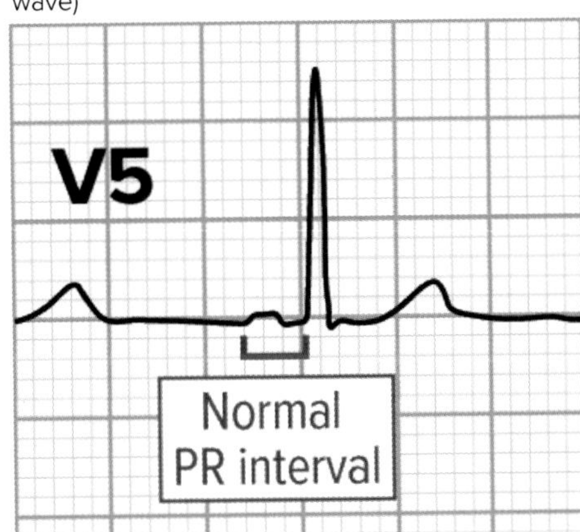

Figure 6.
Lead V6 from the repeat ECG shows no signs of ventricular pre-excitation (ie, normal PR interval, normal QRS complex duration, and no delta wave)

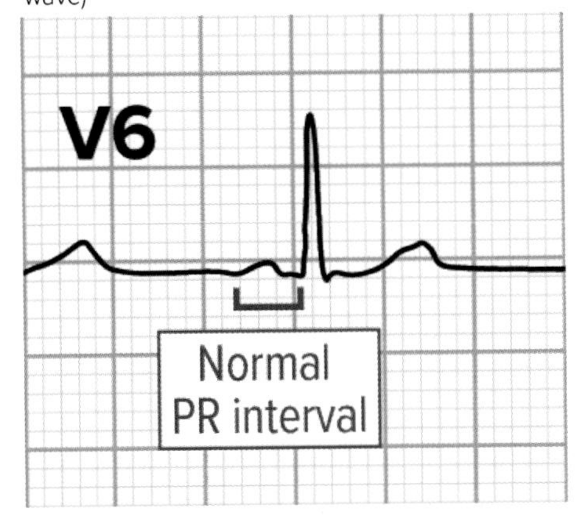

Delta waves represent pre-excitation of a portion of the ventricular myocardium via the AP. The depolarization wave resulting from this portion of pre-excited ventricular myocardium subsequently fuses with the depolarization caused by conduction via the AV node, ultimately creating the characteristic morphology of a QRS complex with a delta wave ***(see Figures 3 and 4)***.

The AV node's intrinsic refractory period prevents ventricular rates from exceeding 220-240 bpm in the absence of any extrinsic factors that increase conduction velocity (eg, catecholamine surge, sympathomimetic toxicity, or hyperthyroidism), so atrial fibrillation with intermittent conduction at rates faster than 220-240 bpm should prompt concern for an AP. The danger of conduction via an AP in atrial fibrillation is due to its short refractory period relative to the AV node. This allows the AP to conduct at much faster rates than the AV node. In atrial fibrillation with WPW, the AV node acts as a brake that tempers the faster AP conduction. Without the protection provided by the AV node, conduction via the AP can lead to extremely rapid rates and related cardiovascular decompensation (eg, ventricular fibrillation). This is why AV nodal blockers should be avoided in atrial fibrillation with known or suspected WPW.

Treatment for atrial fibrillation with WPW includes electrical cardioversion (for stable or unstable patients) and IV procainamide or ibutilide for stable patients.[1] Procainamide and ibutilide reduce conduction velocity throughout the entire cardiac conduction system, including the AP and ventricles. Verapamil, diltiazem, adenosine, digoxin, lidocaine, and intravenous amiodarone should not be used.[1]

This patient was admitted to the cardiology service and an EP study showed an antegrade bypass tract, consistent with WPW, which was successfully ablated.

WPW Learning Points

- Congenital condition involving abnormal conduction pathway between atria and ventricle
  - Most common dysrhythmia is orthodromic AVRT
- ECG findings seen in sinus rhythm include:
  - Shortened PR interval (< 120 msec)
  - Delta wave: slurring of initial portion of the QRS complex
  - QRS complex duration prolonged, usually > 110 msec
  - Secondary ST and T-wave changes
  - Patients with WPW can have baseline ECGs (ie, in normal sinus rhythm) with a normal PR interval, normal QRS complex duration, and/or without delta waves
- Regular rhythm tachycardias in WPW can be narrow (orthodromic conduction via AV node) or wide (antidromic conduction via accessory pathway)
  - WPW with orthodromic AVRT (most common dysrhythmia)- regular NCT, treat like AVNRT (PSVT)
  - WPW with antidromic AVRT- regular WCT, treat like monomorphic VT
- WPW with atrial fibrillation
  - Rapid, irregularly irregular wide complex tachycardia with beat-to-beat variation in QRS complex morphologies
  - Treatment includes electrical cardioversion (for stable or unstable patients) and IV procainamide or ibutilide for stable patients (avoid AV nodal blocking medications)
- In wide-complex atrial fibrillation, ventricular rates > 220-240 bpm suggest anterograde conduction via an accessory pathway

References

1. January CT, Wann LS, Alpert JS, et al. 2014 AHA/ACC/ HRS guideline for the management of patients with atrial fibrillation: a report of the American College of Cardiology/American Heart Association Task Force on Practice Guidelines and the Heart Rhythm Society. J Am Coll Cardiol. 2014;64:e1–76.

NOTES:

Case 82: Presentation

A 54-year-old male presents with chest pain. On exam, he appears pale, diaphoretic, and anxious. What is your interpretation of his ECG?

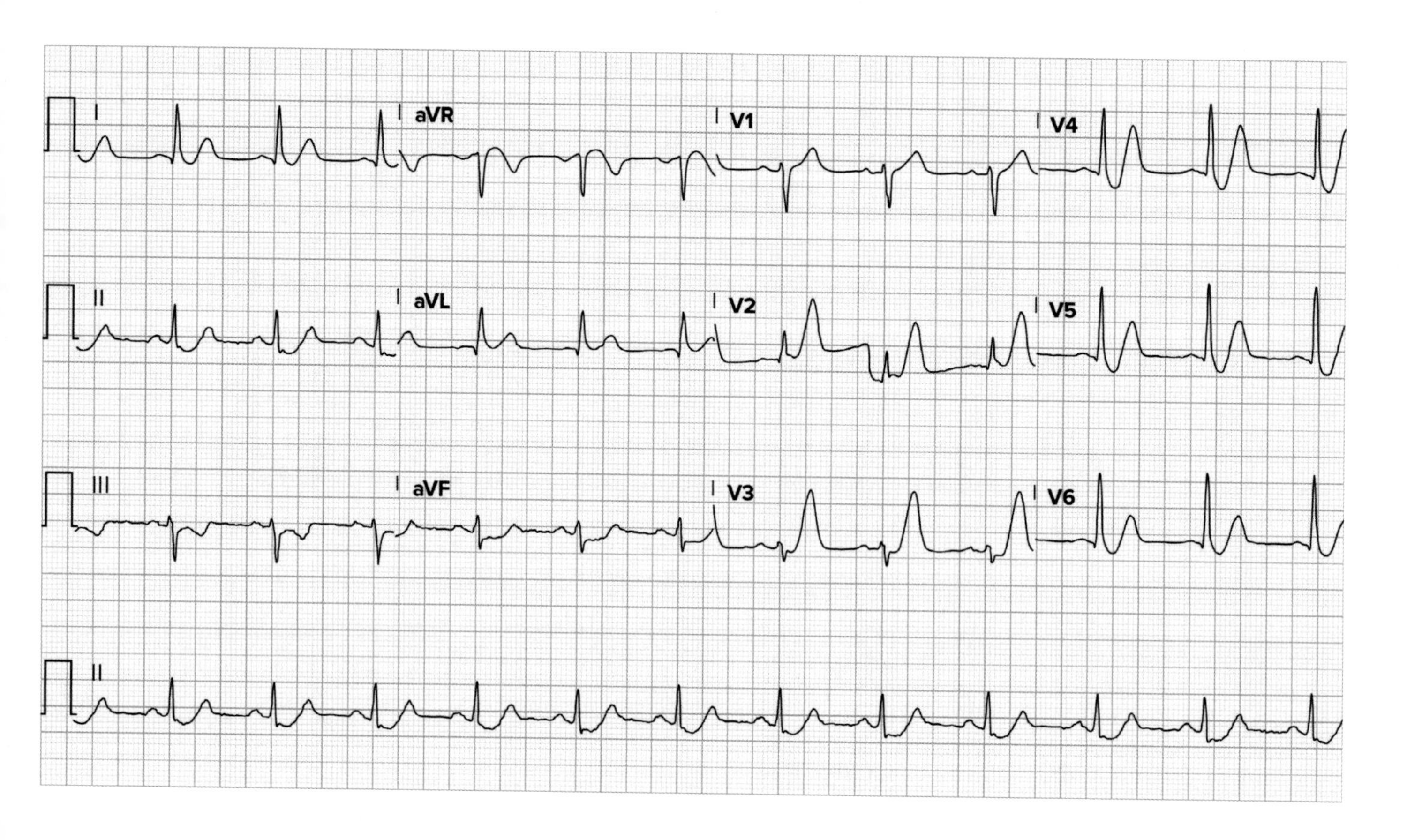

Case 82: Answer

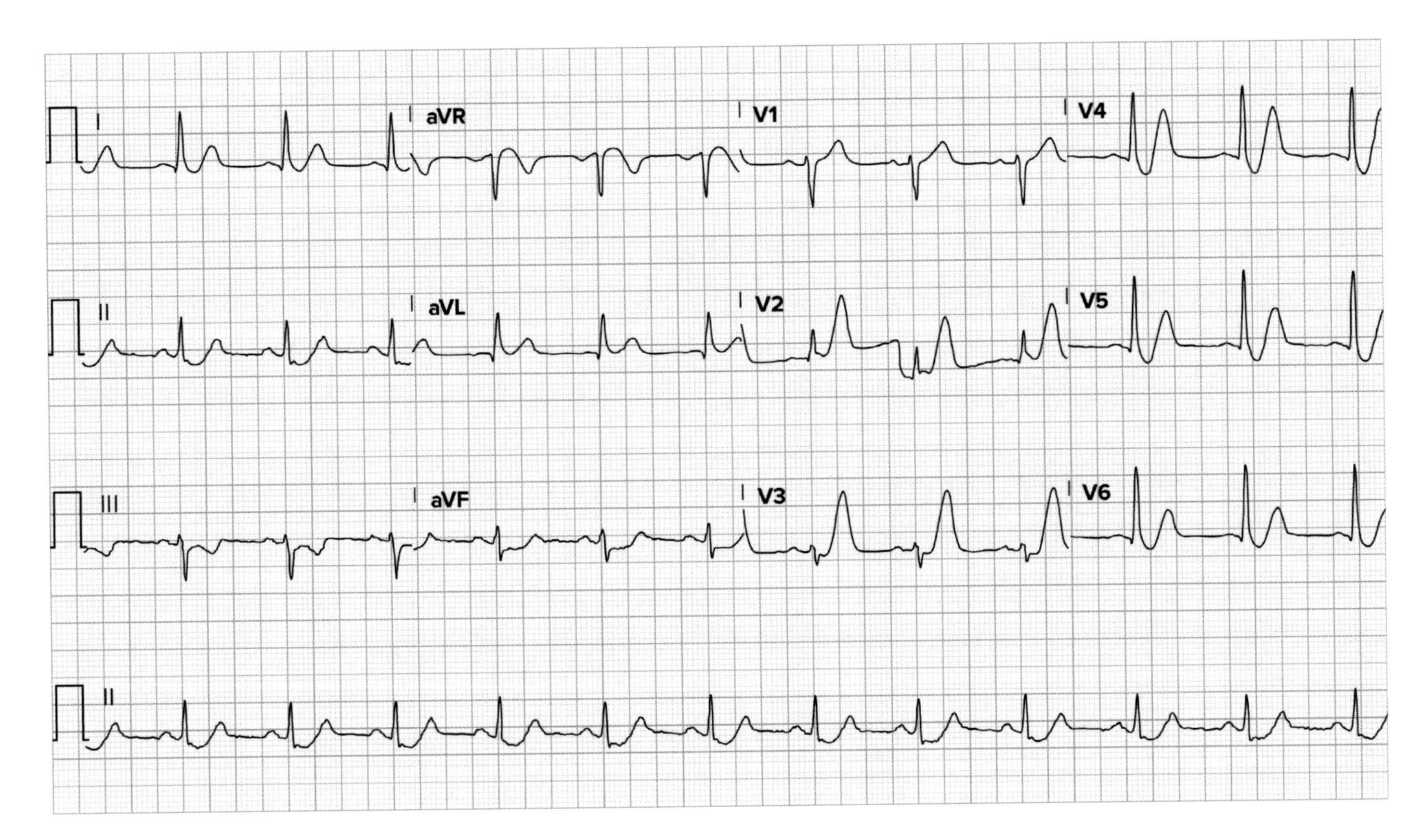

This ECG shows a normal sinus rhythm with ventricular rate of 74 bpm, normal axis, STE in lead aVR, STD in leads II, III, and aVF, hyperacute T-waves in lead V2, and STD with tall symmetric T-waves in leads V3-V6 consistent with de Winter's syndrome.

De Winter's syndrome is a high-risk ECG pattern, first described in 2008 by RJ de Winter who noted it occurred in approximately 2% of LAD occlusions.[1] The syndrome pattern includes tall symmetric T-waves with the ascending limb of the T-wave starting below the isoelectric baseline (ie, the J point is depressed) and > 1 mm of STD ***(see Figure 1)*** with no STE in the mid-precordial leads. These T-waves typically have a hyperacute appearance, suggesting an early, significant ACS event. STE between 0.5-1 mm is commonly seen in lead aVR.

De Winter's syndrome is not included in current STEMI guidelines, but patients with this ECG pattern and a presentation concerning for ACS warrants consideration for immediate revascularization.[2]

Figure 1.
Lead V4 shows tall symmetric T-waves with the ascending limb of the T-wave starting below the isoelectric baseline and > 1 mm of STD, consistent with De Winter's T-wave

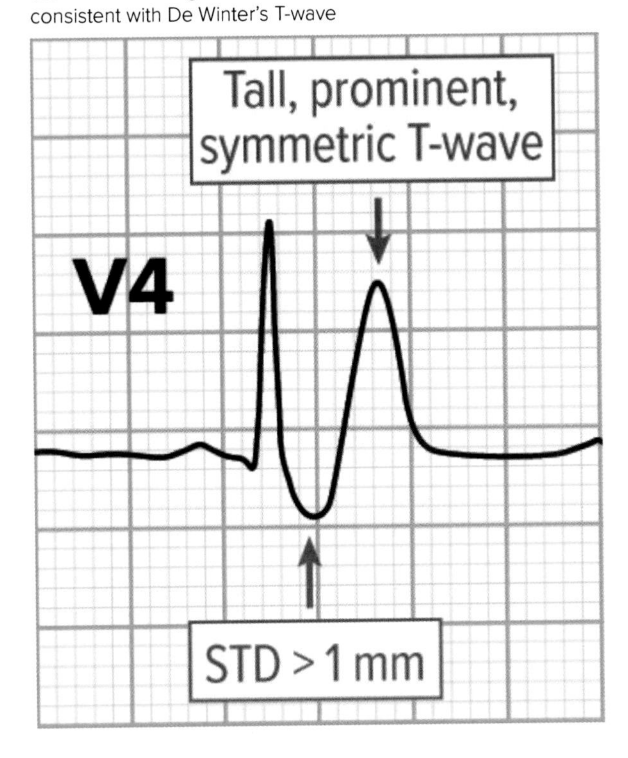

This patient was taken to the catheterization laboratory after an urgent call was placed to the interventional cardiologist. Coronary angiography revealed a 100% occlusion of the proximal LAD which was successfully treated with a stent.

It is important to remember that an ECG is not 100% sensitive for coronary occlusion and that the absence of STE does not rule out an AMI. Remember to treat the patient and not just the ECG, so if the diagnosis is unclear due to non-diagnostic findings, obtain serial ECGs. Also note that the 2014 AHA/ACC Guidelines for Management of Patients with Non-ST-Elevation ACS recommend early (ie, within 2 hours) invasive strategies for patients with hemodynamic (ie, hypotension) or electrical instability (ie, malignant dysrhythmia), signs of acute heart failure, or angina refractory to medical management.

De Winter's Syndrome Learning Points

- Can represent an acutely unstable proximal LAD occlusion and warrants consideration for immediate revascularization
- ECG features include:
  - Tall, prominent, symmetric T-waves in the precordial leads
  - STD > 1 mm at the J point in the precordial leads
  - Absence of STE in the precordial leads
  - STE (0.5-1 mm) in lead aVR is common
  - Typical STEMI morphology may precede or follow the de Winter pattern

Indications for immediate (within 2 hours) invasive strategy for non-STE ACS presentations, including unstable angina and NSTEMI:

- Refractory angina
- Hemodynamic or electrical instability
- Acute decompensating heart failure

References

1. Winter RJ, Verouden NJ, Wellens HJ, Wilde AA. A New ECG Sign of Proximal LAD Occlusion. N Engl J Med. 2008;359(19):2071-2073.
2. Rokos IC, French WJ, Mattu A, et al. Appropriate Cardiac Cath Lab activation: Optimizing electrocardiogram interpretation and clinical decision-making for acute ST-elevation myocardial infarction. Am Heart J. 2010;160(6):995-1003.

NOTES:

Case 83: Presentation

A 69-year-old male presents with worsening chest pain for the past 8 hours.
What is your interpretation of his ECG?

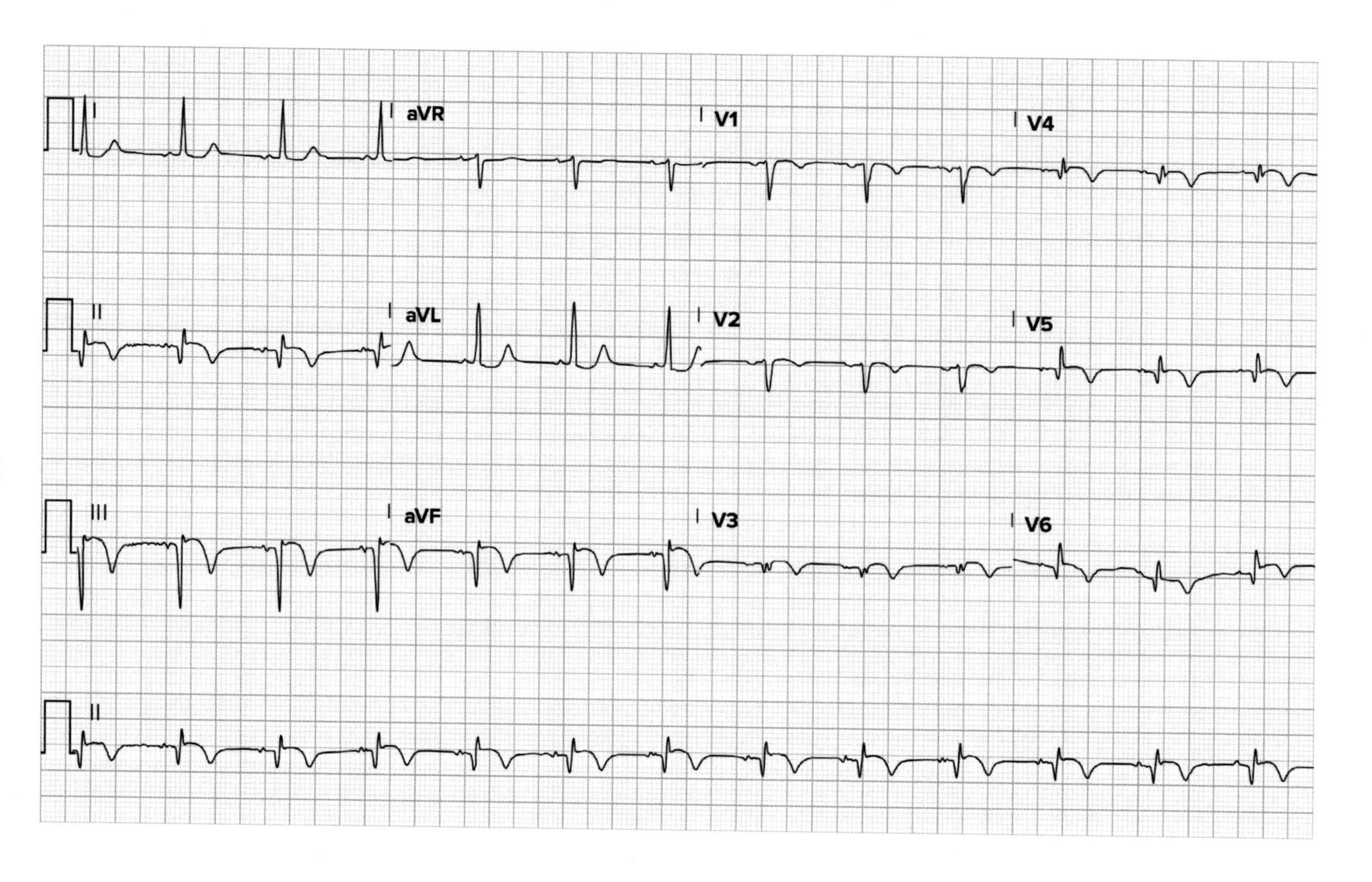

Case 83: Answer

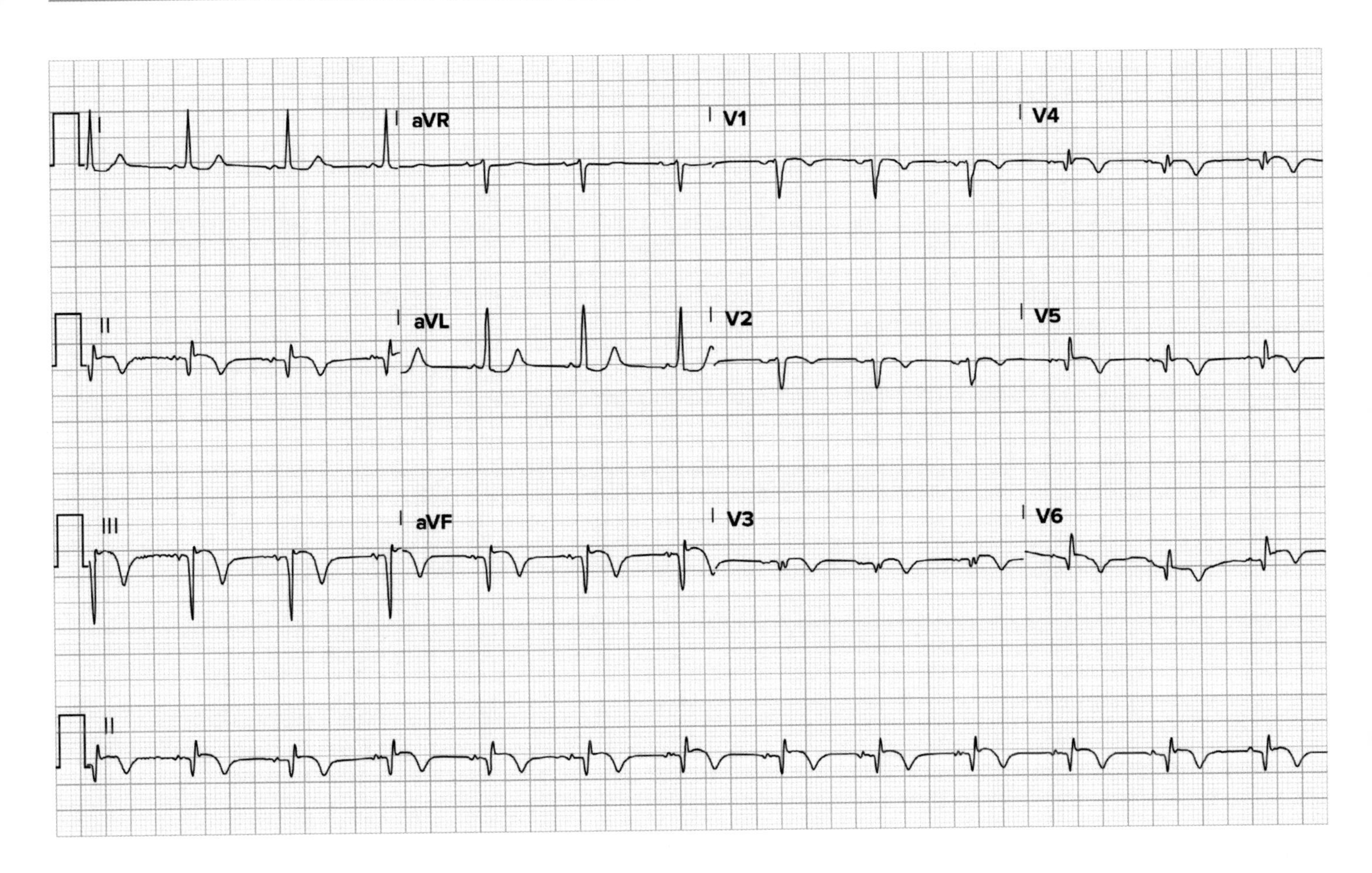

This ECG shows a normal sinus rhythm at 75 bpm, borderline left axis deviation, normal intervals, STE with both Q-waves and TWI in leads II, III, aVF, and V3-V6, and STD in leads I and aVL.

This ECG shows an inferolateral MI with very prominent Q-waves. Q-waves are the initial negative deflection that precede the upright R-wave of the QRS complex and can be pathological or non-pathological (see Learning Points below). Pathologic Q-waves are generally defined as ≥40 msec and/or ≥ 25-33% of accompanying R-wave height ***(see Figure 1)***.

Figure 1.
Pathologic Q-waves are generally defined as ≥40 msec and/or ≥ 25-33% of accompanying R-wave height

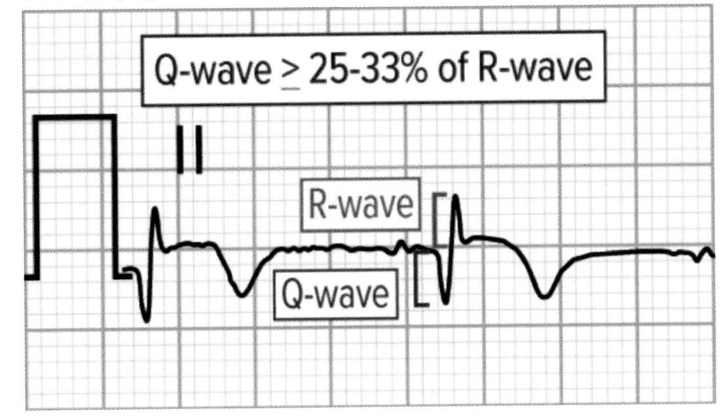

In the past, MIs were classified as Q-wave MI and non-Q-wave MI. Although these terms are no longer used, misconceptions based on this classification system persist. Current cardiology research has shown:

- Q-waves correlate with size or infarction but do not differentiate between transmural and non-transmural/subendocardial infarction
- Q-waves associated with infarction are not permanent and can resolve or diminish over time
- Q-waves do not predict viability of myocardium (a common misconception)
- There is a high risk for LV dysfunction with Q-waves that suggest a large infarction, but LV dysfunction can occur in the absence of Q-waves

This patient was taken urgently to the catheterization laboratory and found to have a 100% occlusion of his RCA extending from the mid-portion back to the origin. An echo showed definite RV involvement, which is important to identify as these patients will be preload dependent and the use of vasodilatory medications can lead to hypotension. RV MIs are often seen concurrently with inferior MI and while there are multiple non-diagnostic findings that can be seen on a standard 12-lead ECG that suggest RV involvement, the diagnosis is made with a right-sided ECG ***(see Figure 2)***. The right-sided ECG is often deferred in order to get the patient to the catheterization laboratory as quickly as possible, so it is not unreasonable to assume RV involvement and avoid medications that decrease preload (eg, nitroglycerin, morphine, etc.) in patients presenting with an inferior MI.

Figure 2.
Recommended placement of right-sided leads

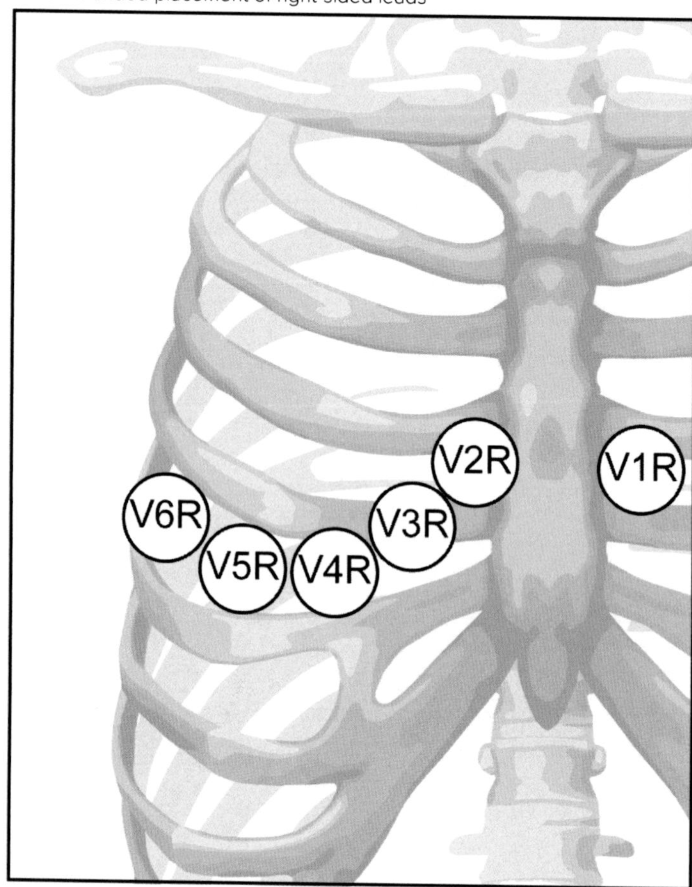

Right Ventricular MI Learning Points

- Consider with any inferior MI
  - RV MI is present in 25-30% of inferior STEMI
- Findings seen with inferior MI that should prompt further evaluation with right-sided leads:
  - STE in lead V1 + STD in lead V2
  - STD in lead V2 + isoelectric ST-segment in lead V1
- Right-sided leads V1R-V6R evaluate for RV MI
  - STE in leads V3R and V4R ≥ 0.5 mm (≥ 1 mm for men ≤ 30 years old)
  - STE in lead V4R > 1 mm most predictive of RV MI
  - STE in lead V4R > STE in leads V1-V3 is highly specific for RV MI
- RV infarct = preload dependent
  - Avoid preload reducing medications (eg, nitroglycerin, morphine, etc.)
  - Consider increasing preload with fluid bolus

Q-waves Learning Points

- Can be pathological or non-pathological (see table below)
- Pathologic Q-waves generally defined as ≥40 msec and/or ≥ 25-33% of accompanying R-wave height
- When due to an MI:
  - Occur in ≥ 2 contiguous leads that also have STE
  - Size correlates with volume of infarcted myocardium
  - Early appearance of Q-waves does not always indicate irreversible myocardial death, particularly with simultaneous STE and/or shorter period of ACS symptoms
  - Tall R-waves in leads V1 and V2 may represent Q-waves due to a posterior MI
- QS complex = single large negative deflection
  - Usually indicates significant irreversible myocardial loss when associated with ischemia
  - QS complex with STE and diminished T-wave should prompt evaluation for LV aneurysm
- Q-waves in leads V1 and V2 can be caused by misplacement of leads in the 2nd or 3rd intercostal spaces

Q-wave Causes	
Physiologic	Normal variant in leads V1, V2, III, and/or aVR
Structural	LVH RVH HCM
Conduction	LBBB Pre-excitation rhythms
Myocardial	Infarct Cardiomyopathy Myocarditis Infiltrative disease

Case 84: Presentation

A 77-year-old male presents with exertional fatigue and near syncope.
What is your interpretation of his ECG?

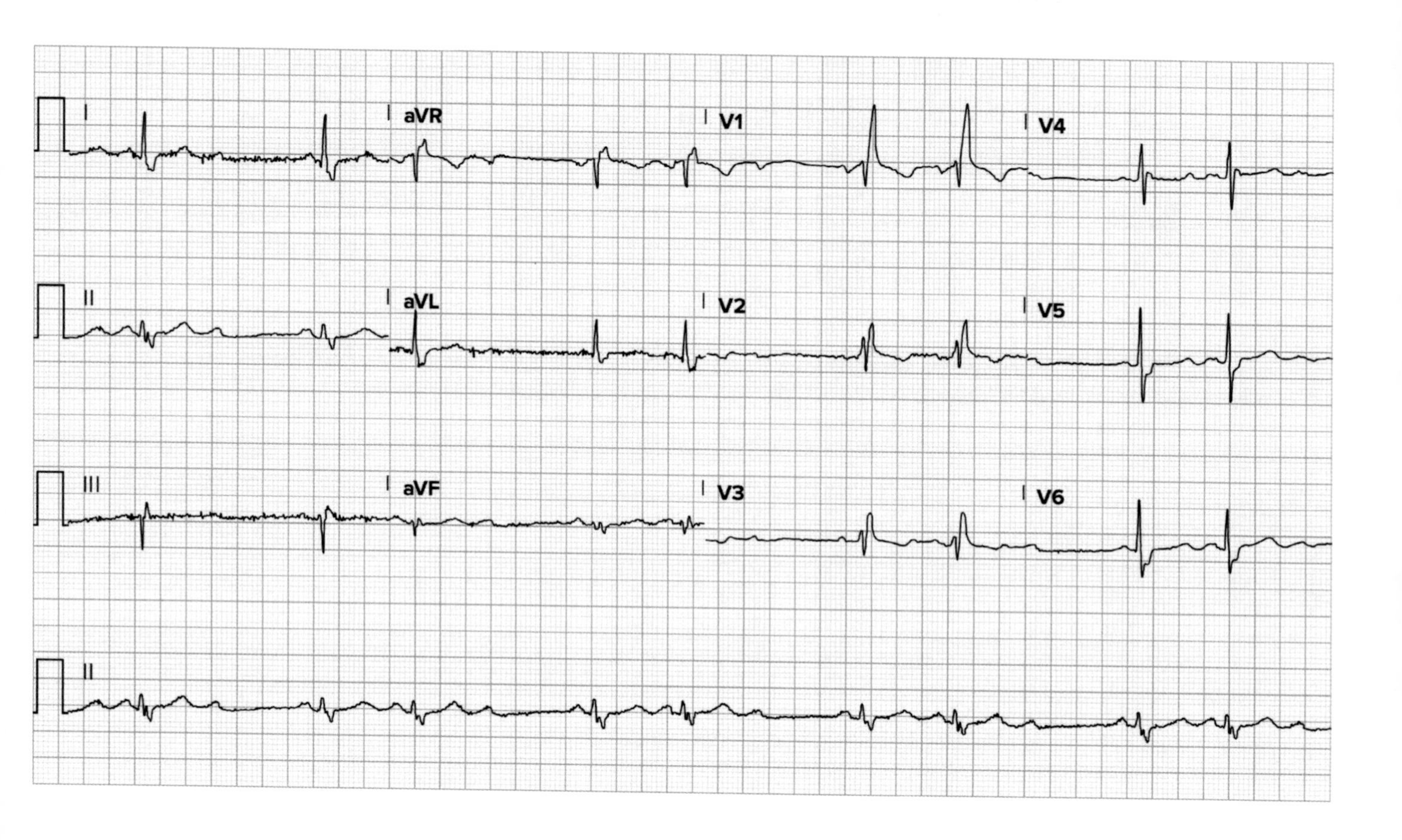

Case 84: Answer

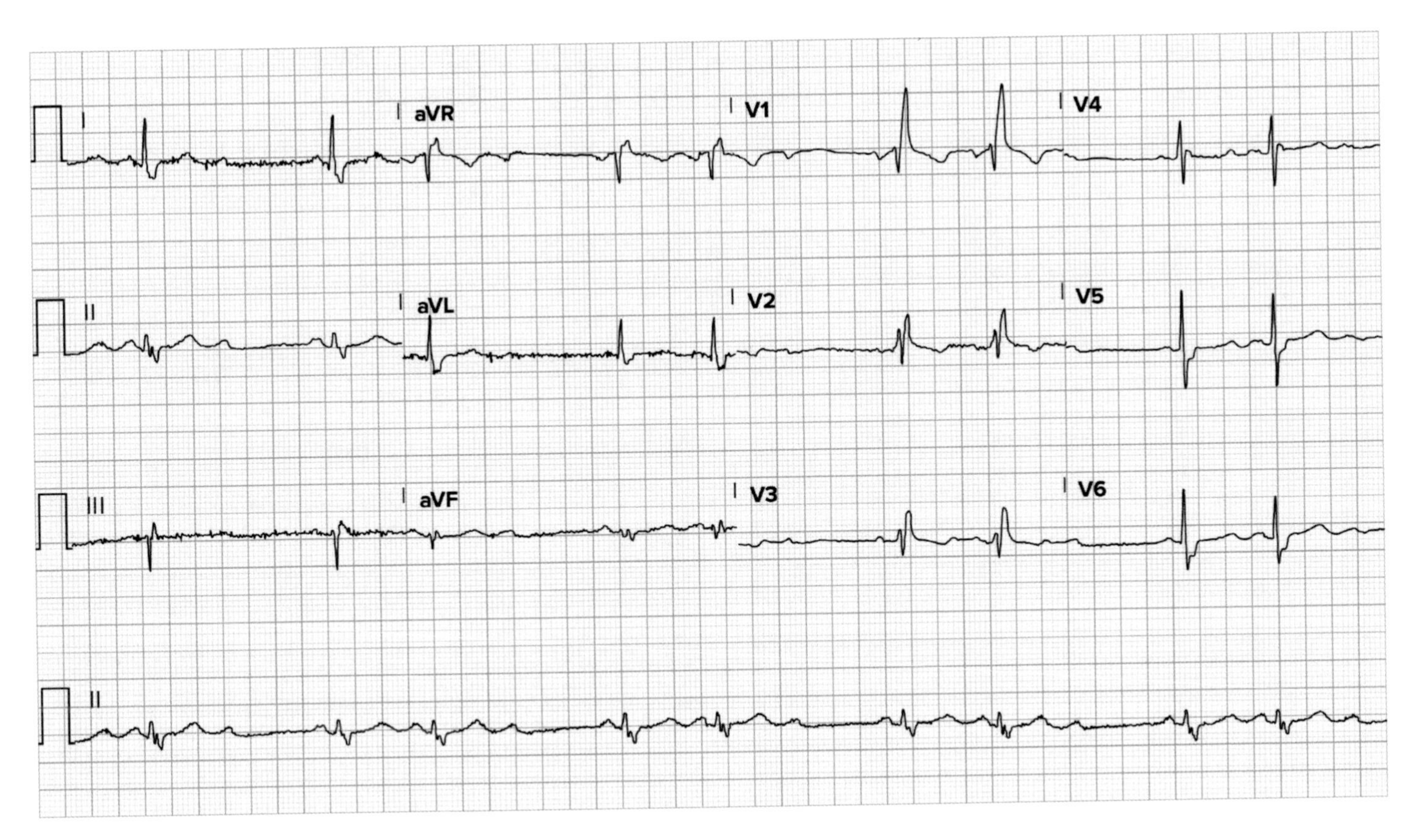

This ECG shows a Mobitz type II 2nd degree AV block with 3:2 conduction and an average ventricular rate of 54 bpm, normal axis, normal PR interval, prolonged QRS complex duration with a RBBB, and prolonged QTc interval.

The differential diagnosis for an irregular wide complex rhythm with bradycardic ventricular rates includes:

- Atrial fibrillation (rate controlled) with aberrant conduction
- Atrial flutter with variable block (rate controlled) and aberrant conduction
- Atrial tachycardia with variable block (rate controlled) and aberrant conduction
- Wandering atrial pacemaker with aberrant conduction
- 2nd degree AV block Mobitz types I and II with aberrant conduction
- Variable high-grade AV block (eg, 3:1, 4:1, etc.) with aberrant conduction
- 2nd degree sinoatrial block with aberrant conduction
- Sinus arrhythmia with aberrant conduction
- Sinus bradycardia, junctional rhythm, or junctional bradycardia with aberrant conduction and irregular pattern of PAC, PJC, and/or PVC
- Sinus bradycardia, junctional rhythm, or junctional bradycardia with aberrant conduction and regular patterns of PAC, PJC, and/or PVC (bigeminy, trigeminy, etc.)
  - Causes of aberrant conduction include fixed or rate-related BBB, metabolic abnormalities, sodium channel blocker toxicity, ventricular-paced rhythm, and ventricular pre-excitation (eg, WPW)

Mobitz type II AV blocks are due to intermittent failure of infranodal conduction but can occur more proximally in the AV node. The distinguishing feature of a Mobitz type II is a constant PR interval (which may or may not be prolonged) followed by a non-conducted P-wave (ie, P-wave without accompanying QRS complex) ***(see Figure 1)***. The PP and RR intervals will be constant and the P-waves will march out. A Mobitz type II AV block is described as a ratio of P-waves to QRS complexes, which is 3:2 in this ECG.

Figure 1.
The lead II rhythm strip shows constant PR intervals followed by a non-conducted P-wave consistent with a Mobitz type II AV block

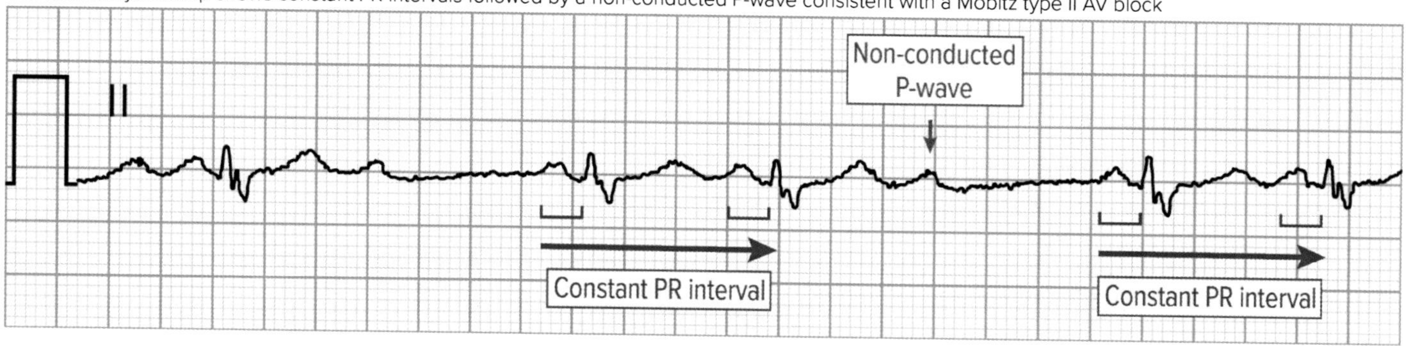

It is essential to differentiate Mobitz type I conduction from Mobitz type II conduction, as the former is typically transient with a more benign course while the latter has a high risk of progressing to a 3rd degree AV block, frequently produces hemodynamic compromise, and is associated with worse outcomes if not treated. The QRS complex duration is typically not useful in differentiating between a Mobitz type I AV block and a Mobitz type II AV block, as a Mobitz type I AV block can have a wide QRS compex if there is aberrant conduction (eg, an intrinsic bundle branch block) and a Mobitz type II AV block can have a narrow QRS complex (ie, duration < 110 msec) if the block is in the AV node. The key to distinguishing between the two is to compare the RR interval that includes the non-conducted P-wave to the PP interval.

In a Mobitz type I AV block, the RR interval that includes the non-conducted P-wave will be less than twice the PP interval. In the example below from a different ECG ***(see Figure 2)***, the RR interval that includes the non-conducted P-wave (1480 msec) is less than twice the PP interval (1680 msec).

Figure 2.
In a Mobitz type I AV block, the RR interval that includes the non-conducted P-wave is less than twice the PP interval (from a different ECG)

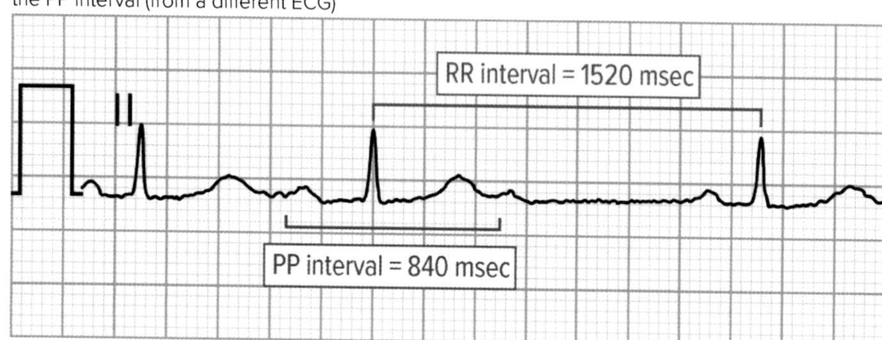

In a Mobitz type II AV block, the RR interval that includes the non-conducted P-wave will be equal to twice the PP interval. This is evident in the lead II rhythm strip from the case ECG ***(see Figure 3)*** where the RR interval that includes the non-conducted P-wave (1440 msec) is equal to exactly twice the PP interval (1440 msec).

Figure 3.
In a Mobitz type II AV block, the RR interval that includes the non-conducted P-wave is equal to exactly twice the PP interval (from case ECG)

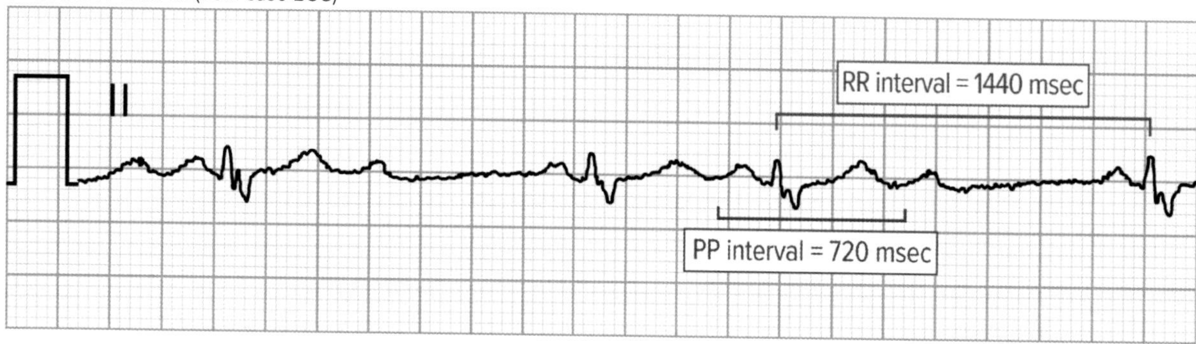

This ECG also shows a RBBB. A RBBB will typically have STD and TWI in lead V1, and if leads V2-V3 have an rsR' pattern present, they will also typically have STD and TWI. Consequently, upright T-waves or STE in those leads with an rsR' pattern is concerning for ischemia, and even isoelectric or minimally elevated ST-segments can be a subtle indicator of early AMI. Otherwise, the presence of a RBBB does not confound the ECG evaluation of ACS as does a LBBB.

The characteristic findings in a RBBB include:

- QRS complex duration ≥ 120 msec
- rsr', rsR', or rSR' pattern in lead V1 +/- V2 ***(see Figure 4)***
  - Variations in lead V1 include qR pattern or broad R-wave that is often notched
  - In lead V1, the initial upward deflection should always be smaller than the 2nd upward deflection ***(see Figure 4)***
- S-wave duration > R-wave or > 40 msec in leads I and V6 ***(see Figures 5 and 6)***
- Normal R-wave peak time in leads V5 and V6 but > 50 msec in lead V1 (only required if broad R-wave +/- notch is present in lead V1)
- Repolarization abnormalities include STD and TWI in lead V1 +/- lead(s) V2-V3 if they have an rsR' pattern, so STE and/or upright T-waves in those leads are concerning for ischemia

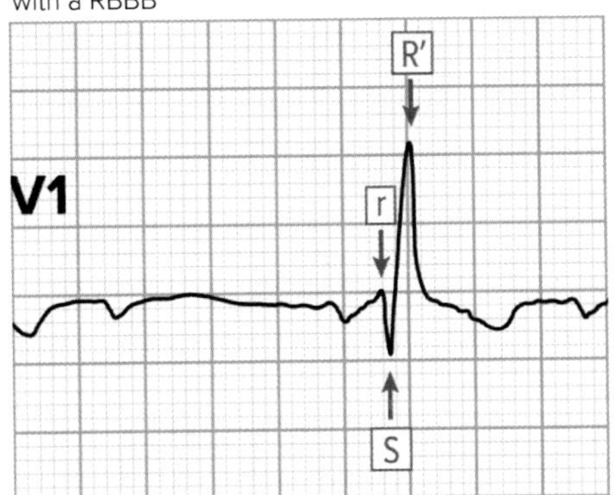

Figure 4.
rSR' pattern in lead V1, consistent with a RBBB

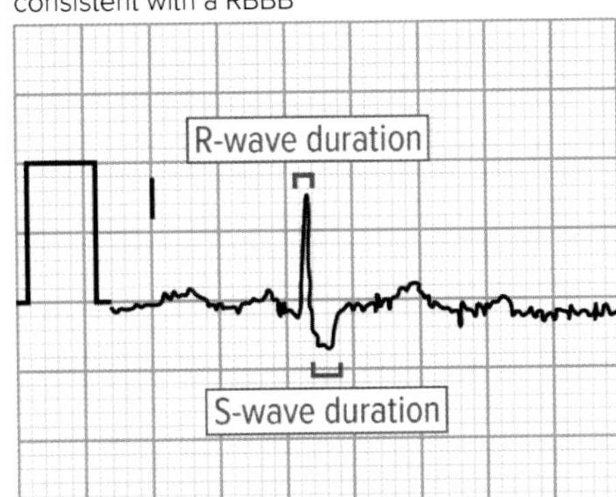

Figure 5.
S-wave duration > R-wave duration in lead I, consistent with a RBBB

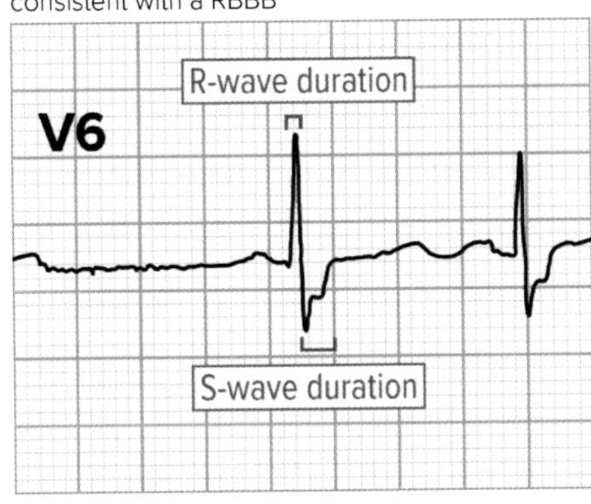

Figure 6.
S-wave duration > R-wave duration in lead V6, consistent with a RBBB

This patient had an unremarkable ED workup and was admitted to the cardiology service for evaluation for pacemaker placement.

Mobitz type I AV Block Learning Points

- Progressively increasing PR interval and decreasing RR interval until a non-conducted P-wave occurs (ie, P-wave without accompanying QRS complex)
  - PR interval immediately after non-conducted P-wave is shorter than PR interval preceding non-conducted P-wave
  - RR interval that includes non-conducted P-wave < twice the PP interval
- Can be normal variant and usually does not produce hemodynamic compromise
  - Typically associated with excess vagal tone and therefore usually responds to atropine when acute treatment is needed
  - Can lead to a more advanced AV block if associated with a pathologic etiology
  - Can be seen with inferior MI

Mobitz type II AV Block Learning Points

- Constant PR interval in conducted beats
  - Described as ratio of P-waves to QRS complexes
  - Typically an infranodal block resulting in a prolonged QRS complex duration
  - RR interval that includes non-conducted P-wave = twice the PP interval
- Never a normal variant and frequently produces hemodynamic compromise
  - High risk of progressing to a 3rd degree AV block
  - Atropine is unlikely to lead to clinical improvement and may lead to a high-grade AV block

High-grade (or advanced) AV Block Learning Points

- 2nd degree AV block with ≥ 2 sequential non-conducted P-waves
  - Most commonly a variant of a Mobitz type II but can be associated with a Mobitz type I
  - PP and RR intervals should have a whole number ratio
- Named as ratio of P-waves to QRS complexes
- Can be seen after anterior MI or with significant pathology of the conduction pathway
- High risk of progressing to a 3rd degree AV block

RBBB Learning Points

- Delayed conduction through right ventricle with normal left ventricular conduction
- In lead V1, the initial upward deflection should always be smaller than the 2nd upward deflection
- Repolarization abnormalities include STD and TWI in lead V1 +/- lead(s) V2-V3 if they have an rsR' pattern, so STE and/or upright T-waves in those leads are concerning for ischemia
  - Otherwise, the presence of a RBBB does not confound the ECG evaluation of ACS as does a LBBB
- RBBB with axis deviation should prompt evaluation for a concurrent LAFB or LPFB

NOTES:

Case 85: Presentation

A 59-year-old male with history of CAD, prior MI s/p coronary stenting presents with chest pain and diaphoresis consistent with his prior MI. What is your interpretation of his ECG? His prior ECG is below for comparison.

Presenting ECG

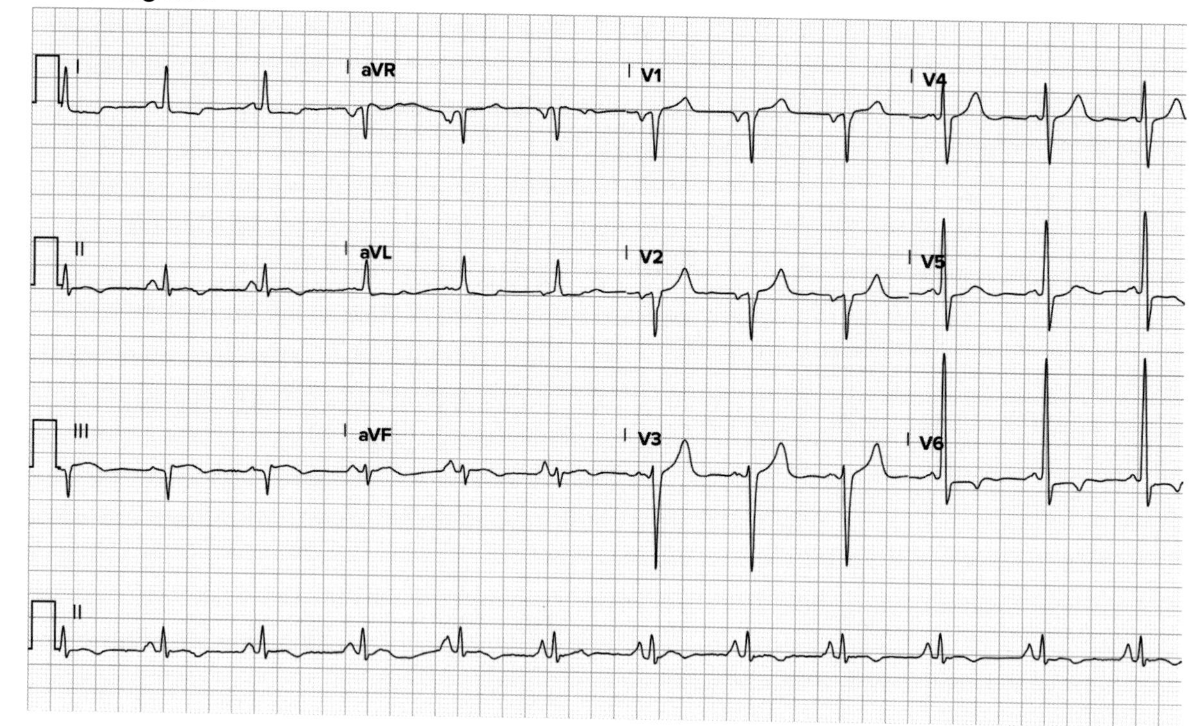

Prior ECG

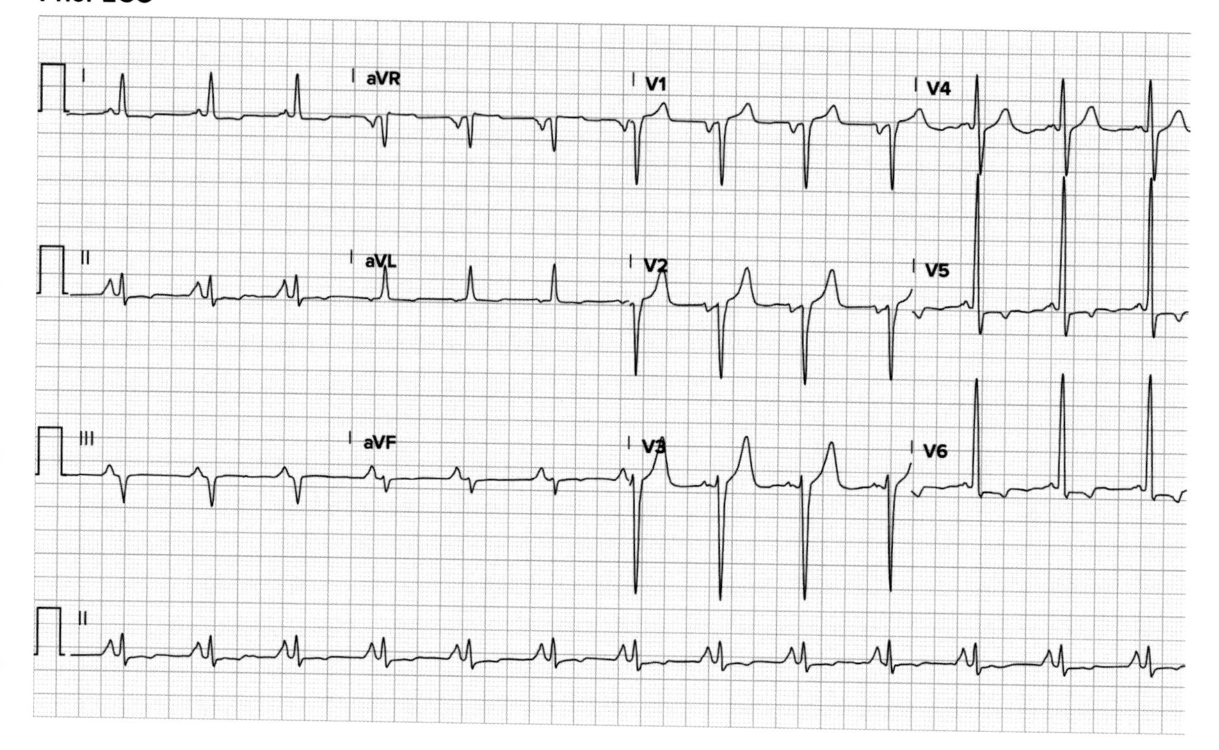

Case 85: Answer

Presenting ECG

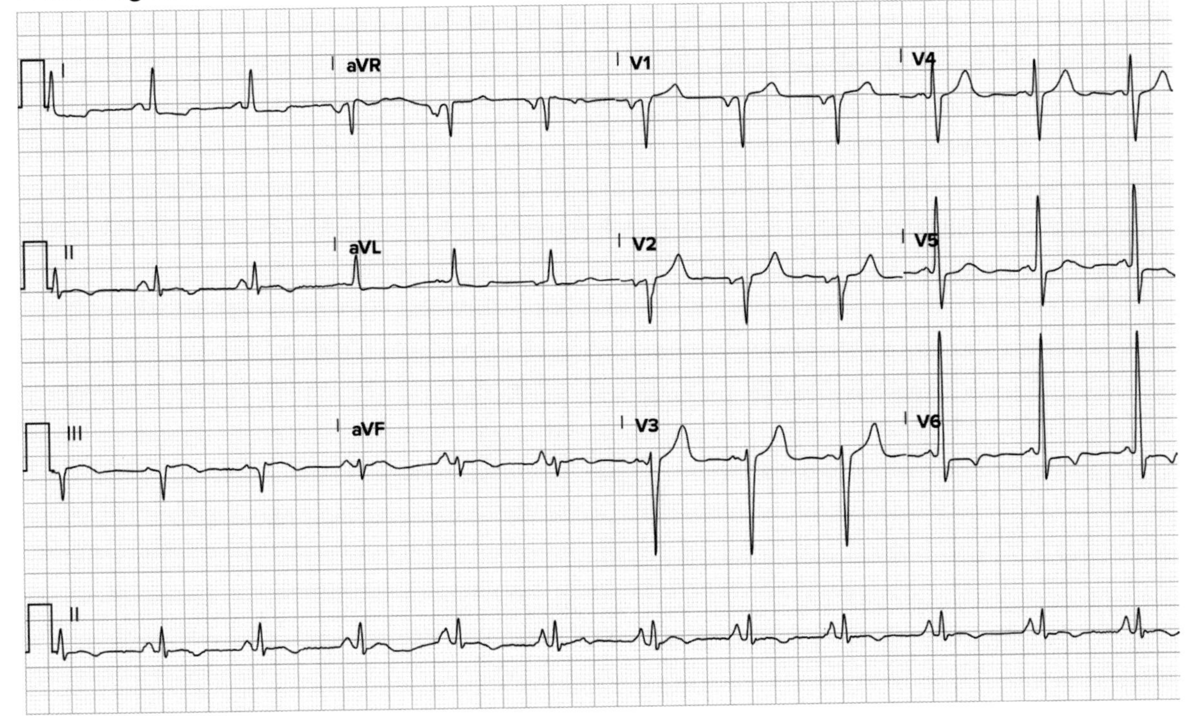

Prior ECG

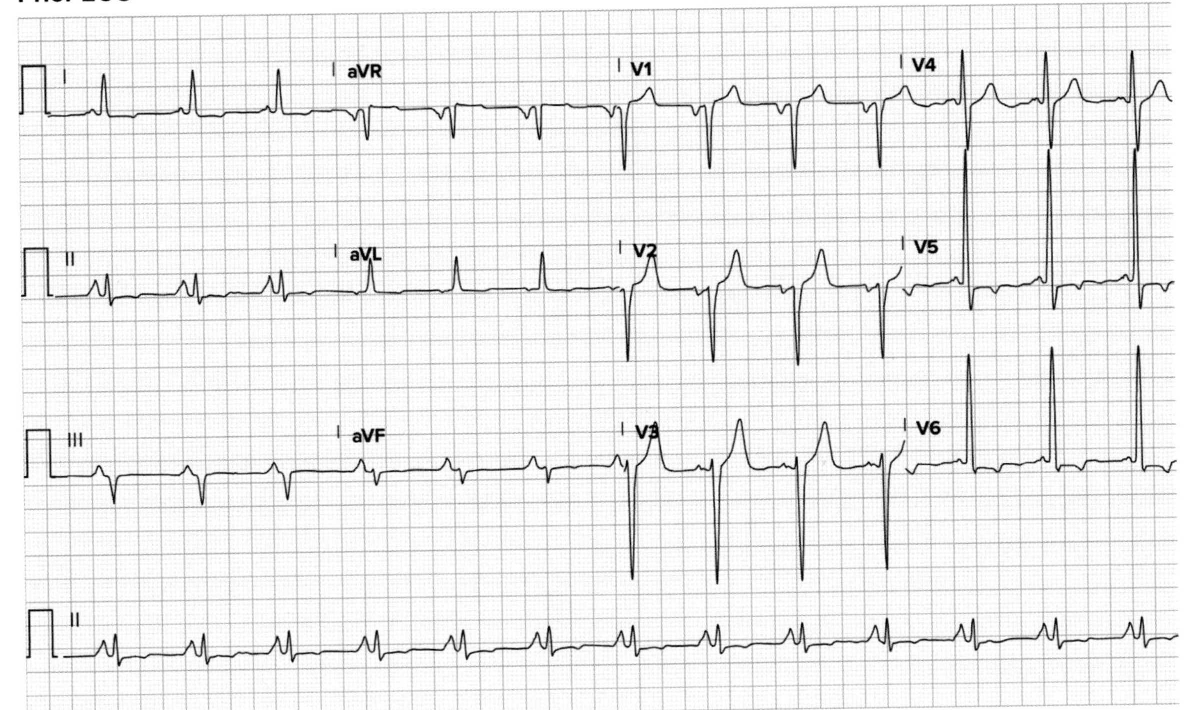

This ECG shows normal sinus rhythm at 70 bpm, normal axis, normal intervals, STE in leads III and aVF, and ST-segment and T-wave abnormalities consistent with LVH by voltage with strain pattern that was present on the prior ECG.

While the ST-segment changes in the inferior leads do not meet STEMI criteria, they are concerning for ischemia/infarct. The ST-segments on the prior ECG are flat in leads III and aVF and depressed in lead II ***(see Figure 1)***. The presenting ECG shows new STE in leads III and aVF but only lead III meets criteria ***(see Figure 2)***. Lead II now has an isoelectric ST-segment which is elevated when compared to the STD seen on the prior ECG.

Figure 1.
Leads II, III, and aVF from prior ECG

Figure 2.
Leads II, III, and aVF from presenting ECG

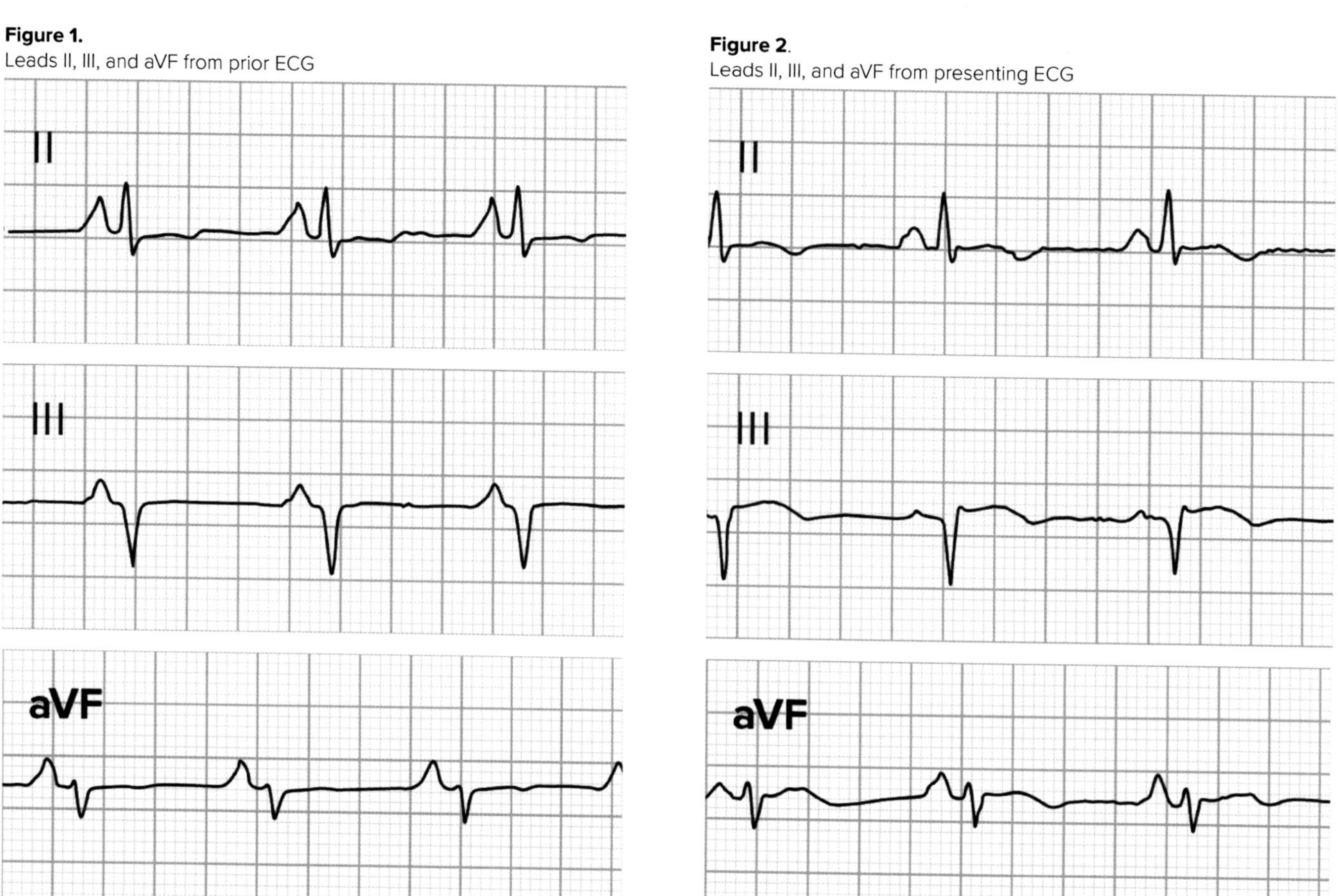

The presence of reciprocal STD supports, but is not required for, the diagnosis of an MI. In fact, the absence of reciprocal STD does not rule out AMI in any instance. In this case, it is impossible to tell whether the STD seen in leads I and aVL are due to ischemia/infarct and/or repolarization abnormalities associated with the LVH strain pattern. The presence of these changes on the patient's prior ECG points against them being acute.

ECG findings seen with the LVH strain pattern include a wide QRS, STE with a concave upward ST-segment morphology and large S-wave in leads V1-V3 ***(see Figure 3),*** and STD with concave downward ST-segment contour and a large R-wave in leads I, aVL, and V4-V6 ***(see Figure 4)***. These ST-segment and T-wave abnormalities can mimic an anteroseptal MI, or in this case, the reciprocal STD expected in an inferior MI. Comparing with prior ECGs and obtaining serial ECGs can help differentiate between ischemia and strain pattern.

Figure 3.
Findings in lead V3 consistent with the LVH strain pattern

Figure 4.
Findings in lead V6 consistent with the LVH strain pattern

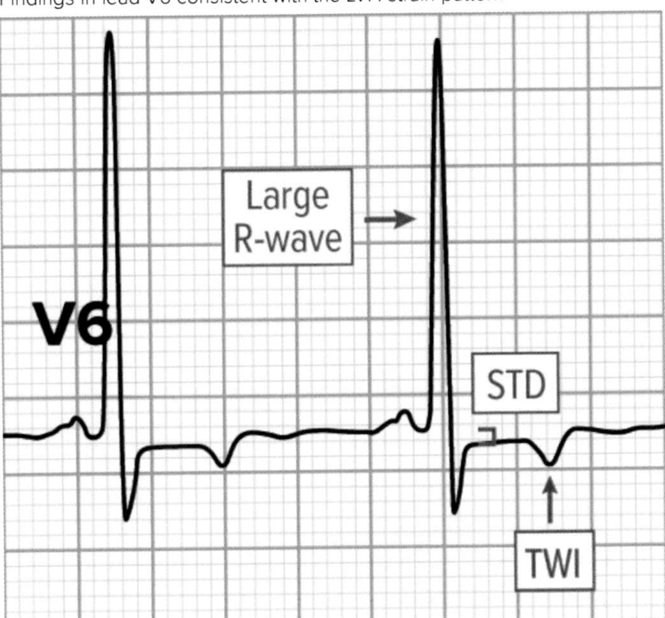

This patient was taken to the cardiac catheterization laboratory and found to have a 100% occlusion of his prior RCA stent.

STEMI Learning Points

- STEMI is defined by new, or presumed new, STE at the J point in ≥ 2 anatomically contiguous leads in the absence of LVH by voltage pattern, LBBB, or ventricular-paced rhythm
  - ≥ 2.5 mm in men < 40 years old and ≥ 2 mm in men ≥ 40 years old in leads V2-V3 (or an increase of ≥ 1 mm when compared to baseline ECG)
  - ≥ 1.5 mm in women in leads V2-V3 (or an increase of ≥ 1 mm when compared to baseline ECG)
  - ≥ 1 mm in all other leads
- ST-segment is measured from the isoelectric baseline, typically the TP segment (see below)
- Reciprocal STD are not required for the diagnosis of STEMI, but their presence does increase the likelihood of the diagnosis of STEMI
  - Reciprocal STD are only present in 70% of anterior MI1
- Posterior MI
  - Consider whenever there is STD in leads V1-V4
  - STE ≥ 0.5 mm in posterior leads V7, V8 or V9 is diagnostic- does not require 2 contiguous leads
- Right ventricular MI
  - Consider with any inferior MI (RV MI is seen in approximately 1/3 of inferior MI)
  - STE in right precordial leads V3R and V4R ≥ 0.5 mm (≥ 1 mm for men ≤ 30 years old)
  - STE in right precordial lead V4R > 1 mm is most predictive of RV MI
  - STE in right precordial lead V4R > STE in leads V1-V3 = highly specific for RV MI
- Significant STE that does not meet the traditional distribution (ie, ≥ 2 anatomically contiguous leads) in a presentation concerning for ACS may still represent coronary artery occlusion and warrant consideration for emergent coronary reperfusion

How to Measure STE per most recent 2018 AHA Guidelines[1]

- The J point is the junction between QRS termination and ST-segment onset and is used to determine the magnitude of the ST-segment shift
- **In patients with a stable baseline, the TP segment (isoelectric interval) is a more accurate method to assess the magnitude of ST-segment shift *(see Figure 5)***, and in distinguishing pericarditis from acute myocardial ischemia
- QRS onset should be used if TP segment does not have a stable baseline ***(see Figure 6)***
- Measurement should be made from the top of the ECG line tracing

Figure 5.
Measure STE from the TP segment if the TP segment is isoelectric (ie, horizontal)

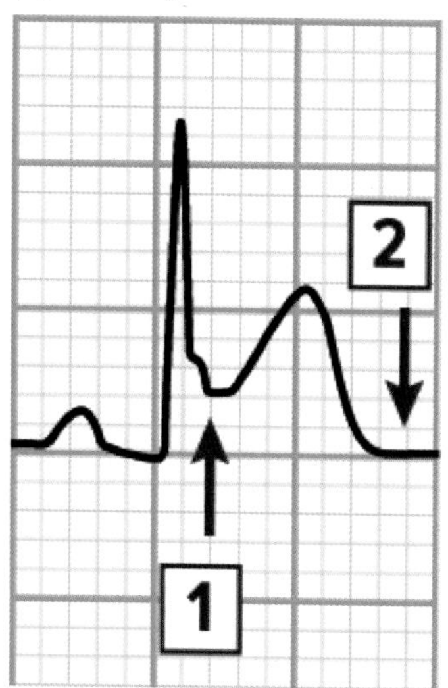

Arrow 1: onset of the ST-segment (ie, J point)
Arrow 2: TP segment

Figure 6.
Measure STE from onset of the QRS complex if the TP segment is not isoelectric (ie, not horizontal)

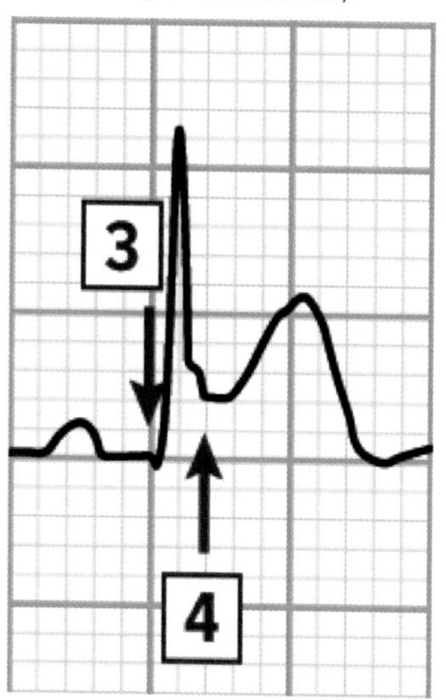

Arrow 3: initial onset of the Q-wave
Arrow 4: onset of the ST-segment (ie, J point)

LVH Learning Points

- ECG is only suggestive of anatomic LVH- echocardiography is the superior diagnostic modality
- ECG findings in LVH are manifested primarily by the increased voltage of the QRS complexes, hence the term "LVH by voltage criteria"
  - No criteria are recommended for use exclusive of other validated criteria
  - Diagnosis of LVH in the presence of intraventricular conduction abnormalities (eg, fascicular blocks, bundle branch blocks) should be made with caution as they may impact the accuracy of the ECG criteria for LVH
- 80% of LVH by voltage patterns demonstrate ST and T-wave abnormalities, termed "LVH with strain pattern," which commonly include:
  - STE in leads V1-V3
  - STD and TWI in leads I, aVL and V4-V6
  - Increased S-wave depth in leads III, aVR, and V1-V3
  - Increased R-wave peak time > 50 msec in lead V5 or V6
  - Increased R-wave amplitude in leads I, aVL and V4-V6
  - Left axis deviation typical, but can occur with any axis
  - Increased QRS complex and/or QT interval duration
- LVH with strain pattern can confound the ECG's ability to detect ACS, particularly anteroseptal MI, and mimics ACS findings

References

1. Thygesen K, Alpert JS, Jaffe AS, et al. 2018 ESC/ACC/AHA/WHF Expert Consensus Document: Fourth Universal Definition of Myocardial Infarction (2018). Circulation. 2018;138:e618-e651.

NOTES:

Case 86: Presentation

A 43-year-old male with history of ischemic cardiomyopathy and AICD placement presents with palpitations. What is your interpretation of his ECG?

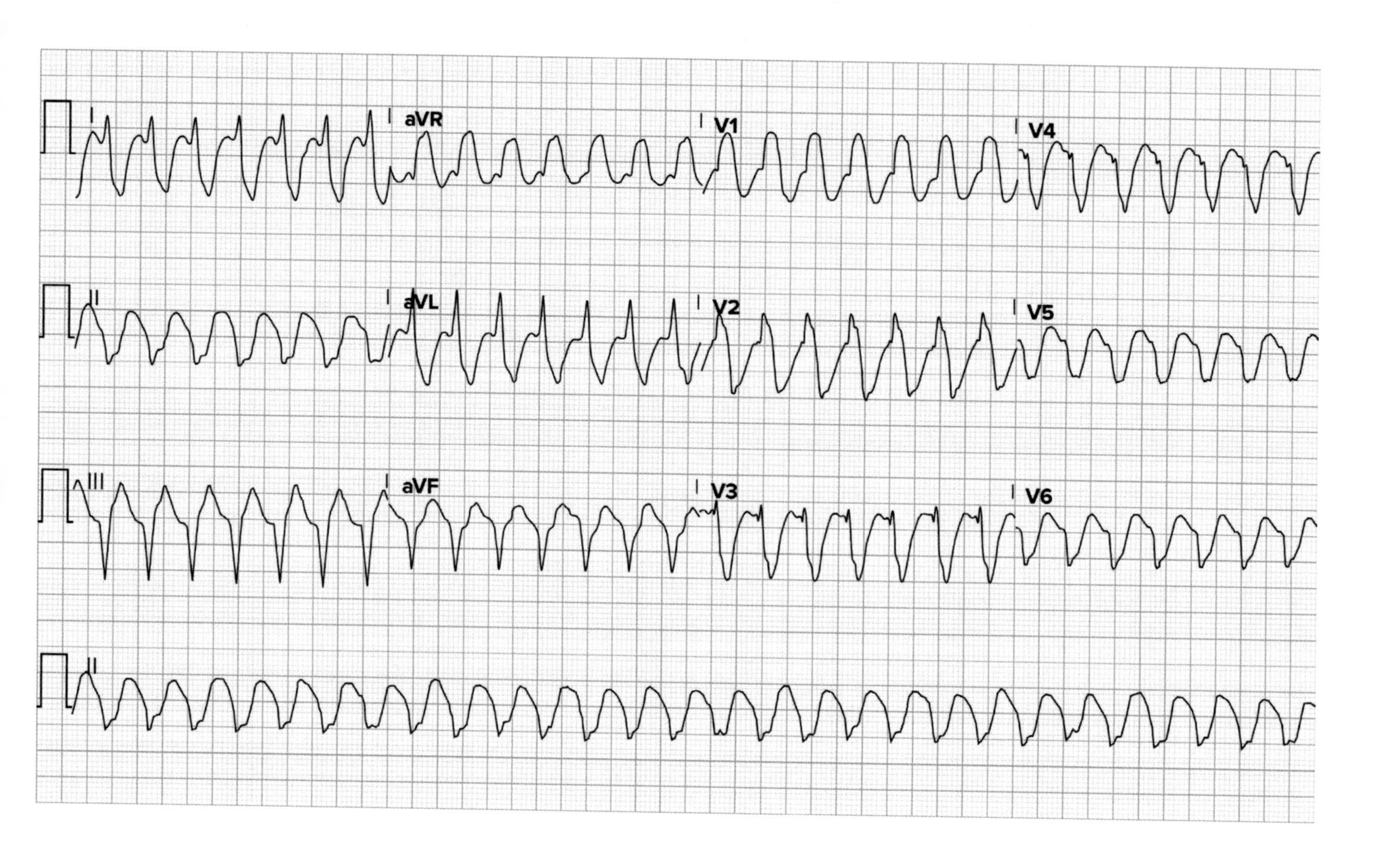

Case 86: Answer

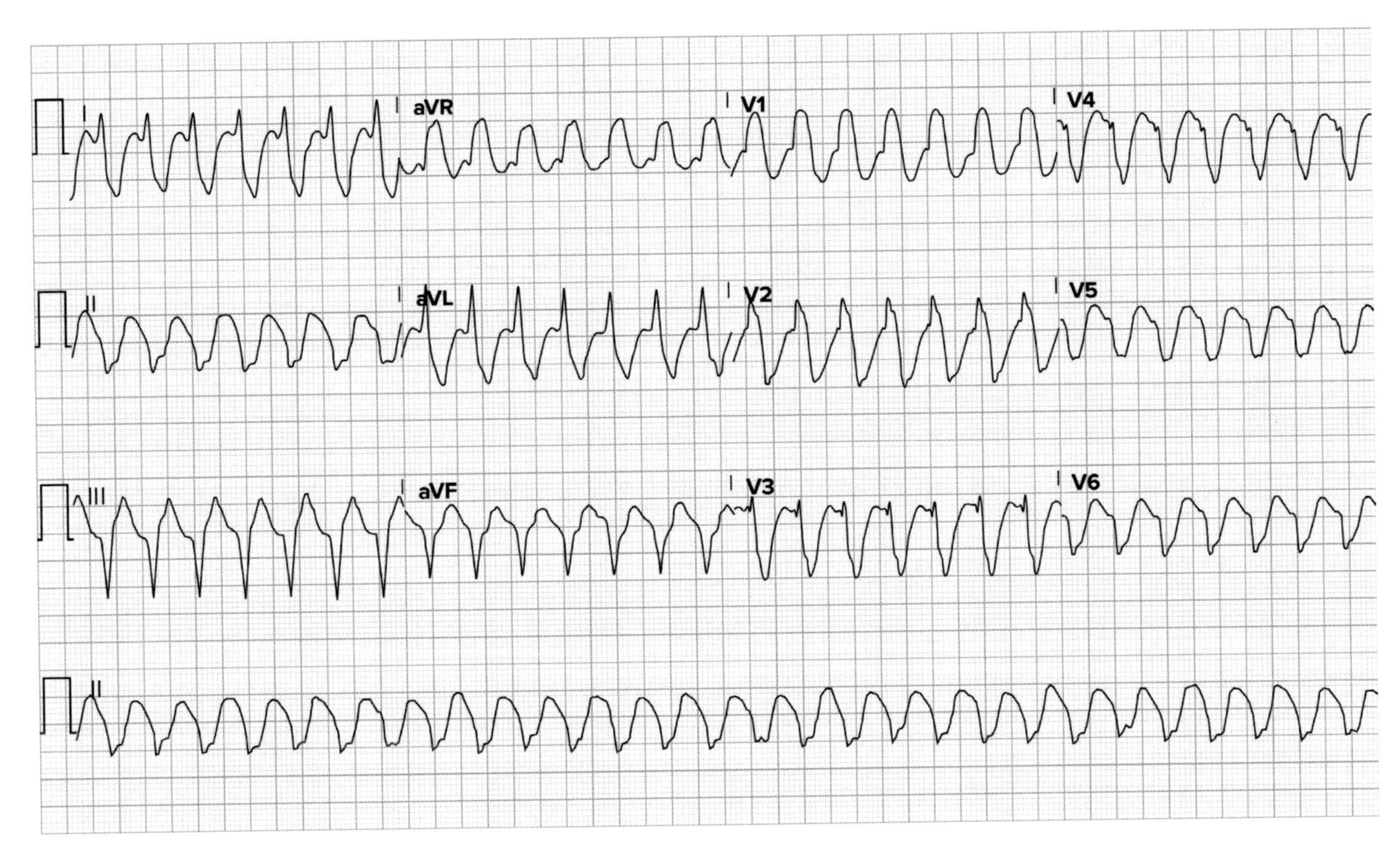

Figure 1.
The R-wave, S-wave, and T-wave are best identified in lead I. The QRS complex in lead II consists of a single large negative deflection which is called a QS complex.

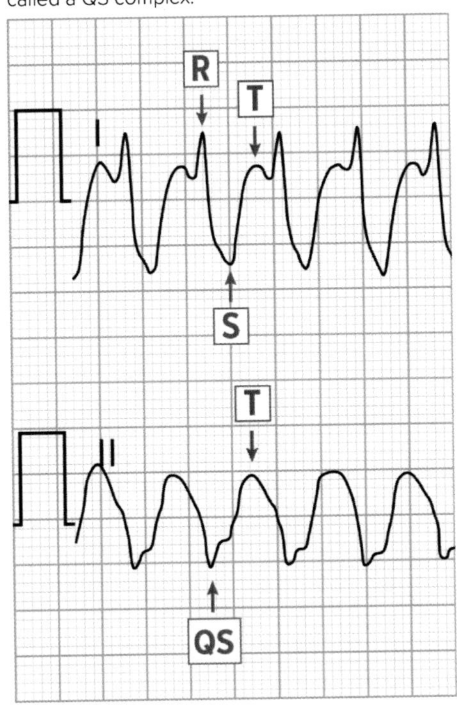

This ECG shows a regular wide complex tachycardia with a ventricular rate of 176 bpm, northwest/extreme axis deviation, and a prolonged QRS complex duration of 200 msec.

The differential diagnosis for a regular wide complex tachycardia includes:

- Monomorphic ventricular tachycardia
- Antidromic AVRT
- Any regular SVT (eg, sinus tach, AVNRT, atrial flutter, etc.) with aberrant conduction
    - Causes of aberrant conduction include fixed or rate-related BBB, metabolic abnormalities, sodium channel blocker toxicity, ventricular-paced rhythm, and ventricular pre-excitation (eg, WPW)

The very prolonged QRS complex duration can make it difficult to distinguish the QRS complex from the T-wave. Lead I has identifiable waves which can be traced down to lead II ***(see Figure 1)***. The lead II rhythm strip can then be used to help identify the waves in any of the other leads. The QRS complex in lead II consists of a single large negative deflection which is called a QS complex.

Based on this patient's history of cardiomyopathy requiring an AICD, this ECG should be assumed to be VT. There are multiple other findings on this ECG which suggest VT, including:

- Prolonged QRS duration > 200 msec (typically associated with VT or hyperkalemia)
- Northwest/extreme axis deviation
- Brugada's sign, best seen in lead V2 ***(see Figure 2)***
- Josephson's sign, best seen in lead V3 ***(see Figure 3)***

Figure 2

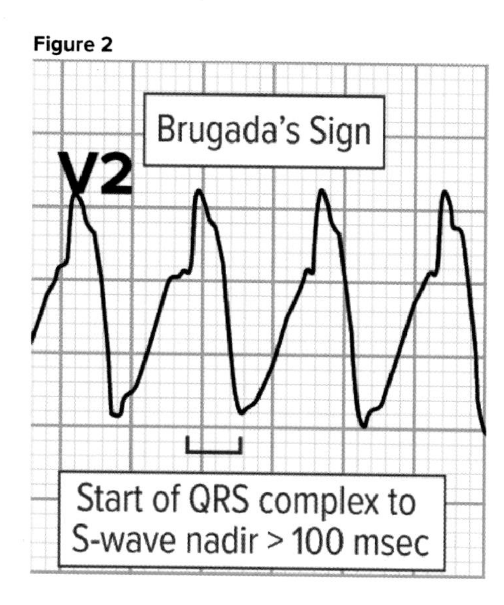

Figure 3

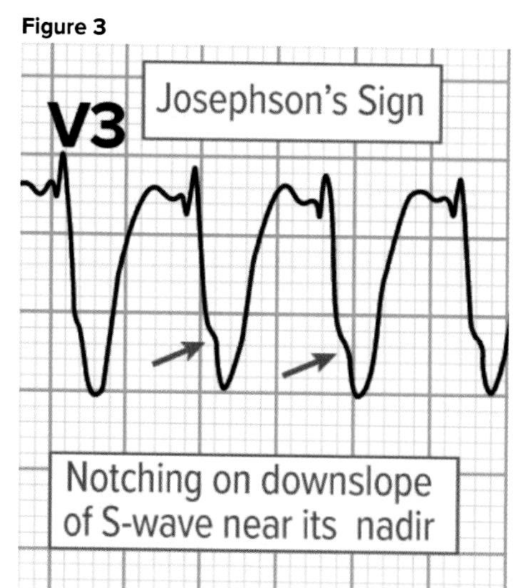

Treatment options for stable VT include synchronized electrical cardioversion and chemical cardioversion with either amiodarone or procainamide. Procainamide should be avoided in patients with long QTc interval or reduced EF. This patient was treated with IV amiodarone as he was already on oral amiodarone for maintenance therapy and has a history of CHF with a reduced EF.

The patient was admitted to the cardiology service and had his AICD interrogated. This patient's AICD could both defibrillate and perform anti-tachycardia pacing (ATP) which works by pacing the ventricle for ~5-15 beats at a slightly faster rate than the VT. This interrupts the circuit of abnormal ventricular conduction and terminates the VT. This patient's AICD was set to perform ATP at ventricular rates > 180 bpm and defibrillate at rates > 200 bpm (or if the ATP didn't work in the 180-200 bpm zone), so his rate of 176 bpm wasn't high enough to trigger the AICD. His AICD was reprogrammed to avoid this by lowering the threshold for ATP to 170 bpm.

Monomorphic VT Learning Points

- ≥ 3 consecutive, regular, wide complex beats with rate > 120-130 bpm
  - Non-sustained: < 30 sec duration with no hemodynamic instability
  - Sustained: ≥ 30 sec duration OR causes hemodynamic instability
- Rates < 120-130 bpm can be seen in patients on chronic antidysrhythmic medications (eg, amiodarone, flecainide, sotalol) or with severe cardiomyopathies
- If rate < 120 bpm, consider mimics:
  - Hyperkalemia
  - Sodium channel blocker toxicity
  - Accelerated idioventricular rhythm (AIVR)
- ECG features that increase the likelihood of VT in a regular WCT:
  - QRS complex duration > 200 msec is almost always VT, hyperkalemia, or sodium channel blocker toxicity
  - AV dissociation (ventricular rate > atrial rate)
  - Positive or negative QRS complex concordance in leads V1-V6 (entirely or predominantly positive or negative QRS complexes from leads V1 to V6)
  - Extreme axis deviation ("northwest axis")
  - The absence of typical RBBB or LBBB pattern suggests VT (ie, normal RBBB or LBBB pattern makes SVT with aberrant conduction more likely)
  - Fusion beats: hybrid QRS complex formed by both supraventricular and ventricular focus
  - Capture beats: sinus QRS formed by transient normal conduction amid AV dissociation
  - Brugada's sign: time from the onset of the QRS complex to the nadir of the S-wave is > 100 msec ***(see Figure 2)***
  - Josephson's sign: notching on the downslope of the S-wave near its nadir ***(see Figure 3)***

NOTES:

Case 87: Presentation

A 67-year-old male with past medical history of CAD presents due chest pain and diaphoresis. He received aspirin and sublingual nitroglycerin by EMS after which his symptoms resolved and this ECG was obtained. What is your interpretation of his ECG?

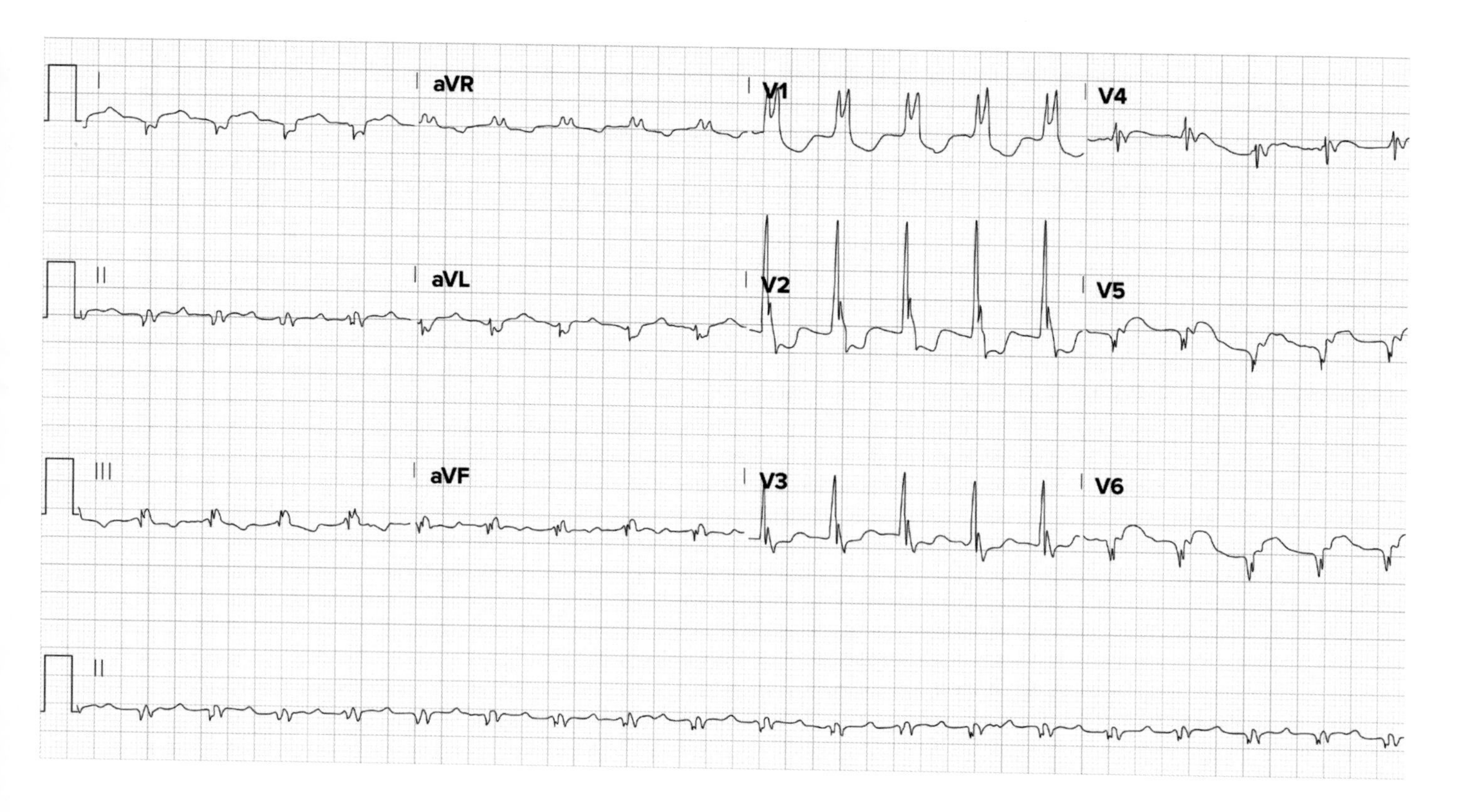

Case 87: Answer

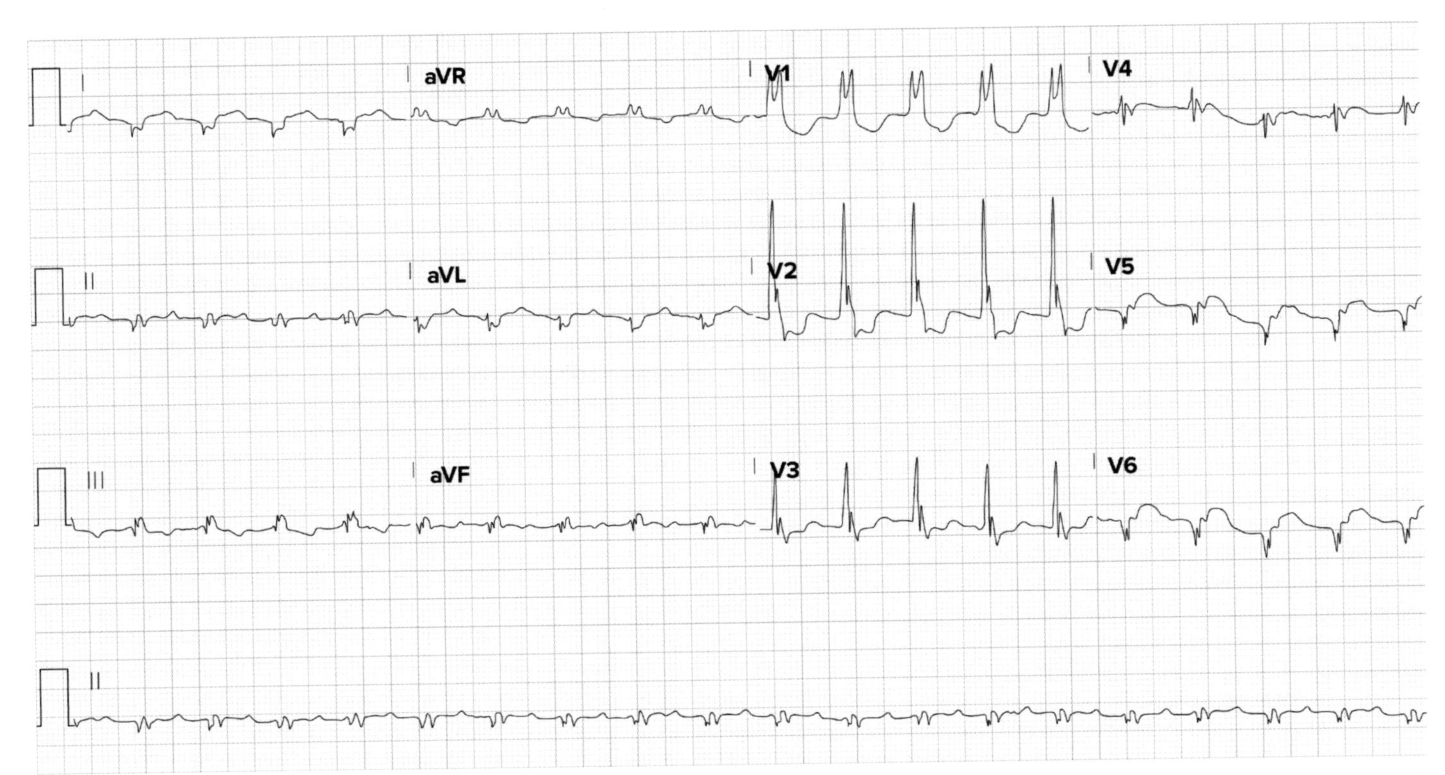

This ECG shows a regular wide complex tachycardia with a ventricular rate of 115 bpm, no P-waves, right axis deviation, and a prolonged QRS complex duration with a RBBB-like morphology. There are ST-segment depressions in leads V1-V3 which can be see with a RBBB.

This ECG could easily be mistaken for "slow" ventricular tachycardia, but the patient's history of recent chest pain that resolved suggests the rhythm is accelerated idioventricular rhythm (AIVR). The classic teaching is that VT has rates > 130-140 bpm and AIVR has rates between 40 and 110 bpm, but these numbers are not strict limits. VT can occasionally be seen with rates as slow as 120 bpm with the exception of patients on chronic oral antidysrhythmic medications (eg, amiodarone, flecainide, sotalol, etc.) or those with severe cardiomyopathies in which slower rates can be seen. Similarly, AIVR can be seen with rates as high as 130 bpm, so it important not to anchor on the ventricular rate as the sole factor to differentiate AIVR from VT. Other considerations for a wide complex tachycardia with ventricular rates < 120 bpm include hyperkalemia and sodium channel blocker toxicity, though there is nothing in this patient's history to suggest either of these causes.

AIVR is a relatively benign dysrhythmia commonly seen after successful reperfusion, partial or complete, of an occluded coronary vessel. The reperfusion can be spontaneous or due to an intervention such as PCI or fibrinolysis. AIVR is typically transient, often lasting only minutes, and unlikely to cause hemodynamic instability. There is no treatment required except for observation.

The danger of mistaking AIVR for VT lies in the treatment. The antidysrhythmic medications used to treat VT (eg, amiodarone, lidocaine, procainamide) can precipitate asystole if given to a patient who actually has AIVR. Conversely, a patient who is in a slow VT is unlikely to be hemodynamically unstable, so mistaking a slow VT for AIVR and observing the patient is unlikely to cause harm.

This patient was seen by Cardiology in the ED. Given the patient's history concerning for ACS and ECG suggestive of spontaneous reperfusion, the patient was taken to the cardiac catheterization lab where a 90% LAD occlusion was successfully treated with a stent.

Accelerated Idioventricular Rhythm Learning Points

- Ectopic focus from Purkinje network or ventricular myocardium
  - Also called ventricular escape rhythm
- ECG shows ≥ 3 consecutive, regular, wide complex beats with no P-waves or AV dissociation if P-waves are present
  - Rates between 40-110 bpm but can sometimes be as high as 120-130 bpm
  - Mimics include hyperkalemia, sodium channel blocker toxicity, and VT in patients on antidysrhythmic medications (eg, amiodarone, flecainide, sotalol) or with severe cardiomyopathies
- Suggests partial or complete reperfusion of an occluded coronary vessel
  - Classically seen in the reperfusion phase of an AMI following fibrinolysis or PCI or peri-arrest (ie, immediately after ROSC)
  - Also seen with digoxin toxicity, cardiac ischemia, electrolyte abnormalities, or can be spontaneous
- Usually well-tolerated, benign, and self-limiting
  - Treating as VT with antidysrhythmic medications can precipitate asystole

NOTES:

Case 88: Presentation

This is the pre-op ECG of a 77-year-old female being admitted for a hip fracture. What is your interpretation of her ECG?

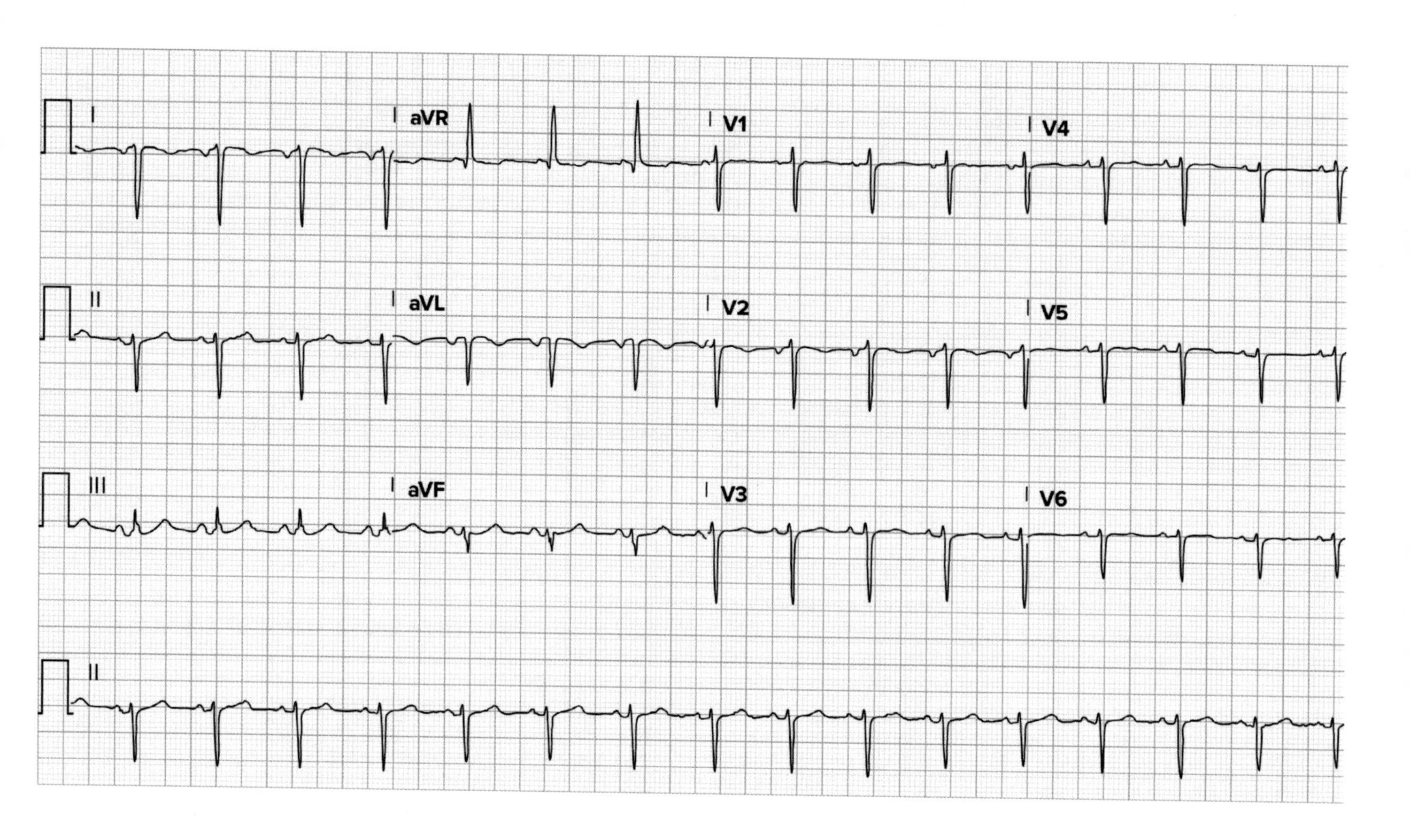

Case 88: Answer

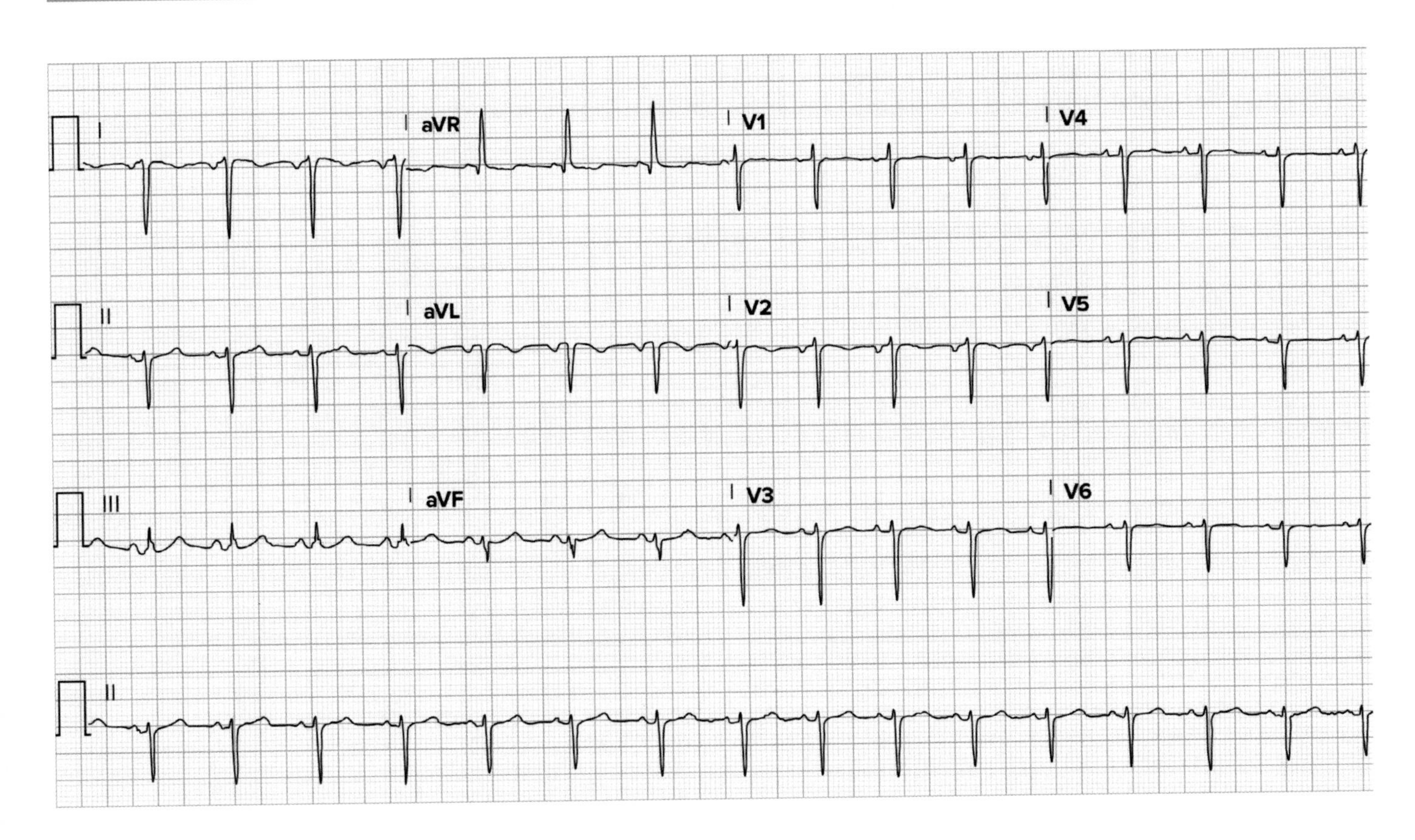

This ECG shows dextrocardia which can be confused for left arm-right arm (LA-RA) lead reversal. The key to interpreting this ECG correctly is found in leads I and V6 which both demonstrate negatively oriented QRS complexes. Both LA-RA lead reversal and dextrocardia will show a negatively oriented QRS complex in lead I and a positive orientation in lead aVR, but LA-RA lead reversal will show normal precordial leads in terms of QRS complex polarities (ie, positively or negatively oriented).

In this ECG, lead V6 has a negatively oriented QRS complex that is consistent with lead I (recall that leads I and V6 image the heart from similar perspectives so should appear similar on the ECG) and there are dominant S-waves with no R-wave progression in the precordial leads. These findings are consistent with dextrocardia which was confirmed on a chest X-ray. ***Figure 1*** is an example of LA-RA lead reversal for comparison purposes.

Figure 1.
An ECG showing LA-RA lead reversal (note the normal R-wave progression)

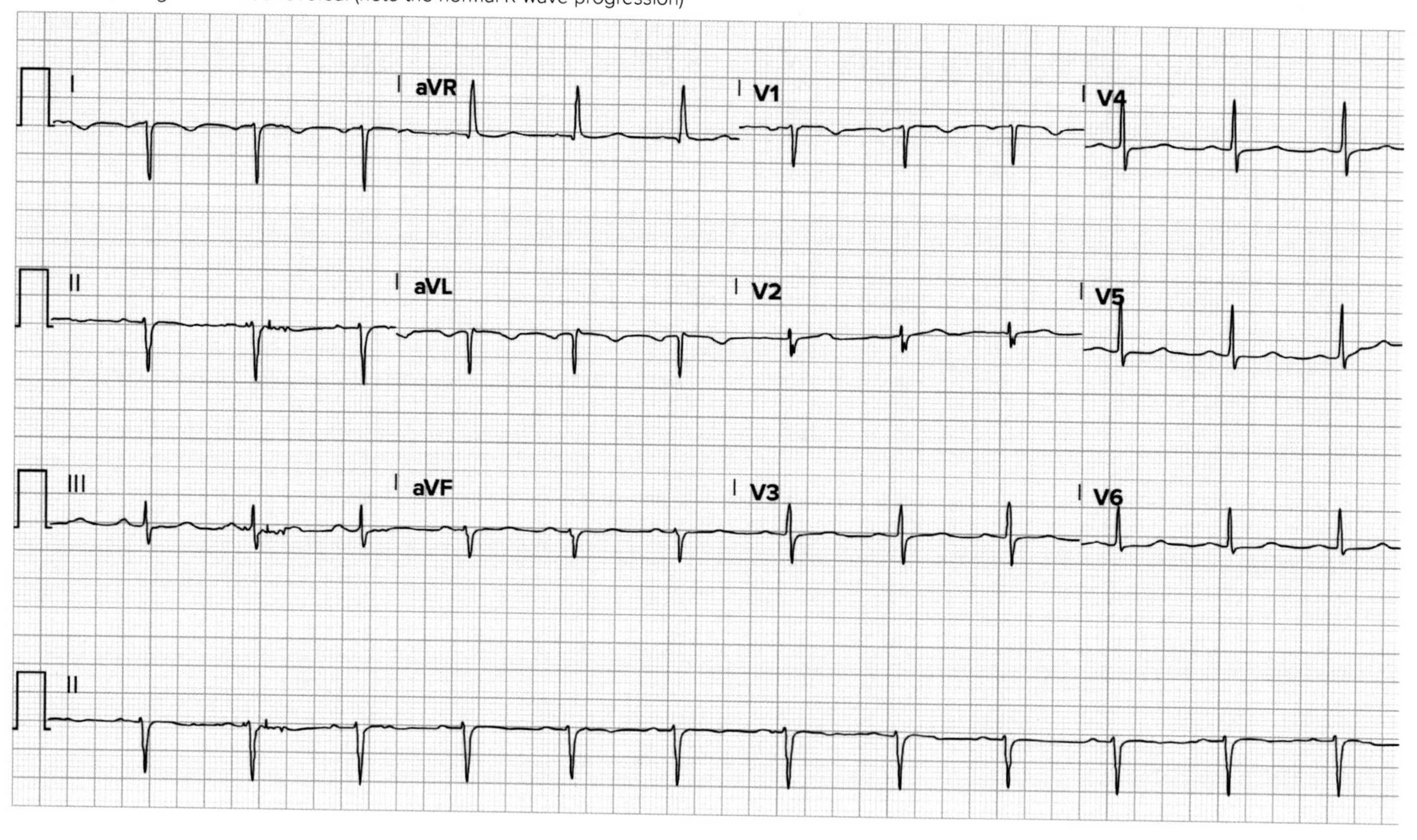

Figure 2.
This patient's ECG showing dextrocardia (note the abnormal R-wave progression)

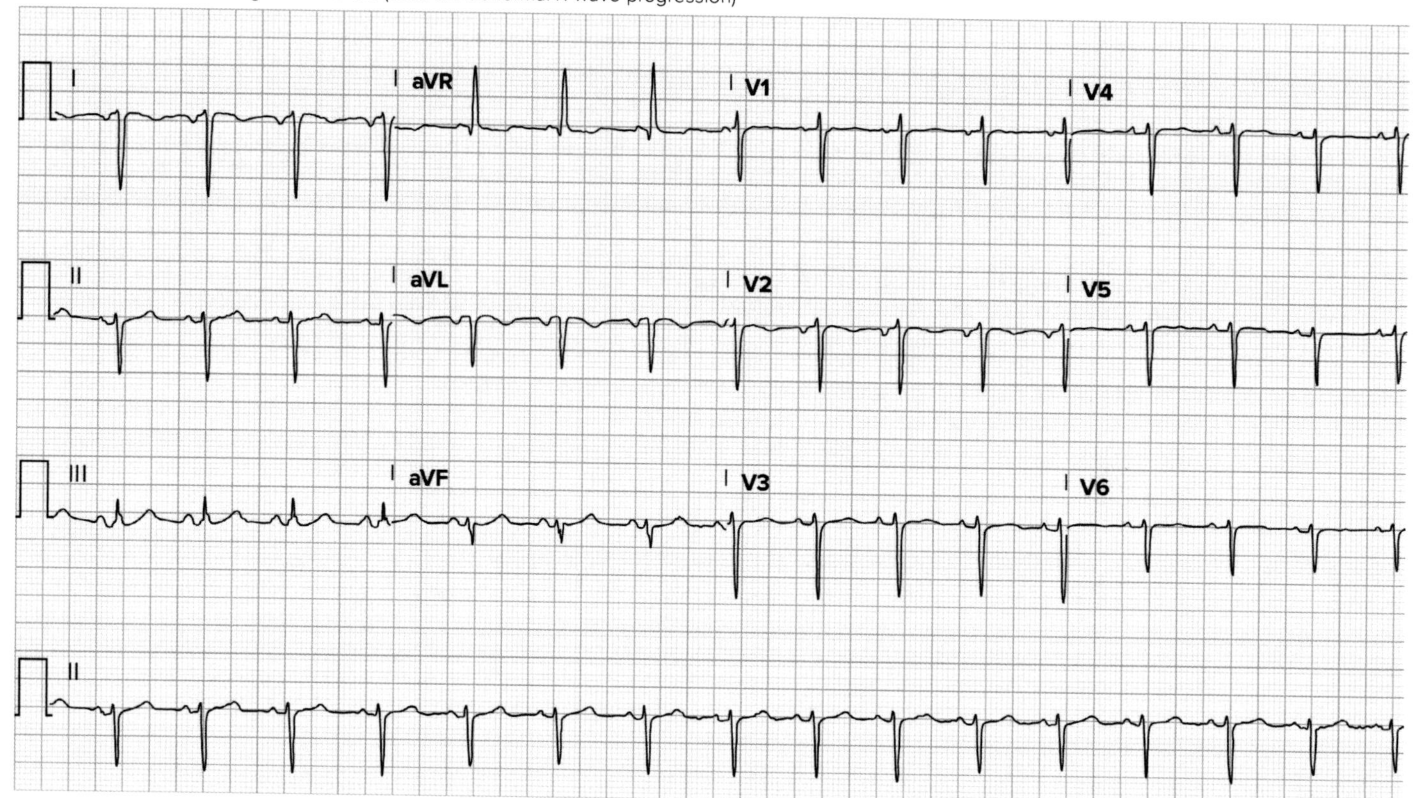

Lead Reversal Learning Points

Lead Reversal Summary							
	I	II	III	aVR	aVL	aVF	V1-V6
LA-RA	Inverted	Switches with III	Switches with II	Switches with aVL	Switches with aVR	No change	No change
LA-LL	Switches with II	Switches with I	Inverted	No change	Switches with aVF	Switches with aVL	No change
LA-RL	Looks like II	Unchanged	Flatline	Looks like inverted II	Looks identical to aVF	Looks identical to aVL	No change
RA-LL	Switches with inverted III	Inverted	Switches with inverted I	Switches with aVF	No change	Switches with aVR	No change
RA-RL	Looks like inverted III	Flatline	Unchanged	Looks identical to aVF	Looks like inverted III	Looks identical to aVR	No change
LA-LL + RA-RL	Flatline	Looks like inverted III	Inverted	Looks identical to aVL	Looks identical to aVR	Looks like inverted III	No change
Dextrocardia	Inverted	Switches with III	Switches with II	Switches with aVL	Switches with aVR	No change	Dominant S-wave and poor R-wave progression

NOTE: *RL is a ground lead, so RL-LL reversal does not result in any significant changes*

Case 89: Presentation

A 57-year-old female presents with exertional chest pain that is now constant and occurring at rest. What is your interpretation of her ECG?

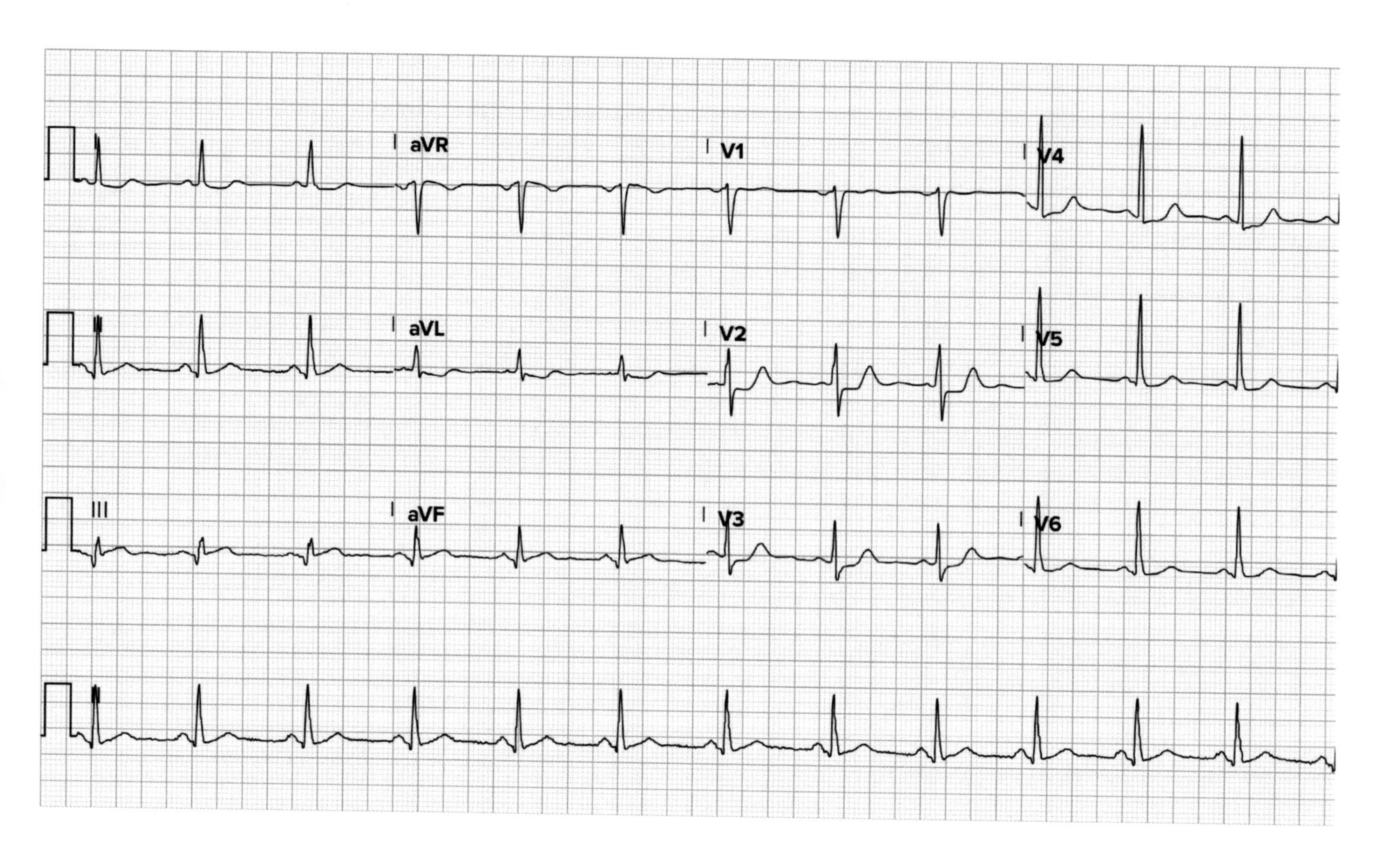

Case 89: Answer

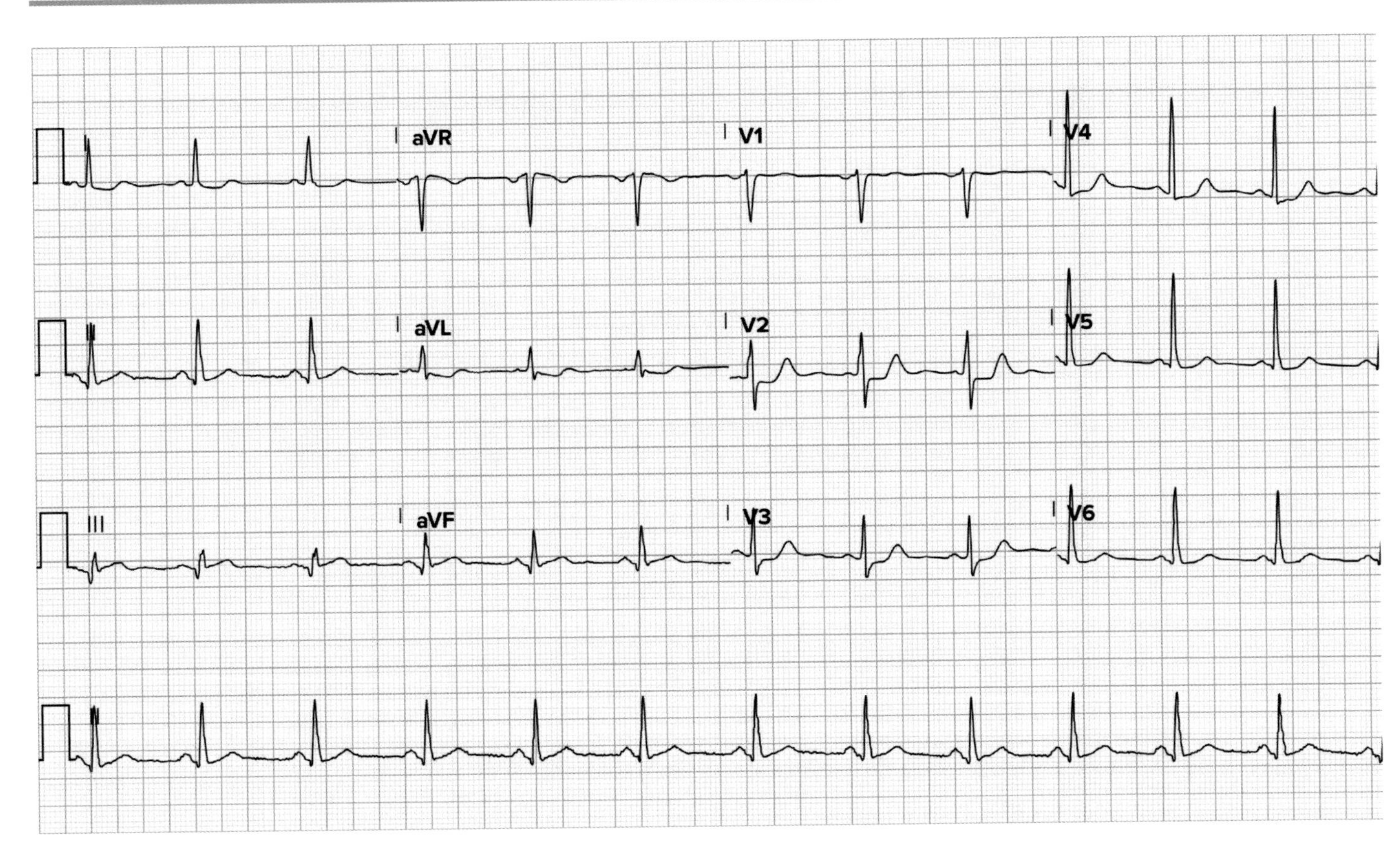

This ECG shows normal sinus rhythm at 73 bpm, normal axis, normal intervals, and STD in leads I, aVL, V2-V6. Lead III has slight STE when measured from the PR segment but not the TP segment. The obliquely straight form of ST-segment elevation in leads III and aVF ***(see Figures 1 and 2)*** is called the checkmark sign[1] or R-T sign and is concerning for early STEMI. The STD in the anterior precordial leads is concerning for an acute posterior MI.

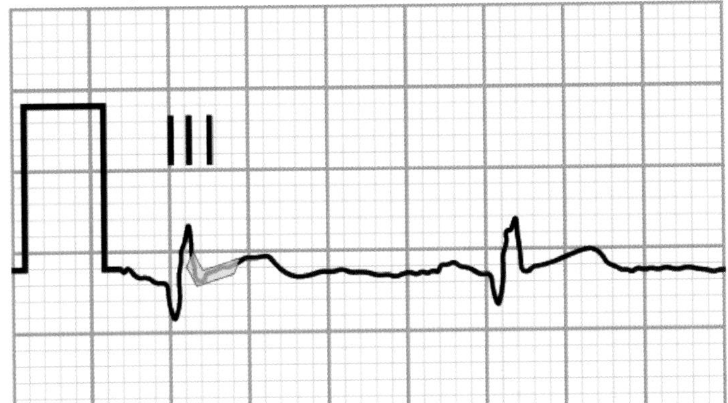

Figure 1.
Lead III shows an obliquely straight ST-segment, sometimes called the checkmark sign

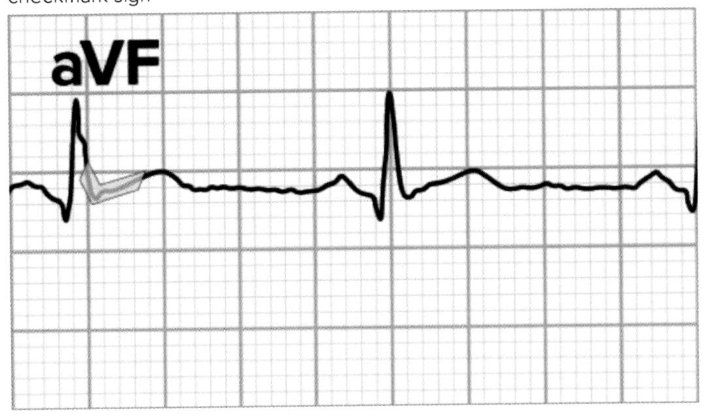

Figure 2.
Lead aVF shows an obliquely straight ST-segment, sometimes called the checkmark sign

The checkmark sign describes the morphology of the ST-segment and T-wave upstroke. In general, concave down STE is usually pathological, frequently related to AMI. Obliquely straight forms of ST segment elevation are analogous to concave down STE in that they suggest AMI if they are new from prior, seen in contiguous leads (especially if there are reciprocal STD), and the patient's presentation is concerning for ACS. It is important to note the absence of reciprocal STD does not rule out STEMI. As well, the presence of concave upward STE is non-diagnostic as it has both pathological and benign causes.

A repeat ECG was immediately obtained ***(see Figure 3)*** and showed STE in leads II, III, and aVF with reciprocal STD in leads I and aVL consistent with a STEMI. If the repeat ECG had been unchanged from the initial, the next step would have been obtaining a posterior ECG given the anterior precordial STD.

Figure 3.
A repeat ECG showing inferior STEMI

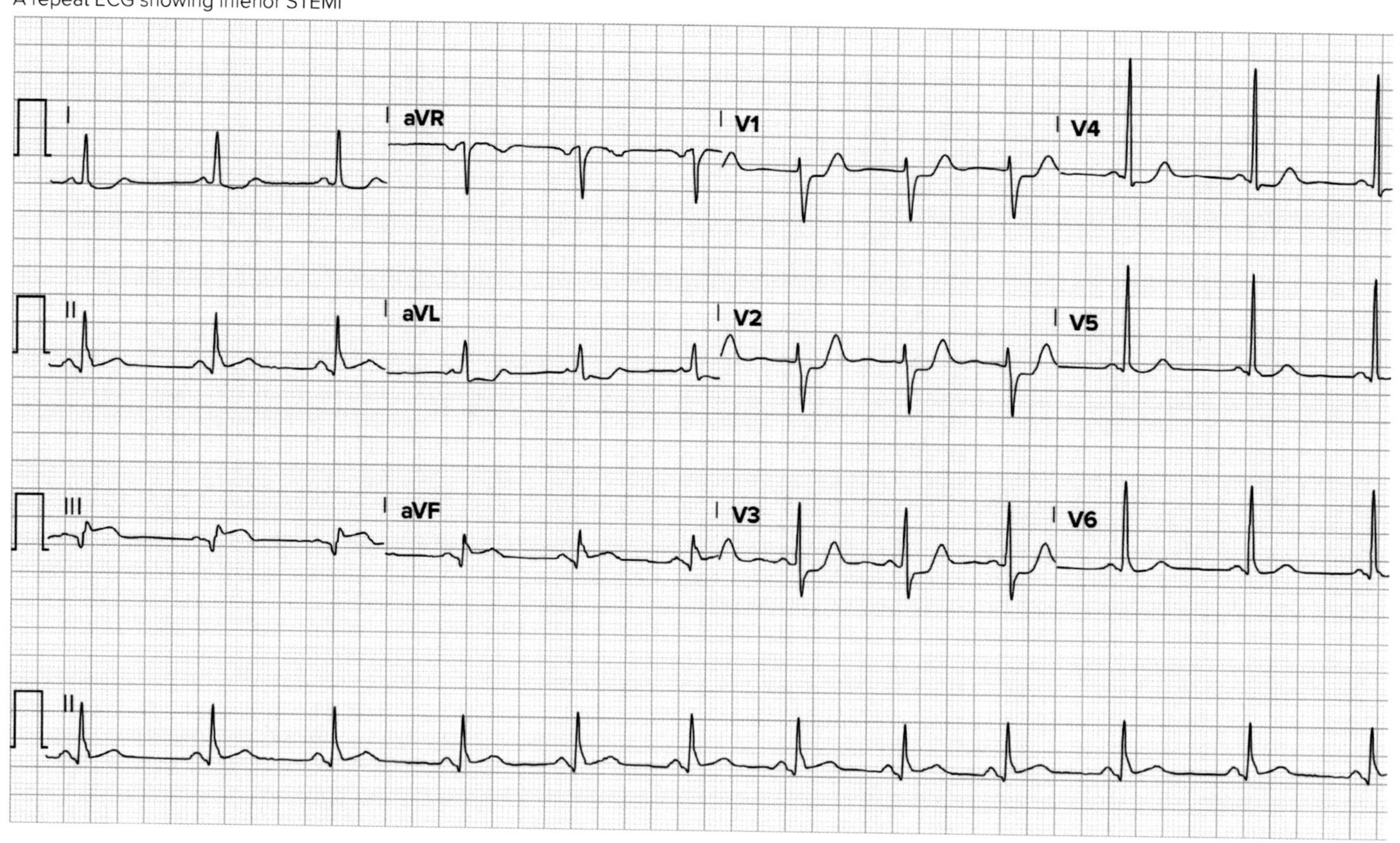

This patient was taken emergently to the cardiac catheterization laboratory where a 100% occlusion of the mid left circumflex artery was successfully treated with a stent.

STEMI Learning Points

- STEMI is defined by new, or presumed new, STE at the J point in ≥ 2 anatomically contiguous leads in the absence of LVH by voltage pattern, LBBB, or ventricular-paced rhythm
  - ≥ 2.5 mm in men < 40 years old and ≥ 2 mm in men ≥ 40 years old in leads V2-V3 (or an increase of ≥ 1 mm when compared to baseline ECG)
  - ≥ 1.5 mm in women in leads V2-V3 (or an increase of ≥ 1 mm when compared to baseline ECG)
  - ≥ 1 mm in all other leads
- ST-segment is measured from the isoelectric baseline, typically the TP segment (see below)
- Reciprocal STD are not required for the diagnosis of STEMI, but their presence does increase the likelihood of the diagnosis of STEMI
  - Reciprocal STD are only present in 70% of anterior MI[1]
- Posterior MI
  - Consider whenever there is STD in leads V1-V4
  - STE ≥ 0.5 mm in posterior leads V7, V8 or V9 is diagnostic- does not require 2 contiguous leads
- Right ventricular MI
  - Consider with any inferior MI (RV MI is seen in approximately 1/3 of inferior MI)
  - STE in right precordial leads V3R and V4R ≥ 0.5 mm (≥ 1 mm for men ≤ 30 years old)
  - STE in right precordial lead V4R > 1 mm is most predictive of RV MI
  - STE in right precordial lead V4R > STE in leads V1-V3 = highly specific for RV MI
- Significant STE that does not meet the traditional distribution (ie, ≥ 2 anatomically contiguous leads) in a presentation concerning for ACS may still represent coronary artery occlusion and warrant consideration for emergent coronary reperfusion

How to Measure STE per most recent 2018 AHA Guidelines[3]

- The J point is the junction between QRS termination and ST-segment onset and is used to determine the magnitude of the ST-segment shift
- **In patients with a stable baseline, the TP segment (isoelectric interval) is a more accurate method to assess the magnitude of ST-segment shift *(see Figure 4)***, and in distinguishing pericarditis from acute myocardial ischemia
- QRS onset should be used if TP segment does not have a stable baseline ***(see Figure 5)***
- Measurement should be made from the top of the ECG line tracing

Figure 4.
Measure STE from the TP segment if the TP segment is isoelectric (ie, horizontal)

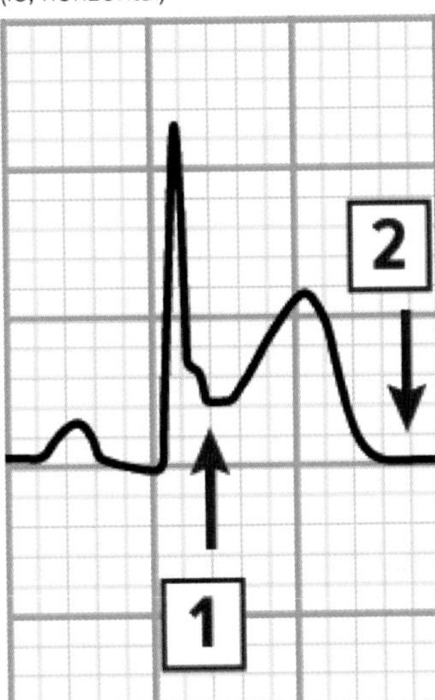

Arrow 1: onset of the ST-segment (ie, J point)
Arrow 2: TP segment

Figure 5.
Measure STE from onset of the QRS complex if the TP segment is not isoelectric (ie, not horizontal)

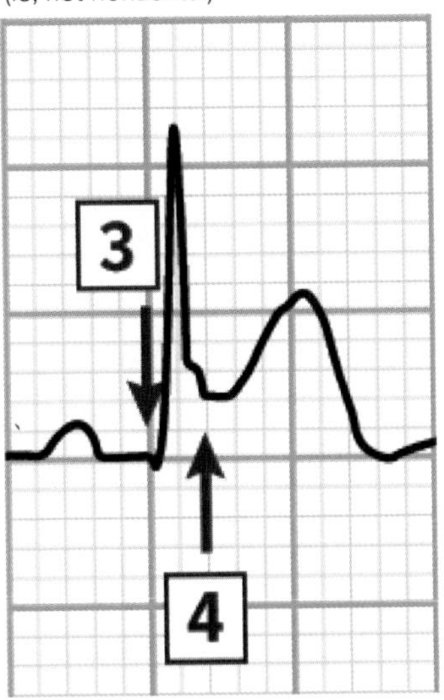

Arrow 3: initial onset of the Q-wave
Arrow 4: onset of the ST-segment (ie, J point)

References

1. Mattu A. ECG Weekly.
2. Knilans T, Surawicz B. Chou's Electrocardiography in Clinical Practice. Philadelphia, PA: Elsevier. 2020.
3. Thygesen K, Alpert JS, Jaffe AS, et al. 2018 ESC/ACC/AHA/WHF Expert Consensus Document: Fourth Universal Definition of Myocardial Infarction (2018). Circulation. 2018;138:e618-e651.

Case 90: Presentation

A 73-year-old female presents with exertional fatigue and near syncope.
What is your interpretation of her ECG?

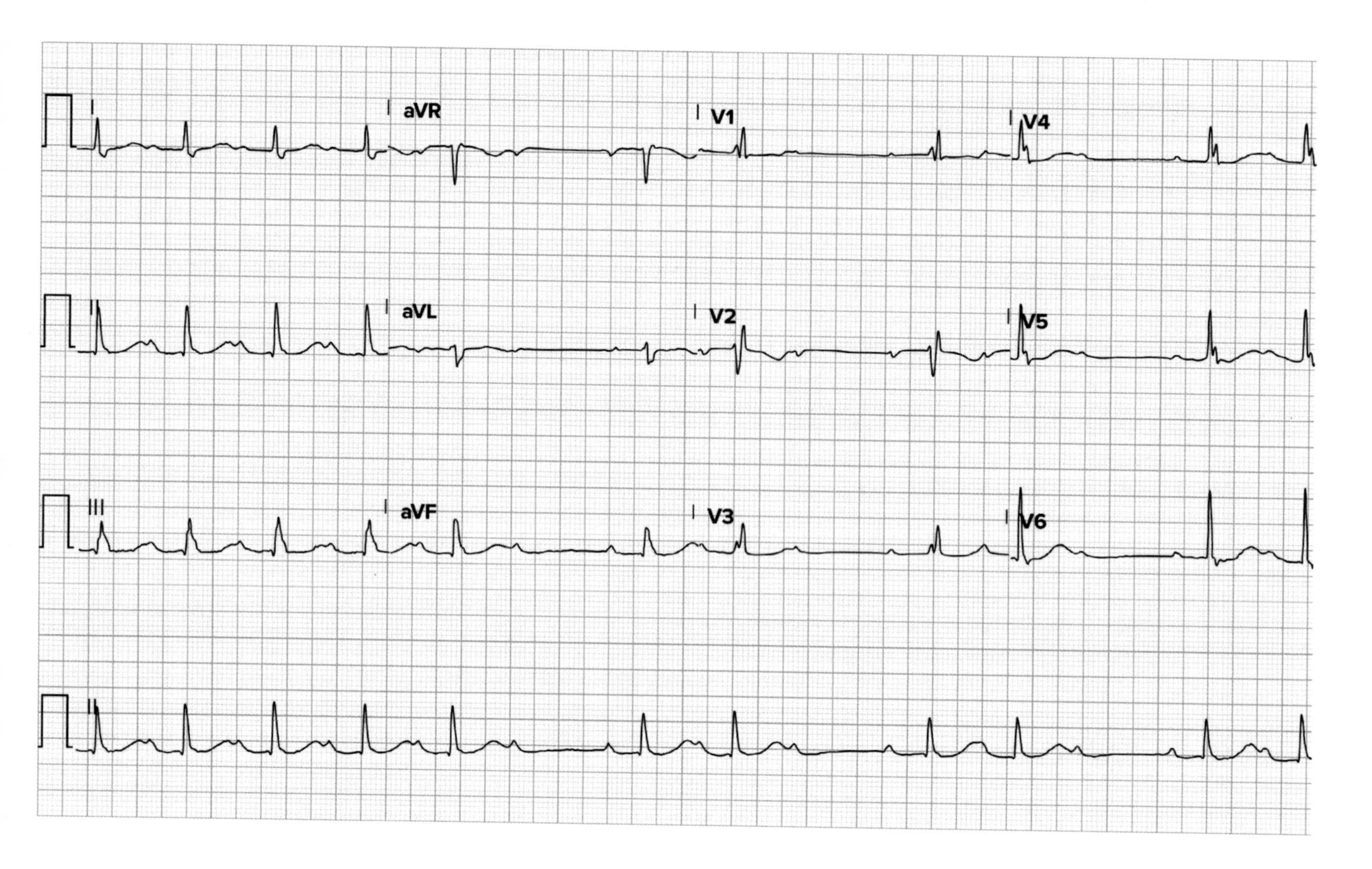

Case 90: Answer

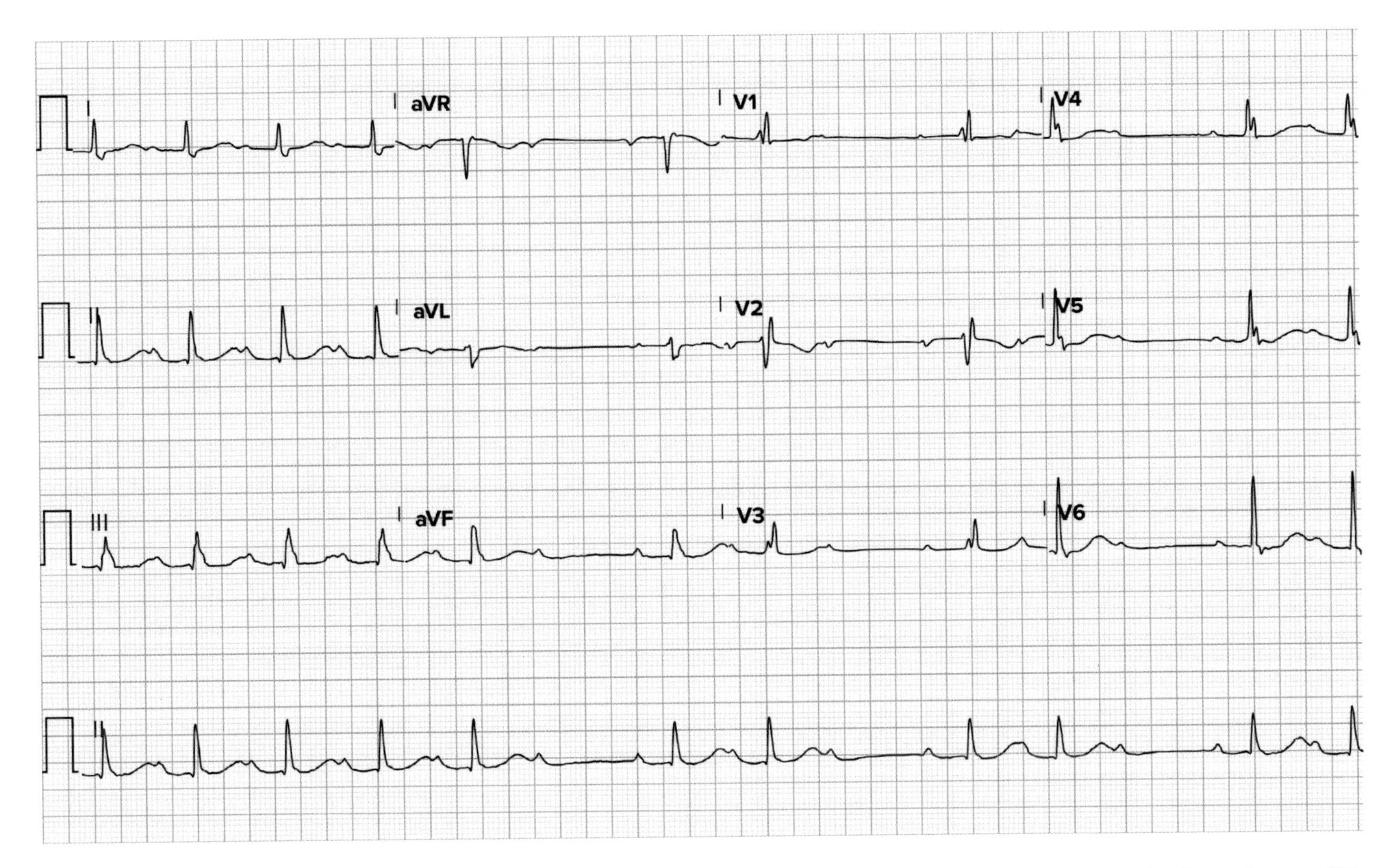

This ECG shows a Mobitz type II 2nd degree AV block with an average ventricular rate of 61 bpm, normal axis, prolonged PR interval, and prolonged QRS complex duration with a RBBB.

The differential diagnosis for an irregular wide complex rhythm with bradycardic ventricular rates includes:

- Atrial fibrillation (rate controlled) with aberrant conduction
- Atrial flutter with variable block (rate controlled) and aberrant conduction
- Atrial tachycardia with variable block (rate controlled) and aberrant conduction
- Wandering atrial pacemaker with aberrant conduction
- 2nd degree AV block Mobitz types I and II with aberrant conduction
- Variable high-grade AV block (eg, 3:1, 4:1, etc.) with aberrant conduction
- 2nd degree sinoatrial block with aberrant conduction
- Sinus arrhythmia with aberrant conduction
- Sinus bradycardia, junctional rhythm, or junctional bradycardia with aberrant conduction and irregular pattern of PAC, PJC, and/or PVC
- Sinus bradycardia, junctional rhythm, or junctional bradycardia with aberrant conduction and regular patterns of PAC, PJC, and/or PVC (bigeminy, trigeminy, etc.)
  - Causes of aberrant conduction include fixed or rate-related BBB, metabolic abnormalities, sodium channel blocker toxicity, ventricular-paced rhythm, and ventricular pre-excitation (eg, WPW)

Mobitz type II AV blocks are due to intermittent failure of infranodal conduction but can occur more proximally in the AV node. The distinguishing feature of a Mobitz type II AV block is a constant PR interval (which may or may not be prolonged) followed by a non-conducted P-wave (ie, P-wave without accompanying QRS complex) ***(see Figure 1).*** The PP and RR intervals will be constant and the P-waves will march out. Accurate measurement of the PR and PP intervals in this ECG is more challenging because some of the P-waves are partially hidden in T-waves. A Mobitz type II AV block is described as a ratio of P-waves to QRS complexes, which is 3:2 in ***Figure 1***. Without more information, it is not possible to determine the ratios for the initial and end portions of this ECG.

Figure 1.
The 6th and 7th P-QRS-T complexes show constant PR intervals followed by a non-conducted P-wave consistent with a Mobitz type II AV block

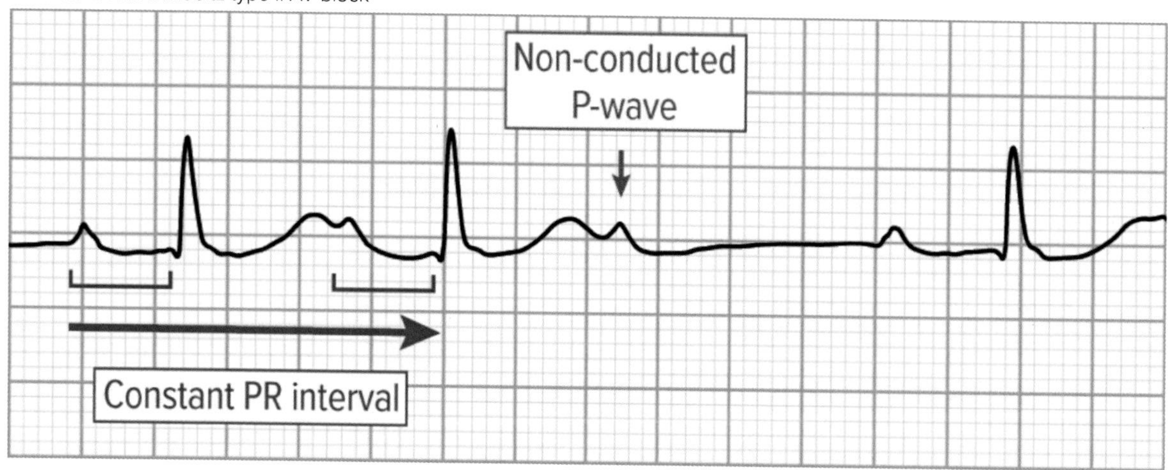

It is essential to differentiate Mobitz type I conduction from Mobitz type II conduction, as the former is typically transient with a more benign course while the latter has a high risk of progressing to a 3rd degree AV block, frequently produces hemodynamic compromise, and is associated with worse outcomes if not treated. The QRS complex duration is typically not useful in differentiating between a Mobitz type I AV block and a Mobitz type II AV block, as a Mobitz type I AV block can have a prolonged QRS complex duration if there is aberrant conduction (eg, an intrinsic bundle branch block) and a Mobitz type II AV block can have a narrow QRS complex (ie, duration < 110 msec) if the block is in the AV node. The key to distinguishing between the two is to compare the RR interval that includes the non-conducted P-wave to the PP interval.

In a Mobitz type I AV block, the RR interval that includes the non-conducted P-wave will be less than twice the PP interval. In the example below from a different ECG ***(see Figure 2)***, the RR interval that includes the non-conducted P-wave (1520 msec) is less than twice the PP interval (1680 msec).

Figure 2.
In a Mobitz type I AV block, the RR interval that includes the non-conducted P-wave is less than twice the PP interval (from a different ECG)

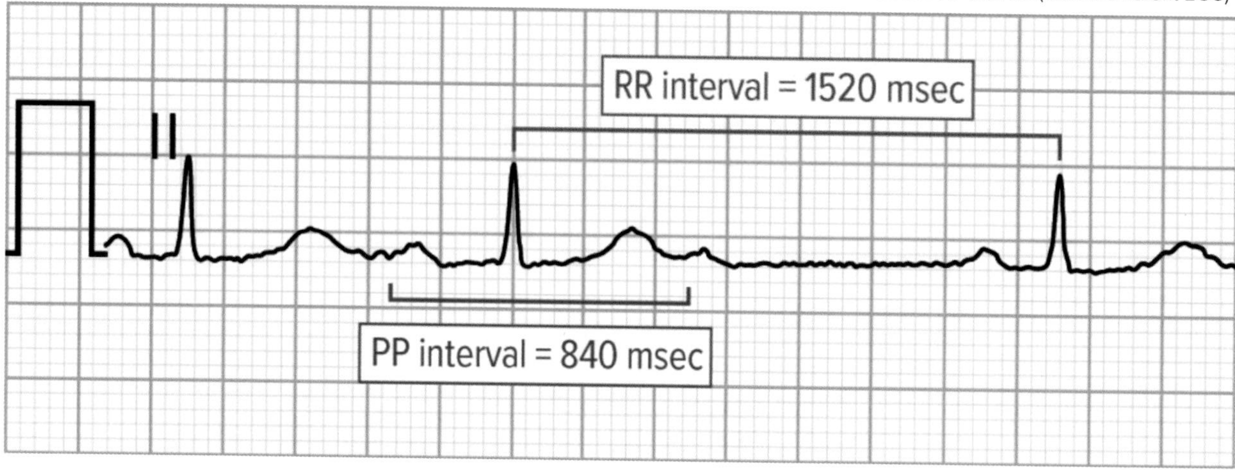

In a Mobitz type II AV block, the RR interval that includes the non-conducted P-wave will equal twice the PP interval. This is evident in the lead II rhythm strip from the case ECG ***(see Figure 3)*** where the RR interval that includes the non-conducted P-wave (1560 msec) is equal to exactly twice the PP interval (1560 msec).

Figure 3.
In a Mobitz type II AV block, the RR interval that includes the non-conducted P-wave is equal to exactly twice the PP interval (from case ECG)

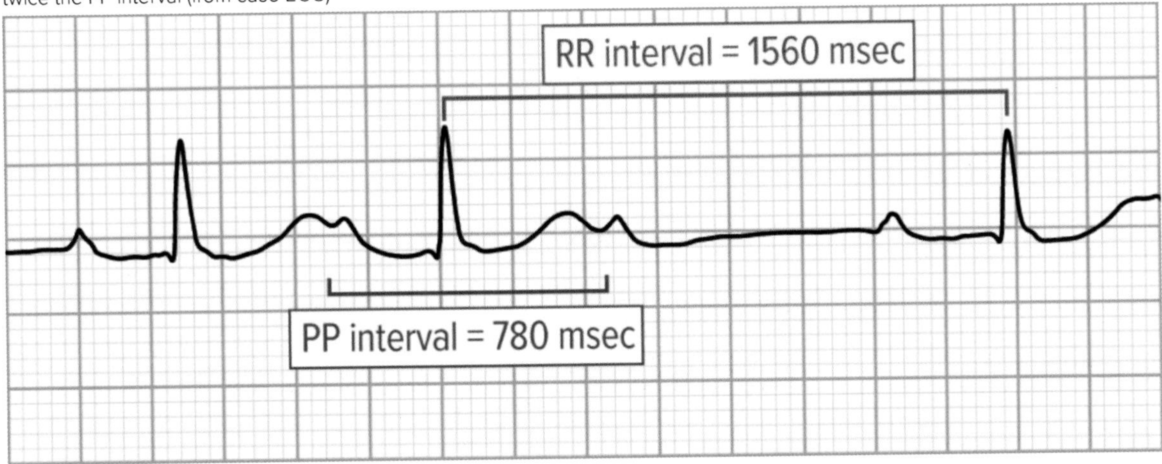

This ECG also shows a RBBB. A RBBB will typically have STD and TWI in lead V1, and if leads V2-V3 have an rsR' pattern present, they will also typically have STD and TWI. Consequently, upright T-waves or STE in those leads with an rsR' pattern is concerning for ischemia, and even isoelectric or minimally elevated ST-segments can be a subtle indicator of early AMI. Otherwise, the presence of a RBBB does not confound the ECG evaluation of ACS as does a LBBB.

The characteristic findings in a RBBB include:

- QRS complex duration ≥ 120 msec
- rsr', rsR', or rSR' pattern in lead V1 +/- V2 ***(see Figures 4 and 5)***
  - Variations in lead V1 include qR pattern or broad R-wave that is often notched
  - In lead V1, the initial upward deflection should always be smaller than the 2nd upward deflection ***(see Figure 4)***
- S-wave duration > R-wave or > 40 msec in leads I and V6 ***(see Figure 6)***
- Normal R-wave peak time in leads V5 and V6 but > 50 msec in lead V1 (only required if broad R-wave +/- notch is present in lead V1)
- Repolarization abnormalities include STD and TWI in lead V1 +/- lead(s) V2-V3 if they have an rsR' pattern, so STE and/or upright T-waves in those leads are concerning for ischemia

Figure 4.
rSR' pattern in lead V1, consistent with a RBBB

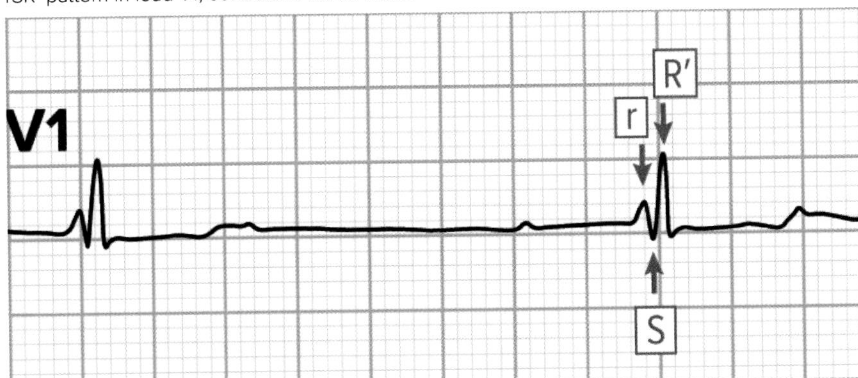

Figure 5.
rSR' pattern in lead V2, consistent with a RBBB

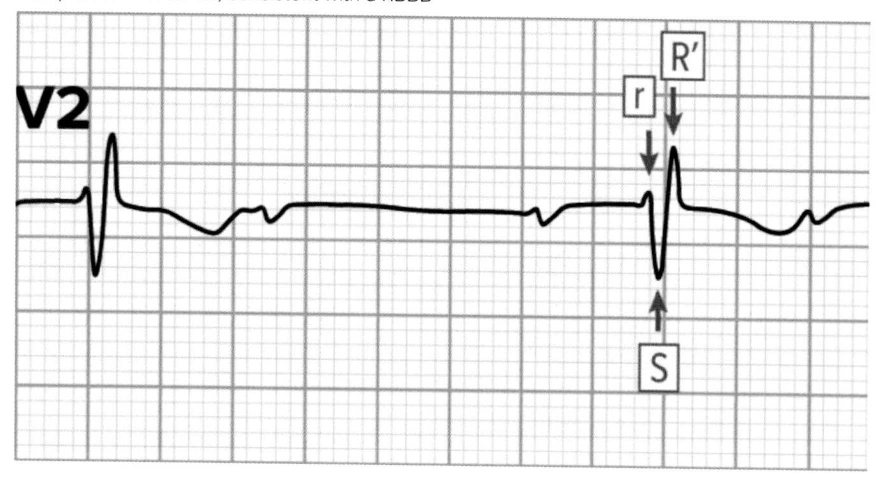

Figure 6.
S-wave duration > R-wave duration in lead I, consistent with a RBBB

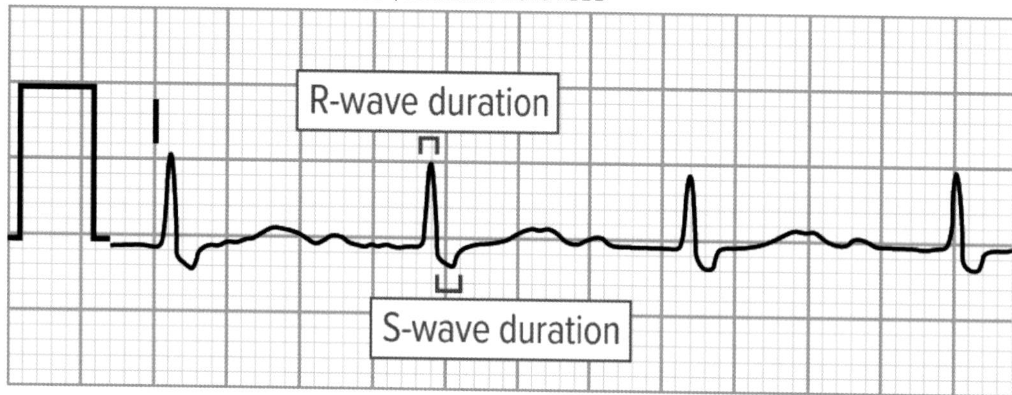

This patient had an unremarkable ED workup and was admitted to the cardiology service for evaluation for pacemaker placement.

Mobitz type I AV Block Learning Points

- Progressively increasing PR interval and decreasing RR interval until a non-conducted P-wave occurs (ie, P-wave without accompanying QRS complex)
  - PR interval immediately after non-conducted P-wave is shorter than PR interval preceding non-conducted P-wave
  - RR interval that includes non-conducted P-wave < twice the PP interval
- Can be normal variant and usually does not produce hemodynamic compromise
  - Typically associated with excess vagal tone and therefore usually responds to atropine when acute treatment is needed
  - Can lead to a more advanced AV block if associated with a pathologic etiology
  - Can be seen with inferior MI

Mobitz type II AV Block Learning Points

- Constant PR interval in conducted beats
  - Described as ratio of P-waves to QRS complexes
  - Typically an infranodal block resulting in a prolonged QRS complex duration
  - RR interval that includes non-conducted P-wave = twice the PP interval
- Never a normal variant and frequently produces hemodynamic compromise
  - High risk of progressing to a 3rd degree AV block
  - Atropine is unlikely to lead to clinical improvement and may lead to a high-grade AV block

High-grade (or advanced) AV Block Learning Points

- 2nd degree AV block with ≥ 2 sequential non-conducted P-waves
  - Most commonly a variant of a Mobitz type II but can be associated with a Mobitz type I
  - PP and RR intervals should have a whole number ratio
- Named as ratio of P-waves to QRS complexes
- Can be seen after anterior MI or with significant pathology of the conduction pathway
- High risk of progressing to a 3rd degree AV block

RBBB Learning Points

- Delayed conduction through right ventricle with normal left ventricular conduction
- In lead V1, the initial upward deflection should always be smaller than the 2nd upward deflection
- Repolarization abnormalities include STD and TWI in lead V1 +/- lead(s) V2-V3 if they have an rsR' pattern, so STE and/or upright T-waves in those leads are concerning for ischemia
  - Otherwise, the presence of a RBBB does not confound the ECG evaluation of ACS as does a LBBB
- RBBB with axis deviation should prompt evaluation for a concurrent LAFB or LPFB

Case 91: Presentation

A 79-year-old male presents with palpitations and chest pressure that resolves during the ECG recording. What is your interpretation of his ECG?

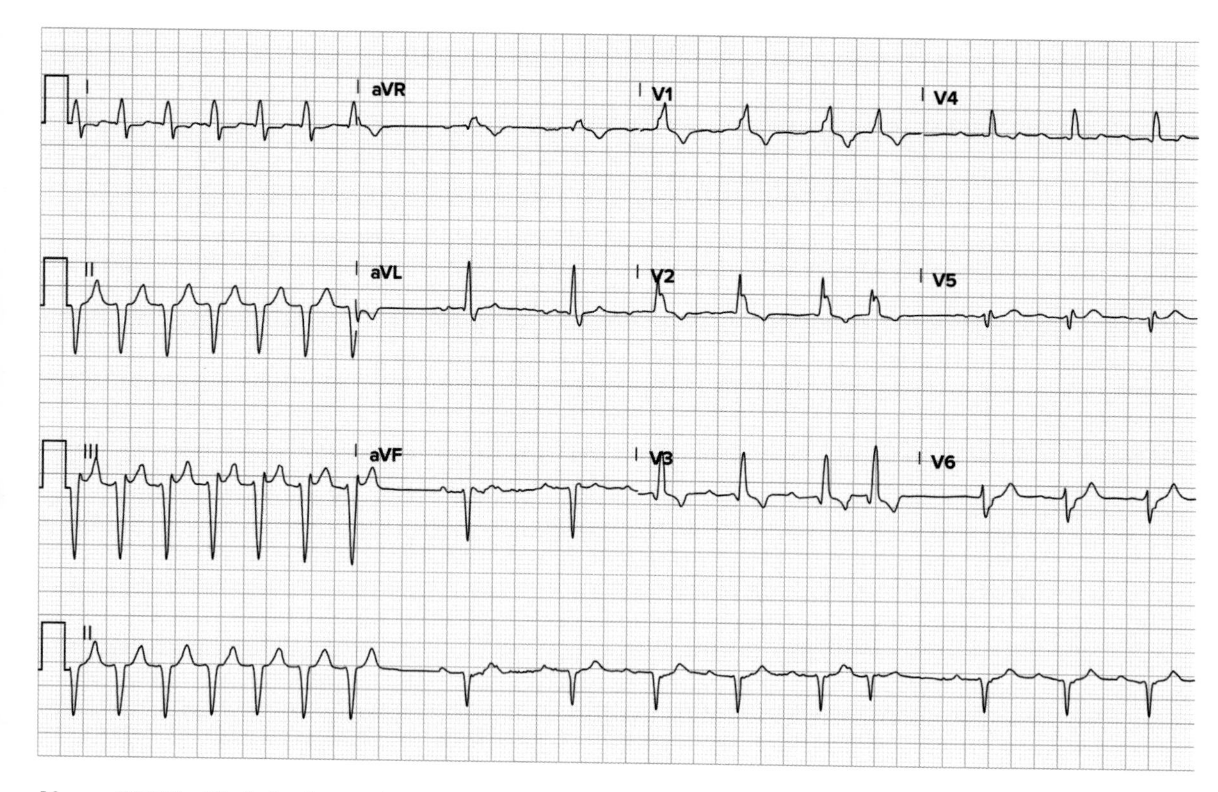

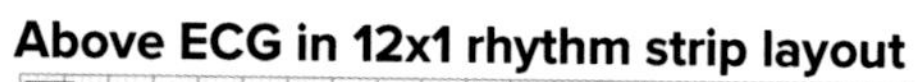
Above ECG in 12x1 rhythm strip layout

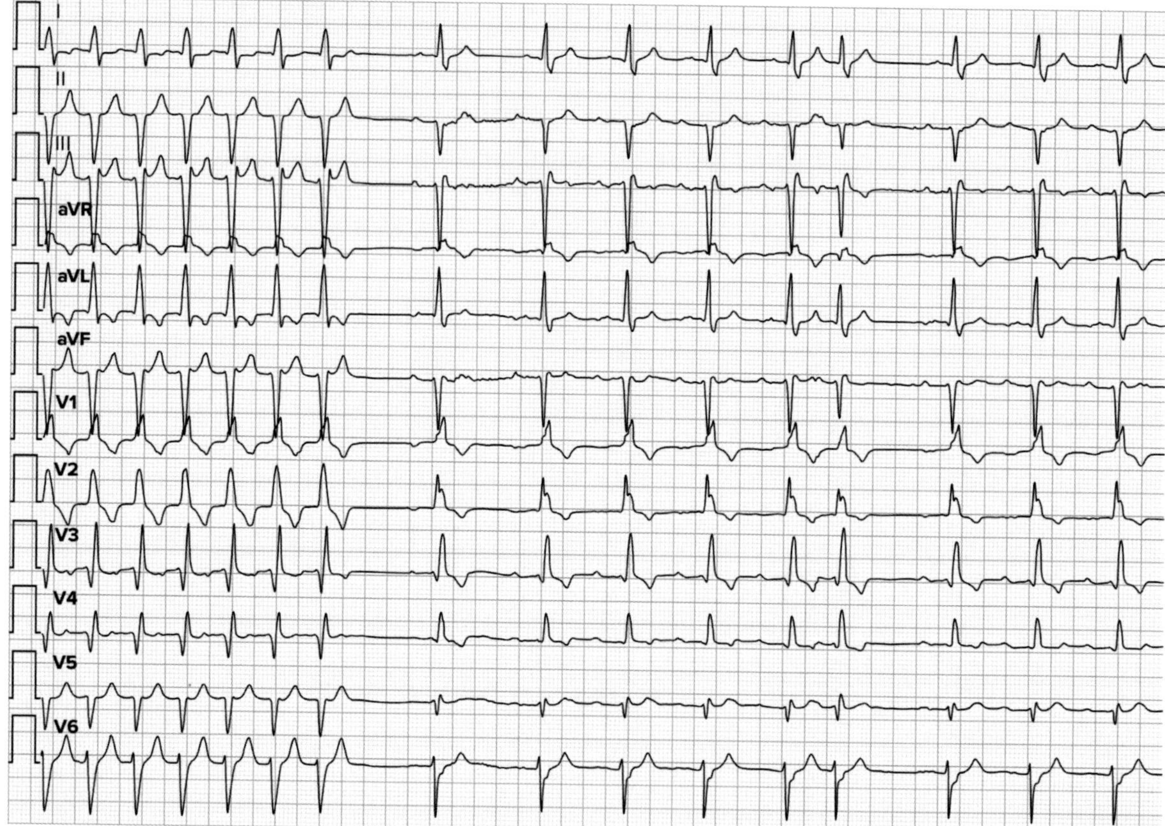

Case 91: Answer

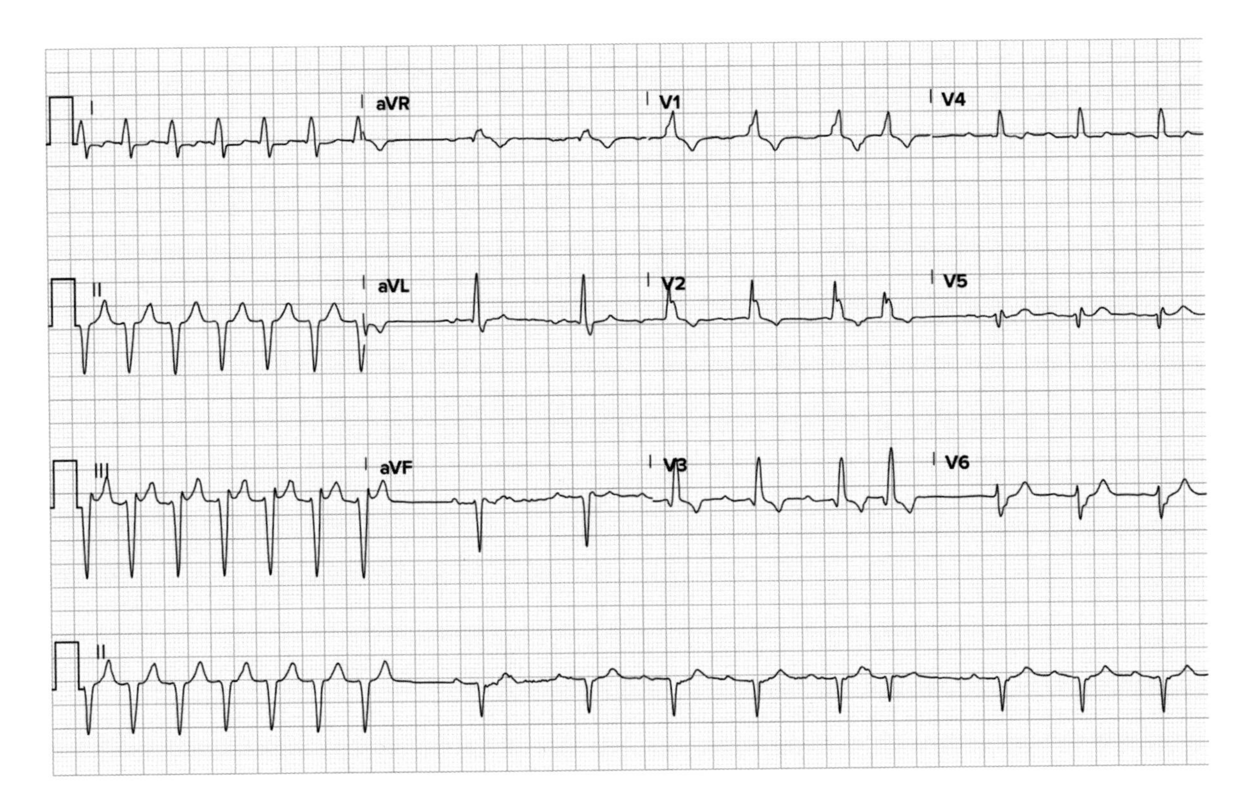

Above ECG in 12x1 rhythm strip layout

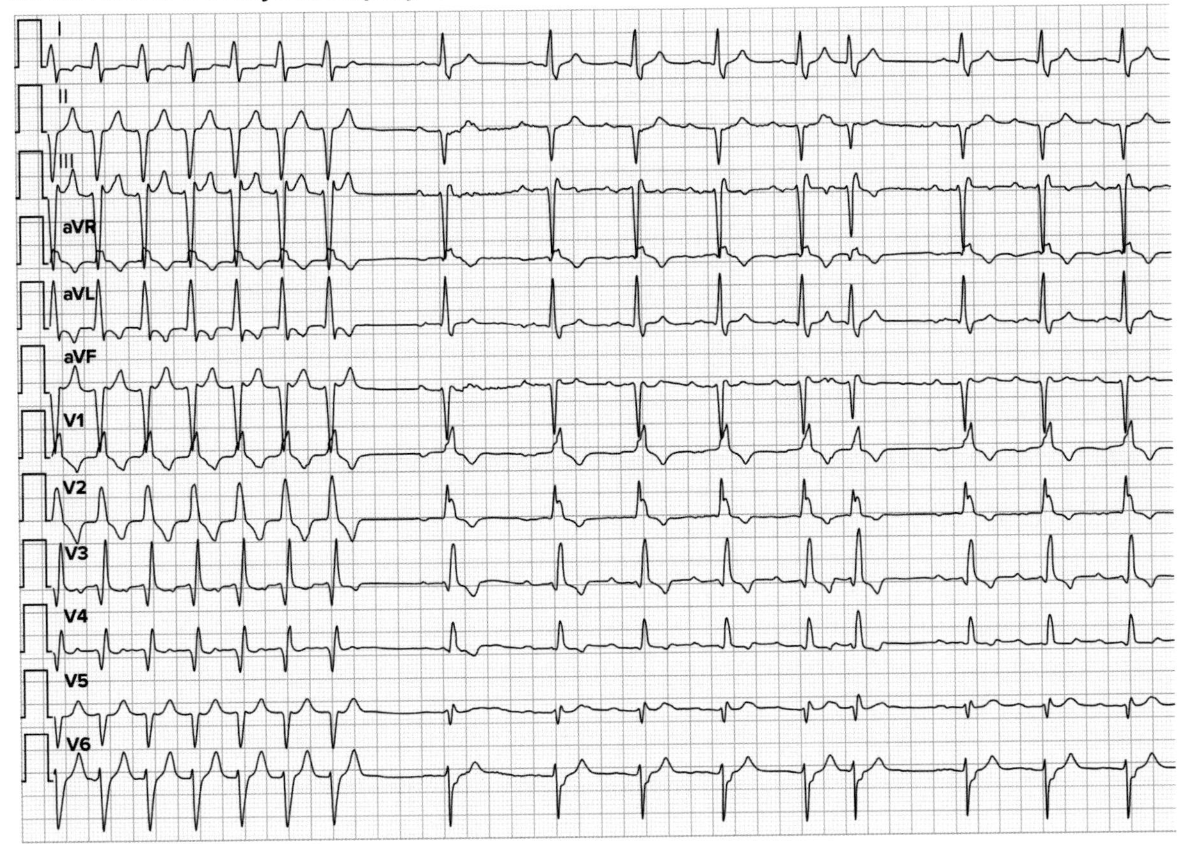

This ECG shows 2 rhythms: a regular wide-complex tachycardia that spontaneously resolves followed by normal sinus rhythm ***(see Figure 1).***

Figure 1.
The lead II rhythm strip shows a regular WCT followed by normal sinus rhythm

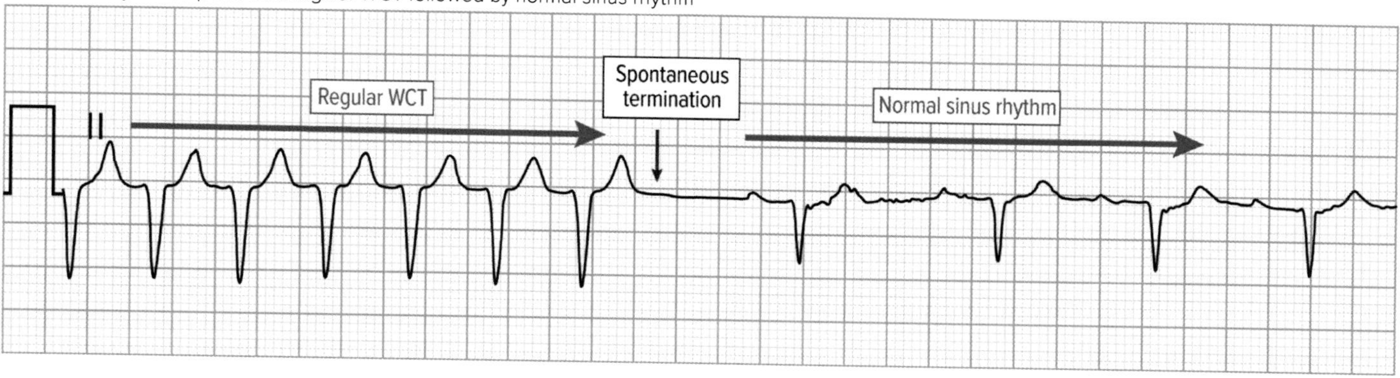

The initial portion of this ECG shows regular wide-complex tachycardia at 150 bpm, left axis deviation, and prolonged QRS complex duration of 130 msec. The QRS complexes have the appearance of a RBBB (ie, a RBBB-like morphology), but whether this represents a true RBBB depends on whether the origin of this rhythm is ventricular or supraventricular. If this rhythm is ventricular tachycardia, the QRS complex appearance cannot be due to a true RBBB as ventricular tachycardia does not utilize the His-Purkinje conduction system. A true RBBB requires a supraventricular or junctional origin that conducts via the normal cardiac conduction system. VT can have QRS complexes that mimic a RBBB with a tall upright R-wave in lead V1, but it's not a true RBBB since there isn't conduction via the His-Purkinje system.

The differential diagnosis for a regular wide complex tachycardia includes:

- Monomorphic ventricular tachycardia
- Antidromic AVRT
- Any regular SVT (eg, sinus tach, AVNRT, atrial flutter, etc.) with aberrant conduction
  - Causes of aberrant conduction include fixed or rate-related BBB, metabolic abnormalities, sodium channel blocker toxicity, ventricular-paced rhythm, and ventricular pre-excitation (eg, WPW)

There is a fixed RBBB (ie, present with all heart rates) seen during the second (sinus rhythm) portion of the ECG, so any of the above are possible. Note that the QRS complex duration is slightly more prolonged in the regular WCT which is probably due to rate-related aberrancy. The rate of 150 bpm is classically associated with 2:1 flutter and AVNRT, and the PAC after the 12th beat is a common trigger for AVNRT. But without more history, a regular WCT in a 79-year-old should be presumed VT until proven otherwise.

The second part of this ECG shows normal sinus rhythm at 83 bpm, left axis deviation, prolonged QRS at 120 msec with a RBBB, and a premature atrial contraction (PAC) followed by a complete compensatory pause.

A PAC is an ectopic atrial beat that captures pacing from the SA node. This frequently happens by the PAC conducting before the SA node is set to fire such that it occurs early in the cycle ***(see Figure 2).*** The PAC is described as interpolated if it occurs at the exact time a sinus beat would be expected (ie, it comes in the middle of the two sinus beats) which is not seen in this ECG.

Figure 2.
The 4th to last P-QRS-T complex in the lead II rhythm strip is a PAC followed by a compensatory pause

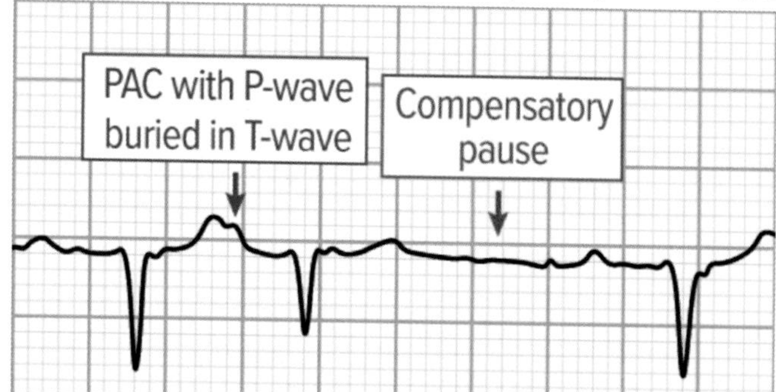

The compensatory pause that follows a PAC can be complete or incomplete. In a complete compensatory pause, the PP interval containing the PAC will be exactly twice the preceding PP interval ***(see Figure 3)***. Another way to look at it is that the P-wave after the PAC will happen right where you'd expect it if you marched them out ***(blue lines in Figure 3)***.

Figure 3.
The lead II rhythm strip shows the PP interval that includes the PAC (purple line) is exactly twice the preceding PP interval (blue line), consistent with a complete compensatory pause

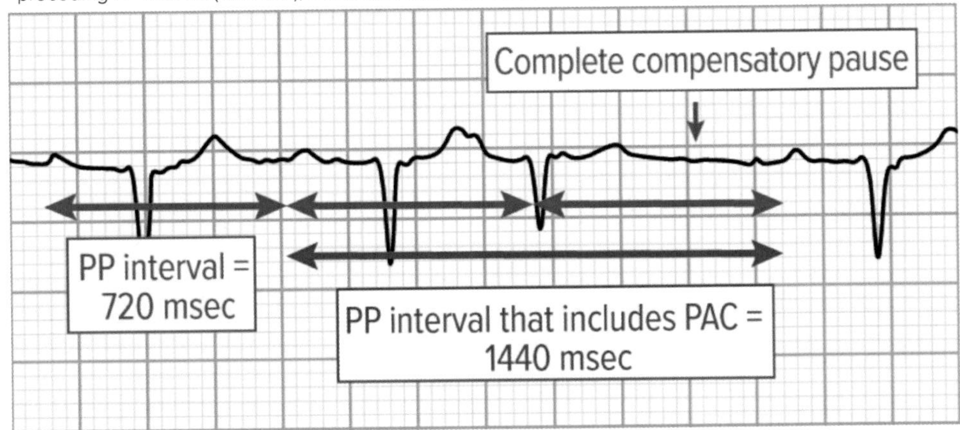

This ECG also shows a RBBB seen during the sinus rhythm portion of the ECG. The characteristic findings in a RBBB include:

- QRS complex duration ≥ 120 msec
- sr', rsR', or rSR' pattern in lead V1 +/- V2
  - Variations in lead V1 include qR pattern or broad R-wave that is often notched ***(see Figure 4)***
  - In lead V1, the initial upward deflection should always be smaller than the 2nd upward deflection
- S-wave duration > R-wave or > 40 msec in leads I and V6 ***(see Figure 5)***
- Normal R-wave peak time in leads V5 and V6 but > 50 msec in lead V1 (only required if broad R-wave +/- notch is present in lead V1) ***(see Figure 4)***
- Repolarization abnormalities include STD and TWI in lead V1 +/- lead(s) V2-V3 if they have an rsR' pattern, so STE and/or upright T-waves in those leads are concerning for ischemia

Figure 4.
Lead V1 shows a broad notched R-wave with an R-wave peak time > 50 msec, consistent with a RBBB

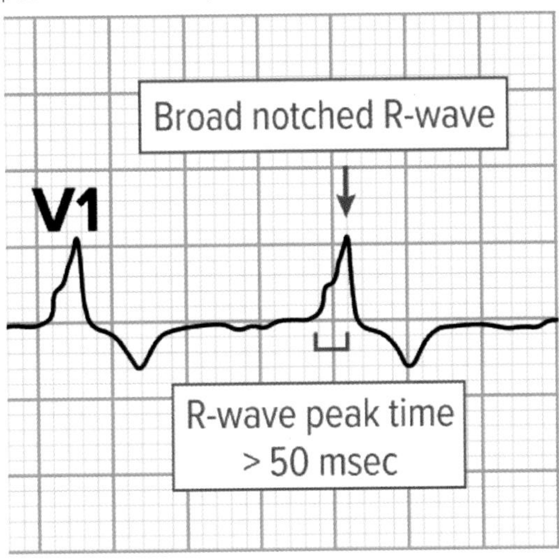

Figure 5.
S-wave duration > R-wave duration in lead V6, consistent with a RBBB

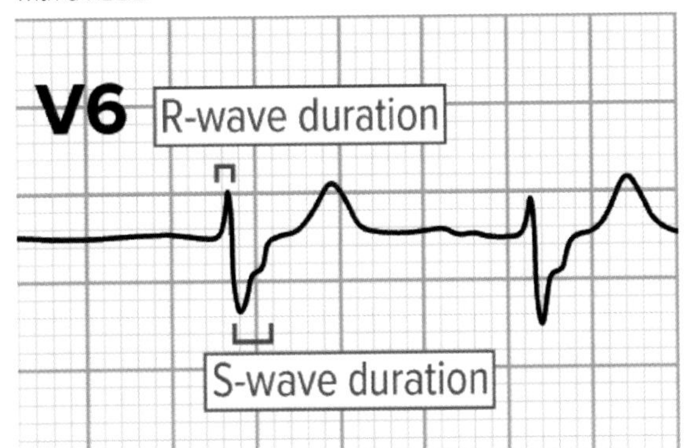

This patient had an unremarkable ED workup and was admitted to the cardiology service. During the course of his hospitalization, he had multiple episodes of regular WCT while on telemetry which was determined to be AVNRT with a RBBB.

Monomorphic VT Learning Points

- ≥ 3 consecutive, regular, wide complex beats with rate > 120-130 bpm
  - Non-sustained: < 30 sec duration with no hemodynamic instability
  - Sustained: ≥ 30 sec duration OR causes hemodynamic instability
- Rates < 120-130 bpm can be seen in patients on chronic antidysrhythmic medications (eg, amiodarone, flecainide, sotalol) or with severe cardiomyopathies
- If rate < 120 bpm, consider mimics:
  - Hyperkalemia
  - Sodium channel blocker toxicity
  - Accelerated idioventricular rhythm (AIVR)
- ECG features that increase the likelihood of VT in a regular WCT:
  - QRS complex duration > 200 msec is almost always VT, hyperkalemia, or sodium channel blocker toxicity
  - AV dissociation (ventricular rate > atrial rate)
  - Positive or negative QRS complex concordance in leads V1-V6 (entirely or predominantly positive or negative QRS complexes from leads V1 to V6)
  - Extreme axis deviation ("northwest axis")
  - The absence of typical RBBB or LBBB pattern suggests VT (ie, normal RBBB or LBBB pattern makes SVT with aberrant conduction more likely)
  - Fusion beats: hybrid QRS complex formed by both supraventricular and ventricular focus
  - Capture beats: sinus QRS formed by transient normal conduction amid AV dissociation
  - Brugada's sign: time from the onset of the QRS complex to the nadir of the S-wave is > 100 msec ***(see Figure 6)***
  - Josephson's sign: notching on the downslope of the S-wave near its nadir ***(see Figure 7)***

Figure 6

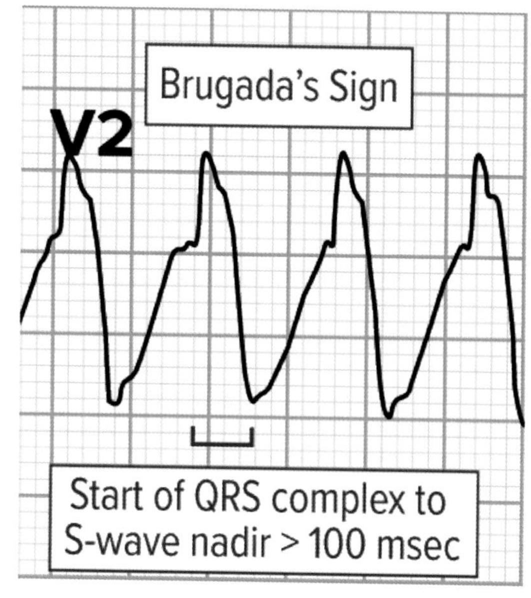

Figure 7

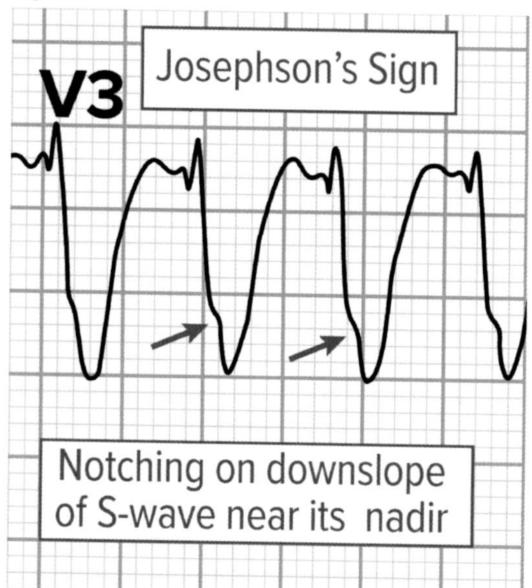

RBBB Learning Points

- Delayed conduction through right ventricle with normal left ventricular conduction
- In lead V1, the initial upward deflection should always be smaller than the 2nd upward deflection
- Repolarization abnormalities include STD and TWI in lead V1 +/- lead(s) V2-V3 if they have an rsR' pattern, so STE and/or upright T-waves in those leads are concerning for ischemia
  - Otherwise, the presence of a RBBB does not confound the ECG evaluation of ACS as does a LBBB
- RBBB with axis deviation should prompt evaluation for a concurrent LAFB or LPFB

NOTES:

Case 92: Presentation

A 57-year-old male with no known cardiac history presents with chest pain and palpitations. What is your interpretation of his ECG?

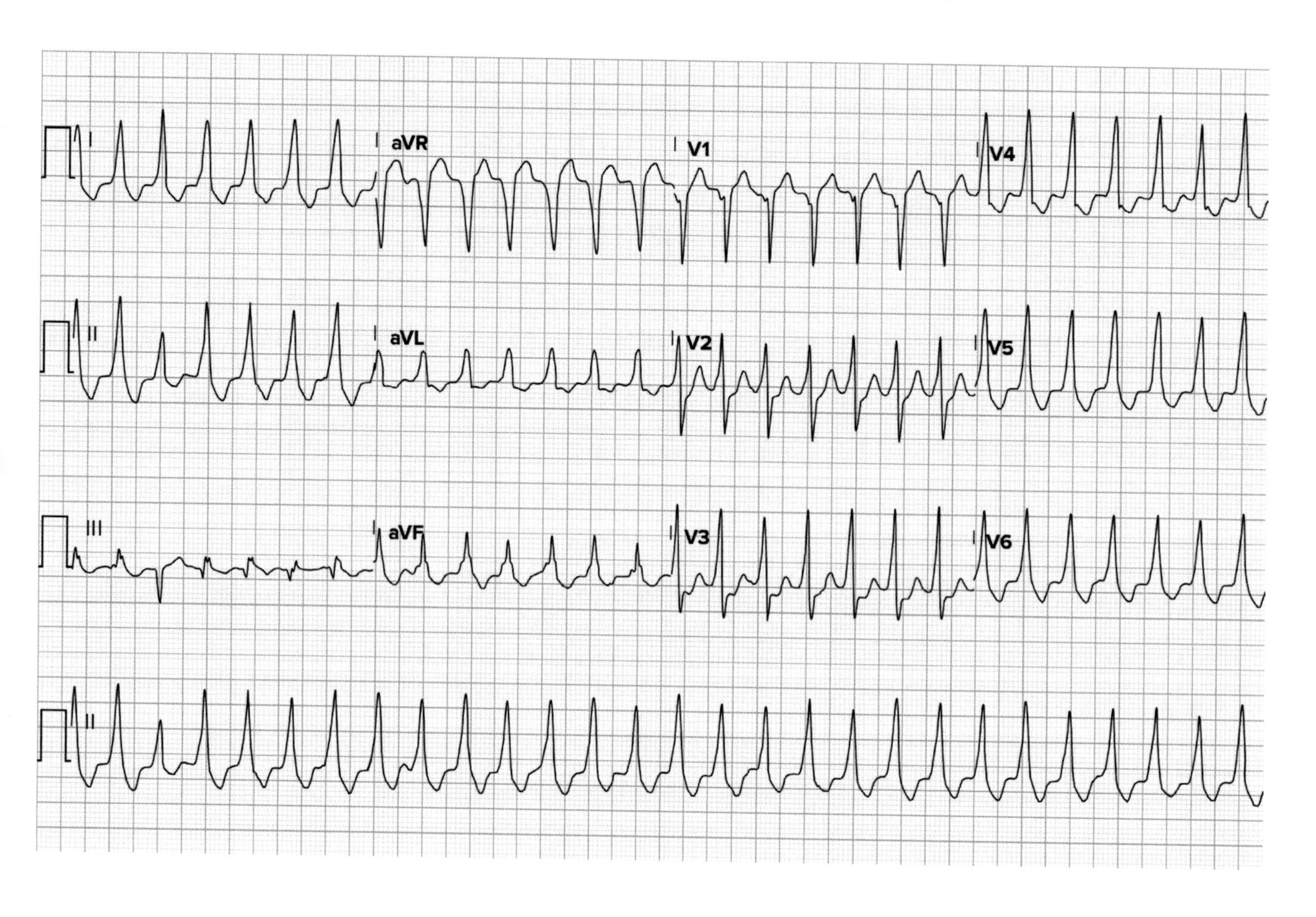

Case 92: Answer

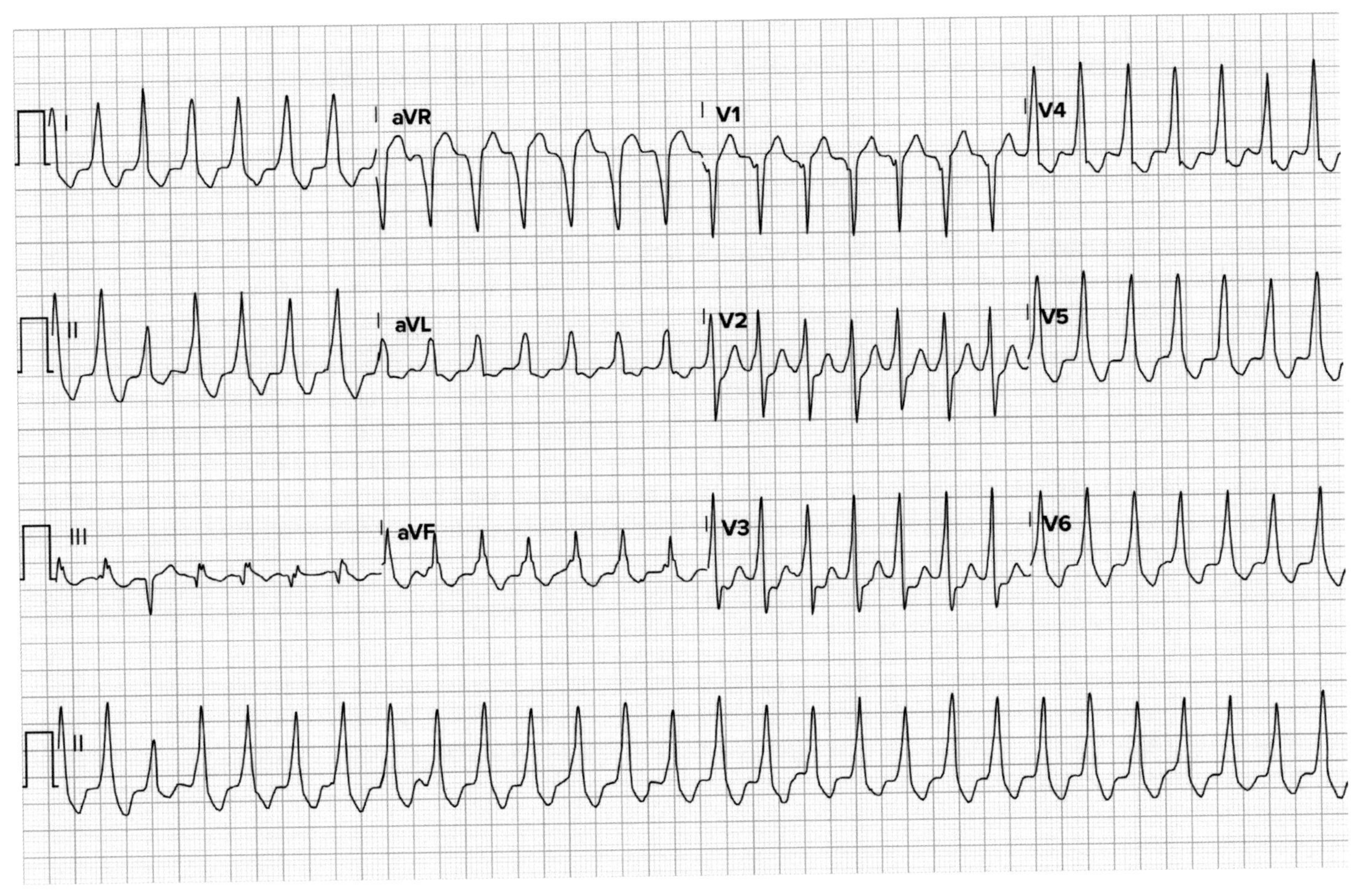

This ECG shows a regular wide complex tachycardia with a ventricular rate of 167 bpm, no P-waves, normal axis, and discordant ST-segments (ie, they point in the opposite direction from the QRS complex).

The differential diagnosis for a regular wide complex tachycardia includes:

- Monomorphic ventricular tachycardia
- Antidromic AVRT
- Any regular SVT (eg, sinus tach, AVNRT, atrial flutter, etc.) with aberrant conduction
  - Causes of aberrant conduction include fixed or rate-related BBB, metabolic abnormalities, sodium channel blocker toxicity, ventricular-paced rhythm, and ventricular pre-excitation (eg, WPW)

There isn't a dominant R-wave or R/S ratio > 0.7 in aVR or a rightward axis, making sodium channel blocker toxicity unlikely. The QRS complex morphology isn't consistent with a typical LBBB or RBBB pattern, but it is possible that there is fixed or rate-related nonspecific intraventricular conduction delay associated with a non-sinus SVT (eg, AVNRT, atrial flutter, orthodromic AVRT).

The key finding in this ECG is the 3rd beat which has a different morphology than all of the other beats ***(see Figure 1)***. This is a fusion beat which is caused by the simultaneous depolarization of the ventricle from both a normal supraventricular focus (eg, a sinus beat from the SA node) and a ventricular focus. The result is a QRS complex morphology that is a fusion of the QRS complex morphology seen in sinus rhythm with the QRS complex morphology seen in ventricular tachycardia. In the setting of a regular WCT with no P-waves, a fusion beat is considered diagnostic of VT. This patient was electrically cardioverted and admitted to the cardiology service.

Monomorphic VT Learning Points

- ≥ 3 consecutive, regular, wide complex beats with rate > 120-130 bpm
  - Non-sustained: < 30 sec duration with no hemodynamic instability
  - Sustained: ≥ 30 sec duration OR causes hemodynamic instability
- Rates < 120-130 bpm can be seen in patients on chronic antidysrhythmic medications (eg, amiodarone, flecainide, sotalol) or with severe cardiomyopathies
- If rate < 120 bpm, consider mimics:
  - Hyperkalemia
  - Sodium channel blocker toxicity
  - Accelerated idioventricular rhythm (AIVR)
- ECG features that increase the likelihood of VT in a regular WCT:
  - QRS complex duration > 200 msec is almost always VT, hyperkalemia, or sodium channel blocker toxicity
  - AV dissociation (ventricular rate > atrial rate)
  - Positive or negative QRS complex concordance in leads V1-V6 (entirely or predominantly positive or negative QRS complexes from leads V1 to V6)
  - Extreme axis deviation ("northwest axis")
  - The absence of typical RBBB or LBBB pattern suggests VT (ie, normal RBBB or LBBB pattern makes SVT with aberrant conduction more likely)
  - Fusion beats: hybrid QRS complex formed by both supraventricular and ventricular focus
  - Capture beats: sinus QRS formed by transient normal conduction amid AV dissociation
  - Brugada's sign: time from the onset of the QRS complex to the nadir of the S-wave is > 100 msec ***(see Figure 2)***
  - Josephson's sign: notching on the downslope of the S-wave near its nadir ***(see Figure 3)***

Figure 1. Fusion beat

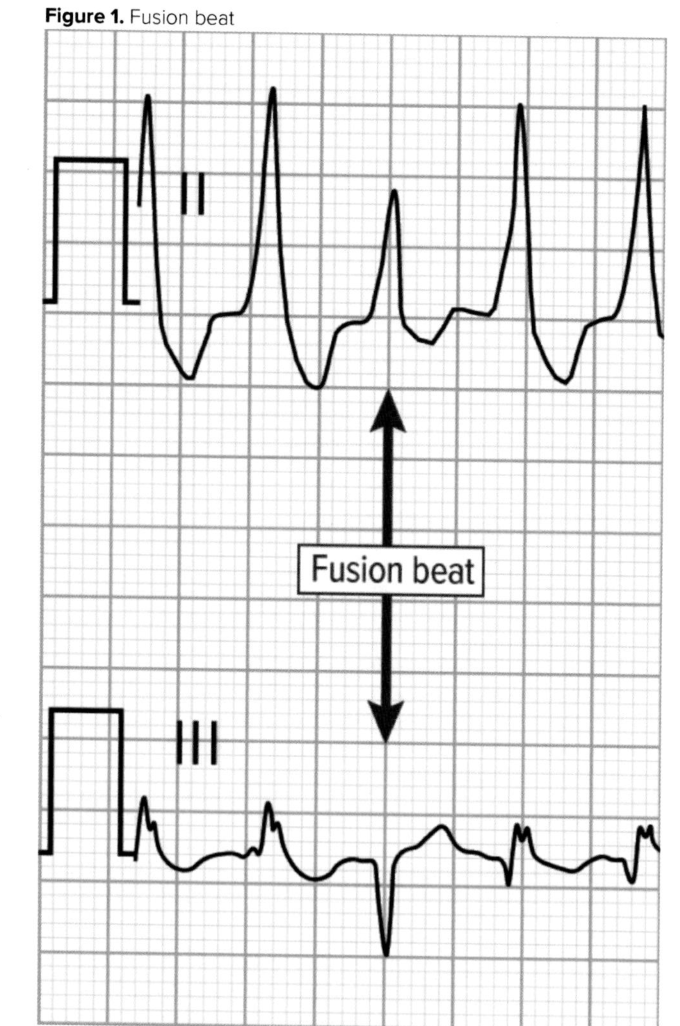

Figure 2

V2
Brugada's Sign
Start of QRS complex to S-wave nadir > 100 msec

Figure 3

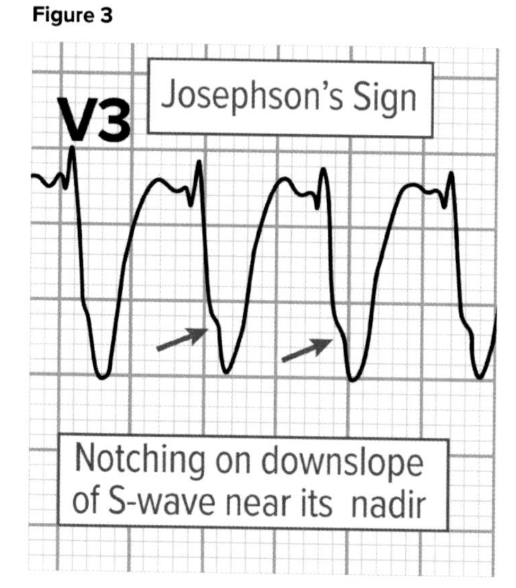

NOTES:

Case 93: Presentation

A 60-year-old female presents with dyspnea on exertion, postural hypotension, and lower extremity edema. What is your interpretation of her ECG?

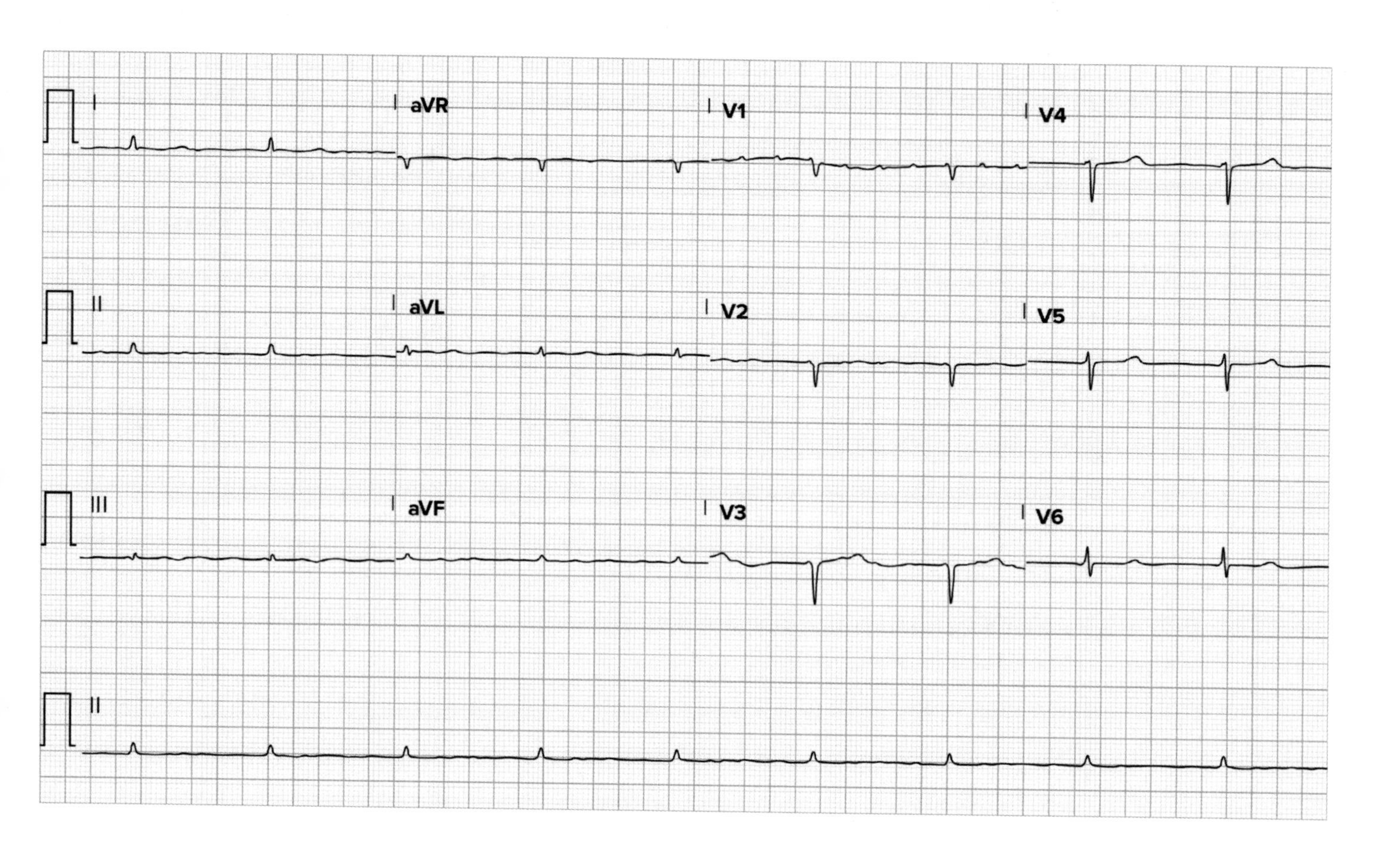

Case 93: Answer

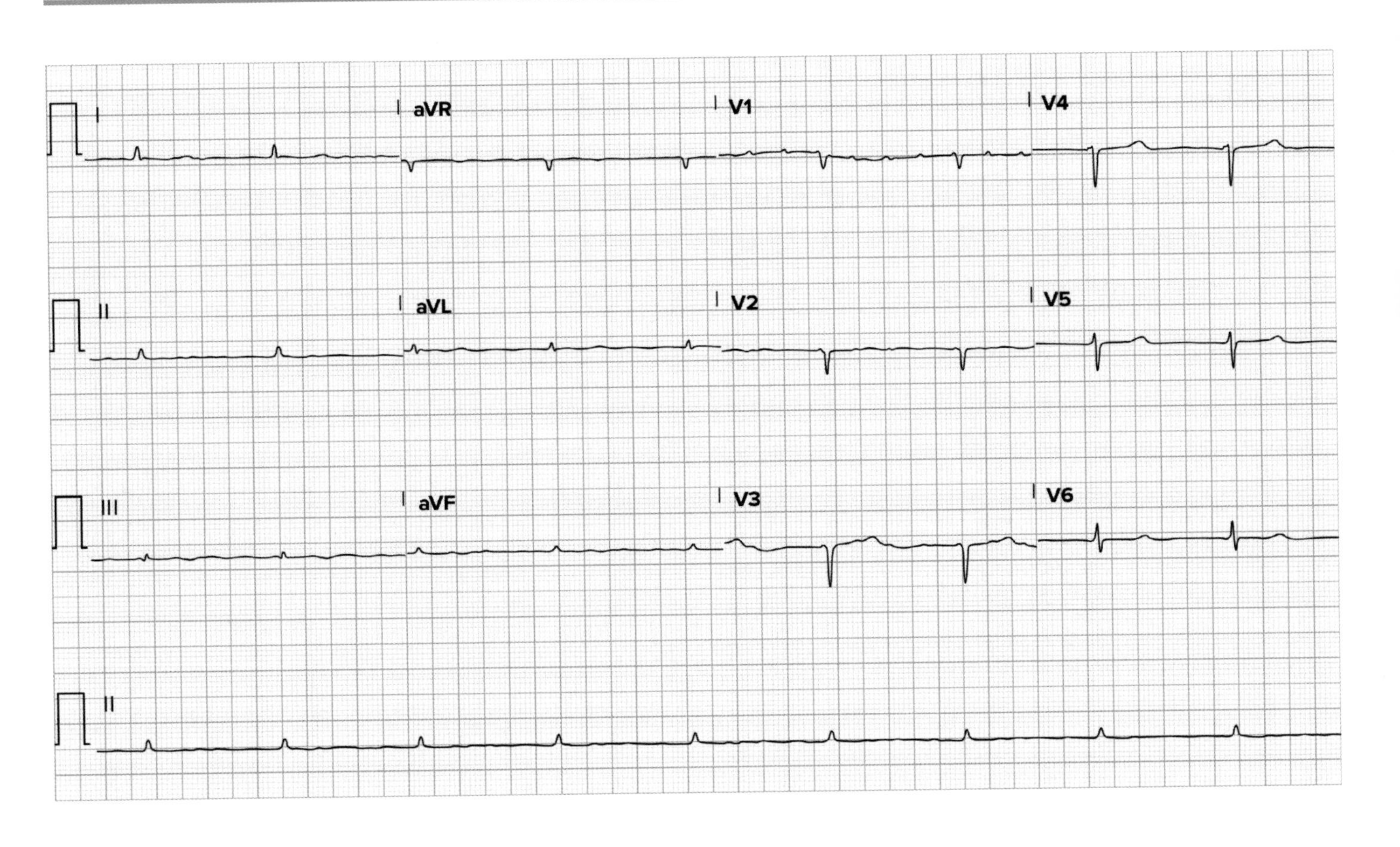

This ECG shows atrial tachycardia with 4:1 conduction and slow ventricular response, atrial rate of 220 bpm, ventricular rate of 55 bpm, normal axis, normal intervals, poor R-wave progression, and low QRS complex voltage.

The differential diagnosis for a regular narrow complex rhythm with bradycardic ventricular rates includes:

- Sinus bradycardia
- Junctional rhythm
- Junctional bradycardia
- Atrial flutter with block (rate controlled)
- Atrial tachycardia with block (rate controlled)
- 2:1 AV block
- High-grade AV block (eg, 3:1, 4:1, etc.)
- 3rd degree AV block with junctional escape rhythm
- 3rd degree sinoatrial block with junctional escape rhythm

The key to correctly interpreting the rhythm in this ECG is found in lead V1. There are distinct P-waves with a regular rate of 220 bpm, though not well visualized in any other lead ***(see Figure 1)***. It is not uncommon for lead V1 to be the best lead, or the only lead, for demonstration of atrial activity. In this case, the low voltage makes the detection of P-wave even more challenging on this ECG. The atrial rate is 4 times the ventricular rate which is consistent with 4:1 conduction (ie, the AV node is conducting every 4th impulse to the ventricles with resultant QRS complex). Atrial flutter is defined by an atrial rate of 250-350 bpm while atrial tachycardia is defined by an atrial rate of 150-250 bpm. The atrial rate seen in this ECG is consistent with atrial tachycardia.

Figure 1.
Lead V1 shows an atrial rate (PP interval) exactly 4 times the ventricular rate (RR interval), consistent with 4:1 conduction

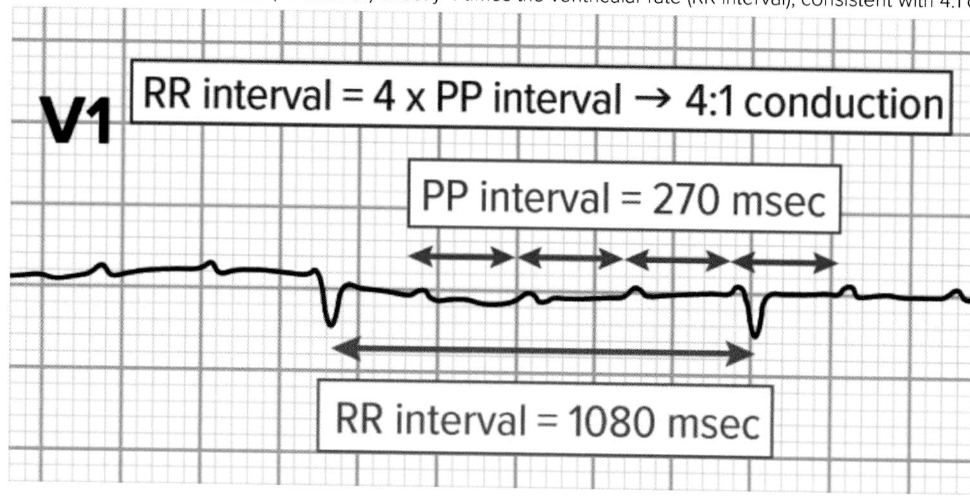

This ECG also shows low voltage, often defined as QRS complex amplitude < 5 mm in the limb leads or < 10 mm in the precordial leads. Some resources say "and" instead of "or" (ie, requiring both limb and precordial lead involvement), but this is academic. The finding of low voltage, regardless of whether it is present in both the limb and precordial leads, should prompt an evaluation for the underlying cause.

The differential diagnosis for low voltage includes:

- Normal variant
- Cardiac etiologies:
    - Hypothyroidism, severe
    - Hypovolemia
    - Infiltrative cardiomyopathies
    - Myocarditis
    - Myocardial infarction
- Extracardiac etiologies:
    - Acute respiratory distress syndrome
    - Anasarca
    - Chronic obstructive pulmonary disease
    - Constrictive pericarditis
    - Obesity
    - Pericardial effusion
    - Pleural effusion
    - Pneumomediastinum
    - Pneumonia
    - Pneumopericardium
    - Pneumothorax
    - Pulmonary edema
    - Subcutaneous emphysema

This patient's symptoms were attributed to right-sided heart failure that were later determined to be secondary to cardiac amyloidosis, which was also the suspected cause of the low voltage seen on her ECG.

Cardiac Amyloidosis Learning Points

- Accumulation of amyloid protein in the heart, eventually leading to cardiomyopathy +/- heart failure
- ECG findings associated with amyloidosis include:
  - Low voltage of all waveforms in the limb leads
  - Left axis deviation typical +/- left anterior fascicular block
  - Changes that mimic infarction (eg, Q-waves, STE/STD, TWI, hyperacute T-waves)
  - Prolonged atrioventricular conduction time (ie, 1st degree AV block)

Atrial Tachycardia Learning Points

- Due to ectopic atrial focus that takes over pacemaker function from the SA node
- Atrial rate is typically 150-250 bpm
- P-wave morphology does not meet sinus criteria
  - (+) P-wave in lead V1 suggests left atrial focus
  - Biphasic P-wave in lead aVL suggests right atrial focus

Atrial Flutter Learning Points

- Due to a re-entrant circuit in the right atrium
- Stereotypical sawtooth pattern of P-waves seen best in the inferior leads
  - Absence of isoelectric baseline (eg, TP segment) in lead II
- Atrial rate is 250-350 bpm and typically fixed over time
  - Ventricular rate is a fraction of atrial rate (ie, for an atrial rate of 300 bpm, 2:1 conduction produces a ventricular rate of 150 bpm, 3:1 conduction produces a ventricular rate of 100 bmp, 4:1 conduction produces a ventricular rate of 75 bpm, etc.)
- Consider atrial flutter when ventricular rate is consistently around 150 bpm
- Vagal maneuvers or adenosine will slow ventricular rate but have no effect on flutter waves

Low Voltage Learning Points

- QRS amplitude < 5 mm in all limb leads or < 10 mm in all chest leads
- Low voltage + electrical alternans = pericardial effusion until proven otherwise

Case 94: Presentation

An 82-year-old female with history of atrial fibrillation and chronic severe heart failure presents with altered mental status. What is your interpretation of her ECG?

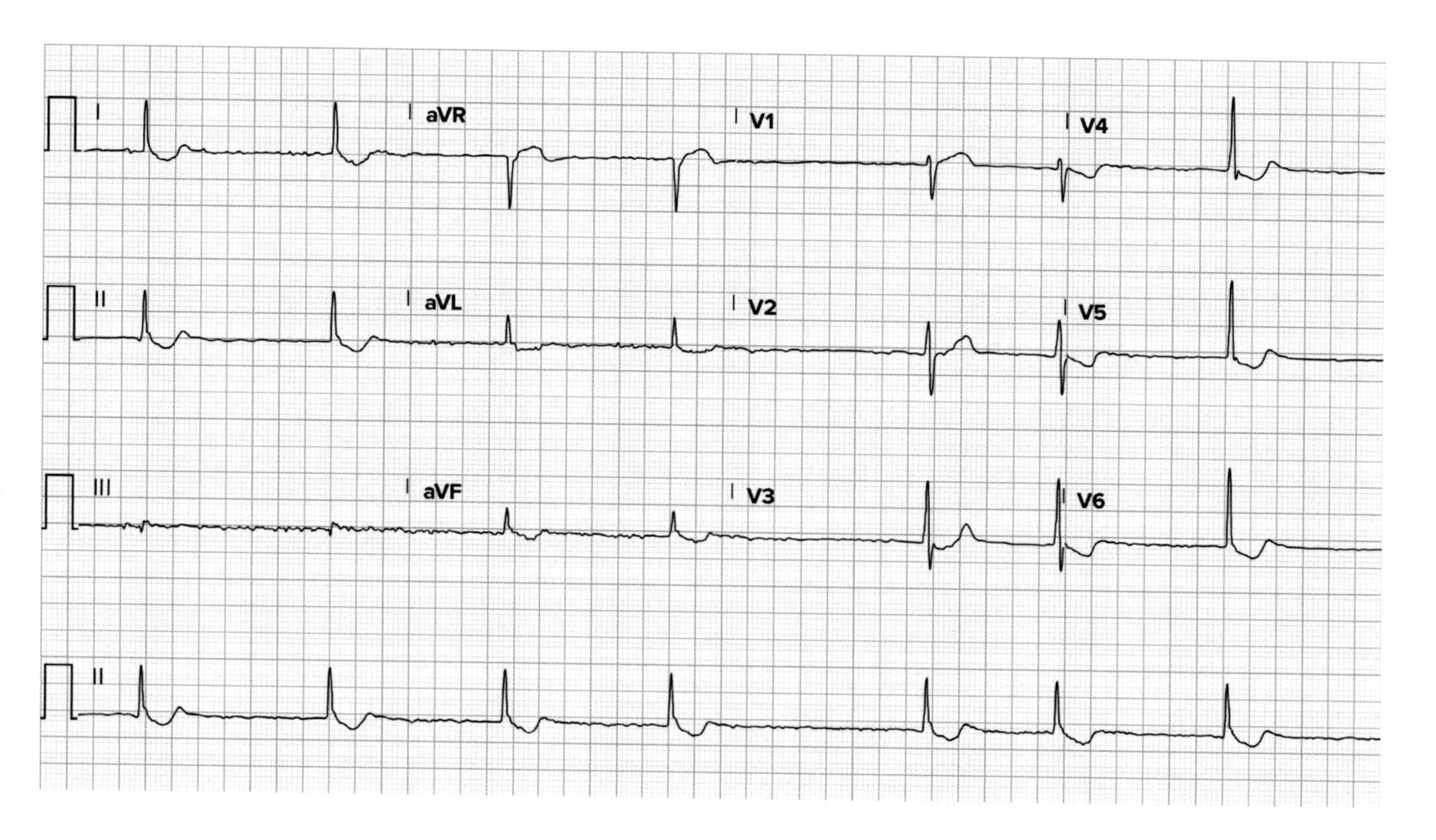

Case 94: Answer

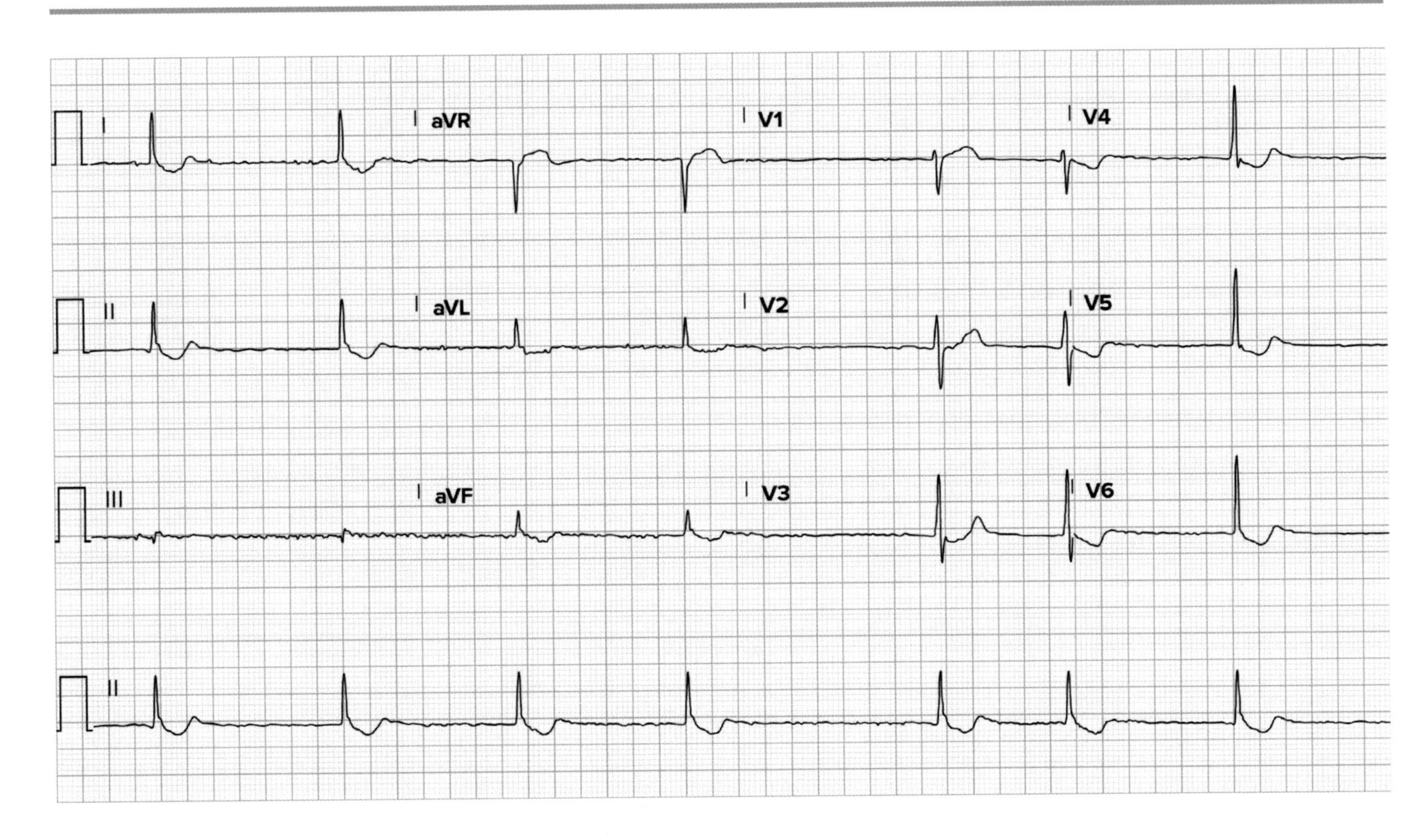

This ECG shows atrial fibrillation with an average ventricular rate of 42 bpm, normal axis, normal intervals, STD with scooped ST-segments in leads I, aVL, II, aVF, and V3-V6, and STE with coved ST-segments in lead aVR.

The scooped ST-segments seen in this ECG are commonly referred to as the digoxin effect ***(see Figure 1),*** or the Salvador Dali sign (in reference to this gentleman's moustache) and is a sign of digoxin's presence with penetration into the myocardial tissues, rather than toxicity. This effect also includes PR interval lengthening and QT interval shortening. These findings are subtle in this ECG and are a testament to the variability in the ECG changes seen with digoxin use and/or toxicity.

Figure 1. The lead II rhythms strip shows scooped ST-segments seen with digoxin use, called digoxin effect or the Salvador Dali sign

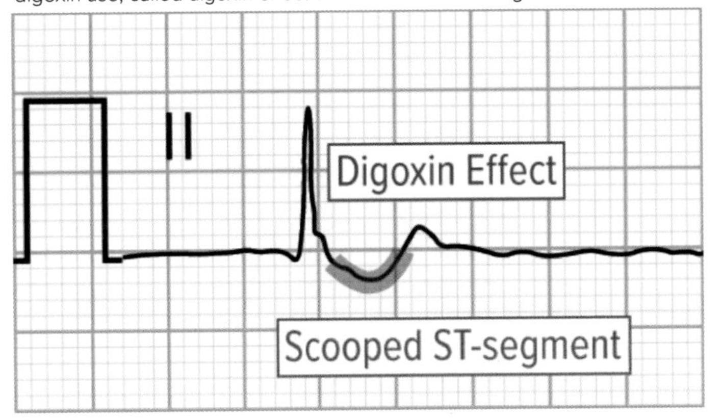

The key to accurately interpreting this ECG is recognizing that atrial fibrillation with slow ventricular response is abnormal and warrants further investigation. Important etiologies to consider include antidysrhythmic medication toxicity (eg, digoxin, nodal blockers such as CCB or beta-blockers, etc.) and electrolyte abnormalities such as hyperkalemia.

Dysrhythmias associated with digoxin toxicity are varied, and if digoxin toxicity were more common, it would certainly compete with hyperkalemia for the title of the "syphilis of electrocardiography."[1] A range of bradycardias, tachycardias, and various blocks can be seen in the patient with digoxin toxicity. Common findings include PACs and PVCs, and dysrhythmias associated with toxicity include paroxysmal atrial tachycardia with variable block and bradycardic rate, accelerated junctional rhythms, bidirectional ventricular tachycardia, and atrial fibrillation with slow ventricular response or a regular bradycardic rate due to the presence of a 3rd degree AV block.

Cardiac glycosides, which includes digoxin, are inhibitors of the sodium-potassium ATPase pump. Other cardiac glycosides include foxglove, oleander, and lily of the valley. Common causes of chronic toxicity include renal disease, electrolyte abnormalities, dehydration, and drug interactions. Common symptoms seen with chronic toxicity include anorexia, abdominal pain, nausea, and CNS symptoms (eg, AMS). Concurrent hyperkalemia is associated with a high mortality rate. Note that patients can have digoxin toxicity clinically with normal serum concentrations, especially in the presence of hypomagnesemia, hypokalemia, and/or hypercalcemia.

First-line treatment for symptomatic dysrhythmias is digoxin immune Fab (eg, Digibind or DigiFab). Other treatments include atropine for bradycardias and AV blocks, and lidocaine or phenytoin for ventricular tachycardias if digoxin immune Fab is unavailable or ineffective. Treatment with digoxin immune Fab will cause potassium to shift into the cells and can lead to clinically significant hypokalemia, so potassium levels should be monitored closely after administration.

This patient's workup in the ED was notable for an acute kidney injury and elevated digoxin level, and it is likely that the former caused the latter. The patient was treated with digoxin immune Fab after which her heart rate normalized.

Digoxin Learning Points

- ECG features seen with therapeutic level (ie, not necessarily signs of toxicity):
  - Scooped ST-segments (ie, digoxin effect) most pronounced in leads with tall R-waves
  - PR interval lengthening
  - QT interval shortening
- "Pathognomonic" dysrhythmias seen with toxicity:
  - Atrial fibrillation with slow ventricular response or a regular bradycardic rate
  - Paroxysmal atrial tachycardia with variable block and bradycardic rate (uncommon)
  - Bidirectional ventricular tachycardia (very rare)
- Acute toxicity may present with hyperkalemia
- Treatment includes:
  - Digoxin-specific antibody (eg, Digibind): causes serum digoxin levels to rise making repeat levels unreliable
  - Atropine for AV blocks
  - Phenytoin or lidocaine for ventricular dysrhythmias

References

1. Mattu A. ECG Weekly.

NOTES:

Case 95: Presentation

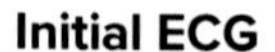

A 60-year-old female presents with chest pain. The initial ECG was obtained when her pain was mild in intensity and a repeat ECG was obtained 10 minutes later when she appeared acutely ill with worsening of her pain. What is your interpretation of her ECGs?

Initial ECG

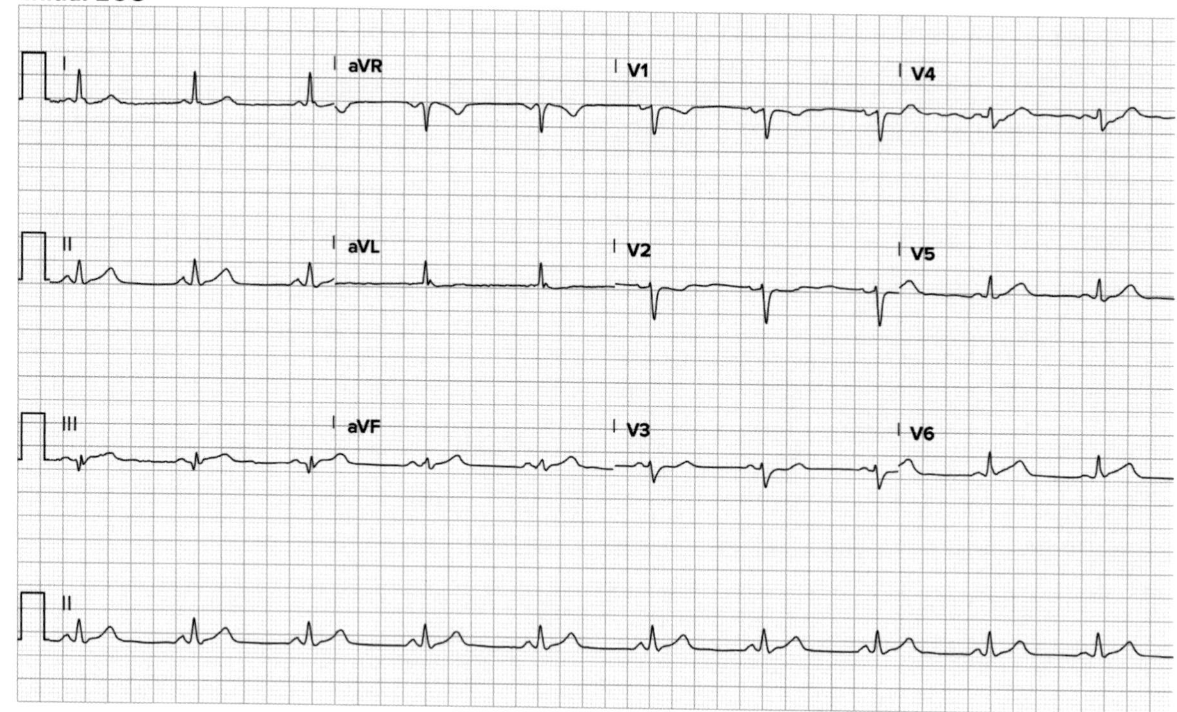

Repeat ECG (approximately 10 minutes later)

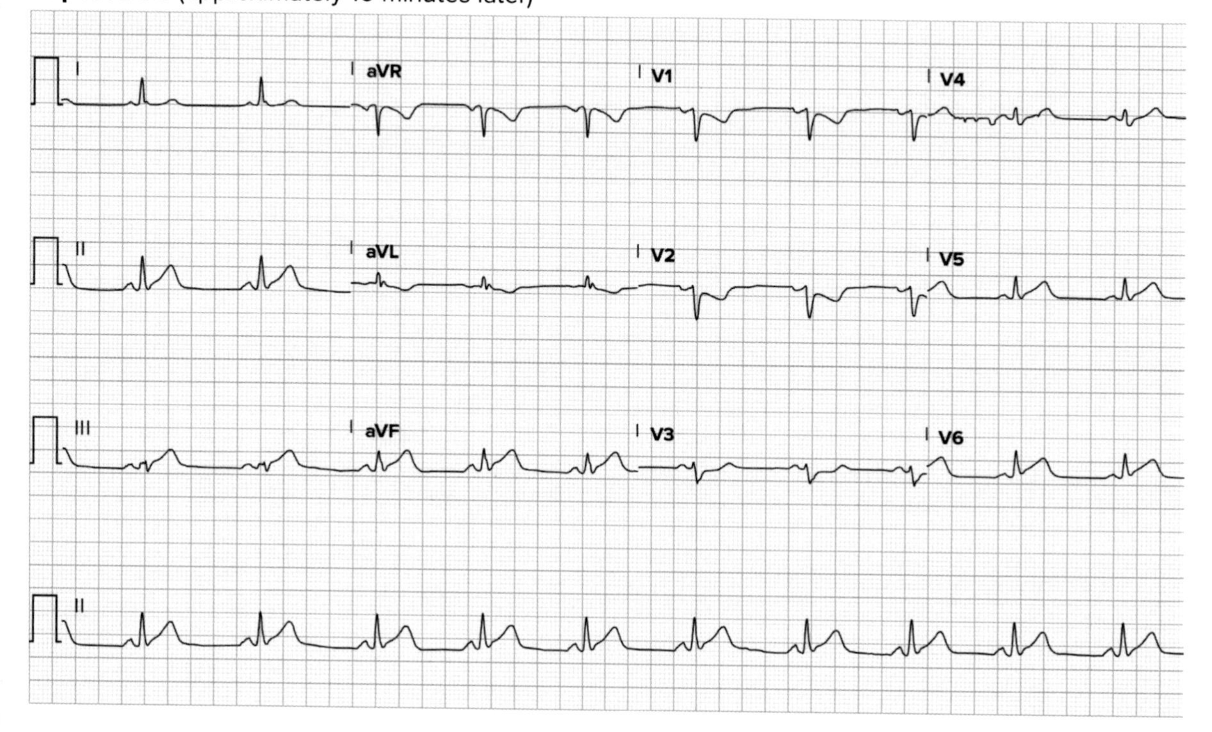

Case 95: Answer

Initial ECG

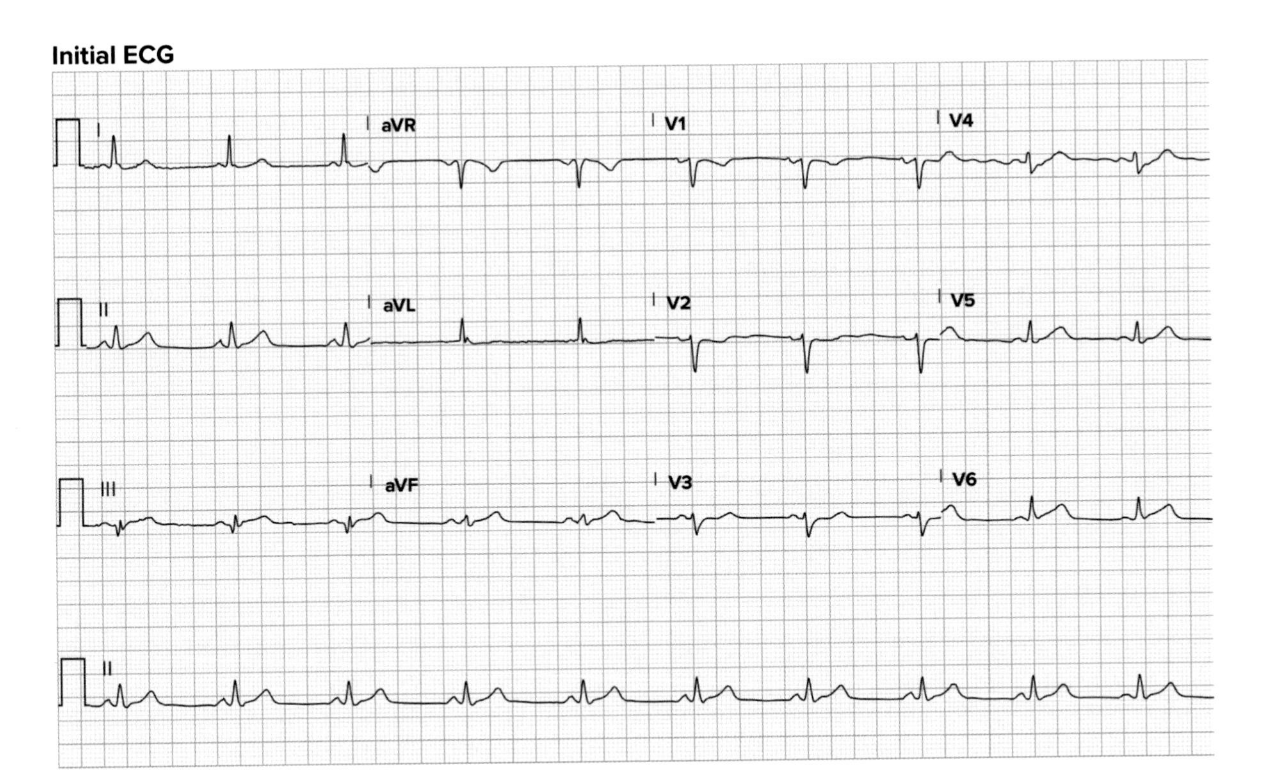

Repeat ECG (approximately 10 minutes later)

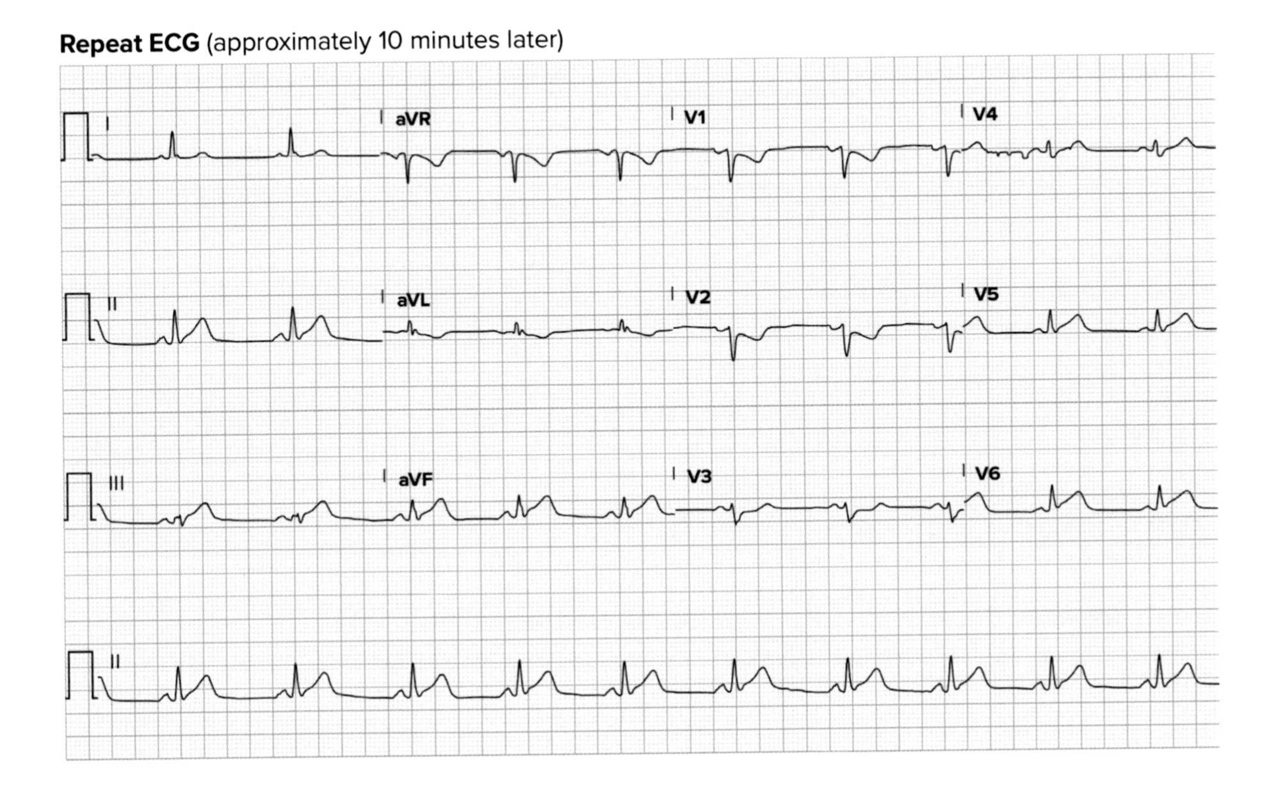

The initial ECG shows a normal sinus rhythm at 60 bpm, normal axis, normal intervals, STE < 1 mm in leads II and III, and STD < 1 mm in leads V2-V4. The T-waves in leads II, III, and aVF appear larger than anticipated and could be considered hyperacute.

There is no universally accepted definition for hyperacute T-waves, but they are generally described as broad based and disproportionately tall. There is no consensus on whether the height of the T-wave should be compared to the amplitude of the preceding R-wave or the entire QRS complex. The hyperacute T-waves in this ECG are not visually impressive, but when considered in light of the relatively smaller amplitude QRS complexes, they are hyperacute.

The repeat ECG shows a normal sinus rhythm at 63 bpm, normal axis, normal intervals, STE in leads II, III, aVF and V5-V6, STD in leads V1-V4, and TWI in lead aVL.

These ECGs demonstrate the importance of obtaining serial ECGs. The STE in the inferior leads on the initial ECG ***(see Figure 1)*** do not quite meet STEMI criteria. The repeat ECG shows increasing STE ***(see Figure 2)*** which meet STEMI criteria. These dynamic changes correlate with the patient's worsening overall condition (ie, signs and symptoms of ACS). It would have been reasonable to obtain a posterior ECG based on the anterior precordial STD seen in the initial ECG.

Serial ECGs, particularly in patients with a high clinical suspicion for ACS who demonstrate an initially non-diagnostic electrocardiogram (ie, no STEMI), can increase the diagnosis of AMI significantly with a corresponding increase in the number of patients who are candidates for emergent reperfusion therapy; this statement applies to patients in which the clinician has a high level of concern for AMI despite a non-diagnostic ECG. Furthermore, short-term dynamic changes in the ST-segment and/or T-wave can suggest AMI in patients with a high clinical suspicion for ACS.

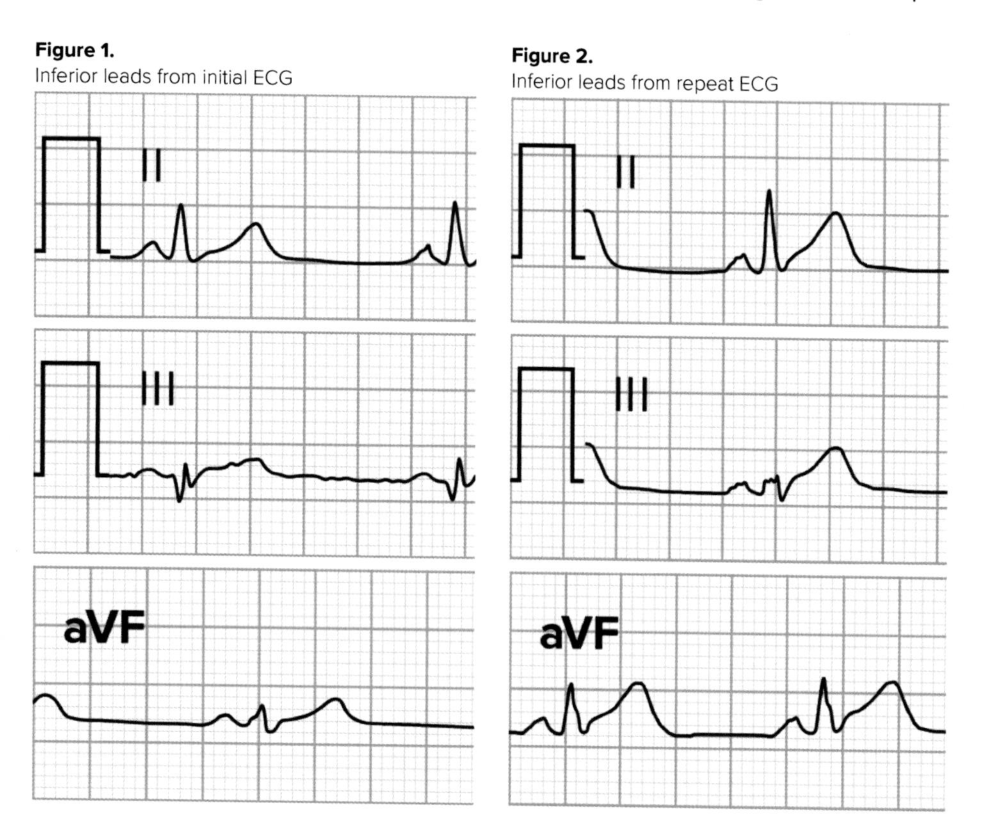

Figure 1.
Inferior leads from initial ECG

Figure 2.
Inferior leads from repeat ECG

This patient was taken to the cardiac catheterization laboratory where a 99% occlusion of the left circumflex artery was successfully treated with a stent.

Hyperacute T-waves Learning Points

- There is no universally accepted definition of hyperacute T-waves (ie, no absolute specific amplitude), but the general characteristics include *(see Figure 3)*:
  - Broad based and disproportionately tall
  - Asymmetric morphology with more gradual upslope and more abrupt return to the baseline
  - J point elevation is common
- Hyperacute T-waves + STD/TWI in reciprocal leads = early AMI
- When in doubt, obtain serial ECGs

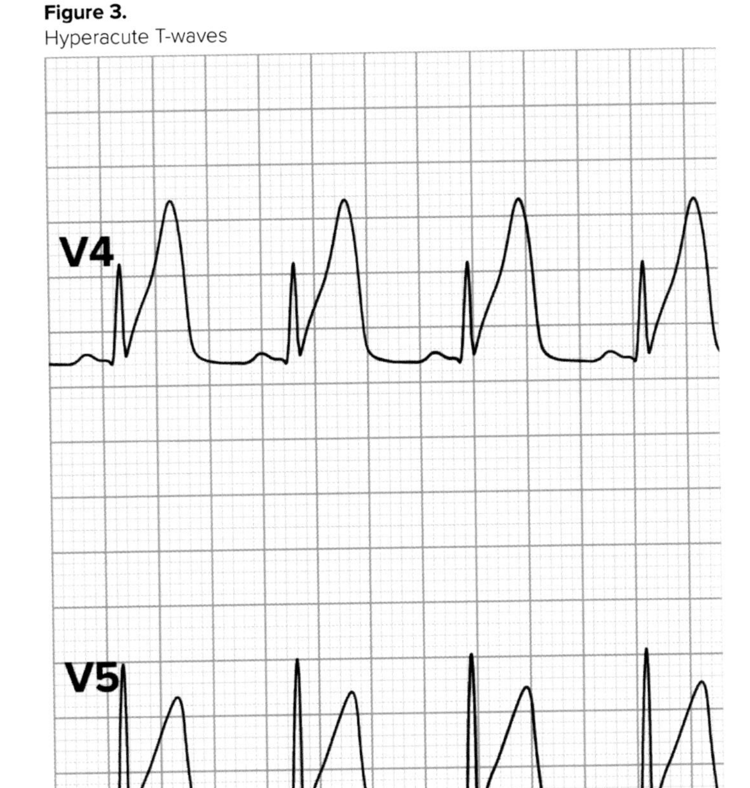

Figure 3.
Hyperacute T-waves

STEMI Learning Points

- STEMI is defined by new, or presumed new, STE at the J point in ≥ 2 anatomically contiguous leads in the absence of LVH by voltage pattern, LBBB, or ventricular-paced rhythm
  - ≥ 2.5 mm in men < 40 years old and ≥ 2 mm in men ≥ 40 years old in leads V2-V3 (or an increase of ≥ 1 mm when compared to baseline ECG)
  - ≥ 1.5 mm in women in leads V2-V3 (or an increase of ≥ 1 mm when compared to baseline ECG)
  - ≥ 1 mm in all other leads
- ST-segment is measured from the isoelectric baseline, typically the TP segment (see below)
- Reciprocal STD are not required for the diagnosis of STEMI, but their presence does increase the likelihood of the diagnosis of STEMI
  - Reciprocal STD are only present in 70% of anterior MI[1]
- Posterior MI
  - Consider whenever there is STD in leads V1-V4
  - STE ≥ 0.5 mm in posterior leads V7, V8 or V9 is diagnostic- does not require 2 contiguous leads
- Right ventricular MI
  - Consider with any inferior MI (RV MI is seen in approximately 1/3 of inferior MI)
  - STE in right precordial leads V3R and V4R ≥ 0.5 mm (≥ 1 mm for men ≤ 30 years old)
  - STE in right precordial lead V4R > 1 mm is most predictive of RV MI
  - STE in right precordial lead V4R > STE in leads V1-V3 = highly specific for RV MI
- Significant STE that does not meet the traditional distribution (ie, ≥ 2 anatomically contiguous leads) in a presentation concerning for ACS may still represent coronary artery occlusion and warrant consideration for emergent coronary reperfusion

How to Measure STE per most recent 2018 AHA Guidelines[2]

- The J point is the junction between QRS termination and ST-segment onset and is used to determine the magnitude of the ST-segment shift
- **In patients with a stable baseline, the TP segment (isoelectric interval) is a more accurate method to assess the magnitude of ST-segment shift** ***(see Figure 4)***, and in distinguishing pericarditis from acute myocardial ischemia
- QRS onset should be used if TP segment does not have a stable baseline ***(see Figure 5)***
- Measurement should be made from the top of the ECG line tracing

Figure 4.
Measure STE from the TP segment if the TP segment is isoelectric (ie, horizontal)

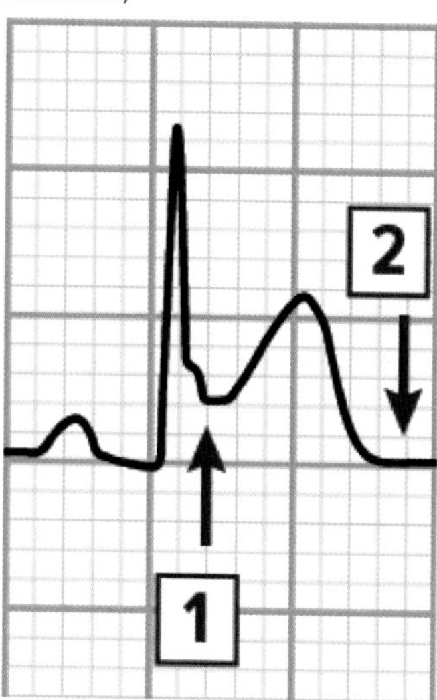

Arrow 1: onset of the ST-segment (ie, J point)
Arrow 2: TP segment

Figure 5.
Measure STE from onset of the QRS complex if the TP segment is not isoelectric (ie, not horizontal)

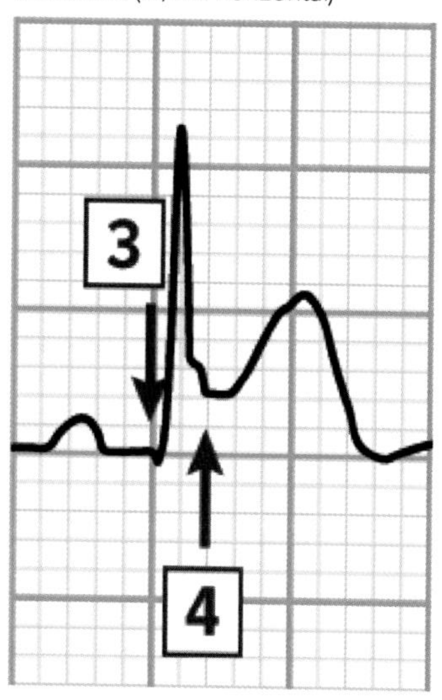

Arrow 3: initial onset of the Q-wave
Arrow 4: onset of the ST-segment (ie, J point)

References

1. Knilans T, Surawicz B. Chou's Electrocardiography in Clinical Practice. Philadelphia, PA: Elsevier. 2020.
2. Thygesen K, Alpert JS, Jaffe AS, et al. 2018 ESC/ACC/AHA/WHF Expert Consensus Document: Fourth Universal Definition of Myocardial Infarction (2018). Circulation. 2018;138:e618-e651.

NOTES:

Case 96: Presentation

A 22-year-old male with no past medical history presents with left sided chest pain for the past 3 days that is worse with lying flat and better with leaning forward. What is your interpretation of his ECG?

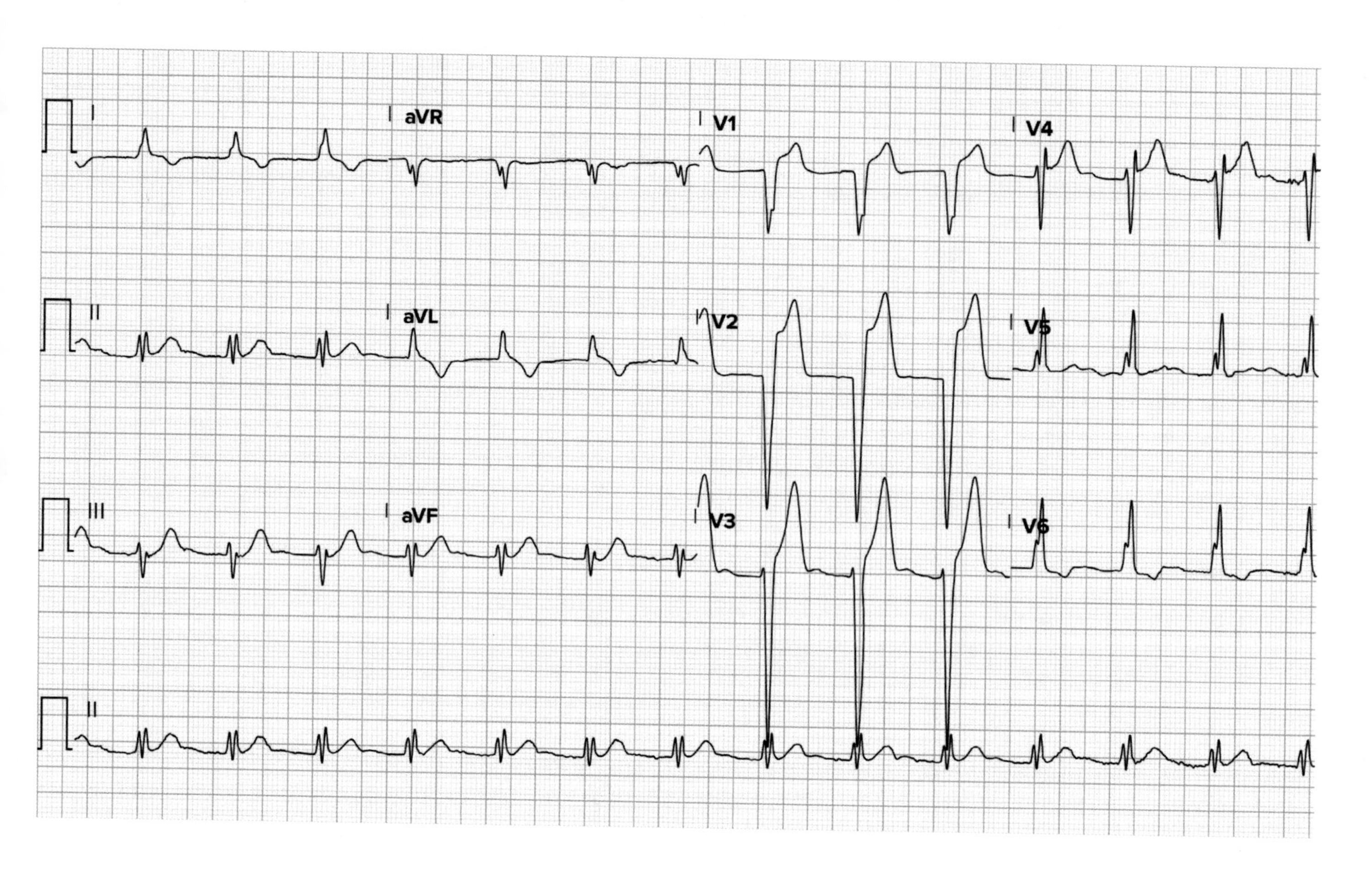

Case 96: Answer

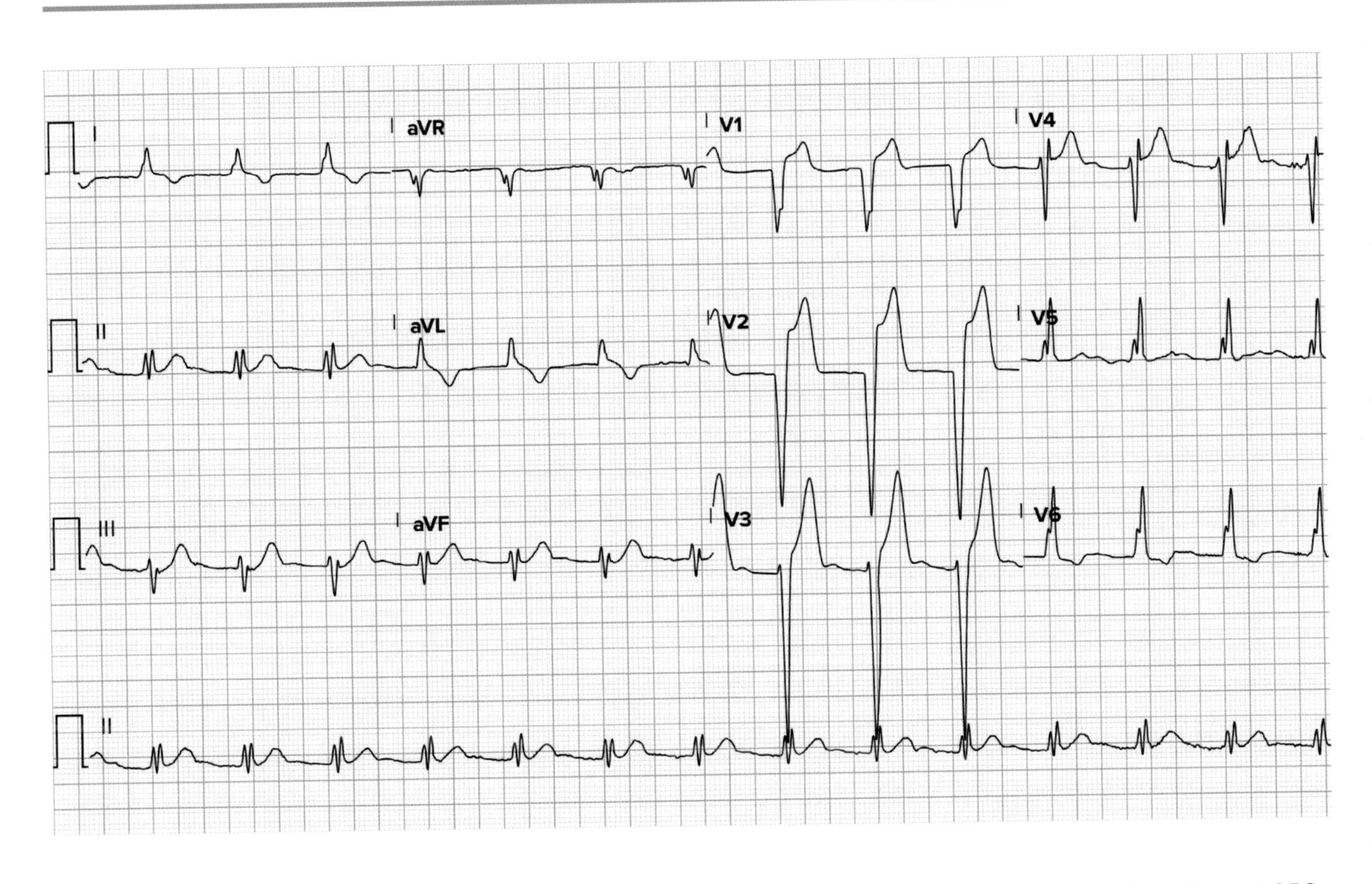

This ECG shows a regular wide complex rhythm with a ventricular rate of 88 bpm, no P-waves, normal axis, prolonged QRS complex duration with a LBBB morphology, U-waves (best seen in leads II, III, aVF, and V3-V5), excessive discordant STE in lead V2, and slight concordant STE in leads I and aVL.

The differential diagnosis for a regular wide complex rhythm with no P-waves (nor flutter waves) includes accelerated idioventricular rhythm and accelerated junctional rhythm with aberrant conduction (eg, fixed or rate related BBB, metabolic abnormalities, etc.). The QRS complexes have the appearance of a LBBB (ie, LBBB morphology), but whether this represents a true LBBB depends on whether the origin of this rhythm is ventricular or supraventricular. If the rhythm in this ECG is an accelerated idioventricular rhythm, the QRS complex appearance cannot be due to a true LBBB as idioventricular rhythms do not utilize the His-Purkinje conduction system. A true LBBB requires a supraventricular or junctional origin that conducts via the normal cardiac conduction system. An idioventricular rhythm can have QRS complexes that mimic a LBBB (eg, a dominant S-wave in lead V1), but it's not a true LBBB since there isn't conduction via the His-Purkinje system. Without more information, it is impossible to determine which of these is present in this patient's ECG.

The characteristic findings in a LBBB include:

- QRS complex duration ≥ 120 msec
- Dominant S-wave in leads V1, V2, and frequently V3 ***(see Figure 1)***
- Broad and notched or slurred R-wave in leads I, aVL, V5, and V6 ***(see Figure 2)***
- Absent Q-waves in leads I, V5, and V6 (can see small Q-wave in lead aVL)
- R-wave peak time > 60 msec in leads V5 and V6 but normal in leads V1-V3 ***(see Figure 2)***
- Axis usually normal or leftward
- ST segments follow the "Rule of Appropriate Discordance"
  - ST-segment deviation in the opposite direction from the QRS complex ***(see Figures 1 and 2)***

Figure 1.
Lead V1 shows a dominant S-wave and appropriate discordance, consistent with a LBBB

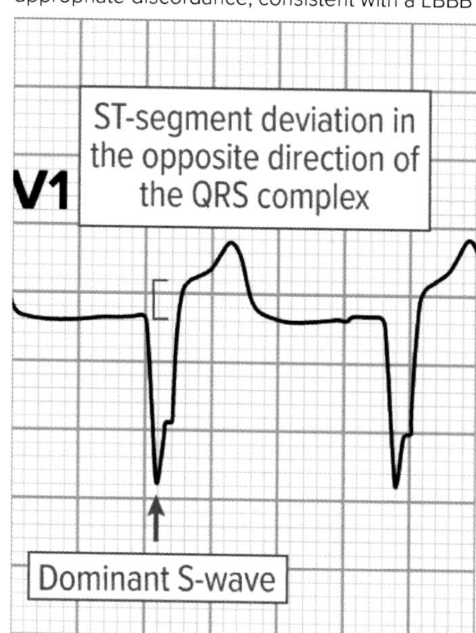

Figure 2.
Lead V6 shows a broad notched R-wave, R-wave peak time > 60 msec, and appropriate discordance, consistent with a LBBB

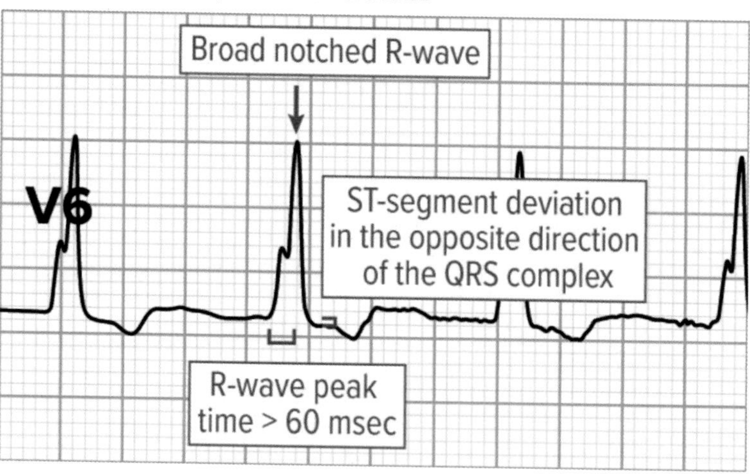

A defining feature of a LBBB is the "rule of appropriate discordance" which describes the relationship between the direction of the QRS complex and its ST-segment. In other words, if the main vector of the QRS complex points up, there will be STD, and if the main vector of the QRS complex points down, there will STE. These repolarization abnormalities confound the ECG's ability to detect AMI and other ACS findings, so interpretation of the ECG with a LBBB in a presentation suggestive of ACS requires using the Sgarbossa criteria to diagnose an MI.

The Sgarbossa criteria are based on the underlying principle that concordance and excessive discordance in a LBBB are abnormal. The criteria assign a point value for any concordant STE ***(see Figures 3a and 3b)*** or excessively discordant STE ***(see Figure 3c)***. A score ≥ 3 is 98% specific for an AMI, so the presence of criteria A or B are considered diagnostic of an AMI. Criterion C is only assigned 2 points, so the presence of just criterion C is not diagnostic of an AMI.

Figure 3a.
Sgarbossa criterion A- concordant STE ≥ 1 mm in ≥ 1 lead (5 points = diagnostic of AMI)

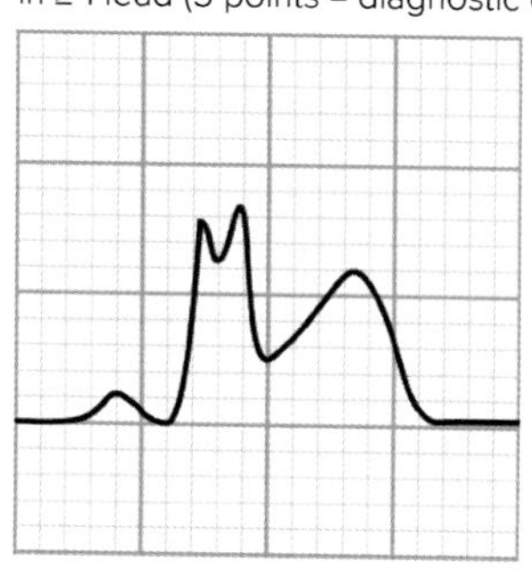

Figure 3b.
Sgarbossa criterion B- STD ≥ 1 mm in leads V1 or V2 or V3 (3 points = diagnostic of AMI)

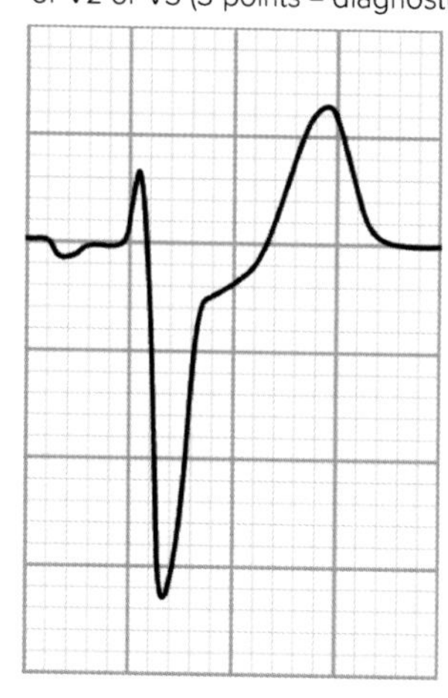

Figure 3c.
Sgarbossa criterion C- discordant STE ≥ 5 mm in ≥ 1 lead (2 points = not diagnostic of AMI)

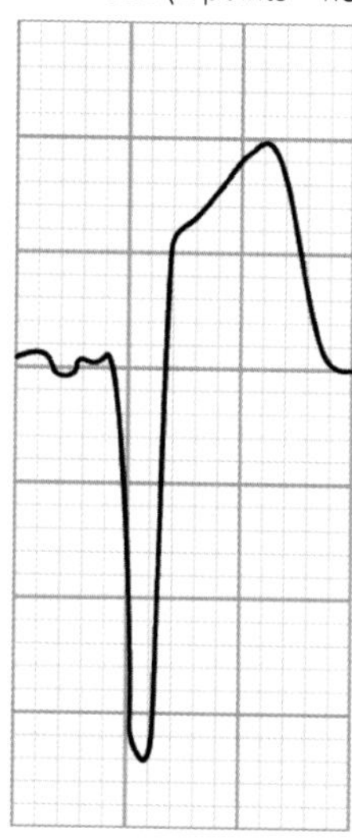

Figure 4.
Modified Sgarbossa criterion C- STE/S ratio ≥ 0.25 in ≥ 1 lead (diagnostic of AMI but not mandated in current AHA/ACC STEMI guidelines)

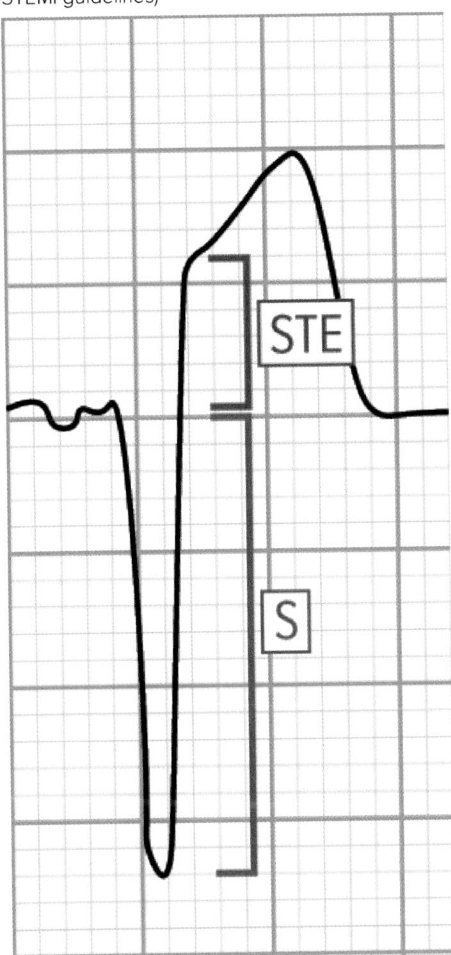

Figure 5.
Lead V2 shows STE that meets both Sgarbossa and Modified Sgarbossa criteria

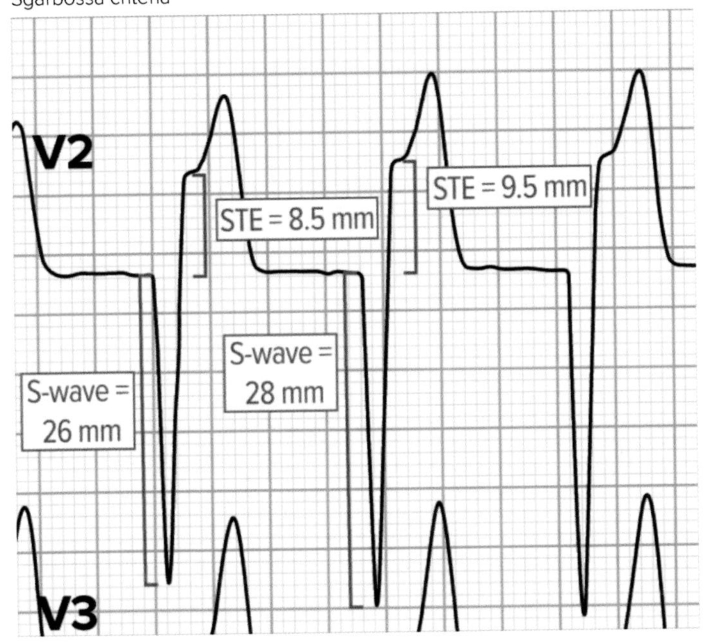

The Modified Sgarbossa criteria includes Sgarbossa criteria A and B with a variation of criterion C. Instead of using a fixed cutoff of 5 mm for discordant STE, it uses a ratio of the STE height to the S-wave depth ***(Figure 4)***. A STE/S ratio ≥ 0.25 in ≥ 1 lead is considered diagnostic of an AMI. This means that more than 5 mm of STE is permissible if there is a large S-wave, and less than 5 mm of STE may be diagnostic if the accompanying S-wave is small. The Modified Sgarbossa criteria are not mandated in the current AHA/ACC STEMI guidelines.

In this patient's ECG, lead V2 shows excessively discordant STE ≥ 5 mm ***(see Figure 5)*** which meets Sgarbossa criterion C, but this not considered diagnostic for an AMI. The STE/S ratio in lead V2 is ≥ 0.25 which is diagnostic of an AMI per the Modified Sgarbossa criteria.

This ECG also showed U-waves in the inferior and mid precordial leads ***(see Figure 6)***. The etiology of these waves is unclear as the patient had normal electrolytes and they were not seen on subsequent ECGs.

This case was discussed emergently with cardiology who evaluated the patient in the ED. A CTA of the chest was unremarkable, and a bedside echocardiogram showed no effusion, right heart strain, nor wall motion abnormalities. The patient's troponin came back slightly elevated. The patient was admitted to the cardiology service and a cardiac MRI later that day was consistent with myocarditis. A formal echo the next day showed a normal EF with a mild septal contraction abnormality.

Figure 6.
The lead II rhythm strip shows U-waves

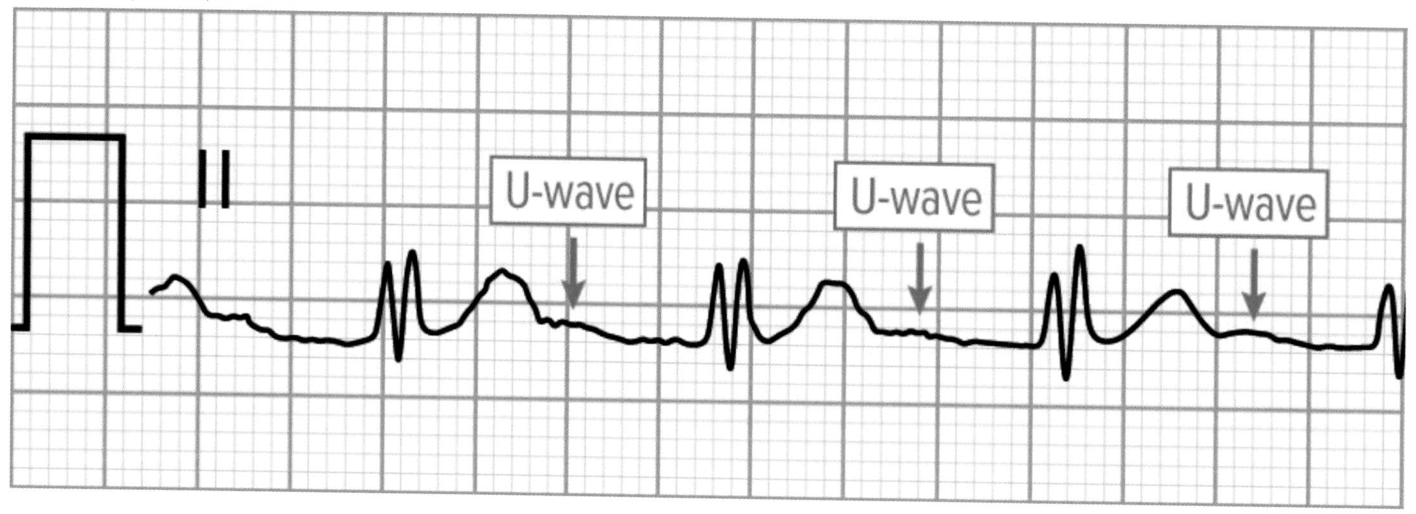

Junctional Rhythm Learning Points

- Ectopic focus from AV node or proximal Purkinje system
  - Also called AV junctional rhythm, nodal rhythm, nodal escape rhythm, junctional escape rhythm, AV nodal rhythm
- ECG shows ventricular rate of 40-60 bpm with normal QRS complex duration unless concurrent conduction abnormality (eg, bundle branch block)
- May have retrograde P-waves that precede (with PR interval < 120 msec) or follow QRS complex, typically best seen in the inferior leads
- Variations include:
  - Junctional Bradycardia: ventricular rate < 40 bpm
  - Accelerated Junctional Rhythm: ventricular rate 61–100 bpm
  - Junctional Tachycardia: ventricular rate > 100 bpm

Idioventricular Rhythm Learning Points

- Ectopic focus from Purkinje network or ventricular myocardium
  - Also called ventricular escape rhythm
- ECG shows ≥ 3 consecutive, regular, wide complex beats with no P-waves or AV dissociation if P-waves are present
- Variations include accelerated idioventricular rhythm (AIVR)
  - Rates between 40-110 bpm but can sometimes be as high as 120-130 bpm
  - Can be seen in the reperfusion phase of a STEMI following fibrinolysis or PCI but can also be spontaneous
  - Also seen with digoxin toxicity, cardiac ischemia, or electrolyte abnormalities
  - Mimics include hyperkalemia, sodium channel blocker toxicity, and VT in patients on antidysrhythmic medications (eg, amiodarone, flecainide, sotalol) or with severe cardiomyopathies
  - Usually well-tolerated, benign, and self-limiting
  - Treating as VT with antidysrhythmic medications can precipitate asystole

LBBB Learning Points

- Ventricular depolarization from right to left (opposite of normal)
- ST segments follow the "Rule of Appropriate Discordance"
  - ST-segment deviation in the opposite direction from the QRS complex
- Confounds ECG's ability to detect AMI and other ACS findings
  - If ACS suspected, must use the Sgarbossa criteria to diagnose AMI
  - A presumed new LBBB in itself is no longer considered a STEMI equivalent, but is a high risk finding in ACS, so if AMI is suspected, urgent reperfusion therapy should be considered

Sgarbossa Criteria Learning Points

- Used to evaluate for STEMI in the presence of LBBB
- Based on "Rule of Appropriate Discordance"
  - In the absence of AMI, LBBB will have ST-segment deviation in the opposite direction from the QRS complex
  - Concordance and excessive discordance in LBBB are abnormal
- Concordant STE ≥ 1 mm in ≥ 1 lead or STD ≥ 1 mm in lead V1, V2, or V3 is considered diagnostic of AMI
- Modified Sgarbossa criteria
  - For discordant STE, a ratio of STE to S-wave depth ≥ 0.25 in ≥ 1 lead is considered diagnostic of AMI
  - Not mandated in current AHA/ACC STEMI guidelines

U-Wave Learning Points

- U-waves are typically low-amplitude deflections that follow the T-wave, best seen in the anterior precordial leads at slower heart rates
- Clinical significance not fully understood
  - Can see U-waves larger than T-waves with moderate to severe hypokalemia
  - Inverted U-waves in leads V2-V5 is abnormal (seen with ischemia and hypertension)
- When measuring the QT interval, exclude U-waves or measure in a lead without U-waves (usually leads aVR or aVL)

Case 97: Presentation

A 67-year-old male presents with chest pain. What is your interpretation of his ECG?

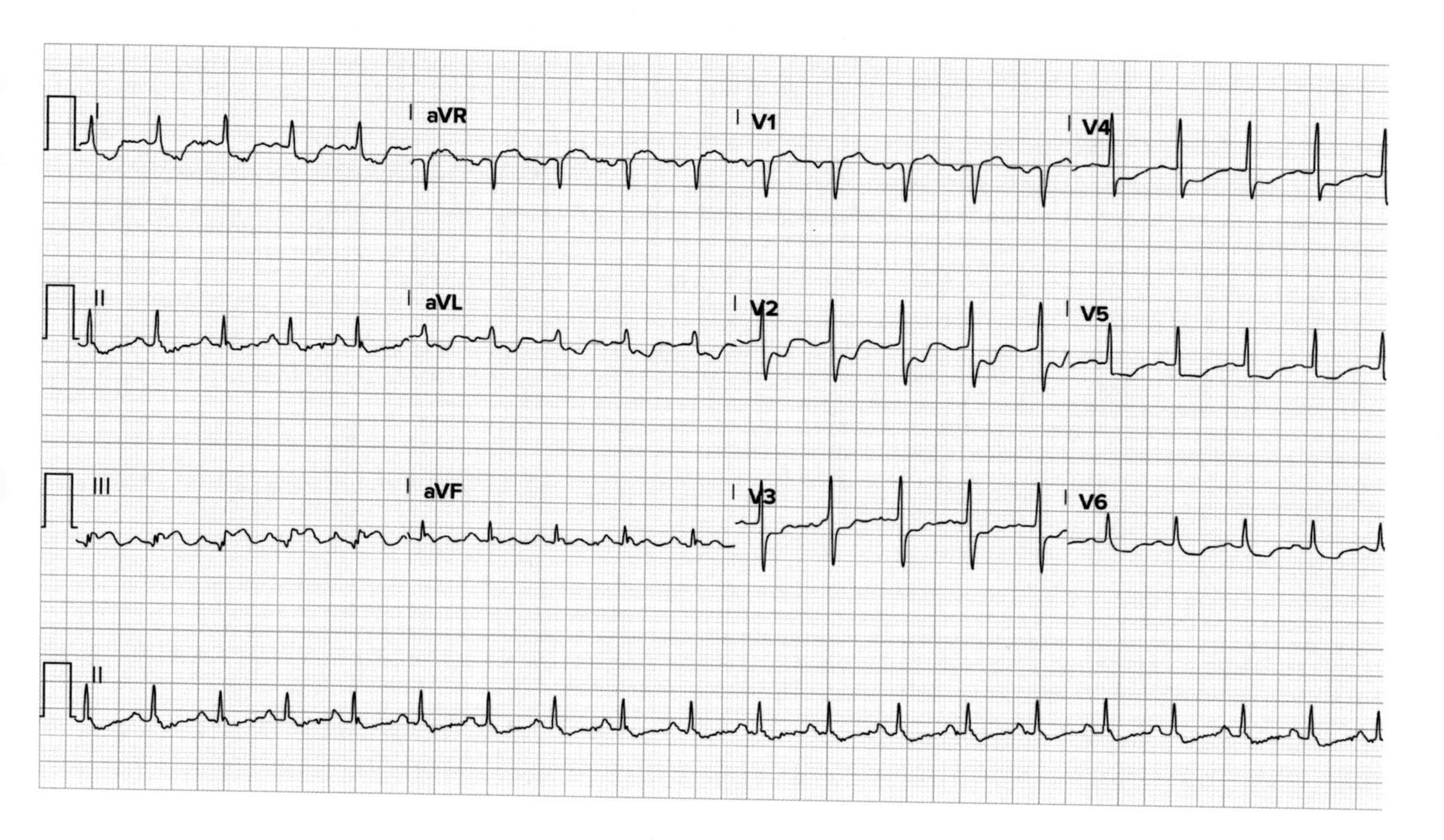

Case 97: Answer

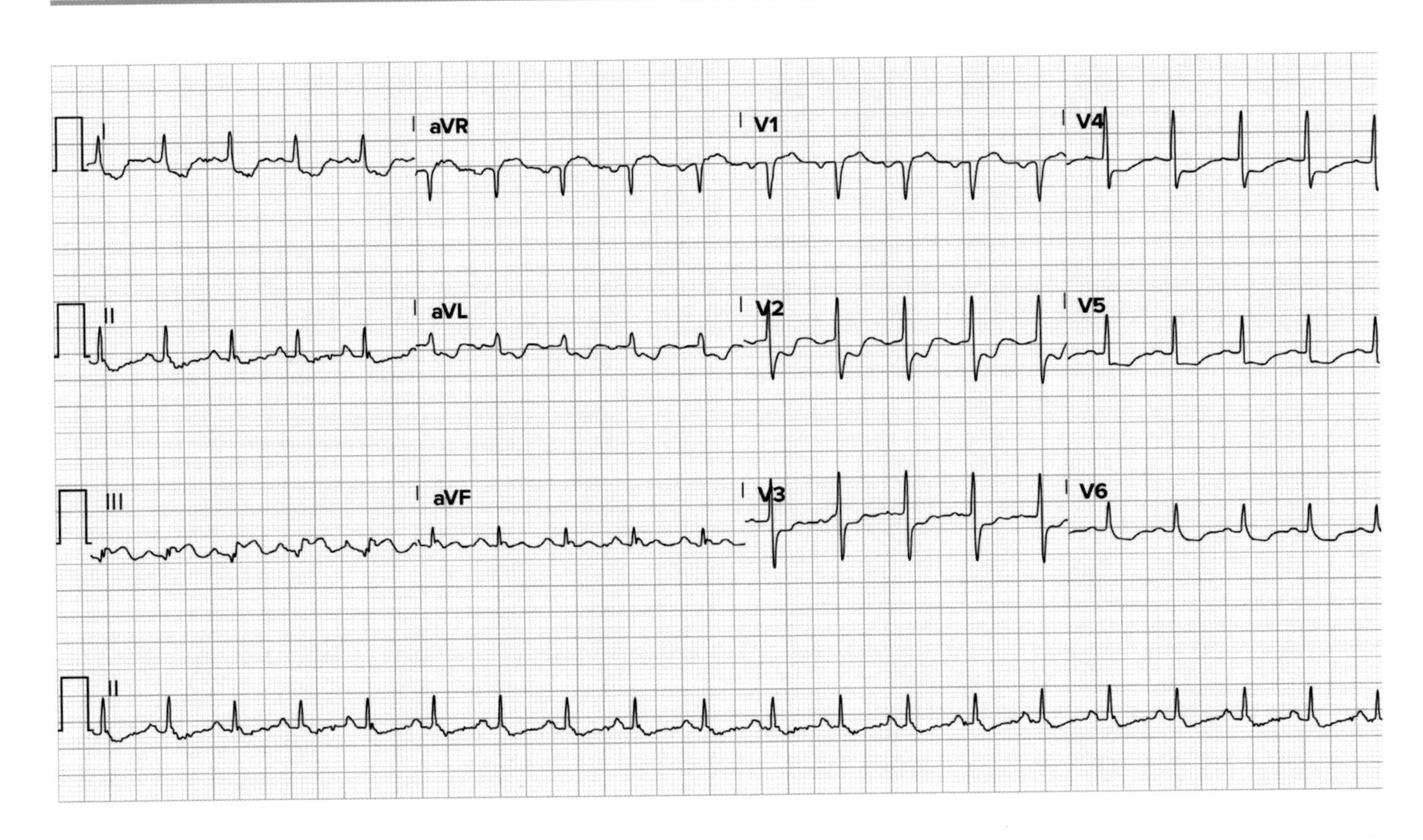

This ECG shows sinus tachycardia at 116 bpm, normal axis, STE in leads aVR, V1, and III with STD in leads I, aVL, II, and V2-V6.

The pattern of STE and STD in this ECG looks a lot like the "aVR pattern" (ie, STE in lead aVR +/- V1 with diffuse STD) and, in the setting of sinus tachycardia, suggests non-ACS etiologies, such as PE or acute blood loss with severe anemia. The key to interpreting this ECG is the STE in lead III which does not fit the "aVR pattern" and should prompt further investigation. Although leads aVR, V1, and III are not considered contiguous leads, they all image the right side of the heart so a repeat ECG was obtained with right-sided leads ***(see Figure 1)***. It also would have been reasonable to obtain a posterior ECG given the STD and tall R-waves in leads V2-V4.

Figure 1.
Repeat ECG with right-sided leads V3R-V6R

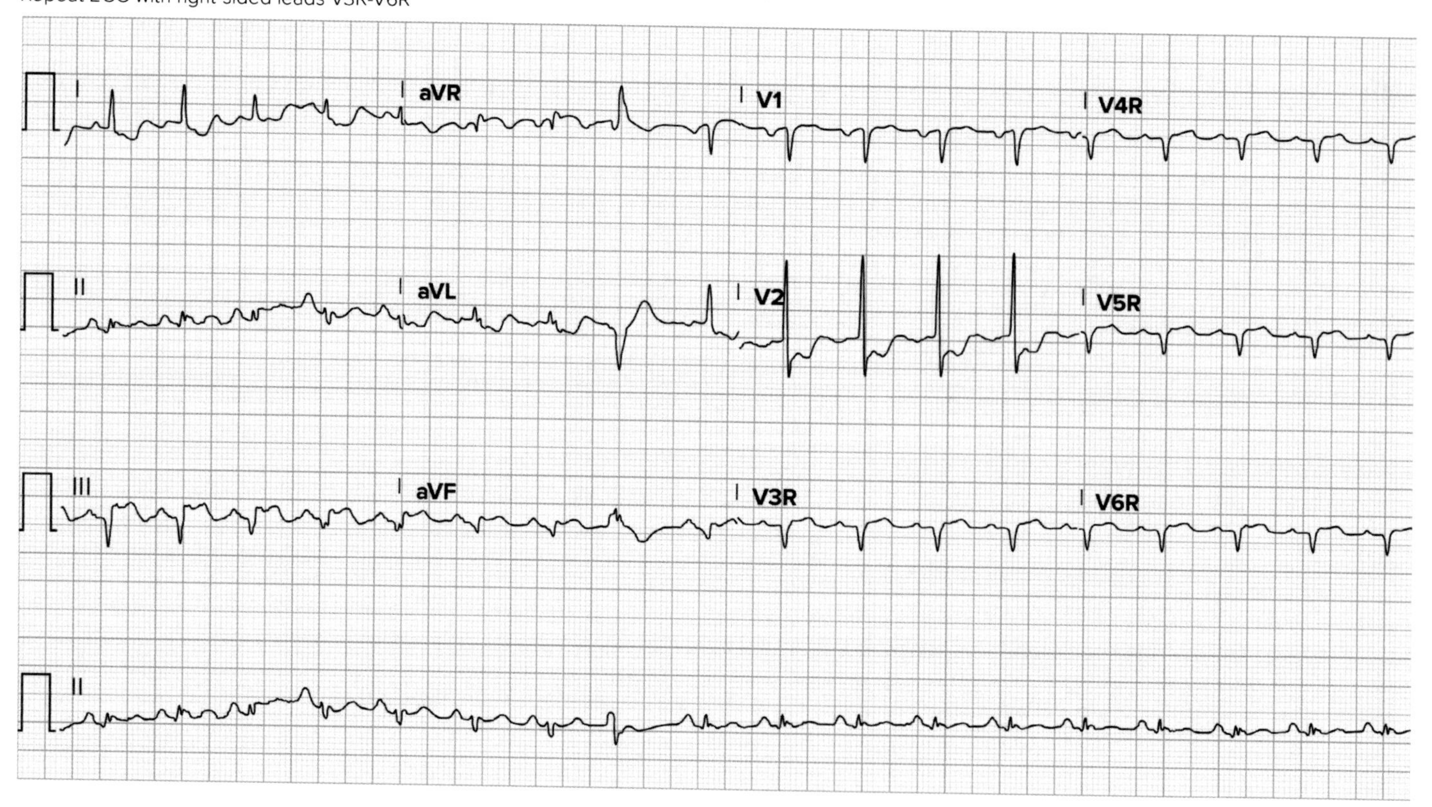

The right-sided ECG shows STE > 0.5 mm in in leads V3R and V4R as well as STE in leads III and aVF that meets traditional STEMI criteria. There are also now pathologic Q-waves and STE in both leads III and aVF.

Figure 2.
Recommended placement of right-sided leads

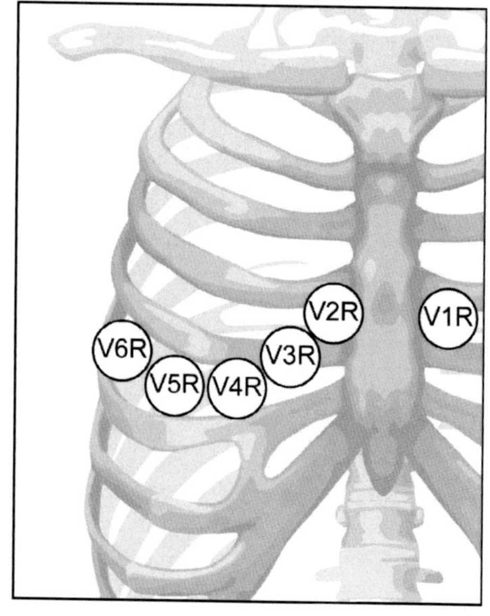

Isolated right ventricular MIs are rare and the criteria put forth in the 2018 Fourth Universal Definition of MI state:

- *In patients with inferior and suspected right ventricular infarction, leads aVR or V1 may exhibit ST-segment elevation ≥ 1 mm. The early recording of right precordial leads V3R and V4R should be performed, since ST-elevation ≥ 0.5 mm (≥ 1 mm in men < 30 years old) provides supportive criteria for the diagnosis.*[1]

There is no further explanation of whether "supportive criteria" warrants activation of the catheterization laboratory and there is no discussion about the utility of the other right-sided leads, such as leads V5R-V6R.

The importance of identifying RV involvement, often seen concurrently with inferior MI, is that these patients will be preload dependent and the use of vasodilatory medications such as nitroglycerin can lead to hypotension.

Q-waves are the initial negative deflection that precede the upright R-wave of the QRS complex and can be pathological or non-pathological (see Learning Points below). Pathologic Q-waves generally are defined as ≥ 40 msec and/or ≥ 25-33% of accompanying R-wave height.

In the past, MIs were classified as Q-wave MI and non-Q-wave MI. Although these terms are no longer used, misconceptions based on this classification system persist. Current cardiology research has shown:

- Q-waves correlate with size or infarction but do not differentiate between transmural and non-transmural/ subendocardial infarction
- Q-waves associated with infarction are not permanent and can resolve or diminish over time
- Q-waves do not predict viability of myocardium (a common misconception)
- There is a high risk for LV dysfunction with Q-waves that suggest a large infarction, but LV dysfunction can occur in the absence of Q-waves

This patient was taken to the cardiac catheterization laboratory where a 100% occlusion of the mid-RCA was successfully treated with a stent.

Right Ventricular MI Learning Points

- Consider with any inferior MI
  - RV MI is present in 25-30% of inferior STEMI
- Findings seen with inferior MI that should prompt further evaluation with right-sided leads:
  - STE in lead V1 + STD in lead V2
  - STD in lead V2 + isoelectric ST-segment in lead V1
- Right-sided leads V1R-V6R evaluate for RV MI
  - STE in leads V3R and V4R ≥ 0.5 mm (≥ 1 mm for men ≤ 30 years old)
  - STE in lead V4R > 1 mm most predictive of RV MI
  - STE in lead V4R > STE in leads V1-V3 is highly specific for RV MI
- RV infarct = preload dependent
  - Avoid preload reducing medications (eg, nitroglycerin, morphine, etc.)
  - Consider increasing preload with fluid bolus

Q-waves Learning Points

- Can be pathological or non-pathological (see table below)
- Pathologic Q-waves generally defined as ≥40 msec and/or ≥ 25-33% of accompanying R-wave height
- When due to an MI:
  - Occur in ≥ 2 contiguous leads that also have STE
  - Size correlates with volume of infarcted myocardium
  - Early appearance of Q-waves does not always indicate irreversible myocardial death, particularly with simultaneous STE and/or shorter period of ACS symptoms
  - Tall R-waves in leads V1 and V2 may represent Q-waves due to a posterior MI
- QS complex = single large negative deflection
  - Usually indicates significant irreversible myocardial loss when associated with ischemia
  - QS complex with STE and diminished T-wave should prompt evaluation for LV aneurysm
- Q-waves in leads V1 and V2 can be caused by misplacement of leads in the 2nd or 3rd intercostal spaces

Q-wave Causes	
Physiologic	Normal variant in leads V1, V2, III, and/or aVR
Structural	LVH RVH HCM
Conduction	LBBB Pre-excitation rhythms
Myocardial	Infarct Cardiomyopathy Myocarditis Infiltrative disease

References

1. Thygesen K, Alpert JS, Jaffe AS, et al. 2018 ESC/ACC/AHA/WHF Expert Consensus Document: Fourth Universal Definition of Myocardial Infarction (2018). Circulation. 2018;138:e618-e651.

Case 98: Presentation

A 46-year-old male with no past medical history presents with cough, subjective fevers, body aches, and palpitations. What is your interpretation of his ECG?

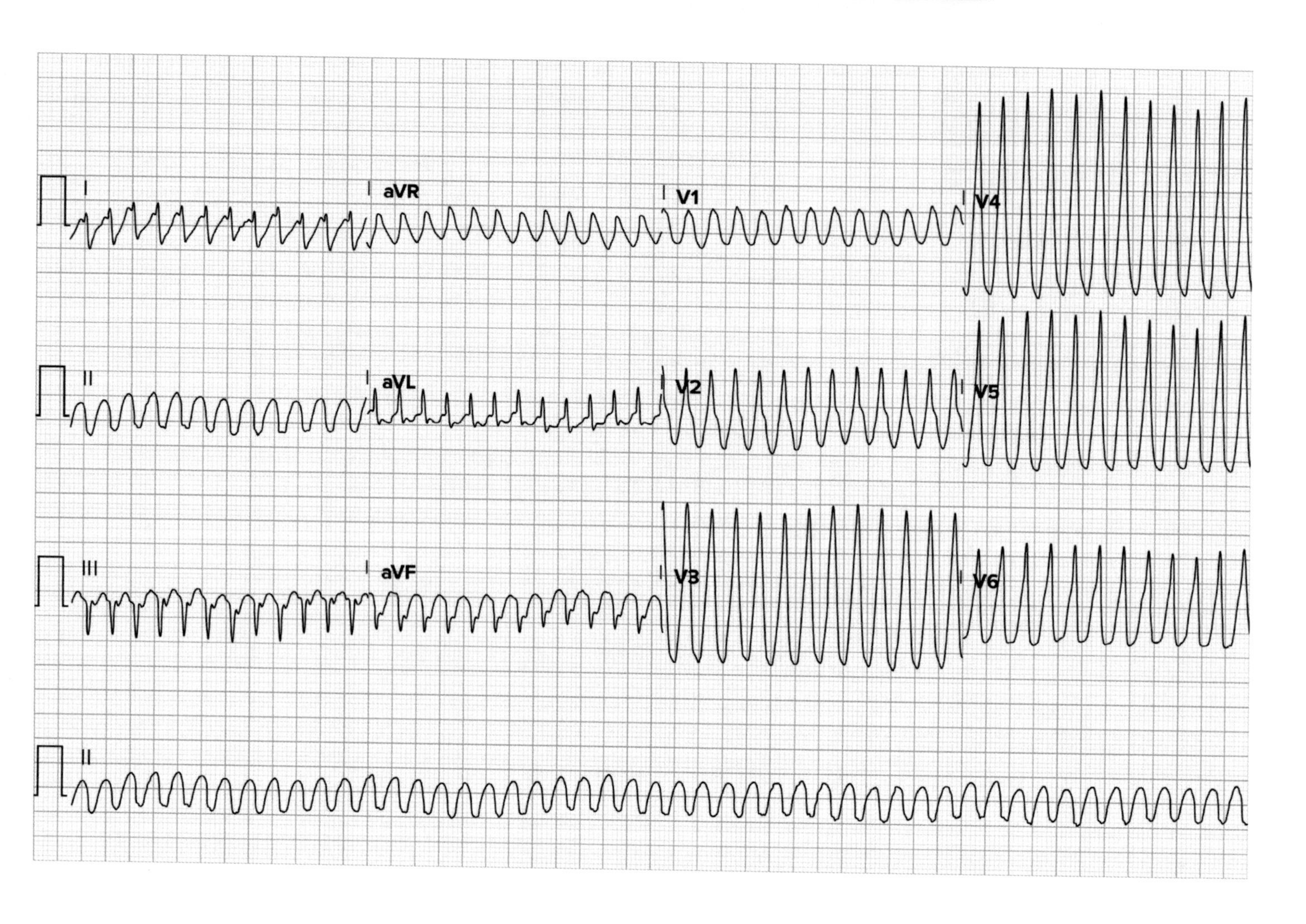

Case 98: Answer

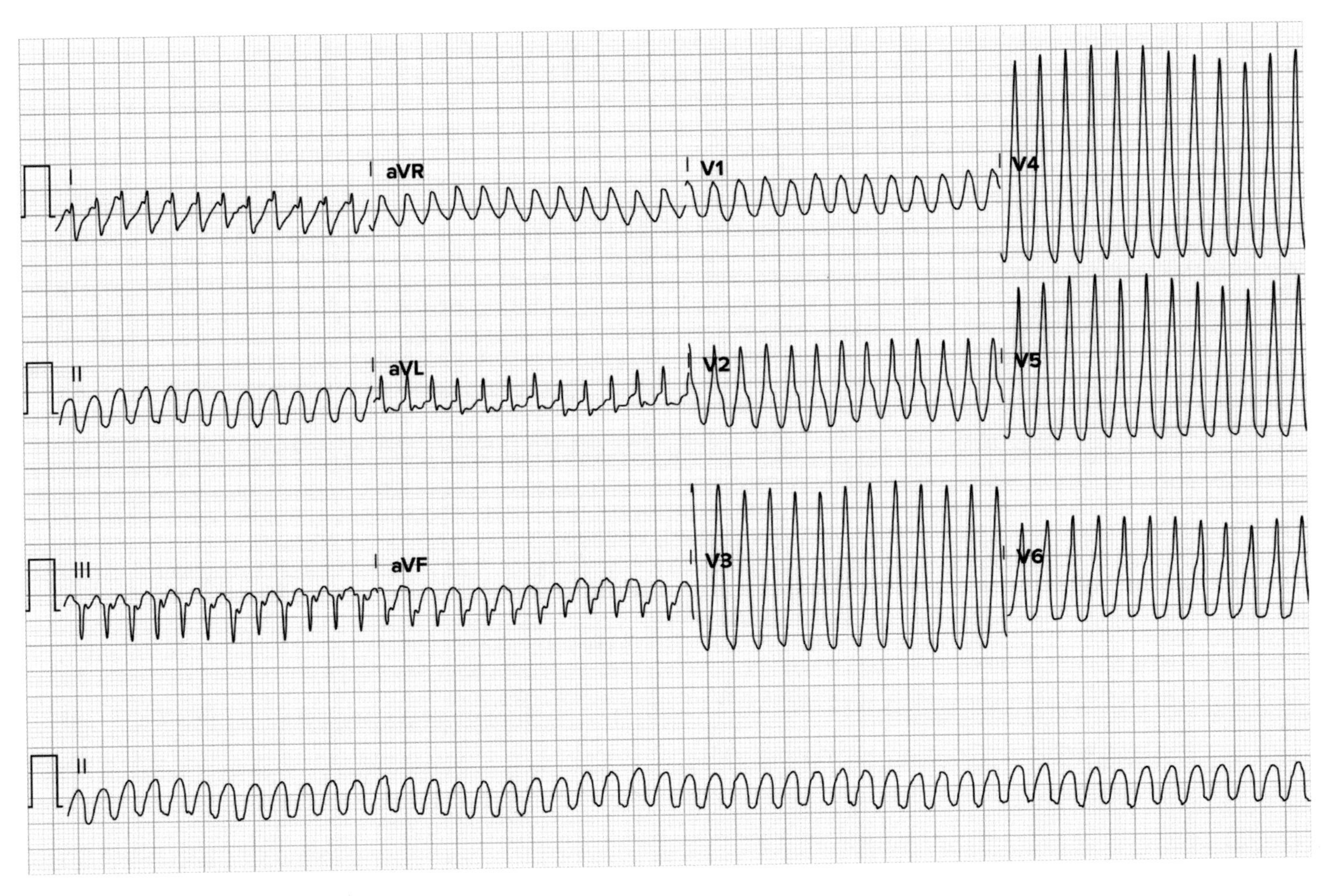

This ECG shows a regular wide-complex tachycardia with a ventricular rate of 297 bpm, northwest/extreme axis deviation, and prolonged QRS complex duration.

The differential diagnosis for a regular wide complex tachycardia includes:

- Monomorphic ventricular tachycardia
- Antidromic AVRT
- Any regular SVT (eg, sinus tach, AVNRT, atrial flutter, etc.) with aberrant conduction
  - Causes of aberrant conduction include fixed or rate-related BBB, metabolic abnormalities, sodium channel blocker toxicity, ventricular-paced rhythm, and ventricular pre-excitation (eg, WPW)

There are multiple findings in this ECG that suggest monomorphic VT, including:

- Northwest/extreme axis deviation
- The absence of typical RBBB or LBBB pattern
- Positive QRS complex concordance in leads V1-V6 (ie, all of the QRS complexes point up) ***(see Figure 1)***

Figure 1.
Positive QRS complex concordance in leads V1-V6

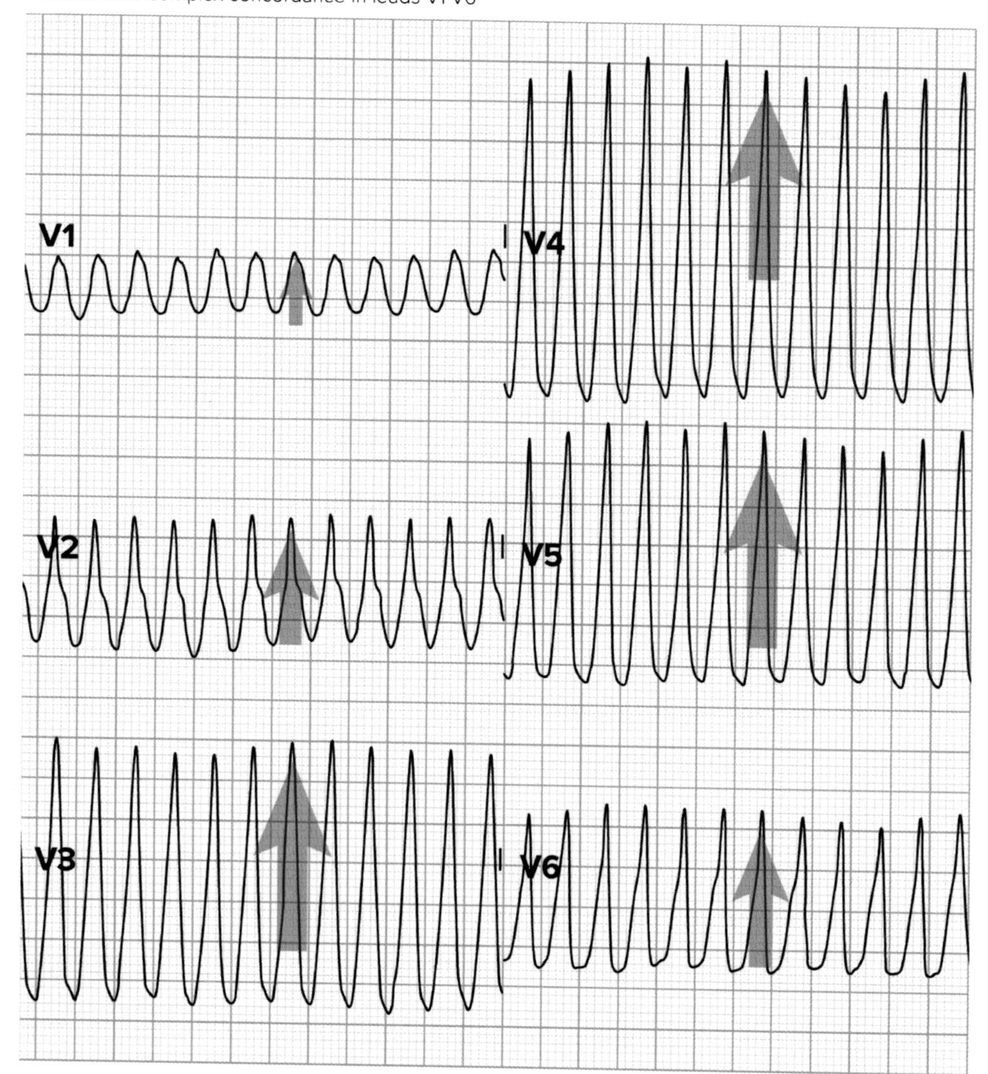

This patient's ED course was complicated by VT storm. VT storm, also called VT/VF storm, electrical storm, or arrhythmic storm, refers to a state of cardiac electrical instability that is generally defined as ≥3 episodes of sustained VT, VF, or appropriate shocks from an ICD within 24 hours.[1] It is most common in patients with an implantable ICD, which makes sense since these patients have an ICD because they are at a high risk for ventricular dysrhythmias. This patient was eventually stabilized on an esmolol drip and was admitted to the cardiac ICU. His workup was unremarkable except for a positive COVID-19 test, which was the suspected trigger of his VT storm.

Monomorphic VT Learning Points

- ≥ 3 consecutive, regular, wide complex beats with rate > 120-130 bpm
  - Non-sustained: < 30 sec duration with no hemodynamic instability
  - Sustained: ≥ 30 sec duration OR causes hemodynamic instability
- Rates < 120-130 bpm can be seen in patients on chronic antidysrhythmic medications (eg, amiodarone, flecainide, sotalol) or with severe cardiomyopathies
- If rate < 120 bpm, consider mimics:
  - Hyperkalemia
  - Sodium channel blocker toxicity
  - Accelerated idioventricular rhythm (AIVR)
- ECG features that increase the likelihood of VT in a regular WCT:
  - QRS complex duration > 200 msec is almost always VT, hyperkalemia, or sodium channel blocker toxicity
  - AV dissociation (ventricular rate > atrial rate)
  - Positive or negative QRS complex concordance in leads V1-V6 (entirely or predominantly positive or negative QRS complexes from leads V1 to V6)
  - Extreme axis deviation ("northwest axis")

- The absence of typical RBBB or LBBB pattern suggests VT (ie, normal RBBB or LBBB pattern makes SVT with aberrant conduction more likely)
- Fusion beats: hybrid QRS complex formed by both supraventricular and ventricular focus
- Capture beats: sinus QRS formed by transient normal conduction amid AV dissociation
- Brugada's sign: time from the onset of the QRS complex to the nadir of the S-wave is > 100 msec ***(see Figure 2)***
- Josephson's sign: notching on the downslope of the S-wave near its nadir ***(see Figure 3)***

Figure 2

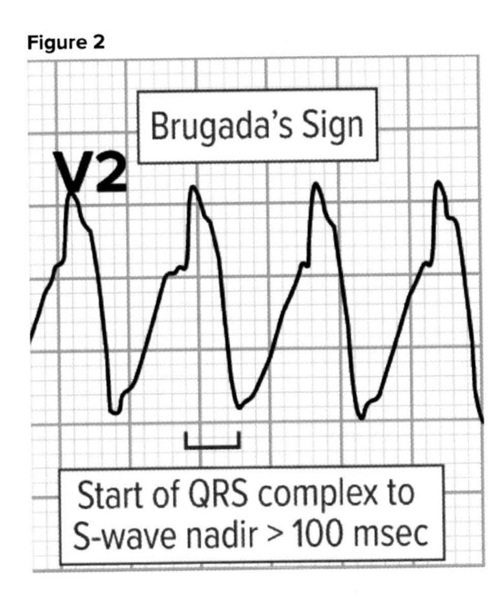

Figure 3

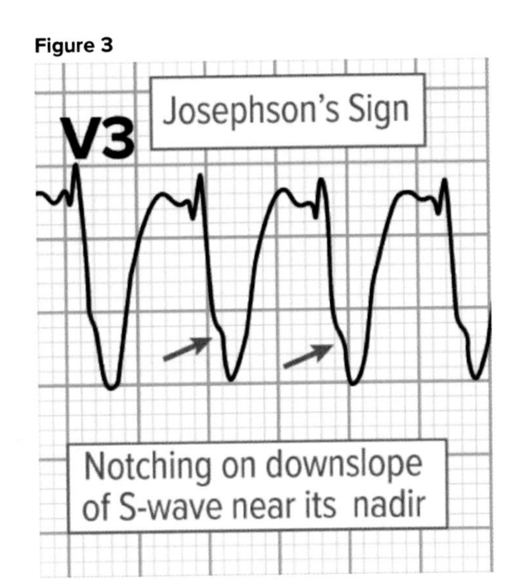

References

1. Al-Khatib SM, Stevenson WG, Ackerman MJ, et al. 2017 AHA/ACC/HRS guideline for management of patients with ventricular arrhythmias and the prevention of sudden cardiac death: a report of the American College of Cardiology Foundation/American Heart Association Task Force on Clinical Practice Guidelines and the Heart Rhythm Society. Circulation. 2018;138:e272–e391.

Case 99: Presentation

A 47-year-old female with history of dual chamber pacemaker due to ischemic cardiomyopathy presents with shortness of breath and orthopnea. Vital sign abnormalities include an oxygen saturation of 87%. What is your interpretation of her ECG?

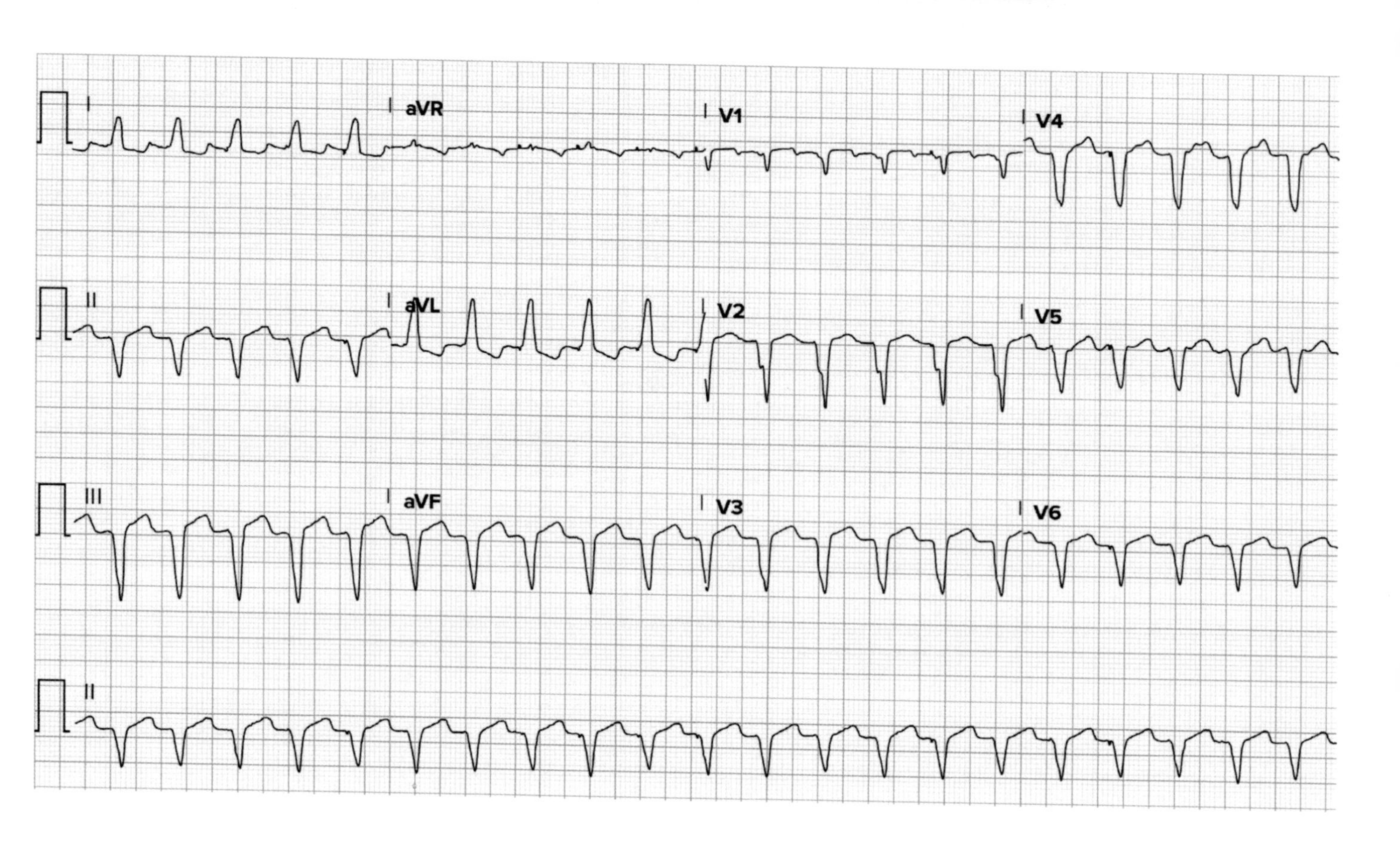

Case 99: Answer

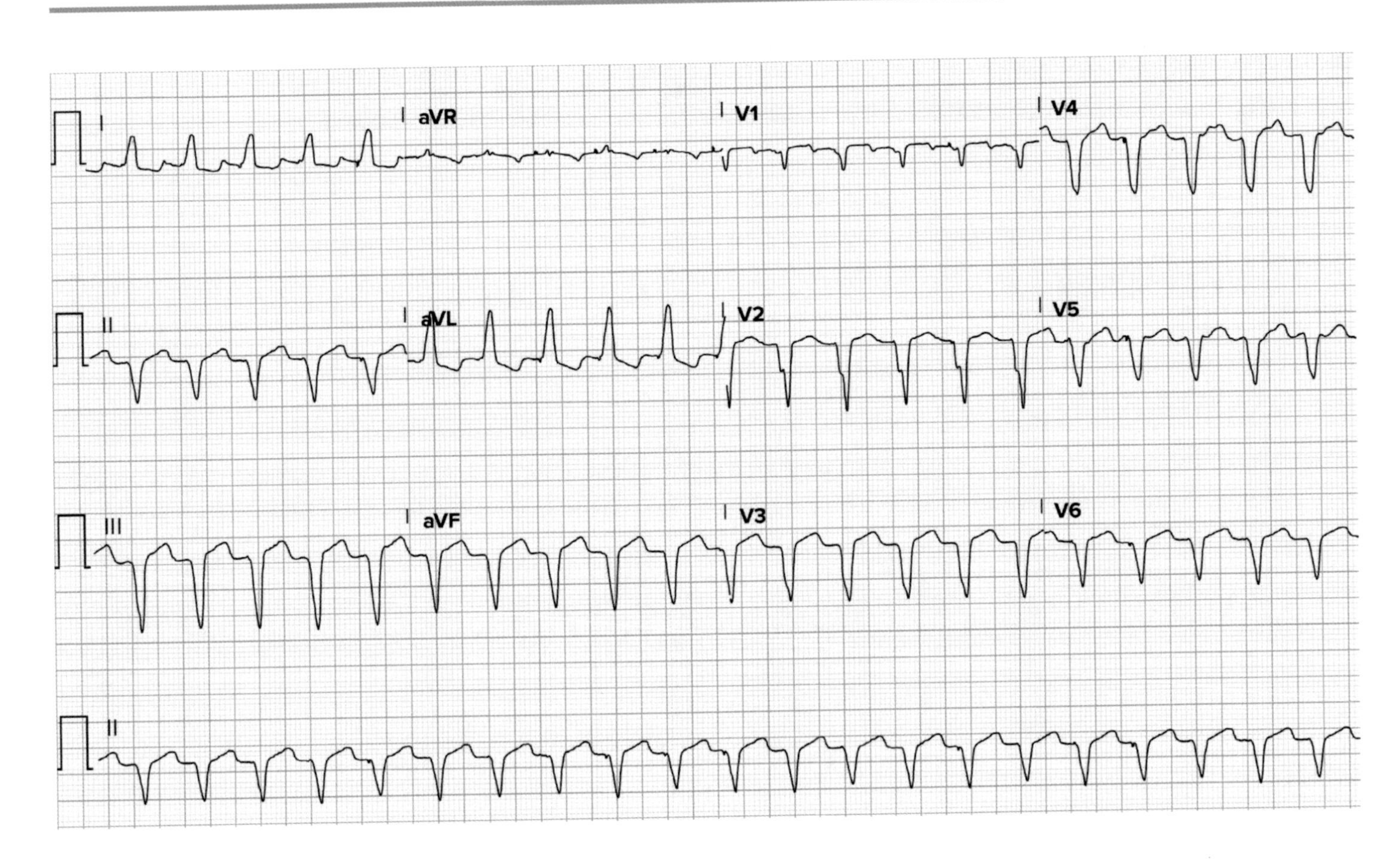

This ECG shows an atrial-sensed, ventricular-paced rhythm with a ventricular rate of 130 bpm, first degree AV block, left axis deviation, and a prolonged QRS complex duration with a LBBB-like morphology. Note that the QRS complex in V6 is negatively oriented which is normal for right ventricular pacing.

The key to interpreting this ECG is in lead V4 which best visualizes the P-waves that are partially hidden in the T-waves ***(see Figure 1)***. The presence of P-waves preceding the QRS complexes suggests that this pacer is appropriately functioning (ie, atrial-sensed and ventricular-paced). There are no downward deflections in the T-waves in leads I, II, and aVF that would suggest inverted P-waves so it is reasonable to assume that the P-waves are sinus in origin. The PR interval is slightly prolonged at 220 msec which is not unusual is AV pacing.

Figure 1.
Native P-waves followed by ventricular pacing, best seen in lead V4, consistent with an atrial-sensed, ventricular-paced rhythm

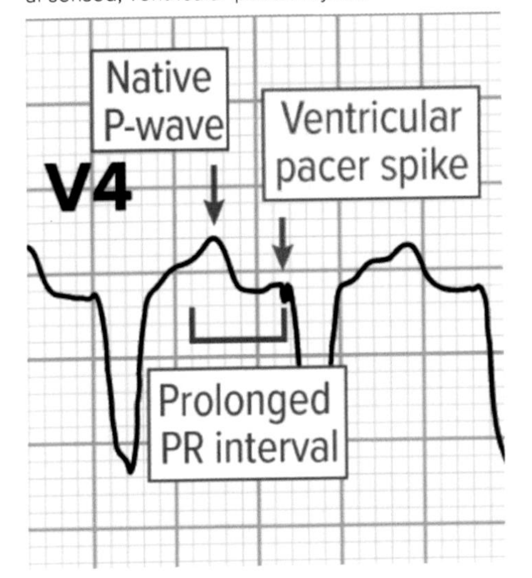

Note that the ventricular pacer spikes are not always apparent before every QRS complex in every lead. In this ECG, the ventricular pacer spikes are best seen on the bottom of the ECG tracing below the lead II rhythm strip ***(see Figure 2)***.

Figure 2.
Ventricular pacer spikes best seen below the lead II rhythm strip

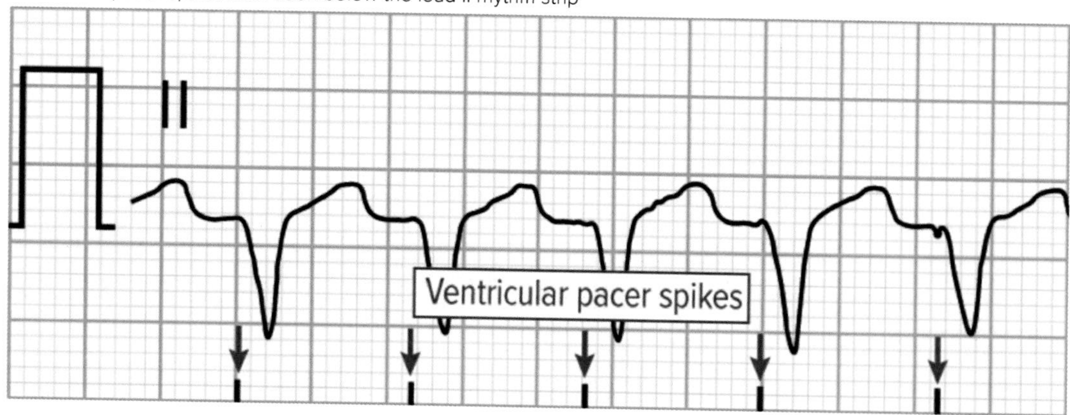

The initial interpretation of this ECG was pacemaker-mediated tachycardia (PMT) which happens when a paced ventricular beat conducts retrograde to the atria. If the atria is outside the refractory period it will depolarize. The pacer senses this and initiates another ventricular beat. This creates a repeating cycle similar to AVNRT with the ventricular pacing lead acting as the antegrade pathway. PMT can be treated with a magnet which will result in the pacer defaulting to the factory set pacing rate (typically 60-70 bpm). It can also be treated like AVNRT with adenosine or nodal blockers.

The importance of distinguishing between PMT and appropriate AV pacing is highlighted in this patient's clinical course. A stat chest X-ray showed pulmonary edema which taken in context of her chief complaint of SOB and orthopnea in the setting of a baseline ischemic cardiomyopathy is concerning for an acute CHF exacerbation. If the patient was in PMT than it would have been appropriate to treat the dysrhythmia in order to improve cardiac function. In this case, the patient's tachycardia was compensatory and inappropriately treating it as PMT could have acutely worsened her clinical condition. The patient was placed on BiPAP and started on IV diuretics and admitted to the cardiology service.

Pacemaker Learning Points

- Pacer spikes are usually visible on the ECG, either at the bottom of the ECG and/or preceding the P-wave and/or QRS complex
  - Atrial pacing: spikes immediately precede P-waves
  - Ventricular pacing: spikes immediately precede QRS complexes
  - Dual chamber pacing: spikes immediately precede both P-waves and QRS complexes
  - Biventricular pacing: 2 spikes immediately precede QRS complexes
- Atrial pacing
  - Pacemaker lead usually implanted in the right atrial appendage
  - Results in P-waves with normal morphology
- Right ventricle pacing
  - Pacemaker lead usually implanted in the RV apex
  - Results in a LBBB pattern in the limb leads and anteroseptal precordial leads
  - The major difference between an intrinsic LBBB and a right ventricular-paced rhythm is that the QRS complex will almost always be negatively oriented in leads V5-V6 with a right ventricular-paced rhythm
- Biventricular pacing
  - Two pacemaker leads usually implanted in the RV apex and the surface of the posterior or lateral LV
  - Typically results in a narrower QRS complex than with right ventricular pacing
  - Dominant R-wave in lead V1 +/- V2 is common
- AICD will have a thick coil that differentiates it from a pacemaker

Pacemaker-Mediated Tachycardia Learning Points

- Re-entry tachycardia with antegrade conduction via the pacemaker and retrograde conduction via the AV node
- ECG will show a paced wide-complex tachycardia (may see retrograde P-waves)
- Treat with magnet, adenosine, or nodal blockers

Case 100: Presentation

A 73-year-old female with history of atrial fibrillation and congestive heart failure presents with generalized weakness. What is your interpretation of her ECG?

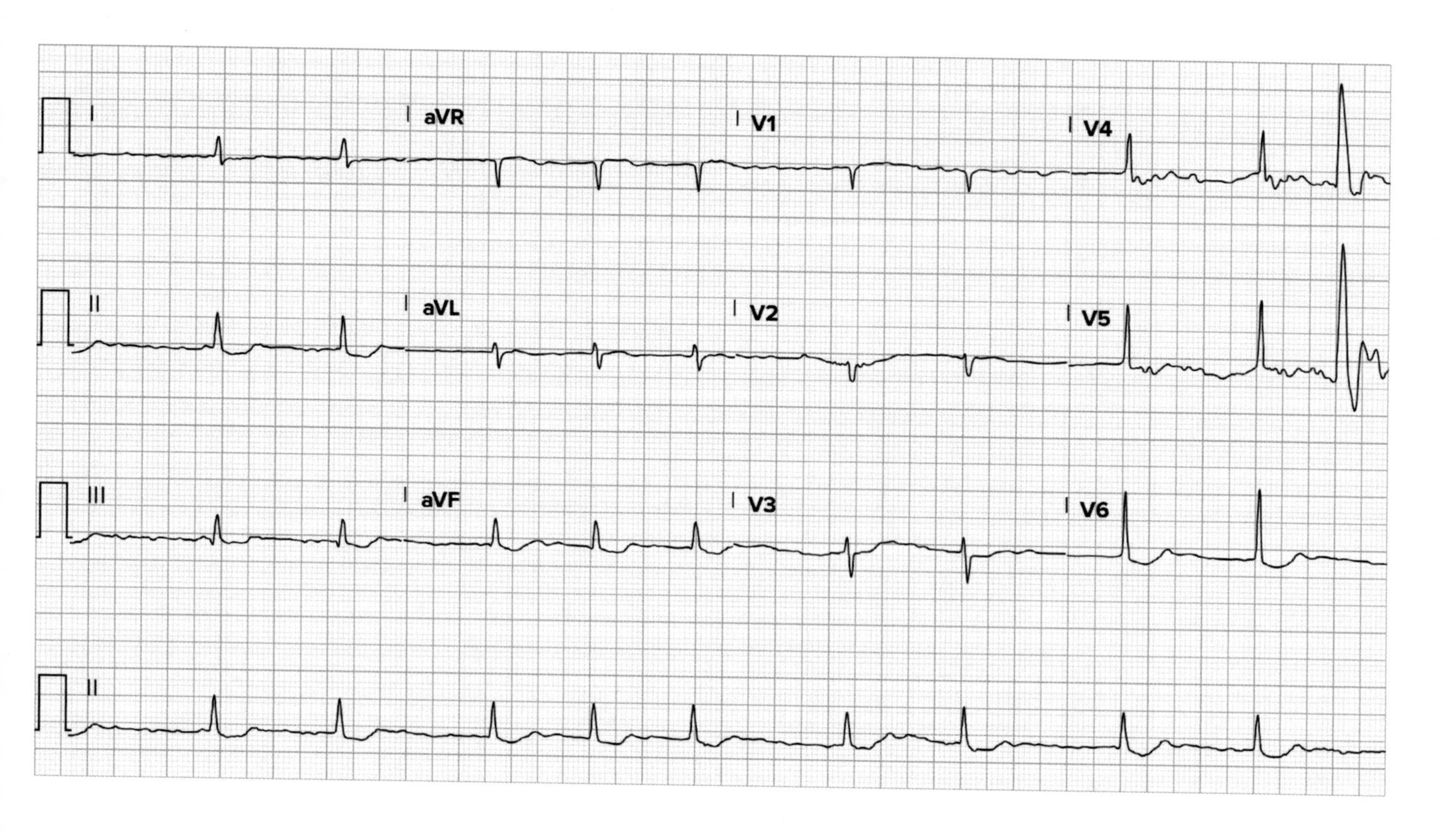

Case 100: Answer

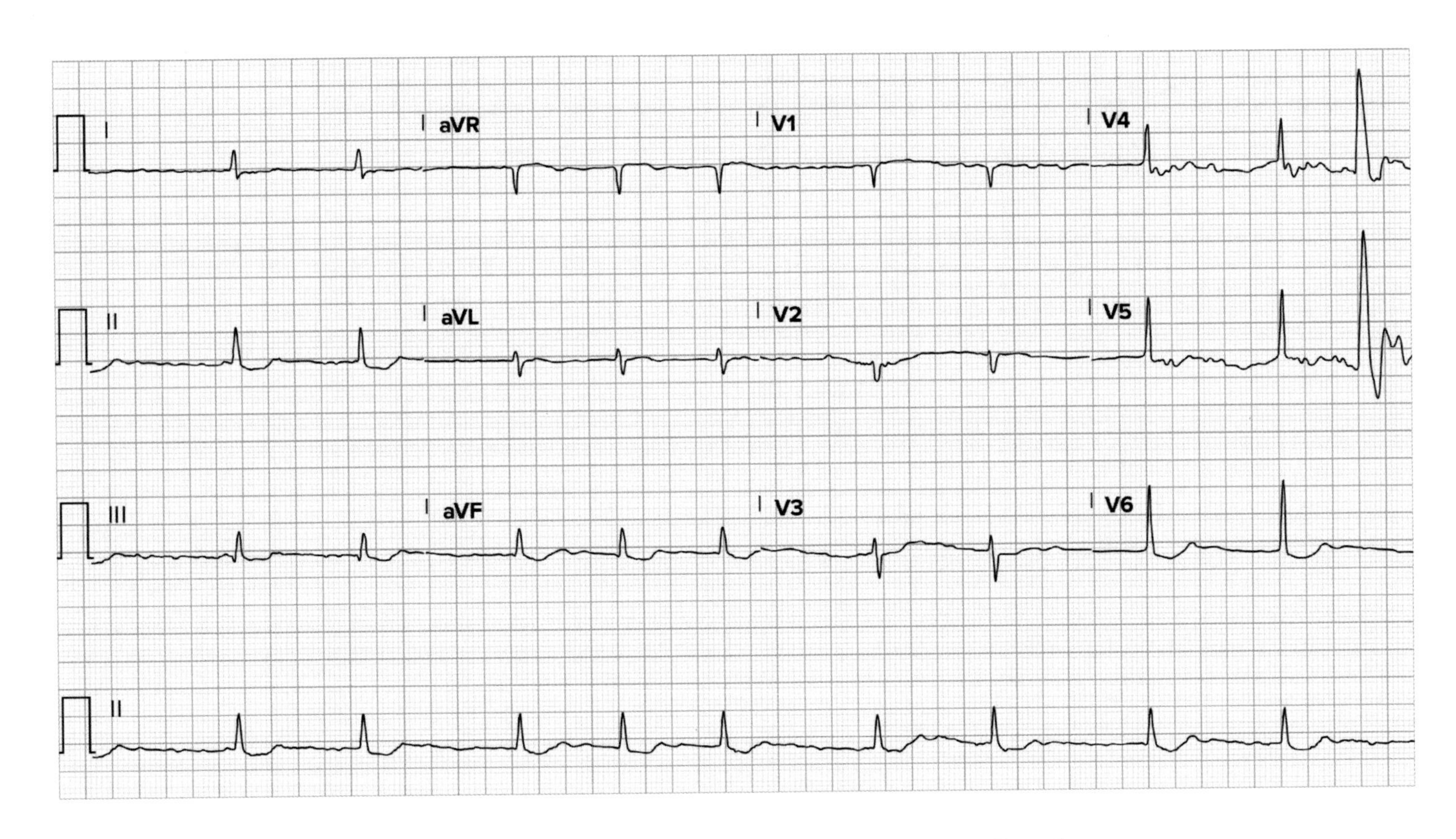

This ECG shows atrial fibrillation with an average ventricular rate of 53 bpm, normal axis, normal intervals, and slight STD with scooped ST-segments in leads II, III, aVF, and V6. Interpretation of leads V4-V5 is confounded by artifact.

The scooped ST-segments seen in this ECG are commonly referred to as the digoxin effect ***(see Figure 1)***, or the Salvador Dali sign (in reference to this gentleman's moustache), and is a sign of digoxin's presence with penetration into the myocardial tissues, rather than toxicity. This effect also includes PR interval lengthening and QT interval shortening.

Figure 1.
Lead V6 shows scooped ST-segments seen with digoxin use, called digoxin effect or the Salvador Dali sign

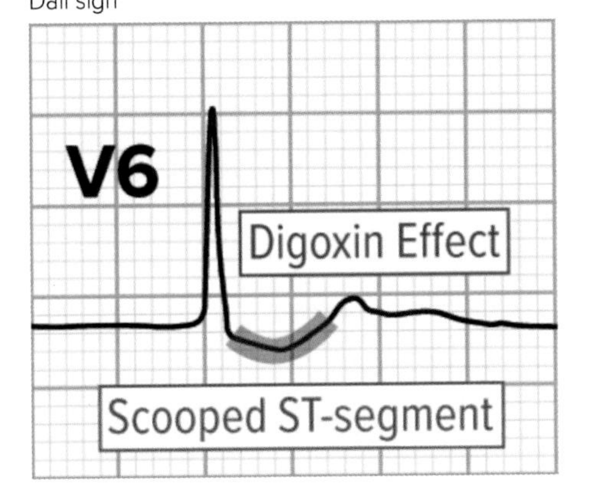

The key to accurately interpreting this ECG is recognizing that atrial fibrillation with slow ventricular response is abnormal and warrants further investigation. Important etiologies to consider include antidysrhythmic medication toxicity (eg, digoxin, nodal blockers such as CCB or beta-blockers, etc.) and electrolyte abnormalities such as hyperkalemia.

Dysrhythmias associated with digoxin toxicity are varied, and if digoxin toxicity were more common, it would certainly compete with hyperkalemia for the title of the "syphilis of electrocardiography."[1] A range of bradycardias, tachycardias, and various blocks can be seen in the patient with digoxin toxicity. Common findings include PACs and PVCs, and dysrhythmias associated with toxicity include paroxysmal atrial tachycardia with variable block and bradycardic rate, accelerated junctional rhythms, bidirectional ventricular tachycardia, and atrial fibrillation with slow ventricular response or a regular bradycardic rate due to the presence of a 3rd degree AV block.

Cardiac glycosides, which includes digoxin, are inhibitors of the sodium-potassium ATPase pump. Other cardiac glycosides include foxglove, oleander, and lily of the valley. Common causes of chronic toxicity include renal disease, electrolyte abnormalities, dehydration, and drug interactions. Common symptoms seen with chronic toxicity include anorexia, abdominal pain, nausea, and CNS symptoms (eg, AMS). Concurrent hyperkalemia is associated with a high mortality rate. Note that patients can have digoxin toxicity clinically with normal serum concentrations, especially in the presence of hypomagnesemia, hypokalemia, and/or hypercalcemia.

First-line treatment for symptomatic dysrhythmias is digoxin immune Fab (eg, Digibind or DigiFab). Other treatments include atropine for bradycardias and AV blocks, and lidocaine or phenytoin for ventricular tachycardias if digoxin immune Fab is unavailable or ineffective. Treatment with digoxin immune Fab will cause potassium to shift into the cells and can lead to clinically significant hypokalemia, so potassium levels should be monitored closely after administration.

This patient's labs were notable for hypokalemia, likely due to over-diuresis, and a normal digoxin level. This patient's heart rate normalized after potassium repletion, illustrating how hypokalemia can lead to digoxin toxicity clinically even with a normal digoxin level.

Digoxin Learning Points

- ECG features seen with therapeutic level (ie, not necessarily signs of toxicity):
  - Scooped ST-segments (ie, digoxin effect) most pronounced in leads with tall R-waves
  - PR interval lengthening
  - QT interval shortening
- "Pathognomonic" dysrhythmias seen with toxicity:
  - Atrial fibrillation with slow ventricular response or a regular bradycardic rate
  - Paroxysmal atrial tachycardia with variable block and bradycardic rate (uncommon)
  - Bidirectional ventricular tachycardia (very rare)
- Acute toxicity may present with hyperkalemia
- Treatment includes:
  - Digoxin-specific antibody (eg, Digibind): causes serum digoxin levels to rise making repeat levels unreliable
  - Atropine for AV blocks
  - Phenytoin or lidocaine for ventricular dysrhythmias

References

1. Mattu A. ECG Weekly.

NOTES:

Case 101: Presentation

A 21-year-old male is brought to the ED by police after he was found with altered mental status, naked outside on a rainy night. What is your interpretation of his EKG?

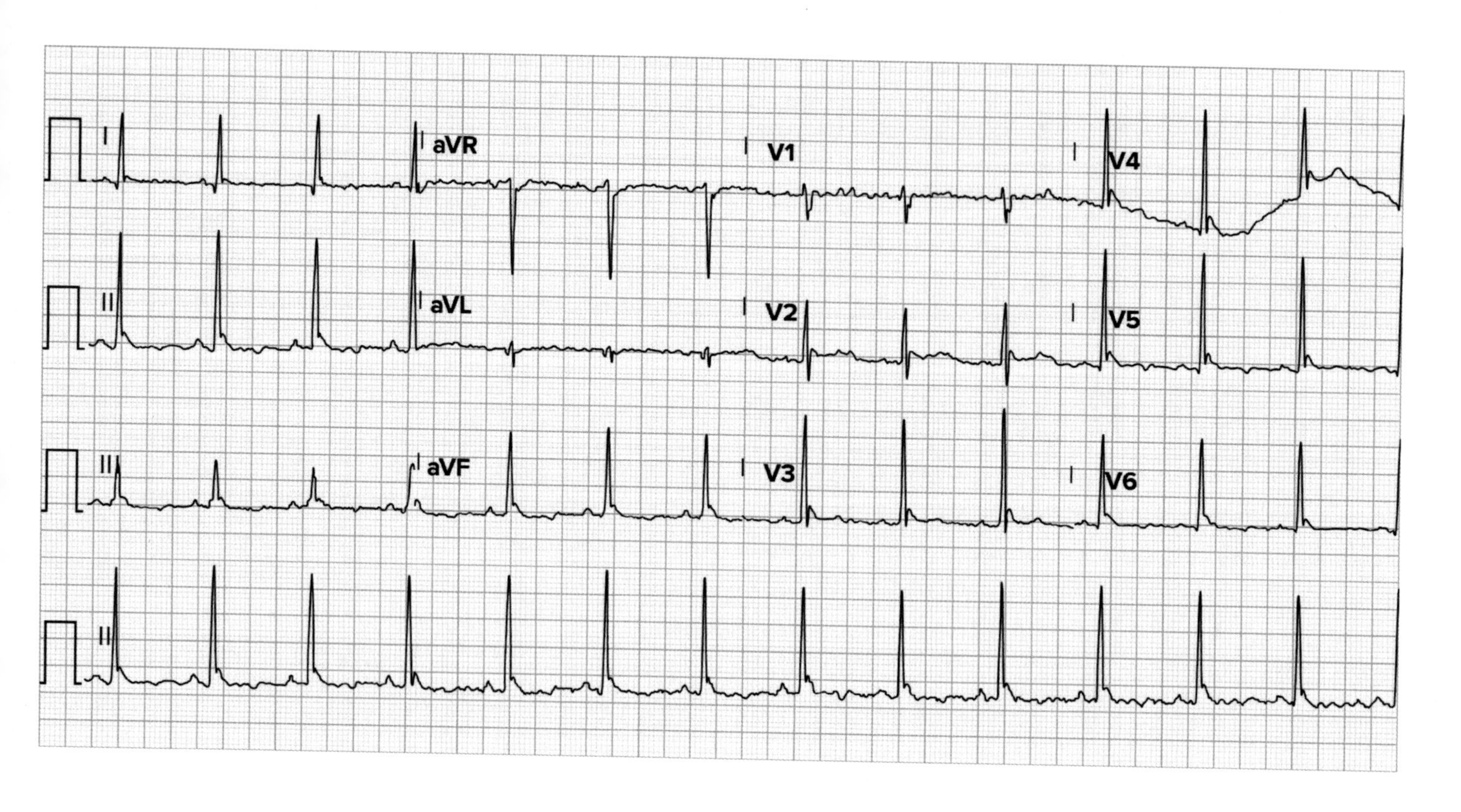

Case 101: Answer

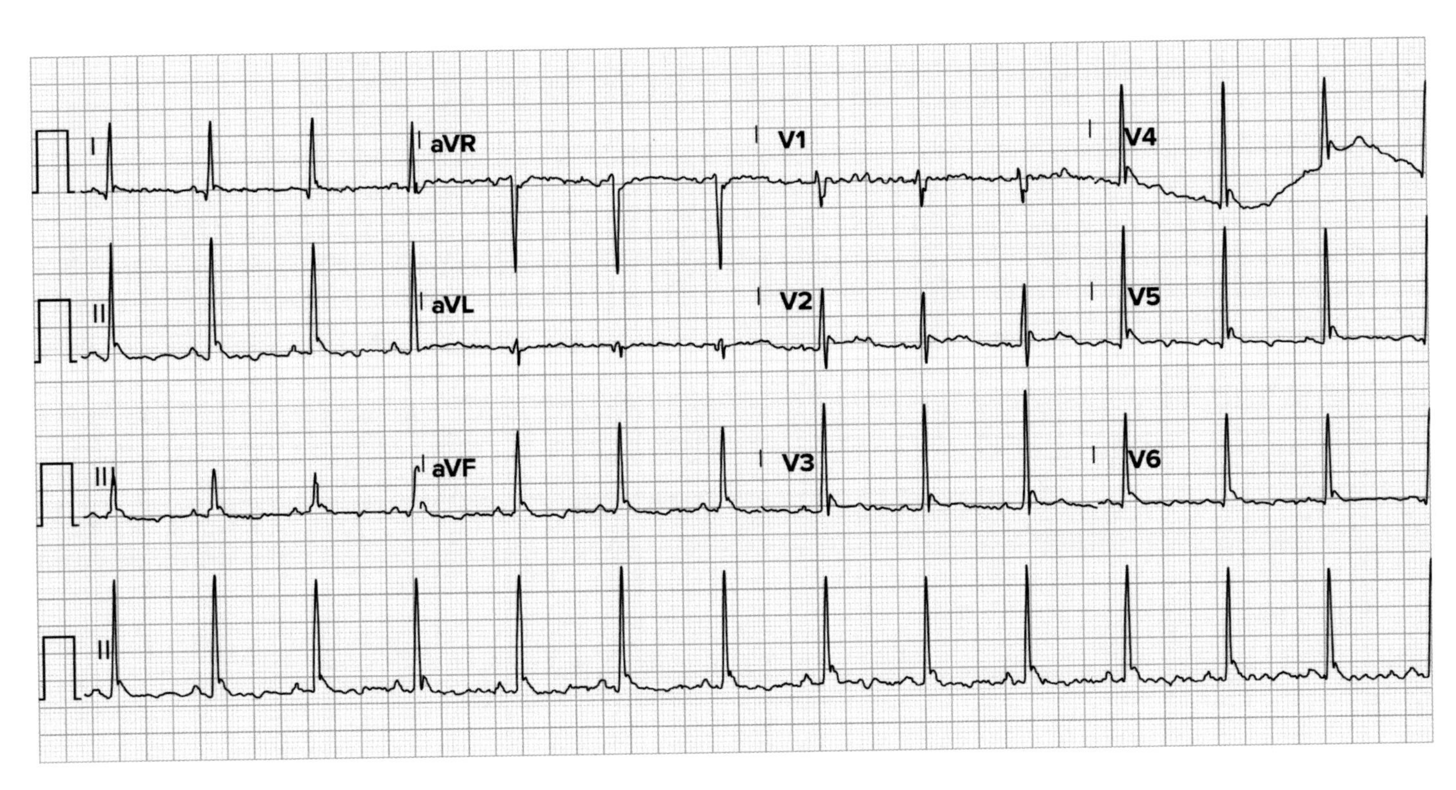

This EKG shows a normal sinus rhythm with a ventricular rate of 80 bpm, a normal axis, prolonged QTc (best measured in lead V2), early R-wave transition in the precordial leads (ie, R-wave amplitude > S-wave amplitude before lead V4), diffuse T-wave flattening and baseline artifact, and J-waves, also called Osborn waves, best seen in leads V2-V6 and the inferior leads.

The differential diagnosis for J-waves (Osborn waves) includes:

- Hypothermia
- Cardiac ischemia
- Intracranial hemorrhage
- Hypercalcemia
- Arrhythmogenic right ventricular dysplasia (with the epsilon wave)
- Normal variant in young healthy patients (eg, benign early repolarization)

J-waves are positive deflections, resembling a dome or hump, at the terminal junction of the QRS complex and the beginning of the ST-segment takeoff ***(see Figure 1).*** When seen in the hypothermic patient, the amplitude and duration have been shown to correlate with the degree of hypothermia, so there will be more prominent J-waves in patients with lower body temperatures (ie, more severe hypothermia). They are most commonly seen in the inferior leads, particularly lead II, and the lateral precordial leads, but can be seen in any or all leads depending on the degree of hypothermia.

Figure 1.
The red arrows point to the J-waves in leads V3-V5

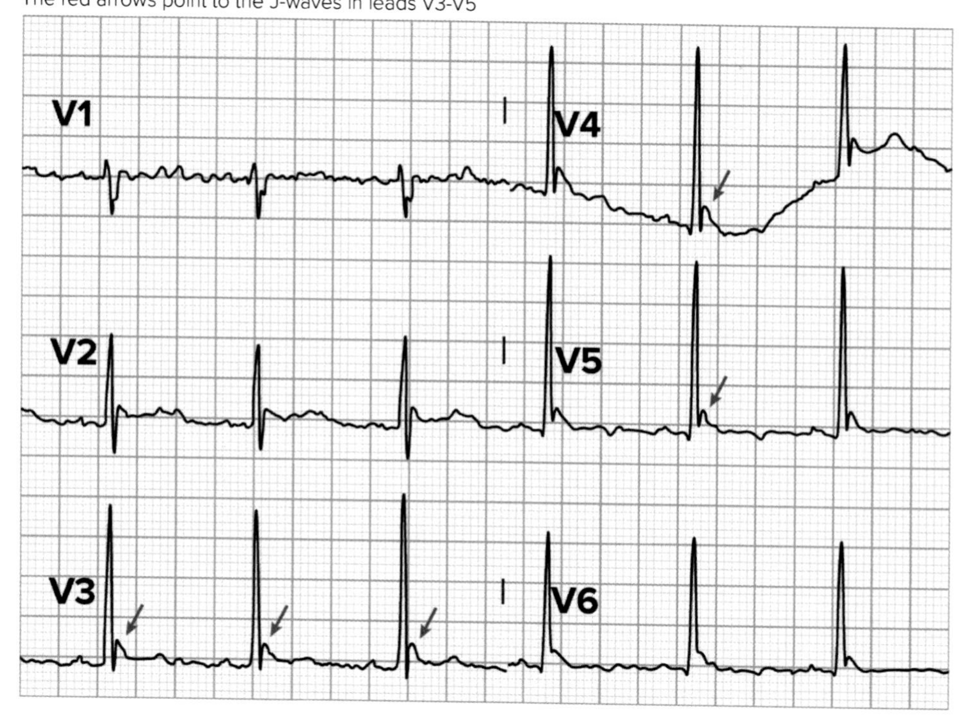

In 1953, Dr. John Osborn described J-waves as an "current of injury" concerning for impending ventricular fibrillation in the setting of hypothermia.[1] Although J-waves had been reported before this notation in hypercalcemia and hypothermia, the J-wave became known as the Osborn wave as a testament to his work. There is no consensus on which name to use, and some use Osborn wave only when seen with hypothermia and J-wave in all other settings. Some clinicians also use the term "Osborn J-wave."

Despite Dr. Osborn's research, the association of J-waves with life-threatening dysrhythmias in the hypothermic patient is unclear. As well, the presence of J-waves is not pathognomonic for hypothermia. J-waves can be seen with hypercalcemia,[2] cardiac ischemia, and CNS injury (eg, SAH). There is even a case report describing J-waves in the setting of Todd's paralysis.[3] Lastly, arrhythmogenic right ventricular dysplasia can also present electrocardiographically with a terminal deflection of the QRS complex, called an epsilon wave, that resembles a J-wave. Accordingly, the presence of J-waves on an ECG warrants a broad differential diagnosis, including environmental exposure, cardiac ischemia, electrolyte abnormalities, and neurologic pathologies.

This patient's core temperature was found to be 29.5°C and his workup was notable for a significantly elevated blood alcohol level along with multiple traumatic injuries. The patient was placed on a rewarming protocol and admitted to the Surgical ICU for further management of his traumatic injuries.

ECG Findings in Hypothermia Learning Points

- ECG changes most commonly seen at temperatures < 32°C and include:
  - Bradydysrhythmias
  - Atrial fibrillation with slow ventricular rate
  - Sinus bradycardia with 1st degree AV block
  - Junctional rhythms
- Prolongation of PR, QRS, and/or QT intervals
- J-waves (also called Osborn waves)
  - Positive deflection at the terminal junction of the QRS complex and the beginning of the ST-segment takeoff
  - Most commonly seen in the inferior and lateral precordial leads
  - Amplitude and duration typically correlate with degree of hypothermia
  - Can also be seen with hypercalcemia, cardiac ischemia, and intracranial hemorrhage
- During hibernation, arctic ground squirrels can survive body temperatures of -3°C without freezing

References

1. Osborn JJ. Experimental hypothermia; respiratory and blood pH changes in relation to cardiac function. Am J Physiol. 1953;175(3):389-398.
2. Morales GX, Bodiwala K, Elayi CS. Giant J-wave (Osborn wave) unrelated to hypothermia. EP Europace. 2011;13(2):283.
3. O'Connell E, Baker N, Dandamudi G, Steinhubl S. Dynamic J point Elevation Associated with Epileptic Hemiplegia: The Osborn Wave of Todd's Paralysis. Case Rep Neurol. 2013;5(1):6-9.

Case 102: Presentation

A 26-year-old female with no past medical history presents with flu-like symptoms including SOB and chest pain. What is your interpretation of her ECG?

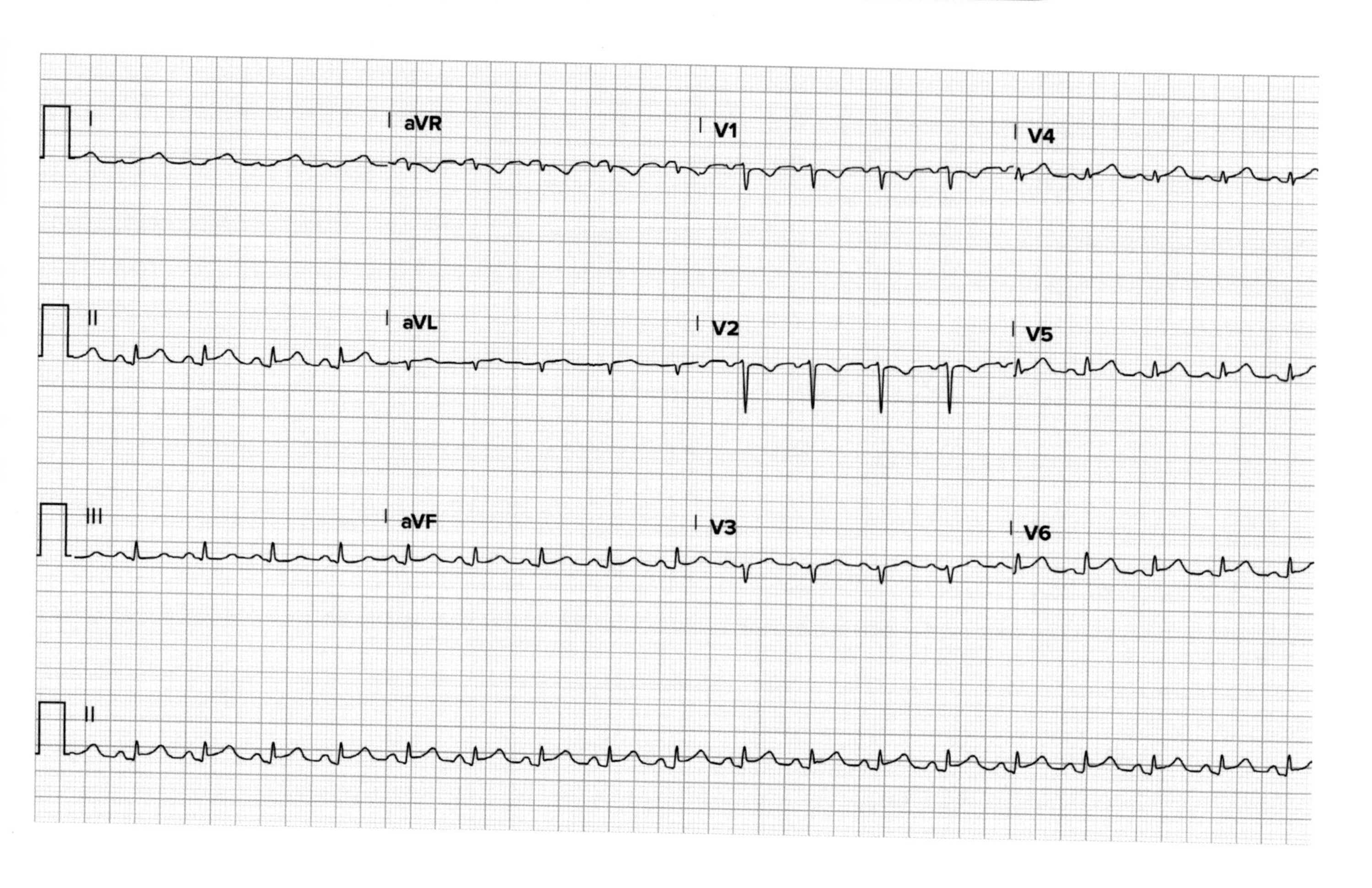

Case 102: Answer

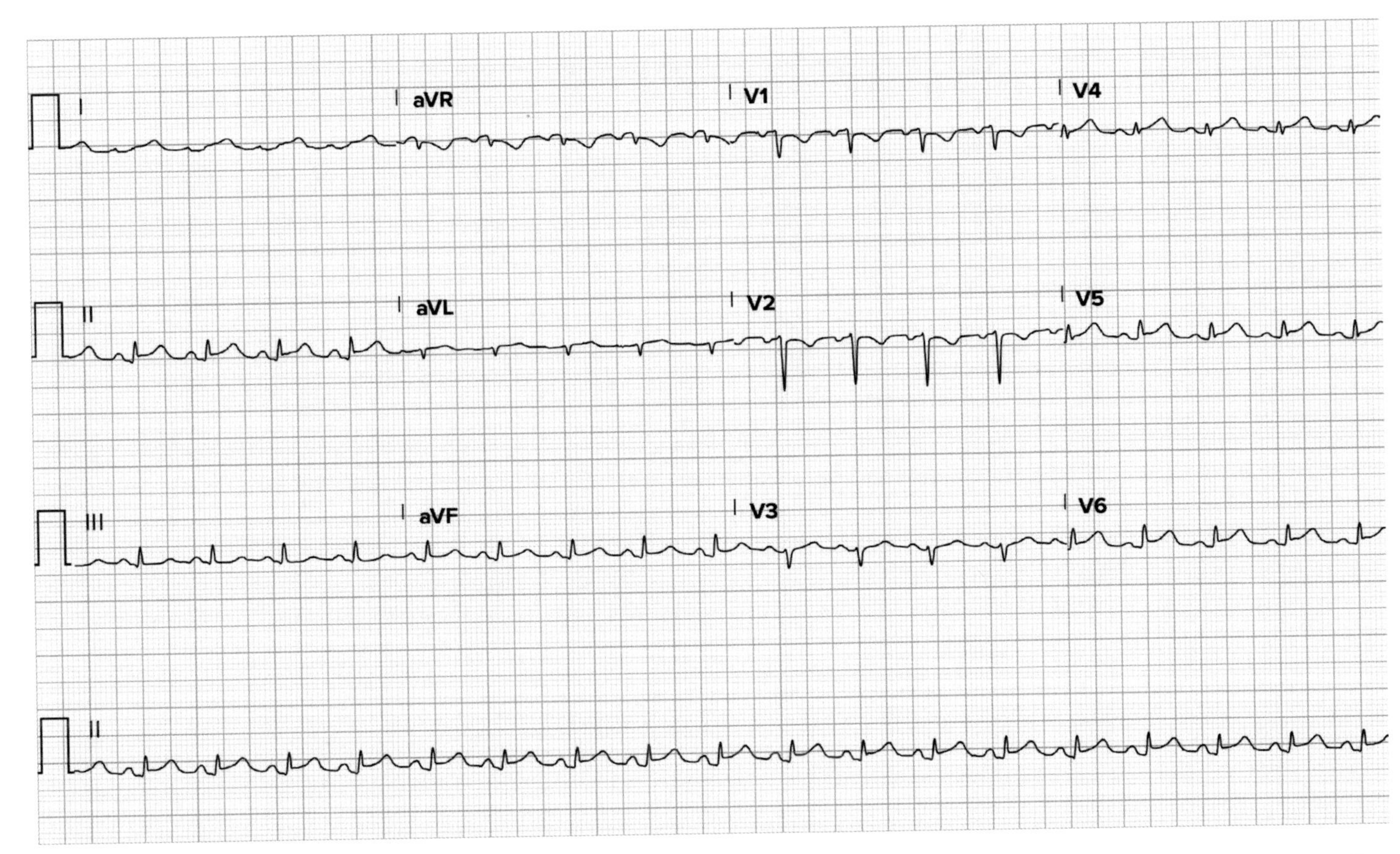

This ECG shows sinus tachycardia with a ventricular rate of 110 bpm, normal axis, normal intervals, STE in leads I, II, III, aVF, aVL, V3-V6, STD in leads aVR and V1, PR segment depression in leads II, aVF, and V3-V6, PR segment elevation in leads aVR and V1, and low QRS complex voltage.

The differential diagnosis for STE includes:[1]	
• Acute myocardial infarction	• Hyperkalemia
• Acute myocarditis	• Hypothermia
• Acute pericarditis	• Left ventricular aneurysm
• Benign early repolarization	• Left ventricular hypertrophy
• Brugada syndrome	• Non-ACS myocardial injury
• Bundle branch blocks	• Pre-excitation syndromes
• Cardiomyopathy	• Post-electrical cardioversion
• CNS injury	• Spiked Helmet Sign
• Coronary vasospasm	• Ventricular rhythms (paced or intrinsic) or ectopy
• Hypercalcemia	

This patient's history, age, and ECG changes are highly suggestive of acute pericarditis, which is an inflammatory process involving the pericardium. Since there are no AHA guidelines on the diagnosis and management of myopericarditis, the European Society of Cardiology guidelines are commonly referenced. The most recent 2015 guidelines[1] are listed below.

The diagnostic criteria for pericarditis include ≥ 2 of the following:

- Pericarditic chest pain: sharp and pleuritic, improved with sitting up and leaning forward
- Pericardial rub: a superficial scratchy or squeaking sound best heard over the left sternal border
- New widespread ST-segment elevations or PR depressions
- New or worsening pericardial effusion

Note that the criteria for pericarditis includes ECG changes, but since the pericardium is electrically silent, these changes are actually secondary to inflammation of the myocardium, often the superficial epicardium. The term myopericarditis is used if there is myocardial involvement appropriate to cause a detectable elevation in cardiac biomarkers but no new LV dysfunction on echocardiogram. The term perimyocarditis is used when there are elevated cardiac biomarkers and new LV dysfunction on echocardiography.

The ECG abnormalities seen in pericarditis classically evolve through 4 stages:

- Stage 1: concave upward STE (typically 2-4 mm) and PR segment depressions diffusely in all leads other than aVR and V1, prominent T-waves, and Spodick's sign (down sloping TP segment)
- Stage 2: normalization of initial abnormalities, most notably the STE
- Stage 3: TWI in the leads that previously had STE
- Stage 4: return to baseline ECG

Stages 1-3 typically develop over hours to days, and Stage 4 may not develop for many weeks. It is important to note that not every patient will have all of these ECG abnormalities nor evolve through these various stages. In fact, there is no time-based understanding of these ECG abnormalities and how they evolve, so it is likely best to disregard the classic stages of ECG abnormalities in the patient with myopericarditis.

PR segment elevations and depressions are due to atrial inflammation and is often described as diagnostic of myopericarditis. PR depression is most often present in leads II, III, aVF ***(see Figure 1)***, and V5-V6. PR elevation is most often seen in lead aVR. In this patient's ECG, the STD in leads aVR and V1 are likely reciprocal to the diffuse STE, but it is important to note that STD in these leads are very non-specific and can be seen in normal patients.

Figure 1.
PR segment depression in lead aVF

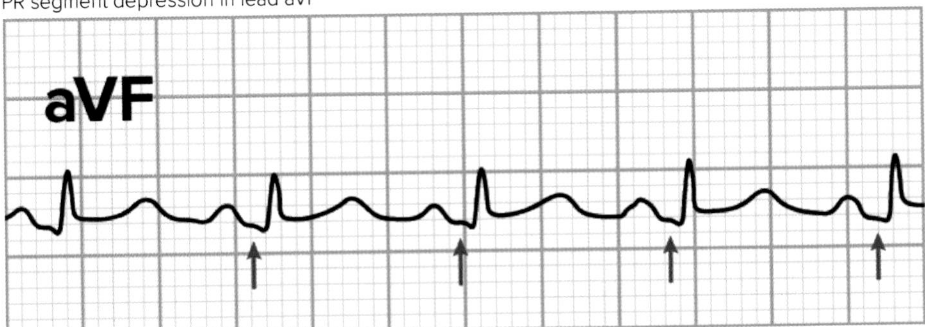

Spodick's sign is used to describe the down sloping TP segment ***(see Figure 2)*** often seen with pericarditis. While it is not present of this patient's ECG, it is important to note that Spodick's sign can also be seen with STEMI,[2] so it should not be considered diagnostic of pericarditis.

Figure 2.
Spodick's sign describes a down sloping TP segment (from the ECG of a different patient with pericarditis)

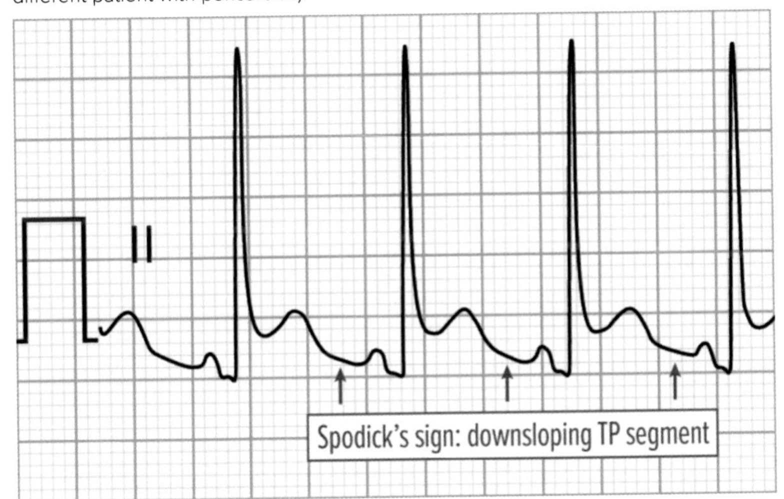

This ECG also shows low voltage, often defined as QRS complex amplitude < 5 mm in the limb leads or < 10 mm in the precordial leads. Some resources say "and" instead of "or" (ie, requiring both limb and precordial lead involvement), but this is academic. In this ECG, the low voltage criterion is met in the limb leads, but not in the precordial leads as the voltage of the first QRS complex in lead V2 is a little greater than 10 mm. Regardless, the finding of low voltage, regardless of whether it is present in both the limb and precordial leads, should prompt an evaluation for the underlying cause.

The differential diagnosis for low voltage includes:

- Normal variant
- Cardiac etiologies:
  - Hypothyroidism, severe
  - Hypovolemia
  - Infiltrative cardiomyopathies
  - Myocarditis
  - Myocardial infarction
- Extracardiac etiologies:
  - Acute respiratory distress syndrome
  - Anasarca
  - Chronic obstructive pulmonary disease
  - Constrictive pericarditis
  - Obesity
  - Pericardial effusion
  - Pleural effusion
  - Pneumomediastinum
  - Pneumonia
  - Pneumopericardium
  - Pneumothorax
  - Pulmonary edema
  - Subcutaneous emphysema

This patient's ED workup was notable for a viral swab positive for influenza B and a bedside echo that showed a large pericardial effusion concerning for tamponade physiology. She was taken to the cardiac catheterization laboratory for a pericardial window and a subsequent cardiac MRI was consistent with myocarditis.

Pericarditis Learning Points

- 4 stages of transient ST and PR segment changes that can mimic STEMI
  - Sequential evolution through various stages is not required
- ECG findings in stage 1 include:
  - Concave upward STE typically 2-4 mm
  - STE and PR segment depressions diffusely in multiple leads other than aVR and V1
  - Prominent T-waves
  - PR segment elevation in lead aVR is very common but not specific for pericarditis
  - Spodick's sign: downsloping TP segment, often seen with pericarditis but not specific as it can be seen in AMI[2]
- Q-waves can be seen with myocarditis but not pericarditis

Low Voltage Learning Points

- QRS complex amplitude < 5 mm in the limb leads or < 10 mm in the precordial leads
- Low voltage + electrical alternans = pericardial effusion until proven otherwise

1. Mattu A. ECG Weekly.
2. Witting MD, Hu KM, Westreich AA, Tewelde S, Farzad A, Mattu A. Evaluation of Spodick's Sign and Other Electrocardiographic Findings as Indicators of STEMI and Pericarditis. *J Emerg Med.* 2020;58(4):562-569.

Bonus Material: ECG Greeting Cards

Electronic cards you won't find anywhere else.

Scan to find downloadable PDFs or access them at
https://www.emra.org/emresident/article/ecg-images-greeting-cards/

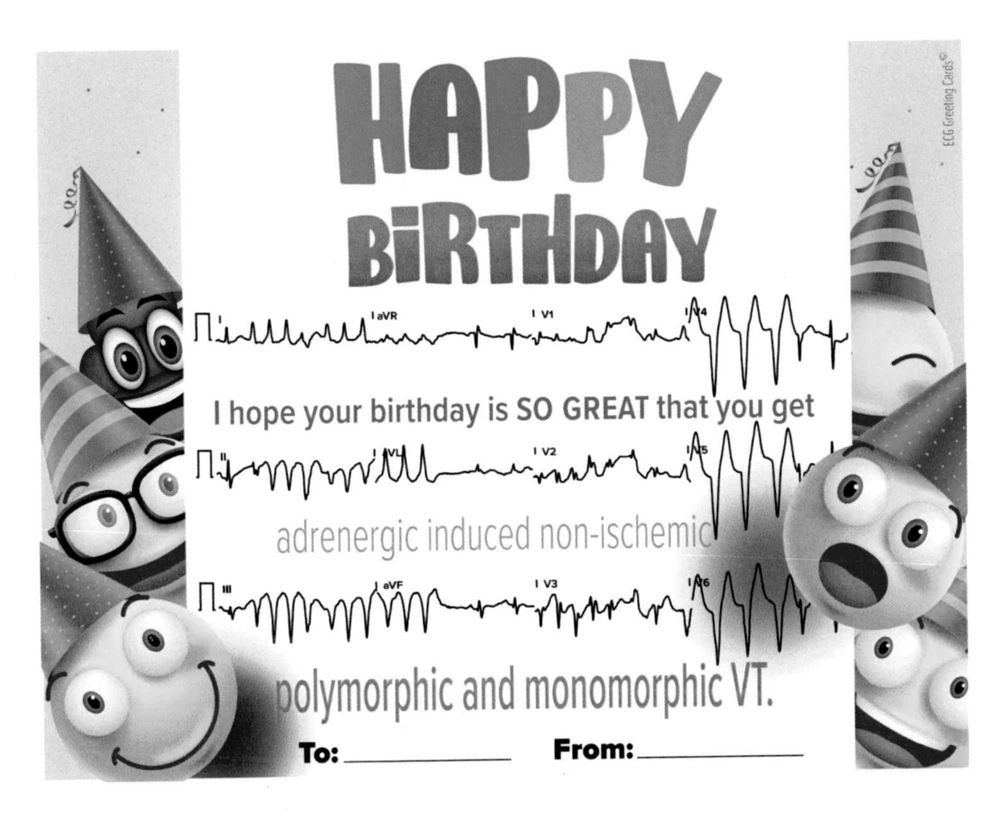

HAPPY
BiRTHDAY
I hope your birthday is SO GREAT that you get
adrenergic induced non-ischemic
polymorphic and monomorphic VT.
To:
From:
ECG Greeting Cards©

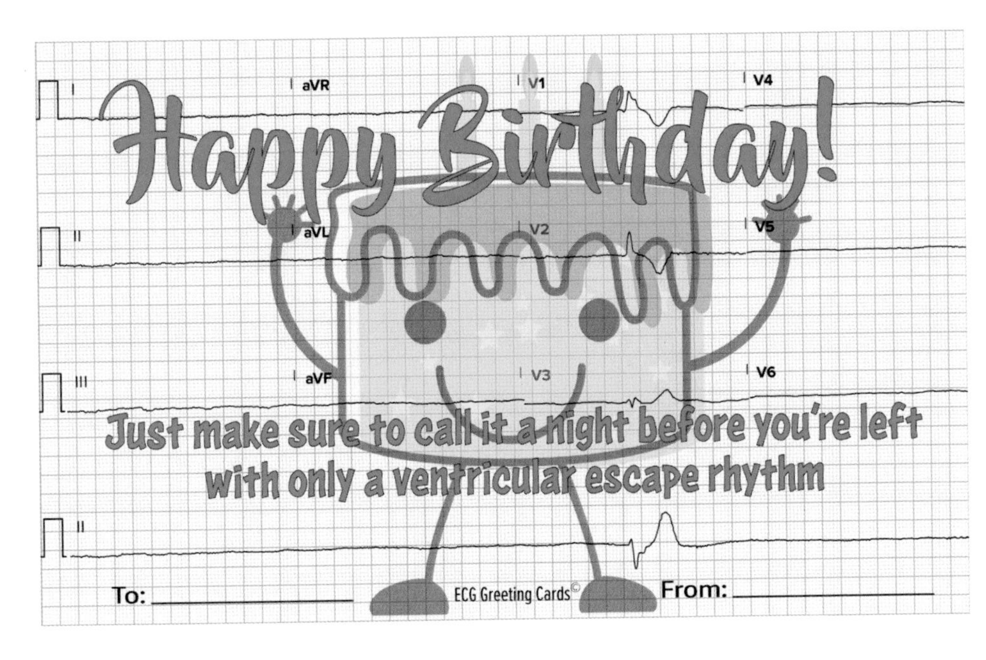

Happy Birthday!
Just make sure to call it a night before you're left
with only a ventricular escape rhythm
To:
From:
ECG Greeting Cards©

EMRA

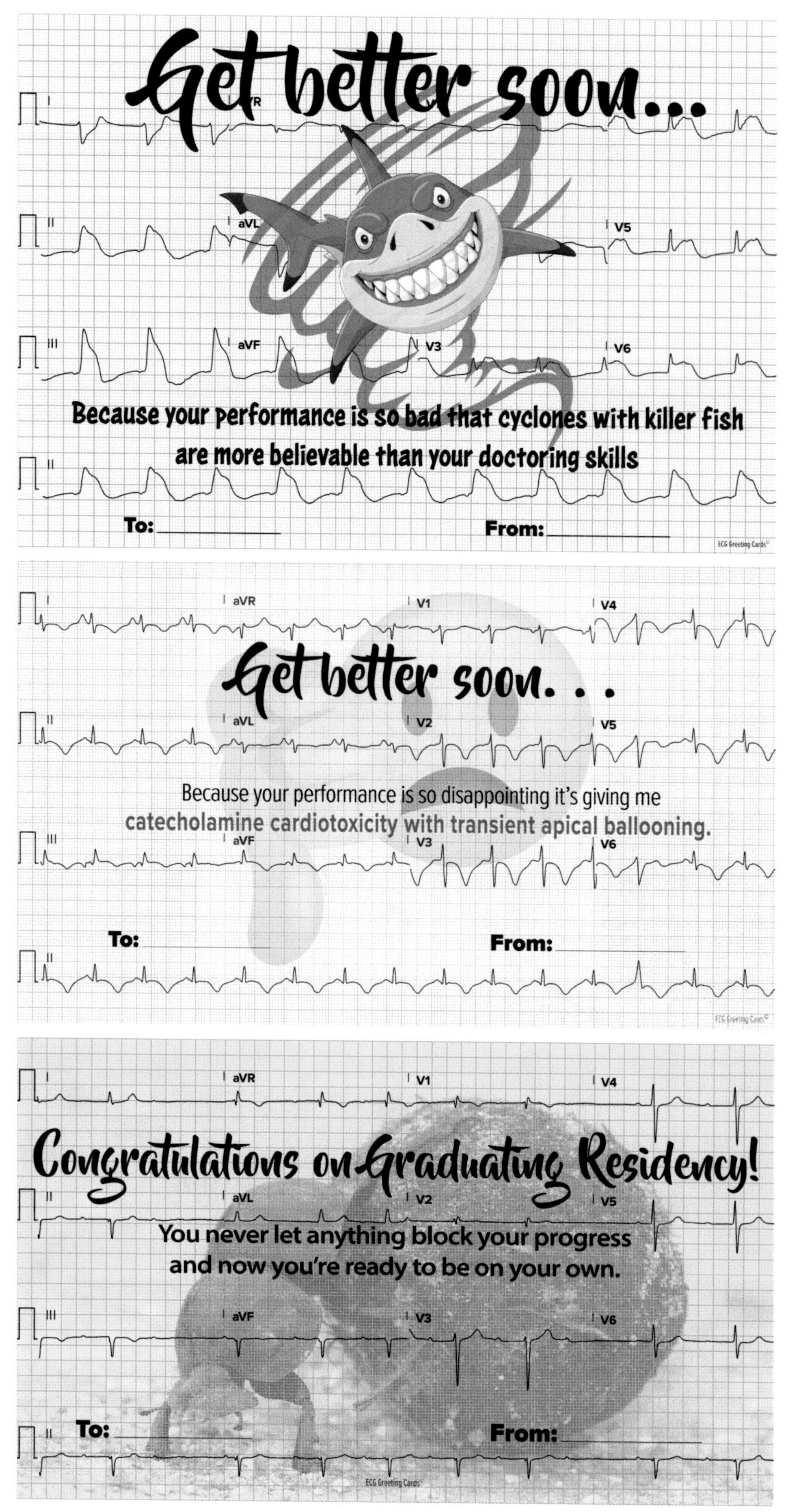
Get better soon...
I
aVR
II
aVL
V5
III
aVF
V3
V6
Because your performance is so bad that cyclones with killer fish are more believable than your doctoring skills
II
To:
From:
ECG Greeting Cards©
I
aVR
V1
V4
Get better soon. . .
II
aVL
V2
V5
Because your performance is so disappointing it's giving me
catecholamine cardiotoxicity with transient apical ballooning.
III
aVF
V3
V6
To:
From:
II
ECG Greeting Cards©
I
aVR
V1
V4
Congratulations on Graduating Residency!
II
aVL
V2
V5
You never let anything block your progress
and now you're ready to be on your own.
III
aVF
V3
V6
II
To:
From:
ECG Greeting Cards©

EMRA

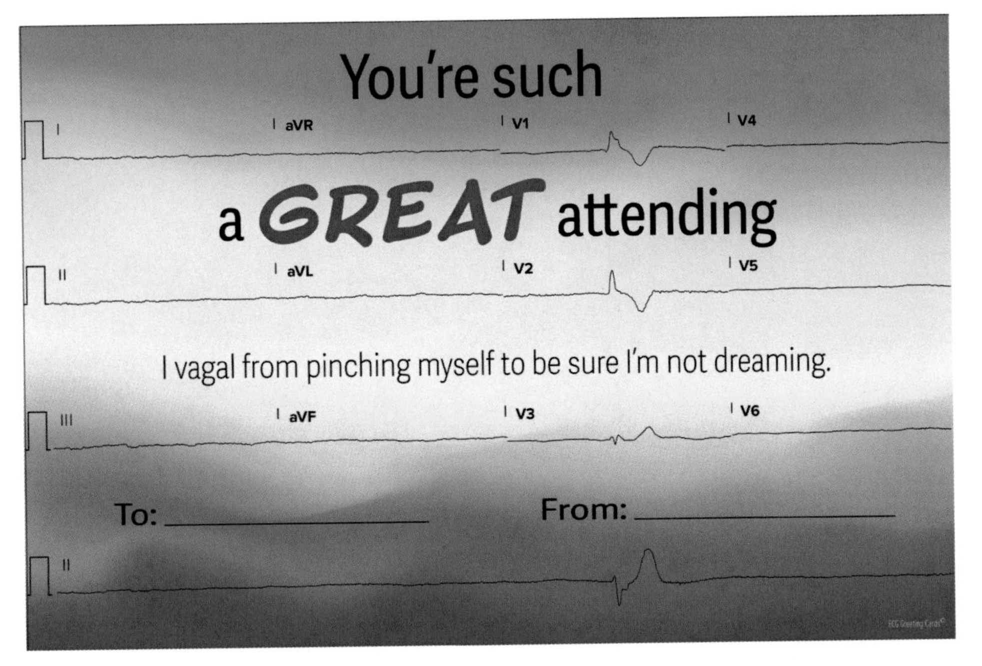
You're such
a GREAT attending
I vagal from pinching myself to be sure I'm not dreaming.
To:
From:
I
aVR
V1
V4
II
aVL
V2
V5
III
aVF
V3
V6
II

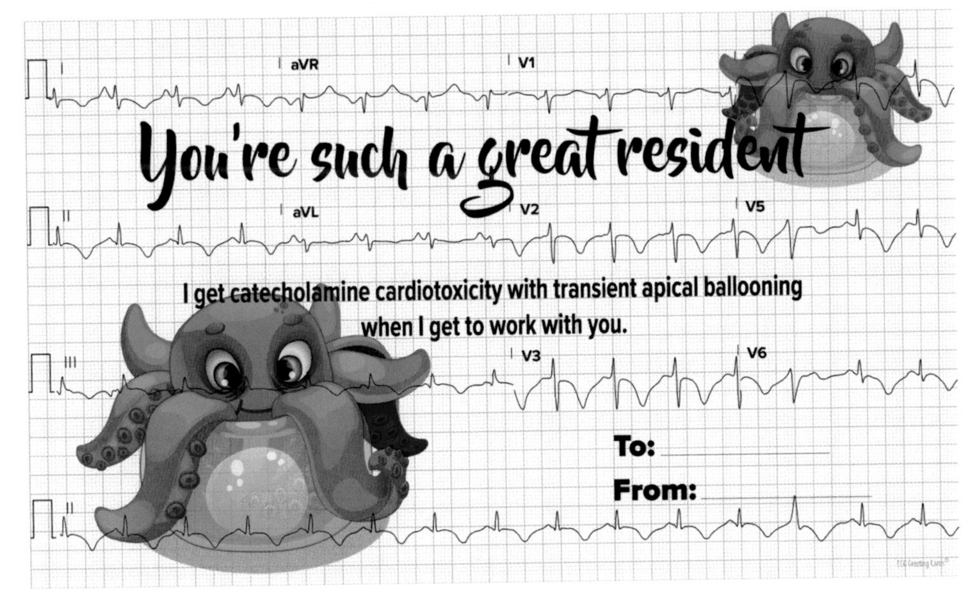
You're such a great resident
I get catecholamine cardiotoxicity with transient apical ballooning
when I get to work with you.
To:
From:
I
aVR
V1
II
aVL
V2
V5
III
V3
V6
II

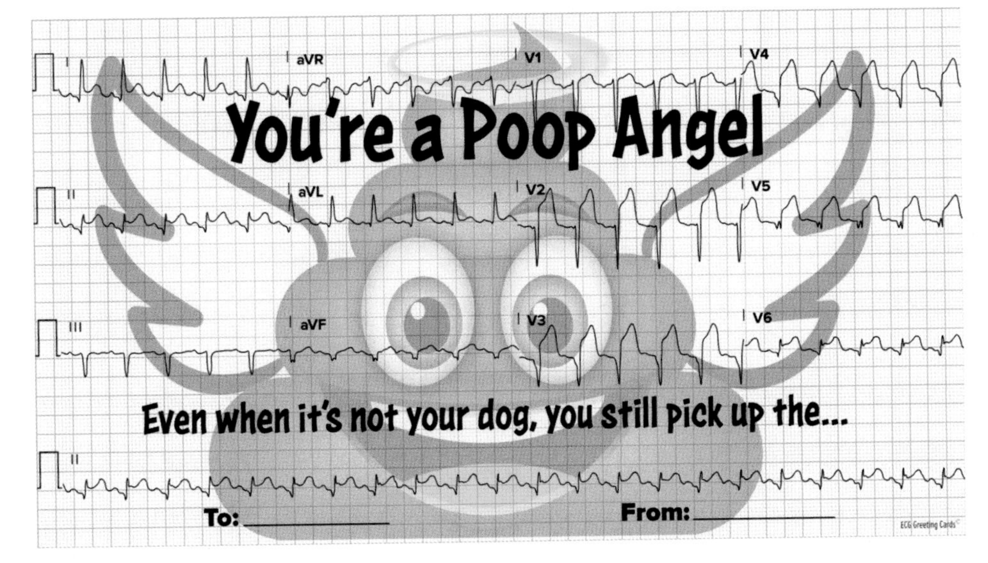
You're a Poop Angel
Even when it's not your dog, you still pick up the...
To:
From:
aVR
V1
V4
II
aVL
V2
V5
III
aVF
V3
V6
II

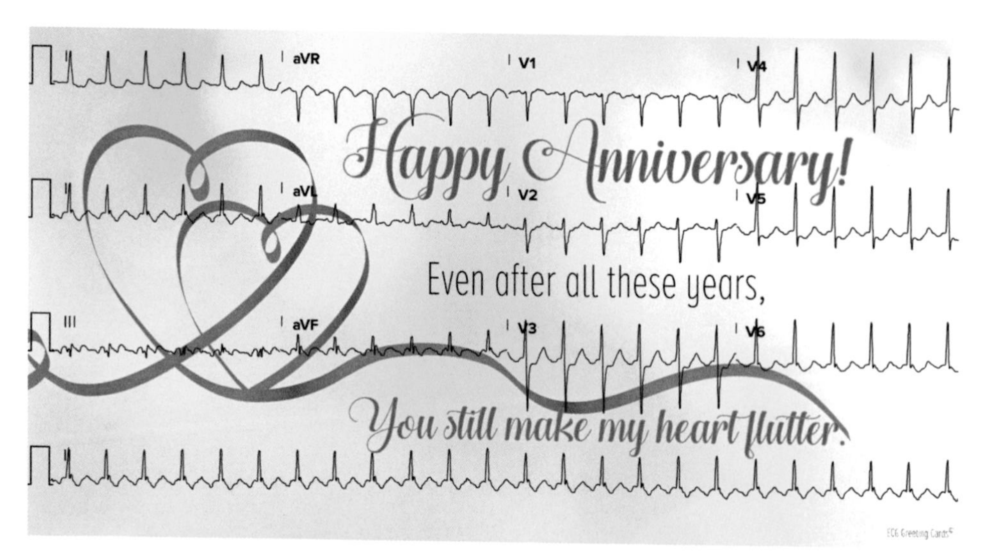
aVR
V1
V4
Happy Anniversary!
aVL
V2
V5
Even after all these years,
III
aVF
V3
V6
You still make my heart flutter.
ECG Greeting Cards©

EMRA

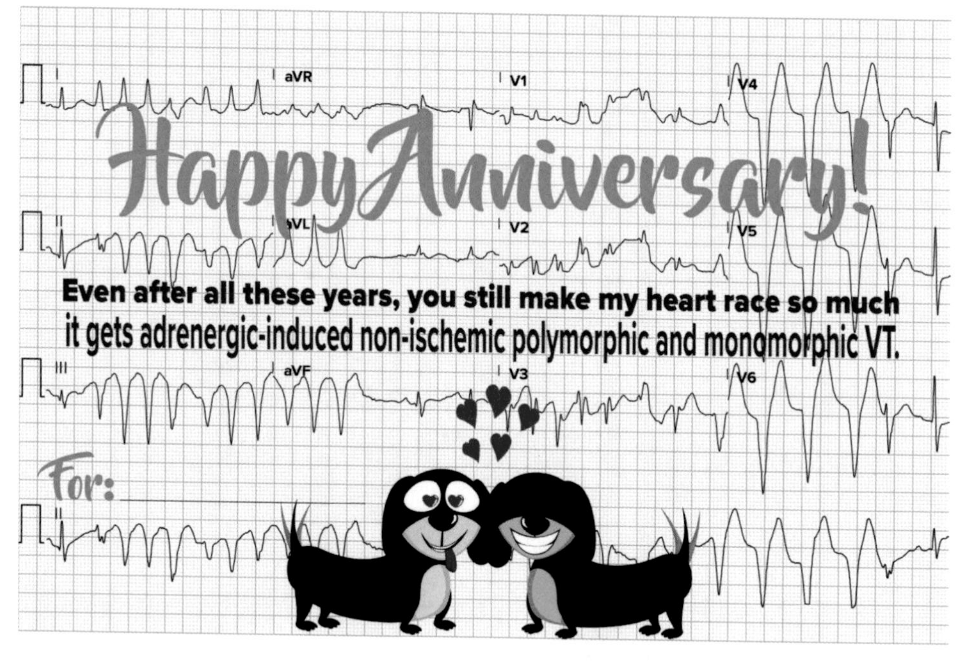
aVR
V1
V4
Happy Anniversary!
aVL
V2
V5
Even after all these years, you still make my heart race so much
it gets adrenergic-induced non-ischemic polymorphic and monomorphic VT.
III
aVF
V3
V6
For:

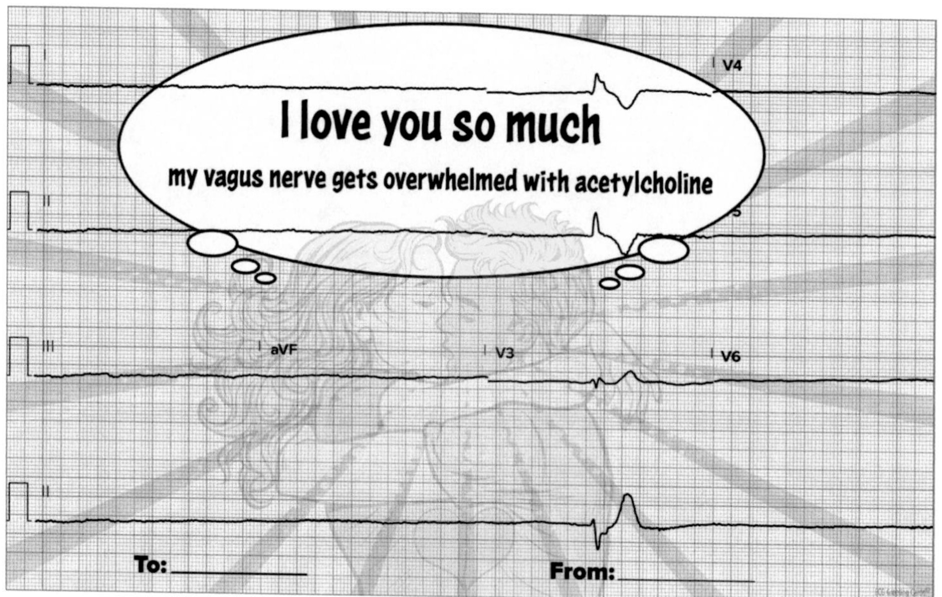
V4
I love you so much
my vagus nerve gets overwhelmed with acetylcholine
III
aVF
V3
V6
To:
From:

EMRA

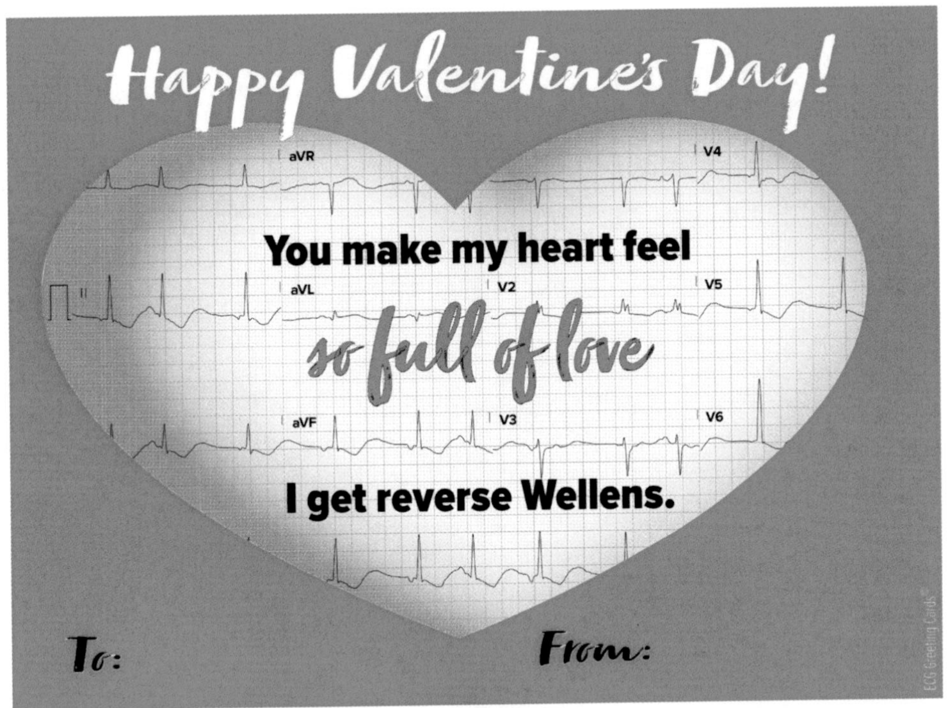
Happy Valentine's Day!
You make my heart feel
so full of love
I get reverse Wellens.
To:
From:
ECG Greeting Cards©

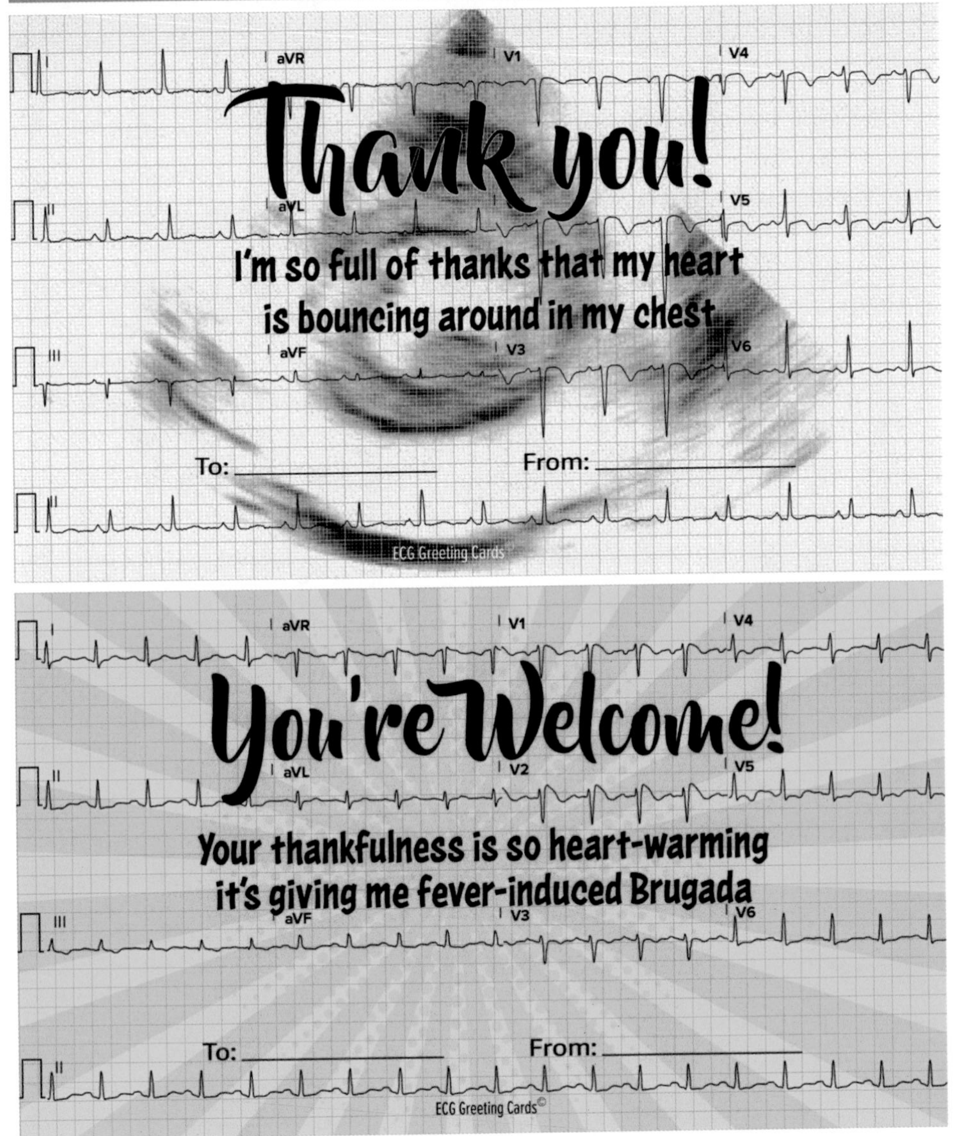
Thank you!
I'm so full of thanks that my heart
is bouncing around in my chest
To:
From:
ECG Greeting Cards
You're Welcome!
Your thankfulness is so heart-warming
it's giving me fever-induced Brugada
To:
From:
ECG Greeting Cards©

Made in the USA
Middletown, DE
04 July 2024